Community Mental Health in Canada

Community Mental Health in Canada

THEORY, POLICY, AND PRACTICE

Revised and Expanded Edition

Simon Davis

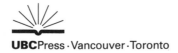

UBCPress · Vancouver · Toronto

21 20 19 18   5 4 3

Printed in Canada on FSC-certified ancient-forest-free paper (100% post-consumer recycled) that is processed chlorine- and acid-free.

Library and Archives Canada Cataloguing in Publication

Davis, Simon, 1956-, author
    Community mental health in Canada: theory, policy, and practice / Simon Davis. – Revised and expanded edition.

Includes bibliographical references and index.
Issued in print and electronic formats.
ISBN 978-0-7748-2699-0 (pbk.). – ISBN 978-0-7748-2700-3 (pdf).

    1. Community mental health services – Canada. 2. Mental health policy – Canada. 3. Mentally ill – Care – Canada. I. Title.

RA790.7.C3D39 2013   362.20971   C2013-906195-9
                                               C2013-906196-7

Canadä

UBC Press gratefully acknowledges the financial support for our publishing program of the Government of Canada (through the Canada Book Fund), the Canada Council for the Arts, and the British Columbia Arts Council.

UBC Press
The University of British Columbia
2029 West Mall
Vancouver, BC V6T 1Z2
www.ubcpress.ca

For Marta, still my hero

WHEN I WAS STILL A TEENAGER, I was admitted for a second time to a psychiatric institution. Although it was the same unit, with the same staff who had been there during my first admission, there was something different about the way they treated me that second time around. In retrospect, I now understand that on my second admission, the staff had lost hope for me. In their eyes I was no longer one of the ones who might leave the hospital and never return. I had returned, and I was now counted among the recidivists. Even the new diagnosis I was given reflected the hopelessness surrounding me: Chronic Undifferentiated Schizophrenia. Perhaps that's why I felt a deep urgency to mobilize all the energy I could muster to get myself out of that place as quickly as possible. Perhaps I was afraid if I fell into the depths of the hopelessness mirrored in their eyes, I might never leave and would be lost forever.

– Patricia Deegan, from the foreword to The Strengths Model (Rapp and Goscha 2012)

Contents

Preface to the New Edition

Community Mental Health in Canada was written to fill a gap in the literature. In addressing for the first time both clinical and structural aspects of mental health practice in Canada, it became a widely used resource for students, practitioners, and policy makers. Since it was first published in 2006, there have been a number of developments in Canada, including the release of a comprehensive Canadian Senate report on the need for system reform, the creation of the Mental Health Commission of Canada in 2007, and in 2012 the publication by the Commission of a national strategy document - the first of its kind in Canada.

This revised and expanded edition of *Community Mental Health in Canada* is a substantial revision of the first. In addition to major updates to the literature cited, the following changes have been made:

- Subjects are covered in more depth, with some given their own chapter rather than being a sub-section of a chapter. New chapters include: "Stigma," "The Recovery Vision," "The Drug Companies," and "Assessment."
- New topics include the two-continua model of mental health/mental illness, models of care, help-seeking, and prevention and health promotion.
- More recent developments, such as the Kirby Report, the creation of the Mental Health Commission, and the commission's 2012 strategy document, are addressed.
- The sequencing of the book's chapters and topics has changed. The intent is to start with broader, more contextual and conceptual issues, then move towards discussion of particular programs (Chapters 9 through 13) and finally towards specific practice approaches (Chapters 14 through 18). In the new edition the topics of recovery and culture are moved up in the sequence since much of the book is seen through a recovery and cultural lens.
- It was decided not to devote a chapter to an overview of the major psychiatric syndromes since there are other more comprehensive sources that

readers should refer to for that purpose, such as the American Psychiatric Association's *Diagnostic and Statistical Manual*. Because of this, readers and instructors should not use the book as a "stand-alone" resource.

The author is appreciative of the feedback provided by reviewers and colleagues who have helped shape this new edition of *Community Mental Health in Canada*.

Introduction

These are indeed "interesting times" to be working in the mental health field. In Canada, as we move through the second decade of the twenty-first century, we have seen the locus of treatment shift from institutions to the community, as the "asylums" – the provincial psychiatric hospitals – downsize and finally close. We have also seen a Canadian Senate report on mental health reform, *Out of the Shadows at Last*, give rise to the Mental Health Commission of Canada, a federal advisory body whose mission is "to promote mental health in Canada, and work with stakeholders to change the attitudes of Canadians toward mental health problems, and to improve services and support."[1] We have seen what is called the *recovery* vision being written about extensively, and its principles adopted by the Mental Health Commission as the basis for a more positive, holistic approach to mental health care, one that moves beyond what has been seen as the narrow confines of the "medical model." We have seen better mental health housing and employment models developed, with persons with serious mental disorders now employed within health authorities as peer workers, committee members, and program leaders.

However, despite these promising developments, problems have persisted. Persons with serious mental disorders are overrepresented among the homeless and in the criminal justice system. Many are not in treatment. Stigma – discrimination from the general public – does not seem to be diminishing. A Canadian Psychiatric Association position paper concludes that: "The promise of deinstitutionalization has not been realized. Hospital bed closures have been too rapid and too extensive. Community resources remain underfunded and limited. Fragmentation in the health care system has meant that no one has taken responsibility for the care of one of the most disadvantaged and marginalized populations" (Chaimowitz 2012, 5). Whether or not this statement is completely accurate, what is noteworthy is that it was written in 2012, yet seems eerily similar to concerns expressed by others in the earlier post-institutional period, thirty, or even forty, years ago.

We have also seen disputes arising about the recovery vision and the new models of care being proposed. As is detailed later, some are concerned about an approach that they see as potentially leading to the abandonment of disabled persons not able to act in their own best interests.

How has this all come about? In attempting to answer this question, *Community Mental Health in Canada* offers an overview of the provision of public mental health services in Canada, looking at their historical development, current manifestation, and future direction. In doing this, the book considers the strengths, limitations, and evidence base of models of care and practice approaches. The services referred to here are the publicly funded programs mandated to meet the needs of persons suffering from the most disabling disorders – schizophrenia, bipolar disorder, and major depression, for example. While some reference is made to children and older adults, the focus is on adult service recipients.[2]

The intention of this book is to address the systemic, or "macro," issues – program philosophies, how services are organized – as well as the clinical aspects of mental health care (i.e., the actual interventions that are used). The notion of covering both systemic and technical concerns in one volume is admittedly ambitious, and perhaps presumptuous. That being said, it has been this author's experience that an appreciation of the political, cultural, and organizational context of mental health care is necessary for clinical interventions to be effective – or for us to understand why they are less than effective. At the same time, in recognition of the breadth of the material being covered, the author has deliberately referenced a large number of published and internet sources, which the reader is encouraged to consult for a more in-depth perspective. Concerning the literature surveyed for this book, wherever possible, an effort was made to use Canadian authors and Canadian data.

It should be said at this point that there are no easy resolutions to some of the challenges that are raised here. Determining how society should respond to the needs of people with mental disorders is a contentious matter that produces strong divisions of opinion and heated arguments. As a Health Canada (2002b, 3) document notes, one of the barriers faced by persons attempting to improve the Canadian mental health system has been the "abundance of ethical dilemmas associated with mental health care that are controversial and actively debated by fractious constituent groups." Areas currently being debated, and covered in more detail in this book, include:

- Whether mental health services are too "illness-oriented," and if there should be more done with respect to prevention and health promotion.

- Whether promoting mental health will mean that the needs of the seriously mentally ill will be neglected.
- Whether it is realistic to talk about prevention in the case of an illness such as schizophrenia.
- How service eligibility is determined and whether some groups are being systematically excluded, and, if so, why.
- Whether the drug companies wield disproportionate influence, engage in "disease mongering," and distort the data from drug trials.
- Whether antidepressant medication is overprescribed.
- How health care professionals themselves may be contributing to the stigma associated with mental illness.
- Whether Western psychiatry is insensitive to the needs of different cultural groups.
- How to address the needs of family members and other informal care providers, and determining the extent to which they should be included in the treatment process.
- How to honour the voice of persons with mental illness when needs and agendas seem so disparate.
- The use of coercion and involuntary outpatient treatment.
- The concept of "recovery" as it is currently being used in mental health: What is it, how does one measure it, is it a safe and realistic goal for persons with a serious mental illness, and what are the implications for the practitioner?
- Whether professional involvement is always necessary for recovery.

When contentious topics are covered in this book the approach is to articulate both (or all) of the competing viewpoints rather than to, in effect, set up "strawpersons."

Community Mental Health in Canada is informed by the author's experiences as a clinician, administrator, and researcher in a large, multi-site community mental health service. This experience has led to an appreciation of the role of medicine and psychiatry in improving the plight of persons with mental health problems. That being said, it is the author's position that our institutional practices have at times been invalidating for service users and, consequently, that new models – described here – that are more holistic and aim for greater inclusion and empowerment are welcome. It should be noted, however, that this is *not* a sociology text. While a social lens is used, the author has been in the privileged position of straddling both the academic and practice worlds, and he is aware of practice realities. The book aspires to the principles of *knowledge exchange*, which is a synthesis of research evidence and an application to real-world situations.

Who This Book Is For

Community Mental Health in Canada evolved out of material prepared for an introductory, one-semester course on mental health practice, given to senior-level undergraduates. Accordingly, it is intended, in the first instance, for those considering or starting a career in health care. The presumed need for this book arose from the author's impression that there was no single text currently available that addressed both clinical and structural aspects of mental health practice in the Canadian context. While *Community Mental Health in Canada* is thus intended for "potential practitioners," the hope is that it is accessible and informative for others, in particular members of stakeholder groups (i.e., service recipients, families, and interested members of the public).

A Note on Terminology

The terms employed in the mental health field have particular connotations, which are not always understood or agreed upon. To begin with, there is the question of what to call the condition itself. "Mental illness" is still used in many settings and is the term preferred in most instances by physicians. Some have suggested replacing "illness" with "disability" to reflect the impact mental disorders have on social and vocational functioning and, in the words of the former Mental Health Advocate of British Columbia, "because successful community living requires more than medical care" (Hall 2001, 10). There is also the question of using the expression "mental health problems" instead of "mental illness," the ramifications of which are substantial enough to warrant a separate discussion in Chapter 1. The Mental Health Commission of Canada (2012) has suggested using "mental health problems and illnesses" as a unitary term. Another term, "mental disorder," is now commonly used in legislation, diagnostic manuals, and other publications, and it is used in this book. Possible limitations of this term must be acknowledged, such as the suggestion by the Anxiety Disorders Association of Ontario (2010) that "condition" would be a less stigmatizing term than "disorder."

What about "community mental health," as per the title of this book? "Community mental health" is a phrase that, at its narrowest, refers to a *location*: persons with mental disorders are now, unlike earlier periods, "in the community," in the sense that treatment and support are provided predominantly in outpatient settings as opposed to in old, remotely located provincial institutions that have either been downsized or closed altogether. "Community mental health," however, has a broader and more complex meaning, one that has antecedents going back to the "moral treatment" approaches used in late-eighteenth-century Europe, approaches that emphasized human dignity, freedom, and potential. Fast-forwarding to mid-twentieth-century

North America, the "community care" movement was one that looked at environmental factors in mental health, which optimistically spoke about, in the words of then president John Kennedy, "the open warmth of community concern and capability," and which emphasized rehabilitation and prevention, beyond simply the management of symptoms (Eaton 2001). More recently, particularly with the development of the earlier mentioned recovery orientation, the importance of *citizenship* for those affected by mental illness has come to the fore; that is, the significance of emphasizing shared humanity rather than "differentness" if we are to combat stigma and achieve inclusion. "Community mental health," then, is both a location and a vision, the vision only partially realized.

Finally, there are the terms that refer to the different participants in the mental health system. "Practitioner" or "clinician" are used here to denote the professionals, such as physicians, nurses, and counsellors. A more contentious issue is how to refer to the users, or recipients, of mental health services (Essock and Rogers 2011; Morrison 2005; Torrey 2011a). One of the earliest terms was "patient," which came out of an era when the treatment and containment of mentally disordered persons was largely hospital-based. This term fell out of favour with a number of non-medical disciplines, in part because the locale of treatment had shifted to the community and in part because of some discomfort with the apparently narrow, symptom-based focus that was implied. During the 1970s and 1980s, the designation "client" came into more common usage, and it is the term used here (except when citing other authors or when referring to hospitalized persons). The use of "client" has, in turn, been criticized because it would seem to indicate choice, or a voluntary relationship, that may not exist. More recently "client" has been replaced by "consumer" in a number of mental health programs, although the limitations of the former term would seem to apply to the latter. "Person with mental illness" is an expression that acknowledges that the individual is a person first. More contentious is the use of "survivor," a designation that has created some unease and defensiveness among practitioners because of the implied anti-psychiatry stance (e.g., Goldbloom 2003). As noted by Covell et al. (2007, 443): "Each of these words carries connotations regarding autonomy versus independence, illness versus health, fiduciary relationships, activity versus passivity, and so forth." While acknowledging the limitations of "client," its use in this book is not intended to carry any particular symbolic or political connotations, as far as that is possible.

It is important for practitioners to be sensitive about the use of language. At the same time, making the "right" decision is not an easy task: there is no clear consensus among practitioners or clients as to preferred terms (Covell et al. 2007; Gibson-Leek 2003; Sharma et al. 2000), and individuals may have different understandings of a particular designation, an example being the woman who told this author that her use of "survivor" referred to surviving depression, not mistreatment at the hands of the mental health system.

Organization of the Book

The intention behind the sequencing of chapters is to start with more contextual and conceptual issues, then move towards discussion of particular programs (Chapters 9 through 13) and finally towards specific practice approaches (Chapters 14 through 18). While the book is intended to be read in this sequence, the chapters can also be read as "stand alone."

The first chapter deals with conceptual issues: what we mean when we refer to "mental health" and "mental illness," and the idea that, while related, these two terms can be seen as representing separate continua. There is discussion of different explanatory models and how these influence our delivery of care. Finally, we look more closely at the "medical model," its ongoing influence, and its limitations.

Chapters 2 and 3 consider the "target populations." Chapter 2 looks at who is served by public treatment programs, which is a function of the way these programs determine eligibility by defining what is "serious," and which is also a function of public help-seeking behaviours. Chapter 3 considers whether public programs should look further upstream and have a greater role in health promotion and the prevention of mental disorders.

Chapter 4 discusses what many believe is the greatest challenge facing community mental health, the impact of *stigma* on help-seeking and on quality of life. It is seen that stigma is created both outside and inside the health care system.

Chapter 5 looks at the *recovery* vision. Twenty-five years or so years after its first articulation we consider its influence and also the challenges in implementing a model of care not always understood or endorsed by all stakeholders.

Chapter 6 looks at *culture* as a powerful influence with respect to explanatory models, how mental disorders are expressed, the coping styles employed, and willingness to seek Western-style treatment, with a particular focus on the situation of Aboriginal persons in Canada. Suggestions are made for service delivery that is more culturally sensitive.

Chapter 7 concerns the "stakeholders": practitioners, clients, and family members – their perspectives and agendas – and the extent to which these interests can be seen as harmonious or in conflict. Chapter 8 considers another stakeholder with considerable interest and influence in the mental health system: the drug companies.

At this point the book starts to look at the service delivery system, with Chapter 9 providing the historical context of mental health reform, from the institutional era to our current version of community care. The chapter ends with the significant arrival of the Mental Health Commission of Canada. Chapter 11 provides an overview of the range of community and hospital-based services in Canada, with Chapter 10 providing a necessary lead-in by describing how these services approach the question of evidence base and whether they can be considered "best practices." Chapter 12 considers what is arguably the most important social determinant of health: housing. The ongoing challenges of inadequate housing and homelessness are described, along with initiatives that have been developed to address these. Chapter 13 deals with the important issue of the overrepresentation of mentally ill persons in the criminal justice system.

At this point, the book moves into the clinical realm. Chapters 14 through 18 describe in greater detail the diagnostic system, the features of the major psychiatric syndromes, and particular areas and aspects of practice: assessment and medical management; education, skills training, and cognitive behavioural treatments; vocational rehabilitation; and the legal and ethical context of practice.

Finally, it will be noted that this book returns on a number of occasions to two key reference points. The first of these is the *recovery vision* (described more fully in Chapter 5): because of its prominence, the recovery vision is necessarily an important basis for comparison in discussions about mental health system reform. The second reference point is the syndrome of schizophrenia itself, which is arguably the most stigmatizing mental disorder and the one with the most impact. If our policies and practices in mental health are to be effective, they need to take into account the particular challenges faced by persons with this condition. That being said, it must be acknowledged that schizophrenia is what is called a "low prevalence" condition and that mood and anxiety disorders have a higher prevalence in Canada and produce more disability on a *population* basis, even if schizophrenia produces more disability on an *individual* basis (see Chapters 2 and 3). Further, persons with mood and anxiety conditions often struggle in anonymity because of the relative "invisibility" of these disorders. Future practitioners need to be acutely aware of this fact and, it is to be hoped, endorse a view of service eligibility based on functional impact rather than on diagnostic category.

Why, then, are the challenges faced by persons with psychotic conditions emphasized in this book? First, they constitute a large proportion of the cases seen in public community mental health settings and represent longer hospital stays than those with other psychiatric diagnoses (see Chapter 3). Second, much of the stigma and rejection associated with mental illness – a major public health issue – is attached to the particular symptoms of this disorder, with public discussion and media reports about mental illness and violence often referencing schizophrenia specifically (e.g., Steinberg 2012). The "other" status of schizophrenia is reflected in a survey by the Canadian Alliance on Mental Illness and Mental Health (2007), which found that respondents saw depression and anxiety disorders as "mental health problems" and schizophrenia as a "mental illness." If we are going to make headway in how society responds to the mentally ill, we need particularly to support those with the most stigmatizing conditions. Third, the book, as noted, uses the recovery vision as a reference point, as a possible model with which to inform and reform mental health practices and services. This is significant because much of the recovery literature *also* uses schizophrenia and psychotic disorders in its examples (see Chapter 5) since, for the recovery vision to have credibility, it must account for those affected by very serious disorders. However, to reassure readers: the interventions described in this book have application across a range of psychiatric syndromes; indeed, as is discussed in greater detail, there is increasing evidence that mental health interventions are not "syndrome specific."

Notes

1   Mental Health Commission of Canada, http://www.mentalhealthcommission.ca/.
2   Chapter 3 provides a discussion on Canada's aging population.

Abbreviations

ACT	assertive community treatment
ADHD	attention-deficit hyperactivity disorder
AIMS	Abnormal Involuntary Movement Scale
APA	American Psychiatric Association
APPN	advanced-practice psychiatric nurse
AUDIT	Alcohol Use Disorders Identification Test
BPD	borderline personality disorder
BPS	biopsychosocial model
CAMH	Centre for Addiction and Mental Health
CAMIMH	Canadian Alliance on Mental Illness and Mental Health
CATIE	Clinical Antipsychotic Trials of Intervention Effectiveness
CBT	cognitive-behavioural therapy
CCPA	Canadian Centre for Policy Alternatives
CCS	Cultural Consultation Service (Montreal)
CFACT	Coalition for Appropriate Care and Treatment for Persons with Serious Mental Illnesses
CLAS	culturally and linguistically appropriate services
CMA	Canadian Medical Association
CMHA	Canadian Mental Health Association
CPG	clinical practice guideline
CTO	community treatment order
DALI	Dartmouth Assessment of Lifestyle Instrument
DALY	disability-adjusted life year
DAST	Drug Abuse Screening Test
DBT	dialectical behaviour therapy
DSM	*Diagnostic and Statistical Manual*
DTC	direct-to-consumer (advertising)
DUP	duration of untreated psychosis
ECT	electroconvulsive therapy

EPI	early psychosis intervention
EPS	extrapyramidal symptom
FDA	Food and Drug Administration (US)
FTE	full-time equivalent (staff)
GABA	gamma aminobutyric acid
GAF	Global Assessment of Functioning
GHPU	general hospital psychiatric unit
GP	general practitioner
GPM	general psychiatric management
GSK	GlaxoSmithKline (drug company)
HALY	health-adjusted life year
HIV	human immunodeficiency virus
HoNOS	Health of the Nation Outcome Scales
HRQOL	health-related quality of life
ICCD	International Center for Clubhouse Development
ICD	International Statistical Classification of Diseases and Related Health Problems
ICM	Intensive Case Management
IMR	Illness Management and Recovery Scale
LLPDD	late luteal phase dysphoric disorder
LOCUS	level-of-care utilization system
MAOI	monoamine oxidase inhibitor
MAST	Michigan Alcoholism Screening Test
MD	major depression
MDS	Minimum Data Set
MHCC	Mental Health Commission of Canada
MHFA	Mental Health First Aid
MHL	mental health literacy
MI	motivational interviewing
MMSE	Mini-Mental Status Exam
MPA	Mental Patients Association
MSE	mental status exam
NAMI	National Alliance on Mental Illness
NCRMD	not criminally responsible on account of mental disorder
NDM	noradrenaline dopamine modulator
NIMBY	not in my back yard
NNT	number needed to treat
NOS	not otherwise specified (diagnosis)
NP	nurse practitioner
OCAN	Ontario Common Assessment of Need

OCD	obsessive-compulsive disorder
ORS	Outcome Rating Scale
OT	occupational therapist
PANSS	Positive and Negative Syndrome Scale
PEPP	Prevention and Early Intervention in Psychosis (London, ON)
PMDD	premenstrual dysphoric disorder
PMS	premenstrual syndrome
PSR	psychosocial rehabilitation
PTSD	post-traumatic stress disorder
RAS	Recovery Assessment Scale
RCMP	Royal Canadian Mounted Police
RCT	randomized controlled trial
ROPI	Recovery-Oriented Practices Index
ROSI	Recovery Oriented Systems Indicators Measure
RPFS	Recovery Promotion Fidelity Scale
RPI	Recovery Process Inventory
RSA	Recovery Self-Assessment
RTMS	repetitive transcranial magnetic stimulation
SAD	social anxiety disorder
SAMHSA	Substance Abuse and Mental Health Services Administration (US)
SAMI	severe addictions and mental illness
SCID	Structured Clinical Interview for Axis I *DSM*-IV Disorders
SDM	substitute decision maker
SE	supported employment
SES	socio-economic status
SSC	Schizophrenia Society of Canada
SRO	single-room occupancy (hotel)
SSRI	selective serotonin reuptake inhibitor
STORI	Stages of Recovery Instrument
TAC	Treatment Advocacy Center
TAU	treatment as usual
TCO	threat, control, override (symptoms causing violent behaviour)
TI	Therapeutics Initiative
TTM	trans-theoretical model of change
WANA	We Are Not Alone
WHO	World Health Organization
WRAP	Wellness Recovery Action Plan

Community Mental Health in Canada

Frames of Reference

1

To offer a context for the rest of the book, this first chapter deals with conceptual issues: what we mean when we refer to "mental health" and "mental illness," different explanatory models that are used to understand mental disorders, and how these conceptions and beliefs – frames of reference – influence our delivery of care. Points of view are shaped by differences in training and orientation, experiences early in life, experiences as a service recipient, and personal belief systems. Because these are not just academic issues – that is, they have significant implications for the way we respond to mental illness and allocate resources – disagreements on these points can be very contentious.

To provide an illustration of the uncertainty with which we approach this subject, the following personal experience is offered. This author once sat on a multi-agency committee whose purpose was to provide a coordinated response to the problem of extreme hoarding, which is the compulsive gathering of objects in a dwelling-place to the point of it becoming a fire, health, or safety hazard. At one of the first meetings, while discussing the terms of reference, a committee member stressed the importance of us having a *common understanding* of what hoarding was, or represented: her view was that it was a "mental health problem." Another member nodded, saying, "Yes, a mental illness." The first speaker was not so sure about the *illness* designation, however. It sounded too severe, and, after all, a number of people in the room had relatives who had minor hoarding behaviours, relatives who otherwise, or prior to the onset of the hoarding, seemed pretty "normal." One committee member had read that hoarding was going to have its own, separate entry in the new edition of the *DSM* – the *Diagnostic and Statistical Manual* of the American Psychiatric Association – which apparently would legitimize its status as a bona fide mental illness. Another person had thought hoarding was a sub-category of obsessive-compulsive disorder (OCD). This prompted the question: Would a hoarder benefit from taking antidepressant medication, which is often used as a treatment for OCD? And another said that, in his experience, hoarding was almost always associated with loss and trauma early in life. There was then some discussion about how to help hoarders, with the committee member most familiar with the issue stating that simply "de-hoarding" – hauling the material out – was no solution and would alienate the hoarder from the helper. A counsellor on the committee offered that building a relationship with the person was the most fundamental task because, without that, nothing could be accomplished. At the end of the meeting, while acknowledging that hoarding was indeed a problem, it was still not clear whether we had agreed either on what sort of a problem it was or on how best to intervene. In speaking about mental health policy more generally, a sociology professor at the University of Saskatchewan voices the fundamental challenge: "the various stakeholders ... don't necessarily agree on *the nature of the problem* ... nor ... on the best solution to it" (Dickinson 2002, 384).

Mental Illness and Mental Health

So, what is a mental illness? The terms "mental health" and "mental illness" are familiar but are not so easily defined. A person may be described as having a mental illness but can also be said to be having "mental health problems." What, if anything, is the distinction here? Are we referring to the same thing – more euphemistically in the case of "mental health problems"[1] – or are we in fact talking about two different areas for possible intervention?

One perspective has been to see mental health as the *absence* of mental illness since it can be hard to imagine someone as being mentally healthy if there are still symptoms of mental illness present. This conception is being challenged, however. The recovery perspective – described in more detail in Chapter 5 – suggests that people can potentially have a good quality of life even if they have residual symptoms of illness. And the World Health Organization (e.g., 2010) has for some time defined mental health as being more than simply the absence of mental illness.

Another perspective is to see mental illness as more serious, and more *biological*, than "mental health problems." This distinction has been endorsed by the general public, as reflected in the findings of a national survey on mental health literacy commissioned by the Canadian Alliance on Mental Illness and Mental Health (2007). In this study, respondents tended to see depression and anxiety disorders as "mental health problems" and schizophrenia as a mental illness. Respondents were also more likely to see the cause of schizophrenia as biological, whereas mood and anxiety disorders were associated to a greater degree with environmental factors such as divorce, problems at work, or relationship difficulties. Significantly, respondents tended to see mental illness – and by extension mentally ill persons – as distinct, or *qualitatively different*, as reflected in the following focus group comments:

- "The more common things, like anxiety and depression, are not mental illnesses. Schizophrenia and bipolar are more mental illnesses."
- "We all have mental health problems, but we are not all mentally ill."
- "We all go through a mild [depression] period from time to time, but there is no [schizophrenia] period in everyone's life" (Canadian Alliance on Mental Illness and Mental Health 2007, 26-27).

This distinction is also supported by family and advocacy organizations, who argue – very reasonably – that the most seriously disabled should be the priority population with respect to the allocation of limited public monies and resources (Treatment Advocacy Center 2012). For example, *Huffington Post* writer D.J. Jaffe (2010), in an article provocatively titled "Mental Health Kills the Mentally Ill," argues that funding should be dedicated to programs for those who suffer from "a biologically based no-fault medical problem that resides in the brain's chemistry" rather than to services that "focus on making the worried well less worried." This cause has been taken up by advocates who believe that the health policy direction in our country – as represented by the Mental Health Commission of Canada – is oriented too much towards mental health issues while neglecting serious mental illness. In a letter to the CEO of the Mental Health Commission, advocate Lembi Buchanan (2011) spoke about the interests of the most vulnerable being downplayed and the need for service providers and others "to be aware that there is a compelling distinction between mild to moderate psychosocial mental health problems that may have a causal relationship with the environment and the severe and complex mental illnesses [schizophrenia and bipolar disorder] that are chronic biomedical brain diseases." Advocate Marvin Ross (2011b) argues further that schizophrenia should not be referred to as a mental health problem at all but – like Alzheimer's – as a brain disease and that we should "stop pretending that these illnesses are ... [due to] stress."

These are strong, sincere convictions being expressed, and certainly one cannot dispute the idea of schizophrenia as a condition that is biologically based, heavily stigmatizing, and potentially very disabling. Notwithstanding this, a few counterpoints to the serious/less serious distinction are offered here. First, seriousness can be applied to conditions other than schizophrenia and bipolar disorder: depression, for example, exists on a continuum and in its most severe form can result in complete social withdrawal and suicide.[2]

Second, the idea that mood and anxiety problems are "non-biological" and psychotic disorders "non-environmental" is a misconception, given that the expression of symptoms is now understood to be the result of a stress-vulnerability interaction (more on this below). Finally, separating some clinical conditions from others is a two-edged sword. Identifying disorders that are more entrenched and disabling may be important in order to protect funding for treatment and research into those conditions. On the other hand, we now know that by emphasizing *differentness* we are creating more stigma and potential isolation for those being identified, even if theirs is "a biologically based no-fault medical problem." The evidence for this is presented in Chapter 4.

At this point we have still not really defined mental health, except as an absence of mental illness or as a less severe condition referred to as "mental health problems." A different perspective is to consider mental health in more *positive* terms:

> Mental health is a state of well-being in which an individual realizes his or her own abilities, can cope with the normal stresses of life, can work productively and is able to make a contribution to his or her community. In this positive sense, mental health is the foundation for individual well-being and the effective functioning of a community. (World Health Organization 2010)

Similarly, the Canadian Mental Health Association (n.d.) defines mental health in terms of resilience, self-actualization, balance (effectively juggling multiple demands), and an ability to enjoy life.

Sociologist Corey Keyes (2002) articulates a conception of mental health that incorporates psychological and social well-being. People are functioning well psychologically "when they like most parts of themselves, have warm and trusting relationships, see themselves developing into better people, have a direction in life, are able to shape their environments to satisfy their needs, and have a degree of self-determination" (Keyes 2002, 208-9). And individuals are functioning well socially "when they see society as meaningful and understandable ... [and] as possessing potential for growth, when they feel they belong to and are accepted by their communities ... and when they see themselves contributing to society" (209). Keyes (2002, 2005, 2009) and others working in this field see mental illness and mental health as influencing each other but as existing on two *separate* continua, or axes (see Figure 1). In this conception an individual may not meet the threshold for mental illness yet still have poor mental health, a condition Keyes terms "languishing."

Figure 1

The two-continua model

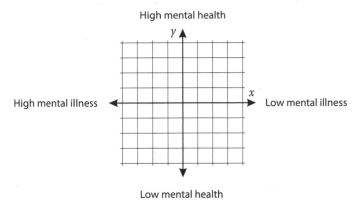

Source: Keyes (2009).

Distinguishing mental illness and mental health in this way carries with it very different implications for intervention. If one is targeting mental illness, then the goals are symptom reduction and prevention of relapse, which have indeed been the focus of public treatment programs in Canada. If, on the other hand, one is targeting mental health, then the goal is health promotion, an area historically outside the scope of practice of clinicians. As we have seen, devoting resources to health promotion is a cause of concern for some who worry that treatment of mental illness will then be neglected – a "zero-sum" situation. In response to this is the argument that health promotion can in fact ameliorate the manifestations of mental illness, both on an individual and population basis (Keyes 2009). By addressing health determinants such as housing, for example, we are reducing the stress load affecting service users, which we know can worsen a mental illness and lead to greater use of other services, such as hospitalization (Thomas 2007). A health promotion perspective can also be seen as consciousness-raising in that it sensitizes clinicians to the social determinants of health. Importantly, clients of the psychiatric system themselves, including persons with schizophrenia, have expressed a desire for more than basic medical management – in other words, for enhanced mental health (Capponi 2003; Fischer, Shumway, and Owen 2002; Gumpp 2009; Pyne et al. 2006). So, where we focus our resources may remain a contentious issue, but it would seem reasonable to suggest that practitioners should, as much as possible, try to both minimize mental illness and maximize mental health.

Explanatory Models

Our conceptions about mental disorder have varied across time and culture. Beliefs about cause and consequence are significant since they shape the interventions, approaches, and models of care adopted. Further, for these interventions to be effective, it is desirable that clinicians and clients be on the "same page" with respect to explanatory models. For example, in reviewing data on the effectiveness of depression treatments Duncan, Miller, and Sparks (2004, 72) note that "congruence between a person's beliefs about the causes of his or her depression resulted in stronger therapeutic alliances, increased duration of treatment, and therefore improved outcomes." However, the survey evidence suggests that disagreement on explanatory models is not uncommon, for instance on the question of whether a mental disorder is a result of stress, an underlying genetic vulnerability, or something else (Pyne et al. 2006; Srinivasan, Cohen, and Parikh 2003). Explanatory models are particularly significant when working with persons from other cultures, a topic explored in Chapter 6.

While there is still considerable uncertainty as to the aetiology of mental disorders (Health Canada 2002a; Marie-Albert 2002), we have increasingly come to understand that they are the product of an interaction between individual vulnerability and environmental factors, in other words, both "nature" and "nurture." Adherence to *monocausation* models, in the words of a professor of psychology, "needs desperately to be abandoned" (Kiesler 1999, 11). That being said, for the sake of clarity, and to provide a historical context, biological and environmental explanations are separated in the following brief review of explanatory models.

Biological Determinants

Currently in North America, the dominant viewpoint in psychiatry is that mental disorders we would consider to be serious – in particular schizophrenia and bipolar disorder – are biological in origin and require biological treatments, a position that is supported by substantial empirical and clinical evidence (Cyranoski 2011; Dincin 2001; Haynes 2002; Kendlar 2004; Kieseppa et al. 2004; Lawrie et al. 2008; Liberman et al. 2008; Paris 2005a; Picchioni and Murray 2007; Torrey 2011b).

The idea that mental disorders have biological origins – the "somatogenic" viewpoint – is not a new one. In 1872 Dr. John Gray, superintendent of the New York State Asylum and editor of the *American Journal of Insanity*, concluded in a conference presentation that "the causes of insanity, as far as we are able to determine, are physical; that is, no moral or intellectual operations of the mind induce insanity apart from a physical lesion" (quoted in Eaton 2001, 272). Similarly, across the Atlantic, German psychiatrist Emil Kraepelin, one of the first to conduct research on *dementia praecox* – an early name for schizophrenia – published a text in 1883 with a classification system that attempted to establish the organic basis of mental disorders. As reflected in the "dementia" designation, Kraepelin saw this condition as having an inevitably deteriorating course. Biological psychiatry was eventually superseded in North America in the early to mid-1900s by psychodynamic approaches (see below), becoming preeminent again in the second half of the century, largely as a consequence of the breakthroughs seen with the use of new psychotropic medications (Healy 2002) – in particular, chlorpromazine, a treatment for psychosis, and lithium, a treatment for mania. Now, well into the twenty-first century, medication has increasingly been the treatment of choice among family physicians and psychiatrists (Ghaemi 2010; Harman, Edlund, and Fortney 2009; Harris 2011; Newman and Schopflocher 2008; Raymond, Morgan, and Caetano 2007; Smith 2011).

Evidence that mental disorders are biological in origin comes from studies of genetic transmission as well as from structural-imaging techniques (Bertram 2008; Cyranoski 2011; Glannon 2008; Kendlar 2004; Kieseppa et al. 2004; Lowry 2011; McGuffin et al. 2003; Picchioni and Murray 2007; Robotham 2011; Torrey 2011b). Concerning genetic determinants, researchers have used twins and/or adopted children as subjects to attempt to tease out the separate contributions of environmental and hereditary factors. In the case of bipolar disorder, for example, in a British study involving identical and non-identical twins (who are, respectively, 100 percent and 50 percent genetically similar), researchers, using a variety of mathematical models, estimated the heritability of bipolar disorder to be 85 percent, with the remaining 15 percent of the variance in illness risk being attributed to unshared environmental factors (McGuffin et al. 2003). In the case of schizophrenia, Finnish researchers compared 190 adoptees considered a "high risk" for the condition, by virtue of having a biological mother with a schizophrenia spectrum disorder, with 137 "low-risk" adoptees, whose mothers did not have the diagnosis, with subjects being followed to a median age of 44 (Tienari et al. 2003). It was found that the mean, age-corrected morbid risk for a schizophrenia spectrum disorder was over five times greater for the high-risk group (22.5 percent) than for the low-risk group (4.4 percent).

The biological paradigm is also supported by evidence from scanning and imaging techniques – EEGs, positron-emission tomography, magnetic-resonance spectroscopy, CT scans, and functional magnetic-resonance imaging – that has enabled researchers to look at the physiological substrate of mental activities, leading a professor of medicine to speculate that "scientists may [now] venture into the frontier of the neural basis of spirituality and feelings" (Pietrini 2003, 1,907). Pietrini (2003, 1908) notes that imaging techniques have effectively eliminated the distinction between what used to be called "organic" psychiatric disorders (ones for which there was a known structural alteration, like dementia) and "functional" disorders (ones like schizophrenia and depression, for which, previously, there were no known alterations), a distinction that "reflected our inability to go beyond what could be visible to the naked eye" (1,908). University of Calgary ethicist Walter Glannon notes: "Thanks largely to structural and functional brain imaging, the neurobiological model of the brain-mind relation has done much to discredit mind-body dualism" (Glannon 2008, 1). As reviewed by Torrey (2011b), a large body of evidence has accumulated showing *differences* in brain structure and function among persons with schizophrenia who have never received treatment,[3] such as enlarged ventricles, neurological abnormalities, and cognitive deficits. Imaging techniques have been able to support "the concept of schizophrenia as a progressive neurodevelopmental disorder with both early and late developmental abnormalities" (Sporn et al. 2003; see also Metherell 2011).

Not everyone has been satisfied with the biological frame of reference, seeing it as narrow and reductionistic, a critique taken up by Toronto author and advocate Pat Capponi (2003, 4):

> If we assume everything is related to physiology then the primary, "sane" response is to treat mental illness with pharmaceuticals – a clean, easy solution, and one we have a lot of comfort with in the twenty-first century. It removes parental guilt and individual responsibility; it pathologizes and medicates behaviours; it elevates a pseudo-science to the big leagues. There is profit in the search for "magic bullets," in the research, development and marketing of newer, better, and costlier medications for the mind. Ultimately, though, this is a soulless and limiting response to pain and distress, however caused. In the rush to study, dissect, and understand the brain, we've forgotten that the whole individual is greater than the sum of her [*sic*] parts.

Psychosocial Determinants

At the other end of the continuum from biological determinism is the view that mental disorders originate in stressful or difficult life experiences. Currently, the strongest expression of this position comes from the work of those involved with the victims of sexual and physical abuse (Briere 2002; Zanarini 2000). Individuals concerned about the psychological impact and sequelae of child abuse argue that pathologizing and applying a medical label to what are, in their view, trauma-induced conditions is not only a misconception but also a form of decontextualizing that has the effect of "blaming the victim" (Simmie and Nunes 2001). This critique is often made by feminist writers such as Lev (1998, 3), who observes: "The unhealthy ways a woman copes with the trauma becomes the avenue for diagnosis, instead of labeling the way she was victimized, or recognizing the healthy ways she has adapted in order to survive."

In reviewing the history of "sociogenic" explanations for mental illness, one can look to theories about the deleterious effects of urbanization and industrialization reflected in the "moral treatment" movement, which started in late-eighteenth-century Europe. As reviewed by Eaton (2001, 271), reformers such as Pinel (in Paris) and Tuke (in England) "recommended maximum freedom for the mentally ill, normal human dignity, and the stabilizing effects of work and religion ... were optimistic about the possibility of cure ... [and believed] that mental disorder was caused by rapid social change, urbanization, and dislocations in society." A century later Emile Durkheim, a French sociologist, published his famous monograph on anomic suicide ("anomie," meaning a sense of dislocation or alienation), which tried to link higher rates of suicide in France with industrialization and social upheaval. In this respect one may also consider theories about the effects of relative deprivation – extremes of wealth and poverty – suggested in the mid-1900s by sociologist Robert Merton as an explanation for differences in crime rates and, more recently, by social psychologists to account for declining self-reported happiness among Americans (Todd 2012). Theories of social cohesion have been used up to the present to explain suicide and self-destructive behaviour among Canadian indigenous peoples, for example by Samson (2009), who revives Durkheim's theory in his analysis of the Innu. For a more recent formulation readers are directed to the writings of Canadian psychologist Bruce Alexander (2008), who attempts to link individual pathologies, such as drug addiction, with social and cultural forces. Unfortunately, these sociological theories are pitched at such a high level of abstraction that they cannot easily be tested empirically.

Interestingly, research conducted up to the present day continues to support an association between urbanization and increased incidence of even biologically based disorders, such as schizophrenia (Abbott 2011; Cantor-Graae 2007; Jarvis 2007; Lederbogen et al. 2011; McGrath 2006; Peen and Dekker 2004). Interpreting these results is made difficult by the high level of analysis and number of complicating factors, and, as an epidemiologist notes, the findings are "ambiguous" (Cantor-Graae 2007, 277; see also Van Os 2004). McGill University researcher Eric Jarvis suggests that this line of inquiry will presumably die out "because of the rise of genetic-biological

paradigms in recent decades" (Jarvis 2007, 287). That being said, the association with social determinants is plausible and explicable if we see schizophrenia as a biological vulnerability potentiated by environmental factors,
a subject discussed in more detail below. A study published in the journal
Nature that used magnetic resonance imaging to look at brain activity found
differences in the ways that urban and rural residents processed social stress,
which the authors hypothesized could contribute to higher rates of mental
disorder among city dwellers (Lederbogen et al. 2011).

Moving from the macro level to the clinical realm, the idea that psychiatric
disorders can have a nonorganic, psychological basis gained momentum in
the nineteenth century with the work of Charcot, a French neurologist, and
the study of *hysteria*, a condition that, for example, caused people to experience paralysis of part of a limb when there was no possible physical basis
for this (in current psychiatric nomenclature, this is referred to as a "conversion disorder"). The work of Charcot and the study of hysteria influenced
Sigmund Freud (1856-1939), who began to study the effect of the *unconscious*
on the manifestation of mental disorders. Articulated about one hundred
years ago, Freud's psychodynamic explanations became very influential in
North America and Europe from the early to mid-1900s,[4] determining to a
considerable extent the nature of psychiatric practice. From this viewpoint,
early childhood experiences, rather than biological predisposition, were
crucial to understanding the genesis of mental disorders. While Freud is
known more for working with persons with neuroses – what we would now
call anxiety disorders – protégés such as American psychoanalyst Harry Stack
Sullivan applied similar techniques in working with individuals diagnosed
with schizophrenia. Increasing criticism of Freudian psychology, which included concerns about theoretical validity as well as clinical utility (e.g.,
Gunderson et al. 1984; Wood 1986), has meant that psychodynamic approaches have now almost completely fallen out of favour in public mental
health settings in North America. Interestingly, Freud did recognize a connection between childhood sexual abuse and adult mental health problems,
but the uproar that this created among his contemporaries led him to subsequently disavow trauma as a causal factor, which he did by interpreting
patients' accounts of incest as mere sexual fantasies (Russell 1986). (Apart
from theoretical considerations, the fact that psychoanalysis is potentially a
long, drawn-out process makes it prohibitively expensive from the perspective of public funding bodies.)

In more recent years there has been greater recognition of the psychological
effects of violence among military and civilian populations. In the 1970s,
American psychologist Lenore Walker made some inroads by proposing the
concept of "battered woman's syndrome," although this still-controversial

diagnosis has not been included in the *Diagnostic and Statistical Manual* of the American Psychiatric Association (some consider it to be an implied subcategory of post-traumatic stress disorder).

In the military, the psychological impact of violence has been documented for some time, including the identification of "shell shock" in the First World War. Sociologist David Pilgrim (2002, 588) suggests that the recognition of the impact of shell shock – given the reality of the large number affected, from all social backgrounds – helped break "the monopoly of bio-determinism" in psychiatry and was a factor in the legitimization of psychoanalytic approaches. Shell shock is what we would now call post-traumatic stress disorder (PTSD), which did not achieve official diagnostic status until 1980 – when PTSD was included in the *DSM* – this largely as a response to the experiences and lobbying of returning Vietnam War veterans in the United States (Yehuda 2002). (The criteria for PTSD in the *DSM* refer to the person's experiencing an event "that involved actual or threatened death or serious injury, or a threat to the physical integrity of self or others," where the person's response "involved intense fear, helplessness, or horror" [American Psychiatric Association 2000, 466]). A high-profile example of the effects of trauma comes from the experiences of Canadians serving as United Nations peacekeepers in the African nation of Rwanda, where, in 1994, 800,000 Tutsi, an ethnic minority, were slaughtered in a civil war by the majority Hutu. A substantial number of the Canadians who witnessed the atrocities later developed PTSD, including the mission commander General Roméo Dallaire, who, in a published memoir, subsequently described symptoms such as distress, insomnia, nightmares, and thoughts of suicide (Dallaire and Beardsley 2003). A decade later, when Canadian forces became involved in more intense combat in Afghanistan in the mid-2000s, there was a concomitant rise in suicides among the troops, to thirty-six in 2007, up from an average of sixteen per year over the previous fourteen years (Hildebrandt 2008). A psychiatrist interviewed about these figures suggested that they were related to the "increased tempo" of the mission and the cumulative stress arising from multiple tours of duty (quoted in Hildebrandt 2008). A report by CTV News ("Military recruiting hundreds to combat PTSD," 2008) found that, around this time, there was a substantial increase in the number of military being identified with a psychiatric condition, in most cases PTSD, with the recruitment of mental health workers to provide support and treatment becoming a major challenge for the Department of Defence.

Notwithstanding the advent of PTSD, it is arguably the case that the psychological effects of trauma and, in particular, child and spouse abuse, have been overlooked or downplayed in clinical practice (Van der Kolk 2002).

Surveys of mental health clinicians have found that, while trauma is recognized as a significant adverse factor, there is, at the same time, a reluctance to address it, this likely being related to staff comfort levels and skill sets (Frueh et al. 2006). In one survey the authors concluded that "trauma has acquired a mystique that leaves clinicians fearful of addressing it, and clinicians have little confidence in their ability to help clients with PTSD" (1,029). Harris and Fallot (2001) talk about the need for a paradigm shift and the need for *trauma-informed* services, arguing that mental health programs still do not adequately screen for trauma histories in new clients, given the high rates of abuse seen in this population. As a consequence, these authors note, appropriate referrals are not made, or, even worse, insensitive responses may result in the client's being re-traumatized. Some have also argued that the under-recognition of trauma is reflected in the use and misuse of the borderline personality diagnosis, which has become pejorative both in the eyes of clients and clinicians and that some claim is actually a misdiagnosis of persons suffering from PTSD (Briere 2002; Simmie and Nunes 2001).

While research has shown an association between early-life trauma and subsequent anxiety, personality, and mood disorders (Lu et al. 2008; Spataro et al. 2004), this relationship is complex, given individual differences in resilience and vulnerability. Not everyone exposed to trauma will develop a clinically significant disorder, and there is some debate as to whether PTSD should be considered a "trait" phenomenon or a "state" phenomenon – that is, whether the manifestation of a disorder should be attributed largely or wholly to the traumatic event itself or to constitutional vulnerabilities (Briere 2002; Kluft, Bloom, and Kinzie 2000). This again speaks to the need for a model that incorporates both "nature" and "nurture," which is the subject of the following section.

The Stress-Vulnerability Model

In this model the manifestation of a mental disorder is the product both of intrinsic factors (vulnerability) and environmental factors (stress). "Manifestation" here can mean either the relapse of an illness or, somewhat more controversially,[5] the initial onset of the illness. "Vulnerability" is often taken to mean genetic endowment, but it can also refer to acquired vulnerability. The assumption here is that more vulnerable individuals will manifest symptoms even in conditions of low stress and will need to compensate for this through medication and lifestyle adjustments (Eaton 2001). A graphic depiction of this, from Zubin and Spring (1977), is given in Figure 2. From this, a person with high vulnerability would be at position "c." In the case of schizophrenia, this could be an individual whose parents both have the disorder and thus genetically is at high risk. In this case a breakthrough of

Figure 2

The stress-vulnerability model

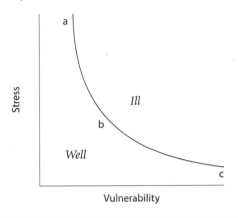

symptoms – such as hallucinations – is possible even in protective environments, that is, it may not require a great degree of stress to cause the person to become unwell. Conversely, the person at position "a" has a low vulnerability to psychosis; while symptoms such as hallucinations are possible, these would only occur if the person was subjected to severe stress, for example, through extreme sleep deprivation.

Empirical support for the model comes from several different lines of research. For one thing, we now clearly understand that stress has physical consequences and can influence the onset and progression of illness (Statistics Canada 2006), this being demonstrated by a number of studies using animal and human subjects that have found that stressful events weaken the immune system (American Psychological Association 2006). Evidence of an interaction between genes and environment comes from a long-term study of 847 patients, in which persons with the "short" form of a gene that affects serotonin metabolism were more likely to report depression in association with an environmental stressor (such as bereavement or job crisis) but no more likely to manifest depression when no stressor was present (Holden 2003). Evidence also comes from epidemiological studies that show variation in the incidence of schizophrenia between different sites and populations, despite earlier beliefs that rates of this illness were "independent of environment" (McGrath 2006, 195). These earlier claims had helped fuel a conception of schizophrenia as very much a "hard-wired" condition, whereas more recent findings support the idea of a vulnerability that is precipitated by environmental factors. Research has also found that the impact of stress appears to be cumulative, or "dose-related." For example, in a Dutch study that followed 140 teens considered at high risk for bipolar disorder (because one parent was so-diagnosed), researchers who looked at the impact of stressful early life events on the onset of a subsequent mood disorder found that the risk of onset increased by 10 percent for each "unit" of stressful life event (Hillegers et al. 2004). Similarly, data from two large community samples in the US and the UK found an association between traumatic life events – such as domestic violence and sexual abuse – and later symptoms of psychosis, particularly when two or more trauma types were experienced (Shevlin et al. 2008).

The epidemiological data, while supportive of a stress-vulnerability model, do not provide an exact mechanism for the activation of a predisposition to illness. For example, researchers following a large (71,165) cohort of persons born in Jerusalem between the years 1964 and 1976 found a significant association between risk of schizophrenia and lower socio-economic status (SES) at birth, the latter assessed by years of parental education, occupational status of the father, and residential area (Werner, Malaspina, and Rabinowitz 2007). These authors note, however, that the measures of SES were *proxies* for factors more directly linked to risk – factors that could not be directly assessed. The findings suggest several plausible hypotheses, including the general observation that adversity and stress are higher among persons with limited resources. As noted in Chapter 3, a potentially fruitful line of inquiry with implications for public health strategies is the connection between maternal health during pregnancy and increased risk for schizophrenia in the offspring, an association that has been found in large-scale studies in China and Europe (Brown and Patterson 2011; Khashan et al. 2008; King, St. Hilaire, and Heidkamp 2010; Sorensen et al. 2011; St. Claire et al. 2005).

In looking at practice applications, it can be argued that the stress-vulnerability model is a more hopeful alternative to the "hard-wired" conception of mental illness since, notwithstanding vulnerability, protective thresholds can be raised by addressing factors such as lifestyle, stress management, and problem-solving skills, with a role for practitioners in the teaching and mentoring of these (Strauss 2008). In describing an education program for clients in the early stages of a psychotic illness, the authors of a practice guidelines document emphasize the importance of the stress-vulnerability model as a framework for presenting information:

> Within this [model], one can present both biological and psychosocial strategies to reduce the risk of psychosis and prevent relapse: complying with medications, avoiding substance use, managing interpersonal conflict, making use of peer support, identifying and managing environmental

stressors, learning the "early warning signs" of the illness, developing and planning proactive coping and help-seeking strategies. By presenting recovery from a first episode as an active process that occurs in recognizable stages, the educator helps both the individual and family to normalize their own experiences and to recognize the value of their own contribution to the recovery. (Mental Health Evaluation and Community Consultation Unit 2002, 14)

Complications and challenges remain. One of these is the difficulty in mitigating stress in a client population that faces considerable socio-economic disadvantage, which becomes a strong argument for a model of care that addresses the social determinants of health. There is also the fact that, while acknowledging psychosocial strategies, clinicians may still place an emphasis on medication adherence as, quoting a practice manual, "the most important protective factor" (Andrews et al. 2000, 339). Clients who are adamantly opposed to medical explanations may find this to be unpalatable. Finally, it should be noted that some family members have expressed concern about a model that emphasizes stress and environmental factors, given what is seen as a potential for blaming caregivers. This subject is covered in more detail later, but, for example, the concept of "expressed emotion," an approach wherein family members are coached in being less critical and emotional when interacting with a mentally ill relative, has been seen by some as effectively blaming caregivers for the relapse of a biologically based disorder (Inman 2011b; Solomon 2001).

Models of Care
How we provide services to persons with mental disorders is influenced by our explanatory models. As noted earlier, the discovery of antipsychotic medications in the 1950s started the shift away from psychodynamic approaches to treatment to what has been called a *medical model*. On this point, University of Calgary professor Walter Glannon (2008, 1) argues that, in the late twentieth century, "a new intellectual framework for psychiatry that emphasized the neurobiological basis of the brain-mind relation ... together with advances in genetics ... [has] helped to establish biological psychiatry as the model for diagnosing and treating disorders of the brain and mind," a model that has "widespread acceptance."

The Medical Model
There is some debate about the "medical model" concept, what it means, and whether it is an accurate depiction of current psychiatric practice (Shah and Mountain 2007), so further explication is necessary. In consulting

dictionaries one will see that "medical model" is defined as a practice used by physicians in the Western world, where through physical examination, diagnostic tests, and patient history an illness is diagnosed, which then forms the basis for treatments that are very often pharmacological. Because it is focused on an illness or defect, the medical approach is considered non-holistic, either in the assessment of cause or in the interventions applied. Mental illness in this model is seen in terms of a physical process that affects people the same way, so that subjective experience and cultural context are often overlooked.

Is this really the way psychiatrists, and, by extension, their colleagues in mental health programs, operate? Obviously – and this comes from the author's own experience – physicians are neither unintelligent nor unsophisticated, so it is almost certainly unfair to characterize them as lacking awareness of psychosocial factors. That being said, in looking at the way mental health services are structured and delivered in North America, there is evidence that it is indeed very "medical."

- As reflected in provincial medical services data, most contacts for mental health reasons in Canada are with a family doctor, not a specialist, particularly when the complaint is depression (Lavoie and Fleet 2002; Picard 2008a; Slomp et al. 2009). Family doctors have less training in psychiatry, and less time in their sessions for patients, a consequence being that the interactions "tend to be shorter in duration, less often include therapeutic listening, and more commonly result in prescription of medication" (Clarke Institute of Psychiatry 1997, 64).
- Psychiatrists themselves have become more biological and less psychological in their treatment approach.[6] A 2005 survey found that only 11 percent of US psychiatrists provided psychotherapy to all of their clients, this driven by the medical model but also by the unwillingness of insurance companies to fund longer counselling sessions – with medications then being the default option (reported in Harris 2011). A *New York Times* report on this notes that this means personal crises are left "unexplored and unresolved," and it quotes a former president of the American Psychiatric Association as saying that psychiatric practice was now "very reminiscent of primary care ... [psychiatrists] check up on people; they pull out the prescription pad; they order tests" (quoted in Harris 2011). In Canada the situation is different with respect to funding psychiatrist services,[7] but access to psychological treatment, in particular to cognitive-behavioural therapies (CBT), remains quite limited (Livingston et al. 2009; Rhodes et al. 2010). Surveys have found that Canadian psychiatrists are

given limited training in CBT and that only a minority are able to offer it in their practice (Goldner, Jones, and Fang 2011; Myhr and Payne 2006).

- The drug companies have been very influential in having mental disorders characterized as biological conditions requiring pharmaceutical treatments. For example, a visitor to the Canadian website "Depression Hurts" (http://www.depressionhurts.ca/en/), sponsored by the drug company Eli Lilly, will be told in the "Frequently Asked Questions" section: "One common theory is that depression is caused by an imbalance of naturally occurring substances called neurotransmitters in the brain and spinal cord." Nowhere in this section is there any mention of the psychosocial determinants of depression. The public is increasingly buying into this, apparently, with one survey finding that that the proportion of the US general population attributing depression to a biological cause increased from 77 percent in 1996 to 88 percent in 2006; the same survey found that respondents endorsing a "biological focus of treatment" increased from 48 percent to 60 percent over the same period (Blumner and Marcus 2009).

- More people than ever are on psychotropic medication, particularly anti-depressants, with the per capita utilization of this class of drugs roughly *doubling* in Canada and the US from the mid-1990s to the mid-2000s (Branham 2003; Newman and Schopflocher 2008; Olfson and Marcus 2009; Raymond, Morgan, and Caetano 2007), this achieved, in part, by more prescriptions being written for young persons (Mitchell et al. 2008).

- Other health care professionals see service delivery as overly medical. For example, a Canadian occupational therapist writes in 2011: "As Canada moves to challenge the *supremacy of the medical model* and incorporate a vision of recovery as a guide for mental health services, significant changes will be required, both in the way services are provided, and in the way they are received" (White 2011, 26, emphasis added).

This conclusion – that changes are needed – was also reached in a 2006 Canadian Senate report arising out of consultations with various stakeholders across Canada. The report, entitled *Out of the Shadows at Last: Transforming Mental Health, Mental Illness and Addiction Services in Canada*, is seen as important because it led to the creation of the Canadian Mental Health Commission and influenced the policy direction of that body. A section of the Senate report asks: "What are individuals living with mental illness asking for?" The replies then refer to the psychosocial determinants of health – and no reference is made, for example, to "more and better medical treatments." The report addresses "the mental and physical dimensions of illness" as follows:

It is important to clarify what "treating mental illness like physical illness" really means. There is nothing approaching universal agreement on how mental and physical factors influence the state of our mental health ... although most people seem to agree that mental illnesses almost always entail some combination of these factors. However, different emphases placed on the role of these four factors can and do lead to very different approaches to mental health policy. For example, someone who believes that the key to "curing" mental illness is an understanding of the underlying functions of the brain, would be much more likely to support *spending scarce research dollars on neurophysiology* than on studies of the impact on individuals of the social determinants of mental health. In the Committee's view, it is essential to recognize that in treating mental illness comparably to physical illness it is not necessary to treat them as if they were identical to one another ... In particular, the Committee believes it is extremely important to stress the significance of what are called the social determinants of health in understanding mental illness and in fostering recovery from it. (Standing Senate Committee on Social Affairs, Science and . Technology 2006, 41, emphasis added)

Not everyone has been happy with this proposed policy direction, particularly when the mental disorder is seen as primarily biological, as is the case with schizophrenia (Brean 2011; Inman 2011b). Commenting on a later Mental Health Commission strategy document, *Globe and Mail* health reporter André Picard (2011) argues that there is "not enough emphasis on brain science":

In fact, reading the draft strategy, one is left with an unpleasant aftertaste: the distinct feeling that psychiatry and medications have no place in Canada's approach to tackling mental illness. There are distinct – and sometimes clashing – views in the mental health field. But the strategy gives too much credence to social science and not enough to neuroscience.

In one of his columns, *Huffington Post* writer Marvin Ross (2011b) similarly speaks about the need to maintain support for research into the physiological underpinnings of schizophrenia: "It's time to put science back into mental illness and to stop pretending these illnesses are [due to]... poor parenting or stress." From this perspective a "medical model" is not necessarily a bad thing: further research will, it is hoped, lead to better pharmacological treatments and a clearer understanding of the genetic basis of disorders such as schizophrenia. Further, as claimed by two British psychiatrists: "Biological

explanations and treatments for diseases have helped to reduce fear, super-
stition and stigma, and to increase understanding, hope and humane
methods of treatment" (Shah and Mountain 2007, 375).

While the argument for a medical model becomes stronger in the case
of very disabling conditions, such as severe psychosis, a few caveats are
offered here.

- A biomedical conception of schizophrenia has not, unfortunately, had the
  desired effect of reducing stigma, and in fact the opposite may be occurring.
  A review of public surveys by Watters (2010) found that persons "who
  adopted biomedical/genetic beliefs about mental disorders were the same
  people who wanted less contact with the mentally ill and thought of them
  as more dangerous and unpredictable." "Differentness" becomes the attributed status: "The biomedical narrative about an illness like schizophrenia carries with it the subtle assumption that a brain made ill through
  biomedical or genetic abnormalities is more thoroughly broken and permanently abnormal than one made ill through life events" (Watters 2010).
- We need to consider the implications of genetic research and our attempts
  to pin down "biomarkers." There is currently no physical test – no blood
  assay or brain scan – that can confirm the diagnosis of schizophrenia, a
  fact that some feel weakens the case for a "medical model" approach to
  the illness.[8] While illnesses of various sorts have been present historically
  before the technology to test for them existed, this "gap" in the medical
  model is concerning for some, and so research on biomarkers continues
  apace, including a group that has identified a "disease signature" comprised
  of fifty-one protein biomarkers to help diagnose schizophrenia (Schwarz
  et al. 2010). Despite gaps in knowledge, health authorities in Canada now
  offer genetic counselling for psychiatric disorders.[9] What if a definitive
  diagnostic test *was* found? Given the stigma and disability associated with
  schizophrenia, would there be concerns about discrimination against the
  diagnosed person should the information of a positive test be leaked to
  others? While they are different syndromes, there may be some parallels
  here between schizophrenia and Huntington's disease, for which a definite
  genetic test exists: researchers have found that most persons at risk for
  Huntington's – 96 percent of Americans and 75 percent of Canadians according to surveys – *do not* pursue predictive testing because of what is
  seen as a poor prognosis (Takeuchi 2012; Walker 2007). Readers may object
  to this comparison on the basis that there are more treatment options for
  schizophrenia than Huntington's. While this is true, it should be noted
  that a significant proportion of persons with schizophrenia, perhaps a

third, achieve only a limited response to antipsychotic medication (Kane et al. 2011). Further, prognosis in schizophrenia is related not only to symptoms but to quality of life, which, in the case of schizophrenia, may suffer because of the stigma and rejection – actual and anticipated – felt by persons with this diagnosis (Stuart and Arboleda-Florez 2001). Other concerns about genetic testing, identified in interviews by Turney and Turner (2000) with health care professionals, include the prospect of pre-natal screening leading to abortions (and what that says about attitudes towards schizophrenia), family members blaming each other for their "bad genes," and persons getting a positive test, then either engaging in denial or feeling hopeless.

- Seeing the problem as a "damaged brain" may not leave the service provider with many options. In working with an advanced Alzheimer's patient, or someone with a severe head injury, the task is less about rehabilitation and more about safety, containment, and providing the basic necessities of life. Schizophrenia has increasingly been categorized as a type of brain damage (e.g. Inman 2010), along with seeing the accompanying lack of insight (lack of awareness that you have a mental illness) as biologically based. Refusing treatment is thus seen as "a symptom of the brain disorder rather than denial ... an unawareness syndrome seen in stroke patients and others with frontal lobe lesions" (Amador 2009, 36). Arango and Amador (2011, 27, emphasis added) suggest that "about 50% of persons with schizophrenia do not know they have an illness, and this unaware-ness typically *does not improve with education, time or treatment.*" Human agency is thus discounted, and from this perspective imposition of treat-ment, involuntarily if necessary, is not only justifiable but an ethical re-sponsibility. Consider the following quote from the Treatment Advocacy Center (2009b), which, according to its website, "is a non-profit organiza-tion dedicated to eliminating barriers to the timely and effective treatment of severe mental illness":

  It is commonly claimed that: if you make the psychiatric services attract-ive enough and culturally relevant, then individuals with serious mental illnesses will utilize them. This appears to not be true ... The greatest reason for non-treatment [according to the study cited] by far was the person's lack of awareness of their illness. Such individuals will not voluntarily utilize psychiatric services, no matter how attractive those services are, because they do not believe that they have an illness.

- The role of the service recipient in a medical model is essentially a passive one. In the "sick role" conception,[10] a person with an illness is exempt from normal social obligations, is not responsible for her/his condition, should try to get well, should seek technically competent help, and should cooperate with the medical professional. This passive role is out of step with a current emphasis in health care on members of the public being informed consumers, and with self-management models being developed for both physical and mental disorders, wherein the service user is a more active participant in care (Bilsker 2003). Proponents of the medical model would argue that people with serious mental illnesses lack the capacity to be "consumers" in this sense (Torrey 2011a); nevertheless, there is still the concern that the medical approach is one that fosters dependency.

Psychosocial Models

In response to the criticism that psychiatry is overly medical, psychiatric practitioners may point out that they are trained in a *biopsychosocial* (BPS) model.[11] For example, Canadian psychiatry residents taking the Royal College exams will be asked to include references to the psychological and social in their assessment formulations. In recounting the history of the BPS model, Pilgrim (2002) notes that it developed in part as a reaction to criticisms of psychiatry, in particular that the discipline's approach was reductionist and thus dehumanizing, with the promise that, through a BPS model treatment, it would become more holistic and acceptable to those receiving services. However, critics argue that the BPS model has never been clearly articulated – an author and psychiatrist refers to it as a "mirage" (McLaren 2002, 701) – and Pilgrim (2002) suggests that if there is a more holistic or "eclectic" approach used in psychiatric practice, this is driven more by convenience and pragmatism than by any underlying theoretical model. When searching websites for psychiatric training programs in Canada, it is in fact difficult to find any detailed references to this concept, although, for example, the *Canadian Journal of Psychiatry* does speak about publishing "psychiatric research on a broad range of biopsychosocial topics" http://publications. cpa-apc.org/browse/sections/. Other writers are sharper in their criticism, arguing that, while lip service is paid to the BPS model, in reality, practice is still very much biological. A psychiatry professor at Yale University, in the book *The Rise and Fall of the Biopsychosocial Model* (Ghaemi 2010, 108-9), concludes that "psychiatry, in practice, is mostly psychopharmacology" and that "this has occurred despite the BPS model, which has not stopped this process, despite its frequent invocation, and never will." Similarly, in referring to the current approach to practice, American psychiatrist Sarah Mourra (2013) notes that "this psychopharmacological myopia is dangerous in that most psychiatrists of my generation pay lip service to the 'psychosocial' part of the biopsychosocial model while failing to put it into practice." In fairness, if psychiatric practice in public mental health programs is less than holistic, this is determined as well by the supply of psychiatrists, funding arrangements, and service delivery structures, all of which mean that contact time with clients is often very limited. Other interventions, if applied, are often provided by allied professionals, and these approaches may include individual counselling, group modalities, and vocational rehabilitation (see Chapters 16 and 17). Concerning a value orientation, while it does not seem unreasonable to suggest that all practitioners should share the same views about client choice and self-determination, physicians and psychiatrists may feel the weight of medical liability more heavily than their colleagues and, consequently, be more cautious and safety-oriented in their actions.

Currently, the best articulation of a biopsychosocial model is the PSR program – Psychosocial Rehabilitation. The PSR approach was developed at Boston University, and PSR curricula and diplomas are offered at several postsecondary institutions in Canada, listed at the website of PSR Canada (http://www.psrrpscanada.ca/index.php). PSR is a strengths-based approach, emphasizing function and ability rather than disability, and, at the PSR Canada website, it is noted that PSR services "focus on helping individuals develop skills and access resources needed to increase their capacity to be successful and satisfied in the living, working, learning and social environments of their choice." While PSR has been associated with the "rehab" disciplines, such as occupational therapy, there is no reason that practitioners of other disciplines could not take this training. Indeed, currently PSR is the curriculum and orientation most in line with the *recovery* perspective – an approach to service delivery endorsed by the Mental Health Commission of Canada and accreditation bodies – and so the assumption would be that all disciplines working in Canadian mental health programs would eventually need to adopt PSR principles in their practice (see box).

In looking at the PSR values listed above, readers may argue that, while laudable, they do not appear to offer any specific guide to action. And, as is seen in Chapter 5, this question of operationalization has been levelled at

PSR Canada Core Principles and Values

- Psychosocial rehabilitation practitioners convey hope and respect and believe that all individuals have the capacity for learning and growth.
- Psychosocial rehabilitation practitioners recognize that culture and diversity are central to recovery, and they strive to ensure that all services and

supports are culturally relevant to individuals receiving services and supports.

■ Psychosocial rehabilitation practitioners engage in the processes of informed and shared decision making and facilitate partnerships with other persons identified by the individual receiving services and supports.

■ Psychosocial rehabilitation practices build on strengths and capacities of individuals receiving services and supports.

■ Psychosocial rehabilitation practices are person-centred; they are designed to address the distinct needs of individuals, consistent with their values, hopes, and aspirations.

■ Psychosocial rehabilitation practices support full integration of people in recovery into their communities, where they can exercise their rights of citizenship and accept the responsibilities, and explore the opportunities that come with being a member of a community and a larger society.

■ Psychosocial rehabilitation practices promote self-determination and empowerment. All individuals have the right to make their own decisions, including decisions about the types of services and supports they receive.

■ Psychosocial rehabilitation practices facilitate the development of personal support networks by utilizing natural supports within communities, family members as defined by the individual, peer support initiatives, and self- and mutual-help groups.

■ Psychosocial rehabilitation practices strive to help individuals improve the quality of all aspects of their lives, including social, occupational, educational, residential, intellectual, spiritual, and financial.

■ Psychosocial rehabilitation practices promote health and wellness, encouraging individuals to develop and use individualized wellness plans.

■ Psychosocial rehabilitation services and supports emphasize evidence-based, promising, and emerging best practices that produce outcomes congruent with personal recovery. Psychosocial rehabilitation programs include program evaluation and continuous quality improvement that actively involve persons receiving services and supports.

■ Psychosocial rehabilitation services and supports must be readily accessible to all individuals whenever they need them; these services and supports should be well coordinated and integrated as needed with other psychiatric, medical, and holistic treatments and practices.

Source: PSR Canada website: http://www.psrrpscanada.ca/index.php?src=gendocs&link=About.

the recovery vision itself. However, as is detailed in this book, tools and resources that can be seen as supporting PSR principles have been and are being developed. For example, well-received cultural competency curricula have been created in Canada (see Chapter 6); more holistic assessment instruments, such as the OCAN, have been implemented (see Chapter 14); and individualized wellness plans have been put into place in a number of settings and are acquiring an evidence base (see Chapter 16).

Is there any way to reconcile a PSR and a biomedical approach? Can they possibly be seen as complementary rather than as competing? In a sense this is already happening: clients of Canadian public mental health programs typically receive what could be called a parallel approach: medical management led by a physician or psychiatrist and rehabilitation-focused services – for example, cognitive behavioural therapy groups – led by allied professionals. While there may be some concern about the coherence of a parallel approach, in such a system the physician can be seen as representing more of the "bio" part of the model, and the allied professional(s) more of the "psychosocial," although to put it this way works against the goal of having a staff that possesses competencies across a range of domains. A somewhat different way of looking at this is to acknowledge that serious mental illnesses are relapsing conditions, but ones in which affected persons are in an acute phase a *minority* of the time – perhaps less than 5 percent of their adult lives (Tondora, Miller, and Davidson 2012). It is during these acute phases that medical management potentially becomes more important, for example, if safety concerns necessitate hospitalization – with the physician then stepping to the forefront. At other times, however, the "medical model," while important for ongoing stabilization, takes a step back as PSR approaches – which include illness self-management – are utilized to move the client further along the road to recovery. This approach, it is hoped, would have the effect of producing better outcomes for clients and, at the same time, promoting and enhancing the skill sets of allied professionals. The latter issue is significant because mental health programs have evolved from a limited, "doctor-driven" model in which the role of the allied professional is largely to support the doctor's medical management of the case. Whether a particular mental health program in the current era is doctor-driven is determined by different factors, including treatment culture and traditions, and also whether the program is in an urban or rural location, with rural workers having to be more self-reliant, simply because of a shortage of physicians (see Chapter 11). In some doctor-driven locales, allied professionals may need to be empowered to broaden their role, which requires sufficient vision and leadership on the part of management.

Notes

1 The Mental Health Commission of Canada (2012, 14) attempts to resolve this by referring to "mental health *problems and illnesses*" (emphasis added), noting that it is not attempting to draw a firm line between "problem" and "illness" but, rather, to be "respectful of a wide range of views."

2 The counterpoint to this counterpoint would be that serious depression, which itself may be more biologically based, should be distinguished from mild-to-moderate forms of the disorder. This is explored further in Chapter 8, which presents the argument that anti-depressant medications are being overprescribed to persons whose problems do not reach the threshold of clinical significance.

3 The "medication naïve" aspect is important in order to rule out the possibility that changes in brain structure are due to the drugs used in treatment (see also Whitaker 2010).

4 While not easily defined, a Canadian psychologist (Ogrodniczuk 2011, 21) refers to psycho-dynamic treatments as those that "focus on identifying recurring patterns in relationships, discussing past experiences, exploring emotions, and [bringing] into awareness mental processes of which the person was not previously aware."

5 There is stronger evidence now that substance misuse may play a significant part in the initial breakthrough of psychotic disorders, as opposed to the view that the illness would have occurred regardless (BC Ministry of Health Services 2008; Degenhardt and Hall 2006; Welch et al. 2011).

6 Writing in 2013, American psychiatrist Sarah Mourra notes the trend of some of her colleagues who refer to themselves as "psychopharmacologists."

7 *Psychologist* services, however, are not generally publicly funded in Canada. "Medically necessary" services are mandated by the Canada Health Act, with this referring mainly to hospital and physician services.

8 One famous critic was American author Thomas Szasz, who, in books such as *The Myth of Mental Illness*, argued that the apparent lack of a neurological basis in schizophrenia meant that the involuntary medical treatment of persons so diagnosed was unsupportable.

9 In 2012, a genetic counselling program for psychiatric disorders was opened in Vancouver, described in an e-mail to this author as a service for persons "interested in learning about what might have contributed to the development of their own mental illness or that of their child/sibling/parent etc.," and one that would "really help people with issues around guilt and stigma."

10 Attributed to American sociologist Talcott Parsons. See also Hewa (2002).

11 A conception attributed to American psychiatrist George Engel (1977).

Priorities and Needs: Who Is Being Helped?

2

The mandate of public mental health programs in Canada is to help persons with mental disorders. This may seem to be an obvious point, but it raises the question: How do we determine who needs help? This question is exceedingly complicated and, since health care resources are not unlimited, has to do with how programs define the "priority population" and what constitutes a "serious" disorder. Answering this question also takes into account help-seeking behaviour and whether public programs have a greater role to play in prevention and health promotion. As will be seen, it has been difficult to reach a consensus definition of the priority population, and there is a parallel concern about stretching the inclusion criteria for mental health services so broadly that the most vulnerable mentally ill end up being displaced. At the same time, we see that there are vulnerable persons who are experiencing considerable distress, as evidenced by perceived need for support, who may be diagnostically excluded from public mental health programs.

Determining Program Eligibility

In considering the provision of services to persons with mental health problems, it is crucially important to be able to identify those most in need of help, the group for whom "it is medically and morally unjustifiable to limit care" (Satel and Humphreys 2003). On this point, McEwan and Goldner (2001, 25) note that "accountability within the sphere of publicly funded mental health services and supports is determined, in part, by how well priority populations are served." This becomes an imperative given that there are apparently a large number of persons with mental health concerns and limited resources to respond to them.[1] Thus, the mandates of public mental health programs usually refer to targeting persons with "serious" or "severe" mental disorders.

So, how do we define "serious?" Newcomers to the field of mental health may be forgiven for thinking that there is a clear consensus among mental health professionals and administrators as to how the priority population is identified. Unfortunately, this has not historically been the case. A Health Canada report concludes that "investigations of the usage of the term 'serious mental illness' amongst service providers and administrative organizations have found little consistency and no clear definition" (McEwan and Goldner 2001, 25). Another government document notes that attempts to define the "target population" have been confounded by the fact that inclusion criteria "are either vaguely defined or not defined at all, permitting a wide variation in practice" (British Columbia Ministry of Health 2002c, 33). An earlier American study on this subject determined that at least seventeen different definitions of severe mental illness could be found, resulting in widely varying prevalence rates, depending on which one was applied (Schinnar et al. 1990).

Diagnosis

Historically, diagnosis has been a key criterion in determining service eligibility. There has been general agreement that two syndromes in particular, schizophrenia and bipolar disorder (manic-depressive illness), constitute serious conditions (British Columbia Ministry of Health 2002e). In some schemes the criteria for "serious" or "severe" are limited to these two disorders exclusively. For instance, in a study of substance misuse among mentally disordered persons, Brunette and colleagues (2003) classified only those persons diagnosed with schizophrenia spectrum disorders or bipolar disorder as suffering from a "severe mental illness." In another example, in arriving at subcategories of the client population, a Health Canada (2001a) report on concurrent mental health and substance use disorders excludes anxiety disorders, personality disorders, eating disorders, and mood disorders other than bipolar from the category of "serious, persistent mental disorders."

Why are schizophrenia and bipolar disorder considered serious by definition? In looking at the acute phase of schizophrenia, persons with the disorder can experience delusions, hallucinations, disordered thinking, and may exhibit bizarre speech and behaviour – symptoms that are collectively called *psychosis*, a "break with reality." Persons in the acute stages of bipolar disorder may similarly experience psychosis, or mania, which can manifest as excessive energy, racing thoughts, and grandiose plans; when in this speeded-up state, individuals can be very impulsive and engage in overspending or reckless sexual activity. In these examples, behaviour is apparently *non-volitional* – out of the person's control. As well, attempts to reason with acutely psychotic people are often unsuccessful, and in these instances

affected persons usually require professional attention, including hospitalization and psychotropic medication. Medical involvement is appropriate
for conditions that are considered biological; on this point blogger and
advocate D.J. Jaffe suggests succinctly that "mental illness is a biologically
based *no-fault* medical problem that resides in the brain's chemistry or
neuroanatomy" (Jaffe 2010, emphasis added). Finally, schizophrenia and
bipolar disorder may be considered serious because of their *duration*: there
may be an ongoing impact of the disorder lasting for a period of years
(Andrews et al. 2000).

It is noteworthy that the acute manifestations of schizophrenia and bipolar
disorder are very much congruent with *lay* definitions of mental illness, with
what the public views as "crazy" behaviour. On this issue, a survey commissioned by the Canadian Medical Association (2008) found that 71 percent
of the general public considered schizophrenia to be a "serious mental illness" – compared to only 36 percent for depression. In the survey, 90 percent
of respondents agreed that mental illness was a *non-volitional* state (you can't
"snap out of it"), with a similar number agreeing that a mental illness required treatment by a health professional, as opposed to self-management.[2]
A different national survey (*n* = 1,000) commissioned by the Canadian
Alliance on Mental Illness and Mental Health (2007) produced similar results; when asked what "mental illness" was, respondents used terms such
as "crazy," "out of control," and "unpredictable," and usually referenced
schizophrenia:

> People made a clear distinction between common mental disorders (such
> as depression and anxiety) and serious disorders (such as schizophrenia
> and bipolar disorder). The former are seen as "mental health problems",
> which are situational, transitory, and not requiring of medical treatment.
> The participants reserved the term "mental illness" for serious mental
> disorders, which are chronic, impair capacity to function in life, and call
> for medical intervention. Most agreed that anyone could suffer from mental
> health problems but fewer people would be at risk for a mental illness.
> (Canadian Alliance on Mental Illness 2007, 25)

While practitioner and lay conceptions of mental illness do not entirely
coincide, one cannot assume that the former are not influenced by the
latter.

Family support and advocacy organizations have also argued that the
designation of "serious" should be applied to schizophrenia and bipolar disorder in particular.[3] The concern here is that, if the definition of mental
disorder is stretched too far, then resources will end up being devoted to

those least in need – the "worried well" rather than the most vulnerable and helpless (Jaffe 2010). This concern was reflected in a letter to the Mental Health Commission of Canada by an advocate who argued that the commission's national strategy focused too much on persons with less serious conditions: "There is a compelling distinction between mild to moderate psychosocial mental health problems that may have a causal relationship with the environment and the severe and complex mental illnesses that are chronic biomedical brain diseases" (Buchanan 2011).

Disability

Diagnostic categories do not necessarily tell us about the degree of disability produced by the disorder. Two Canadian authors note that "a wide spectrum of symptom severity and functional disability is associated with specific mental disorders; any particular diagnosis ... does not, in and of itself, provide enough information to make a determination regarding the presence or absence of *serious* mental illness" (McEwan and Goldner 2001, 26, emphasis added). Diagnostic prevalence rates may in some cases *over-rate* the illness burden and the associated need for mental health services in the general population.[4] "Diagnostic inflation" can occur for different reasons. In some instances this can be the over-diagnosis of a recognized condition, an example being the contention, which is admittedly controversial, that PTSD is being over-diagnosed in the US military, possibly as a means to accessing medical benefits for veterans (Dobbs 2009; see also Merskey and Piper 2007). In other cases, it has been argued that psychiatry is expanding into the realm of normal, as opposed to pathological, conditions, a tendency referred to as "disease mongering" (and discussed in more detail in Chapter 8) (Kleiner 2011). An example here would be, arguably, the inclusion of the condition "premenstrual dysphoric disorder" in the *Diagnostic and Statistical Manual* of the American Psychiatric Association (Moynihan and Cassels 2005).

The fact that diagnosis alone does not tell us about the severity of symptoms, or the degree of functional impairment, can create problems in several respects. First, the assumption that a particular condition, by definition, is or is not serious means that some populations will always be underserved. An example here is anxiety disorders, which have tended historically to be considered "less serious" as a group and consequently underserved by public mental health programs, even though for some people they can be profoundly disabling. This also means, conversely, that schizophrenia will always be considered pervasively disabling, despite studies that show that people with this diagnosis often see an improvement in perceived quality of life, symptoms, relapses, and self-management later on in the course of illness (Jeste, Wolkowitz, and Palmer 2011).

Diagnosis as a guide to action is notably unclear with respect to major depression (MD). Depression exists on a continuum, and for some it is a very serious condition, resulting in social withdrawal and suicidal thinking. For others, it may be painful but transitory, relating more to a traumatic social event than to a biological vulnerability. Some persons may experience a longer-term but milder form of depression known as *dysthymia* (referred to in the 2013 edition of the *DSM* as "persistent depressive disorder"). In reviewing this subject, Canadian psychiatrist Scott Patten (2008) notes that, as defined by the *DSM*, MD is extremely common, with lifetime prevalence rates estimated to be at least 20 percent and possibly as high as 50 percent. Taken at face value, these numbers would have considerable implications for the fiscal and human resources needed to deal with the problem. The author concludes, however, that "the *DSM* ... definitions capture such a broad spectrum of morbidity that they should not be regarded as de facto indicators of need, at least not in community populations" (411). Rather, "in many instances [of MD] these episodes are brief, preceded by losses and stressors, often not treated, and later not remembered" (417). For milder or more transient forms of depression, co-management along with a family doctor, who may or may not prescribe medication, may be a viable alternative to specialized mental health care (Meredith et al. 2007).

How is disability established? In clinical settings, client disability is established through the collection of collateral information, history-taking, and professional judgment. Greater numbers of psychiatric hospitalizations, a greater duration of unemployment, and other factors (such as homelessness) are taken into account, although not necessarily in a systematic fashion. Concerning assessment scales, prior to 2013 the *DSM* provided a rough guide to functional levels called the Global Assessment of Functioning (GAF), which was a scale running from zero to 100. The GAF could be used during hospitalization to get a sense of improvement from the time of admission. The GAF was in fact dropped in the 2013 revision of the *DSM* because of concerns about validity and reliability (Keyes 2005; Söderberg, Tungström, and Armelius 2005; Vatnaland et al. 2007). A scale coming into wider use in Canada is the Health of the Nation Outcome Scales (HoNOS), on which a problem rating of 2 or higher on a 0-4 scale item is considered to require some form of intervention (Spaeth-Rublee et al. 2010). Another instrument used in some mental health and addiction settings is the Outcome Rating Scale (ORS), on which the client rates his or her own levels of distress and well-being (Duncan, Miller, and Sparks 2004). The HoNOS and ORS have not typically been used as screening instruments for program eligibility, but they may be useful in this respect. As this book went to press, the Vancouver Coastal Health Authority was piloting an American level-of-care utilization system called LOCUS (American Association of Community Psychiatrists 2010), to determine if it could more systematically determine appropriate care levels for clients.

At the *population* level, epidemiologists establish disability rates through public surveys that attempt to address functional impairment as well as diagnosis. Researchers may use health-adjusted life years (HALYs), which are calculated by combining (1) the years of life lost due to premature death and (2) reduced functioning associated with the illness (Ratnasingham et al. 2012). It has been found that prevalence rates indeed change when an assessment of illness severity is applied. For example, Narrow and colleagues (2002) used the data from a large-scale US public survey (n = 20,861), comparing the one-year prevalence rates for different mental disorders with and without the application of "clinical significance" questions. Subjects for whom it was determined that the thresholds for diagnosis had been met were additionally asked: whether they had contacted a doctor or other professional about this; whether they were taking medication for the symptoms; or whether the symptoms interfered with their everyday life. Significance was counted if the participant answered "yes" to any of the three questions. It was found that, by including clinical significance questions, the one-year prevalence rates dropped as follows: for "any mood disorder," from 9.5 to 5.1 percent; for major depressive episode, from 5.8 to 4.5 percent; and for dysthymia (the least severe mood disorder), from 5.5 to 1.7 percent. Consistent with the understanding that schizophrenia is on average more disabling than other mental disorders, the difference in the two rates for this diagnosis was minimal, ranging from 1.1 to 1.0 percent. The data here suggest that psychotic disorders are less prevalent but have more impact on an individual basis. On the other hand, given their considerably higher prevalence rates, mood and anxiety disorders still represent a significant impact on a *population* level with respect to disability; for example, a study of the Ontario population found that anxiety disorders produced a larger number of HALYs across the general public than schizophrenia (Ratnasingham et al. 2012).

Substance Misuse and Personality Disorder

Whether substance misuse or personality disorders should be included as serious mental illnesses, or even mental illnesses at all, remains a contentious issue. A survey of the Canadian public found respondents split on this topic, with 45 percent claiming that drug addiction was not a mental illness and 51 percent claiming that it was; 26 percent of the sample considered it to be a serious mental illness (Canadian Medical Association 2008). This ambivalence has been reflected among mental health practitioners as well (Campbell 2003; Potter 2011; Satel 1999). At the same time, addiction services are being increasingly integrated with mental health programs in Canada, and epidemiologists – if not clinicians – are now including persons misusing substances in their priority population definitions, referring, for example, to severe addictions and mental illness (SAMI) (Centre for Applied Research in Mental Health and Addiction 2007a).

There are several issues to consider here. One is the ongoing concern that limited mental health resources will be stretched thinner by including persons with addictions in the mandate. Another has to do with learning different treatment models, with mental health practitioners being typically less familiar with the philosophies and interventions that are applied in addictions practice (or in working with persons with severe personality disorders) (El-Guebaly 1997). A partial response to this is to note that a number of clients have *both* a mental illness and an addiction and that having one of these has often meant being excluded from services designed to treat the other. Instead, it can be argued that a more effective and coherent approach is to treat both conditions in parallel fashion at the same program, if not necessarily with the same worker (Minkoff 2001).

An even more fundamental problem, however, has to do with our belief systems. Recall our discussion above about mental disorder, at least from a lay perspective, being a *non-volitional* state – out of the individual's control. From this viewpoint someone with schizophrenia who has frightening delusions can, compellingly, be seen to be suffering from a serious illness and to be in need of help. What about drug addiction and personality disorder? Persons with these conditions may be having – and causing – a lot of problems but, nonetheless, seem to have control over their actions. They are, in other words, being *willful*. Since, as Calgary physician William Campbell notes, "acts of will or volition are usually not accepted as diseases" (Campbell 2003, 673), many practitioners have been uncomfortable with the idea that alcoholism and drug addiction, for instance, should be considered mental disorders. But are drug addicts really exercising free will? In a position paper on this topic, a group of psychiatrists notes that, in fact, "the role of biological factors in addiction is supported by increasingly compelling evidence" and that "certain individuals seem more vulnerable to developing alcoholism because of their genetic background" (Committee on Addictions of the Group for the Advancement of Psychiatry 2002, 708). These authors conclude that, "if we recognize that an individual with an addiction may not be fully able to exercise free will, then society's obligation to intervene becomes stronger" (712). Other practitioners have suggested that addicts still have the ability to make choices and should not be given the "illness excuse." A Yale University psychiatrist writes: "To reduce addiction to a slice of deranged brain tissue vastly underplays the reality that much of addictive behavior is voluntary ... During those times [of sobriety] it is the individual's responsibility to make himself [sic] less vulnerable to relapse. The person, not his autonomous brain, is the instigator of relapse and the agent of recovery" (Satel 1999, 861).

Similar reasoning may follow with respect to personality disorders. Clients diagnosed with borderline personality disorder (BPD) are often a challenge for practitioners, who may see their behaviour as manipulative, bullying, and divisive (Potter 2011). What is important for our purposes here are the attributions made by clinicians in these cases: Potter (2011, 10) notes: "The difficult behavior of the patient with BPD is often seen as 'bad' and 'deliberate' rather than as 'sick.' The schizophrenic patient, on the other hand, is not seen as having this control." The perception seems to be that, "unless a patient is deluded or hallucinating ... she [sic] knows what she is doing and is therefore responsible for what she does [and] since she is responsible ... she is to blame for it" (3). Queens's University professor Heather Stuart concludes that "people [in this case, staff] who hold moral models of mental illness ... who believe that the illness is controllable ... are more likely to respond in an angry and punitive manner" (Stuart 2008, 185). Whether persons suffering with BPD are really exercising free will, or are really "in control," is questionable, however (Williams 1998). If nothing else, clinicians should consider the acute distress and turmoil being experienced by these individuals and whether anyone would freely choose this state. The idea that personality disorders are clinically less serious is also reinforced by the fact that, in 1980, the *DSM* of the American Psychiatric Association started classifying these conditions on a separate axis from schizophrenia and bipolar disorder. While this was not intended to give personality disorders an inferior status – Axis I vs. Axis II – this in fact has been the result (Paris 1998). (The multi-axial system was dropped in the 2013 edition of the *DSM*.) Persons with BPD, even if not considered "priorities," are nonetheless seen in community mental health programs and in some cases are referred to in agency mandates (see below). This may come about because of their high profile in the community or simply because they meet the eligibility criteria by having another "serious," co-occurring diagnosis – often depression or bipolar disorder.[5]

Defining "Serious"
Attempts have been made to come up with a population-based definition of "serious" that draws from the different dimensions discussed above (see Lesage 2010). These dimensions usually include:

- *Diagnosis*, which, as we have seen, includes psychotic disorders such as schizophrenia and bipolar disorder.

- *Disability*, which can refer to number and length of hospitalizations, unemployment, living on income assistance, and requiring help with activities of daily living such as food preparation and money management. Disability days may be used, for example determining the number of days an individual was "out of role" over a period of time, this referring to the ability to work, get out of the house, interact with and care for others, or manage self-care (Gonzalez et al. 2010).
- *Duration*, which overlaps with disability in that it can refer to the length of the presumed impact, reflected, for example, in time spent in treatment (inpatient or outpatient) or supervised residential care. Some epidemiological surveys have used "more than two years of contact with support services" as a threshold for duration (Ruggeri et al. 2000). Some programs explicitly include "persistent" in the definition of "serious," while others do not. "Duration" is problematic as an inclusion criterion for clinical programs in that it does not deal with first episodes of mental illness or people who have been coping poorly but "below the radar" of the service system. It also seems to imply that a short-term condition is not serious. In addressing this, some community mental health programs have two tracks: one for assessment and treatment of shorter-term conditions and one for assisting persons with established longer-term disability.

In addition to the above, some surveys have used suicidal behaviour with lethal intent in the past twelve months as an indicator of "seriousness." Because of differences in the criteria used, estimates of the prevalence of serious mental illness arising from one study may be difficult to compare with another.

A national population survey conducted in the US illustrates an attempt to quantify the twelve-month prevalence of serious mental disorders by incorporating both diagnostic and functional criteria (Kessler et al. 2007). In this scheme, anyone diagnosed with a psychotic or bipolar disorder, regardless of functional impairment, was counted as "severe." Substance dependence (the most serious form of misuse) was also counted if there was "serious role impairment." Any mental disorder that resulted in role impairment or work limitations was also counted, as was anyone who made a significant suicide attempt in the previous year (regardless of diagnosis). Using these criteria, the authors came up with a one year prevalence rate of severe mental disorder of 5.8 percent among the population sampled.

How does this translate into eligibility criteria for treatment programs? In the box below is an example of a Canadian adult community mental health program mandate.[6] The term "serious and persistent" is used, and, in this case, major depression is included with schizophrenia and bipolar disorder as qualifying diagnoses. Substance misuse and personality disorder are included but only as co-occurring conditions. The functional aspect is referred to in the bulleted statements. The reference to "risk for medical conditions" is an acknowledgment of the higher rates of mortality and physical illness among the seriously mentally ill. And the statement that the individual "needs the services of an interdisciplinary team" refers to the possibility that some persons meeting the diagnostic criteria may be coping well enough to be supported through a private psychiatrist or general practitioner.

"De Facto" Criteria: Visibility and Treatability

Before leaving the subject of program eligibility, some comments should be made on "the extra-clinical" factors that impinge on decision making, in particular *visibility* and *treatability*. "Visibility" is used here to refer to the fact that treatment programs will respond to the most manifest examples of mental illness, such as the psychotic man who is causing a disturbance in a corner store, the tearful client who in a counselling session reveals plans to

Example of an Agency Mandate

The mental health program provides service to individuals who suffer from a serious and persistent mental illness and whose functional impairment requires a broad range of coordinated services provided by an interdisciplinary team.

Diagnostically, clients primarily fall into one of two categories:
(1) schizophrenia and other psychotic disorders, and
(2) mood disorders, i.e., bipolar and major depressive disorders.

Services are also provided to individuals who have co-occurring disorders such as personality disorders, substance abuse/misuse, mental challenges, etc.

Characteristics that generally describe the above population include:
- history of multiple psychiatric hospitalizations
- unstable housing and/or relationships
- difficulties with activities of daily living
- high risk for co-occurring medical conditions
- refractory treatment history
- high risk of causing harm to self or others

kill herself, or the rooming-house tenant who has covered his windows with aluminum foil and is screaming at night about alien invasions. These are "demand characteristics" that require some action on the part of the authorities, in some cases first-responders, and, subsequently, treatment providers in inpatient and outpatient settings. In these cases the community mental health program does not have to engage in case-finding: the referral comes to it, via a concerned citizen, relative, or hospital clinician. If the community profile of a prospective client is very high – that is, an individual is "out there" in terms of publicly visible, bizarre behaviour – the demand to "do something" may trump diagnostic exclusion criteria. For example, a program may normally exclude persons with fetal alcohol syndrome from their service but may be persuaded to take some action if there is publicly visible self-neglect or harmful behaviour. And this may well be a good thing, hinging on the self-reflection: "If our program can't help the individual, who will?"[7]

The flip side of the visibility factor is that some people may be suffering from a mental illness but may not seek help themselves and are otherwise "under the radar." Their appearance seems normal; the authorities are not alerted; and, if there are involved friends or family, these persons may not recognize the situation as one in which help should be provided. This can happen in the early stages of schizophrenia, before symptoms clearly break through, and it certainly could apply to depression, in which case an individual may appear quieter and more withdrawn than usual but otherwise "appear normal." Persons who are depressed may believe, or have been told, that "we all feel this way" at times and that the proper response is to carry on and not dwell on it (an attitude that is even more pronounced among some minority cultures). What is, or should be, the role of the health authorities in these cases? Should the mental health system be more proactive in educating such persons and helping engage them in treatment? While this has for some time been the vision of community care (Eaton 2001), publicly funded treatment programs have not, historically, seen this as their role, in part because of a lack of dedicated resources. There are also some ethical concerns about proactive interventions: What if an individual has symptoms of psychosis that could be treated but is otherwise coping adequately and not bothering anyone else? Do we need, at times, to acknowledge the right of individuals to be left alone? Or is this a form of negligence?

Then there is the question of treatability, which is used here to mean *medically* treatable since, as was discussed in the previous chapter, a biomedical conceptualization of mental disorder has been very influential in most public mental health settings in Canada (Boydell, Gladstone, and Crawford

2002; Ghaemi 2010; Rae-Grant 2002; Smith 2011). As we have noted, this approach is consistent with the lay understanding of serious mental illness: a medical condition to be treated by a health professional. And certainly, in the case of psychosis and mania, medication has proven to be effective in remitting symptoms. However, conditions such as anxiety disorders are most effectively managed when psychological approaches are provided as well (Ehlers et al. 2003; van Minnen et al. 2003). While the situation is changing (and described in more detail later), historically, community programs have not offered these cognitive-behavioural treatments (Mood Disorders Society of Canada 2011b), and this has influenced program mandates. Persons employed as case managers in mental health settings, such as nurses and social workers, may not be trained in cognitive-behavioural methods (Newton and Yardley 2007), which have been seen as the domain of clinical psychology. Further, how the work is organized (read: compressed) in mental health programs – thirty-minute appointments every two to three weeks, for example – does not lend itself to the type of contact needed to treat persons with anxiety disorders. Consequently, persons with these problems may be referred for treatment at specialized clinics (which may not exist in all areas or may have private-pay arrangements). Clinical situations in which community mental health may lack expertise, or in which effective interventions are not fully developed, include persons with drug addictions, personality disorders,[8] hoarding behaviours, eating disorders, and brain injury conditions such as fetal alcohol syndrome. In sum, eligibility decisions may be driven by client needs, but they are also determined by the tools that clinicians have or do not have at their disposal.[9]

A Concluding Example

As we have seen, eligibility for public mental health services is determined by: (1) diagnosis, with "seriousness" applied particularly when the condition is perceived as non-volitional; (2) functional impairment; (3) the visibility of the condition; and (4) the treatment tools available. These determinants are helpful in understanding why persons with anxiety disorders have historically not been "a good fit" with public treatment programs. First, they are less visible, both with respect to appearing "normal" or non-bizarre and also because the very symptoms of the disorder may cause them to withdraw from the social world. Second, there may be some question about "seriousness," especially if we reserve that term mainly for people who are psychotic and "out of control." In anxiety conditions, symptoms may be intermittent or present only in certain situations. (The older term for a person with an anxiety disorder, "neurotic," also fails to connote seriousness.) Finally, the cognitive-behavioural methods shown to be beneficial with anxiety disorders have not historically been included in the skill set of community mental health workers, one more reason for the "disconnect" with public treatment programs. In response to this apparent under-recognition, it is noteworthy that the Anxiety and Depression Association of America has as a running subtitle on its website (http://www.adaa.org) the statement: "Anxiety disorders are real, serious and treatable." Similarly, in response to the "low visibility" of a condition like PTSD, the Mood Disorders Society of Canada (2012) issued a report entitled *Out of Sight, Not Out of Mind.*

Help-Seeking and Perceived Need

As we have just seen, answering the question, "Who is getting help?" takes into account program eligibility requirements – that is, how mental health services define "serious mental illness." Two other important considerations are whether a potential service user *perceives* a need for support and whether she or he actually seeks help. Help-seeking is an evaluative process, wherein the individual weighs potential costs and benefits, basing this at times on incomplete information (Afifi, Cox, and Sareen 2005). Some generalizations can be made. We know that women tend to seek health services to a greater extent than men (Johnson 2010; Rhodes and Bethell 2008). And, in psychiatry, we know that help-seeking is deterred by the embarrassment and stigma associated with mental illness (Lim, Jacobs, and Dewa 2008), a stigma that is felt even more acutely among some ethnic minority groups (Chen et al. 2010; Kirmayer et al. 2007). A national Canadian survey addressed this issue by asking participants, in response to a vignette, "Why people might not seek help for a mental illness" (Canadian Alliance on Mental Illness and Mental Health 2007, 26):

> The most frequent response was denial or an inability to recognize having a mental health problem. Being too ashamed or uncomfortable asking for help was in second place ... a response [that] was slightly higher for the male character in the vignette, suggesting that men are perceived as having a harder time asking for help. Concerns over the stigma associated with mental illness came third and ... not knowing where to go for help ranked fourth. [However] if shame and stigma are combined, they become the main reason for not seeking help.

Prior to help-seeking is the question of whether or not there is a "need," and determining this is a complicated matter. In some cases, individuals simply lack awareness that there may be a problem; we know that a significant proportion of individuals with a psychotic illness are unlikely to perceive need or seek help because they lack the basic awareness that they are affected by this condition (Arango and Amador 2011; Kessler et al. 2001; Olfson et al. 2006b). In this case, the argument for a more assertive approach by service providers becomes stronger. In other cases, despite the presence of a mental illness, or despite being exposed to considerable trauma, some individuals seem to experience less impact, are more resilient, and cope better (Bowman 1999). Conversely, there are those who seem to have neither a significant trauma history nor symptoms of a "serious" mental illness, yet are apparently more vulnerable and cope poorly. Why this happens is not well understood, but, in any event, it further complicates the argument that service eligibility be driven primarily by diagnosis. Druss (2007, 295) notes that, while "the most common method of defining a need is based on prevalence of a mental disorder ... diagnosis is a crude proxy for need. Some people with diagnoses of mental disorders may not need professional care; others without formal diagnoses may benefit from treatment."

Perceived need and help-seeking have been studied in a number of settings in population-based surveys, which, as noted above, are representative samples of the general population. One of these is a study in Western Europe in which the sample (n = 8,796) consisted of persons who had screened positive for mood and anxiety symptoms and then were further interviewed to try to establish diagnosis and degree of functional impairment (Codony et al. 2009). "Service use" was defined as visiting a health professional. Among those who met the threshold for diagnosis of a mood or anxiety disorder in the previous twelve months, only 33 percent had perceived need; among those who met the diagnostic threshold *and* were considered to be disabled by the condition, only 44 percent had perceived need. Not surprisingly, perceived need was a major predictor of help-seeking: respondents with perceived need and a disabling twelve-month mental disorder were eight times more likely to seek help than those in the same category but without perceived need. Concerning demographic factors, it was found that men, younger persons, and persons living alone were less likely to seek help.

Perceived need and help-seeking have been studied in Canada as well, and what follows draws from two reports authored by Sareen and colleagues (2005a; 2005b), with data derived from large-scale population-based surveys of the Canadian public, which involved interviews conducted with residents of private dwellings, aged fifteen and older. Past-year prevalence of mood, anxiety, and substance use disorders was assessed using the Composite International Diagnostic Interview; as with the European study above, the presence of psychotic disorders was not assessed. "Help-seeking" was defined as respondents having seen a professional about their emotions, mental health, or use of alcohol or drugs in the past twelve months. "Perceived need without help-seeking" was defined as endorsing the question: "During the past 12 months, was there ever a time when you felt that you needed help for your emotions, mental health, or use of alcohol or drugs, but you didn't receive it?" The study authors found that, while diagnosis was associated with perception of need, help-seeking, and disability, persons *not* meeting the diagnostic threshold nonetheless could be in considerable distress. Findings included the following:

- Concerning the care required, persons with perceived need most frequently asked for "therapy or counseling," and much less frequently endorsed "medication" (a finding that has been made in other studies, for example, Raue et al. [2009]).
- The three most common reasons for not seeking help when there was perceived need were "preferred to manage by self," "did not get around to it," and "did not know how to get help."
- Substance use disorders were less likely to be associated with help-seeking, compared with perceived need.
- Among persons not meeting the threshold of diagnosis, women were more likely than men to perceive need.
- Younger persons were less likely to perceive need or to seek help even with a diagnosable condition.
- Perceived need, even without diagnosis, was associated with increased levels of distress, suicidality, and disability (see also Rhodes and Bethell 2008). This was examined with a cohort of 8,116 Ontario residents, by making within-group comparisons on the basis of six measures of functioning: (1) current perception of emotional status, (2) current dissatisfaction in life domains, (3) past thirty days dysfunction, (4) past year suicide attempt or ideation, (5) past year score on General Well-Being Schedule, and (6) self-reported disability in activities of daily living. It was found, not surprisingly, that persons who met the threshold of diagnosis *and* had perceived need fared the poorest on these measures. More interesting, however, was the finding that persons with *no* diagnosis and perceived need fared worse than those with diagnosis but no perceived need on five of the six measures of functioning.

What do these data tell us? For one thing, persons not meeting the threshold of diagnosis but perceiving need were coping poorly in a number of instances. For example, in the Ontario cohort almost 10 percent of those perceiving need without diagnosis had considered or attempted suicide in the previous year, and 46 percent had expressed dissatisfaction with quality of life (compared to 18 percent of those with no perceived need or diagnosis). Thus, perception of need appears to reflect real distress and problems in coping, independent of diagnosis. The significance of this is that, without an established diagnosis, these individuals would potentially not be considered eligible for public treatment programs.

In qualifying these findings it is important to note that the Canadian researchers did not screen for all psychiatric conditions, and personality disorders, significantly, were excluded (Sareen et al. 2005b). Poor coping, distress, and suicidality are often the hallmarks of these conditions, borderline personality disorder in particular, so their exclusion may explain, in part, the finding of perceived need among persons who apparently did not meet a diagnostic threshold. The question of whether this category of psychiatric disorders *should* be excluded, from population based surveys and agency mandates, remains unanswered.

Concerning help-seeking, the most common reason respondents gave for not seeking help was that they preferred to "manage it by themselves." It would be important to further explore what was meant by this, given the possibility that some may have simply been unaware of resources or felt too embarrassed to seek professional help. Taking the response at face value, however, there are implications for the wider implementation – through schools, workplaces, and family doctors – of self-management tools, available in print form and, increasingly, online (Reger and Gahm 2009).

Persons with perceived need most commonly asked for an intervention that took the form of "therapy or counselling." In explaining this, Sareen and colleagues (2005a, 649) note that "the most common professionals to be contacted for emotional symptoms are primary care physicians [family doctors], who are more likely to be able to meet the need for medications but may be less skilled in providing psychological treatments." This observation is almost certainly accurate (and is an issue covered in more detail in Chapter 7) and speaks to the frustration experienced by persons in need who find that there is no time for caregivers to explore the nature of their problems and that there seems to be a rush to reach for the prescription pad.

Finally, the data show that, in many cases, even those disabled by a diagnosable psychiatric condition did not perceive need. This finding cannot be explained by the impaired awareness that is associated with psychotic illnesses since the screening addressed only mood, anxiety, and addictive disorders. This may have to do with the "visibility" issue, referred to above, that is, that depression and anxiety are not necessarily seen as "serious" and that people struggling with these conditions should just "get on with it." On this point it may be noted that the public survey sponsored by the Canadian Medical Association (2008), referred to earlier, found that only 19 percent of the general public considered "panic and anxiety attacks" a "serious" condition.

There are a number of policy and practice implications that flow from the apparent under-recognition of mental disorders, the key one being that mental health services should focus not just on the casualties that arrive at their doorstep but should also look further "upstream" and consider ways of reaching and educating the public and, thereby, intervening earlier in the trajectory of a potential mental disorder – *prevention*, in other words. Further, there is the matter of health *promotion*, of enhancing resilience, coping, and mental health among the public. These topics are discussed in the next chapter.

Notes

1 This argument is taken up by some advocacy organizations who suggest that estimates of mental illness prevalence are inflated. For example, the Treatment Advocacy Center (2012) in the United States, in commenting on a survey finding that 20 percent of the American public have a mental illness, argues that this figure is arrived at by including persons with "mild, transient mental health issues," a group that should not, in its view, be included with those suffering from schizophrenia and bipolar disorder. For an argument that mental health programs should address the needs of persons with less severe mental disorders, see BC Ministry of Health Services (2010) and Dewa et al. (2003).

2 Lim, Jacobs, and Dewa (2008, 31) suggest that the idea that a mental condition is non-volitional, or "personally uncontrollable," is potentially more attractive to program funders, apparently by making the target population appear more sympathetic.

3 For example, see http://mentalillnesspolicy.org, http://www.cfact.ca, and http://www.treatmentadvocacycenter.org.

4 The rubric of "mental illness" has been expanded in some instances to include a very wide range of conditions. An example of this comes from the report of a large-scale European survey with the headline: "Nearly 40 Percent of Europeans Suffer Mental Illness" (Kelland 2011), a claim that is both alarming and seemingly implausible. The high rates of "mental disorder" captured in the survey are explained by the researchers including – among other conditions – dementia, insomnia, epilepsy, Parkinson's disease, and multiple sclerosis.

5 It is this author's impression that referring agencies, concerned about whether a borderline diagnosis will be accepted by the community team, will include an additional diagnosis such as major depression or bipolar disorder – even when it is not clear if the client meets the criteria for those disorders. This may sound surprising to some, but using diagnosis expediently is not an uncommon practice in the health care system. Another interesting example of this concerns the disorder autism, specifically, the fact that the number of new cases increased dramatically in the US in the 1990s, too fast to plausibly claim a "true" increase in incidence, with the speculation that diagnosis was being used strategically with mentally handicapped persons since individuals diagnosed with autism may be eligible for more services through the educational and health care systems (Shattuck 2006; Stobbe 2007).

6 See: http://mentalhealth-policies.vch.ca/Policy/301.pdf.

7 While perhaps a separate issue, visibility and demand characteristics may also come about when an individual or her/his relative or advocate complains loudly to various officials that service should be offered, even when the person in question does not meet the agency's mandate. Administrators may find it politically expedient in some of these cases to give in to the "squeaky wheel" and have the person seen – if for no other reason than to contain the situation.

8 Woollaston and Hixenbaugh (2008, 708) found from interviews with psychiatric nurses that the negative perceptions about clients diagnosed with borderline personality disorder were, in part, related to the feeling of being "unable to help."

9 Treatability may apply to psychotic disorders as well since not all psychoses are responsive to medication. If there is no evidence of pharmacological benefit, and if the client will not voluntarily attend the program and imminent harm to self or others has been ruled out, there may be no choice but to discharge the individual.

Illness Burden and Prevention

3

In its framework document, *Toward Recovery and Well-Being*, the Mental Health Commission of Canada (2009, 38) makes the case for prevention and promotion (one of its seven goals for a reformed mental health system):

> A strategy that is based on a comprehensive approach to mental health and mental illness cannot focus only on assisting people who are already experiencing the symptoms associated with mental health problems and illnesses. It also must promote the mental health and well-being of all people living in Canada, help to keep people from becoming ill in the first place, and strive to minimize the impact that mental health problems have on individuals, on communities and on society as a whole ... It is becoming increasingly clear that there are limits to what can be done to reduce the impact of mental illness through treatment alone.

In a later strategy document the commission reiterates the need for a promotion/prevention approach, making the promotion of mental health across the lifespan, and the prevention of mental illness and suicide, one of its six key strategic directions (Mental Health Commission of Canada 2012). This is clearly an ambitious agenda, one that would require an expansion in the scope of public mental health services to a "whole population approach," whereby interventions would target not just those meeting the threshold of mental illness but at-risk populations as well, and even the well population (e.g., Government of Manitoba 2011).

The rationale for moving beyond treatment to a model of care that includes prevention comes from several directions:

- As noted in the quote above, that existing psychological and pharmacological treatments cannot reduce the burden of illness beyond a certain point, in the case of depression by 35 percent according to one review (Cuijpers et al. 2008).

- As noted by Cuijpers et al. (2008, 1,272), "duration of [a mental] disorder is inversely related to outcome, so that by the time cases come to the attention of practitioners they are harder to treat," supporting the need for early intervention.
- The finding that the earlier the exposure to illness or trauma (e.g., the first trimester of pregnancy), the greater the potential for subsequent developmental impact (Khashan et al. 2008). Evidence from the field of neuroscience concerning brain plasticity suggests that brain development – synapse formations and neural refinement – is responsive to both stimulation and deprivation in childhood years, supporting preventive interventions with this age group (Beardsley, Chien, and Bell 2011; Lawrie et al. 2008).
- The finding that improved mental health is associated with better outcomes with respect to both physical and mental illnesses (Keyes 2007; Prince et al. 2007).
- The evidence that poor health outcomes are related to socio-economic determinants (Standing Senate Committee on Social Affairs, Science and Technology 2002).
- The argument that prevention measures are cost-effective in that they would reduce the need for inpatient treatment, which is the most expensive component of health care budgets (Canadian Mental Health Association 2001).

How are prevention and promotion defined? Perhaps the most succinct definition comes from the World Health Organization (2002, 9): "Prevention is concerned with avoiding disease, while promotion is about improving health and well-being." A Canadian Senate report elaborates: "Mental health promotion ... emphasizes positive mental health, as opposed to mental illness. It addresses the determinants of mental health – the many personal, social, economic and environmental factors that are thought to contribute to mental health" (Standing Senate Committee on Social Affairs, Science and Technology 2006, 411). The prevention/promotion distinction relates well to the two-continua model discussed earlier, which proposes that mental health and mental illness are related but are on two separate axes. That being said, the implications for intervention – public health strategies – are similar whether one is talking about prevention or promotion (with the exception of what is called *tertiary* prevention, discussed further below). At this point it is necessary to consider what a whole population approach is trying to prevent. The following section considers the adverse outcomes related to mental illness.

The Impact of Mental Illness

Because of health care costs as well as lost employment and productivity, mental disorders have a substantial impact on the quality of life of affected individuals, their families, their loved ones, and on society in general. The great tragedy is that serious mental disorders interrupt an individual's life trajectory in early adulthood, just when education is being completed, careers are being started, and families and significant attachments are being formed. While in many cases the impact of a mental disorder will be similar across subsections of the population, there are some notable differences, such as the higher rates of suicide seen in some First Nations communities (see Chapter 6). Fairly consistent gender differences have also been seen; for example, depression, eating disorders, and borderline personality disorder are all diagnosed more frequently in women (Davidson 2008; Gucciardi et al. 2004; Proudfoot 2007; Romans and Ross 2010). These differences may reflect the differential impact of socio-cultural factors as well as gender-specific patterns in seeking help.

One way to look at the impact of mental illness is to estimate its economic consequences. Lim, Jacobs, and Dewa (2008) note that economic impact refers to direct costs (use of services), indirect costs (lost productivity), and the monetary value that a mental illness has on a person's health-related quality of life (HRQOL). A study by Jacobs et al. (2008) determined that, in Canada, the provinces spent about $6 billion on mental health and addiction services (in 2006 dollars). Add to this the $1.7 billion spent on pharmaceuticals and the estimated $44 billion in indirect costs and you arrive at a figure for the economic burden of mental disorders in Canada of $52 billion for 2006 (Lim, Jacobs, and Dewa 2008).

A considerable proportion of these direct costs come from hospital expenditures (Canadian Institute for Health Information 2008b; Kendall 2010; Picard 2008a):

- About one in seven hospitalizations in Canada are related to treatment of a mental illness.
- Psychiatric admissions tend to be longer than those for medical reasons and make up about one-third of all bed days in Canadian hospitals (although length of stay for psychiatric reasons continued to drop during the early 2000s). Persons diagnosed with schizophrenia and psychotic disorders have longer stays than those with other psychiatric diagnoses.
- Mental illnesses make up the largest portion of acute care inpatient costs. For example, for the 2004-05 fiscal year, mood disorders, schizophrenia, and other psychotic conditions combined represented 12.9 percent of

inpatient costs (almost $650,000,000). The next two largest categories were acute myocardial infarction (9.5 percent) and stroke (9.5 percent).

Another way to look at illness impact is through the World Health Organization's Global Burden of Disease methodology, which uses disability-adjusted life years (DALYs), also referred to as health-adjusted life years (HALYs) (Lim, Jacobs and Dewa 2008). DALYs are calculated by combining years of life lost to premature mortality (due to suicide in the case of mental illness) and years of life lived with a disability (of specified severity and duration). As reviewed by Lim, Jacobs, and Dewa (2008), mental illnesses accounted for 13 percent of the disease burden worldwide (measured in DALYs) in 2002, with estimates that this figure would increase to 15 percent by 2010. Unipolar depression was the fourth leading cause of disease burden in 2002 and was estimated to become the second leading cause worldwide by 2030, behind ischemic heart disease. In *developed* countries unipolar depression is projected to be the leading cause of disease burden by 2030. Concerning the impact of mental illness and addictions, a study sponsored by Public Health Ontario (Ratnasingham et al. 2012) found that, in that province, as measured by DALYs:

- The burden of mental illness and addictions was more than 1.5 times that of all cancers and more than seven times that of all infectious diseases.
- The five conditions with the highest impact were (in order) depression, bipolar disorder, alcohol use disorders, social phobia, and schizophrenia.
- Alcohol misuse was by far the greatest contributor to premature mortality.

There has been increasing concern expressed about the association between mental illness and poor physical health outcomes (Jones et al. 2004; Lawrence, Kisely, and Pais 2010; Mental Health Commission of Canada 2012). Persons with mental disorders have a much higher mortality rate than the general public, due to suicide, accidents, reckless behaviour, and premature death from medically treatable conditions (Daumit et al. 2006; Hall 2001; Health Canada 2002a; Miller, Paschall, and Svendsen 2006; Seeman 2007; Vahia et al 2008). As reviewed by Kisely (2010), the death rate for persons with mental illness is about 70 percent higher than that for the general population even after controlling for demographic and socio-economic factors. Persons with schizophrenia on average die many years earlier than their counterparts in the general public, with most of these deaths due to common illnesses such as heart disease, cancer, and chronic lung diseases. Cardiovascular disease is the single most common cause of death for persons with schizophrenia and other categories of mental disorder (Lawrence, Kisely, and Pais 2010). In British Columbia, a study was conducted on the mortality rate of persons discharged from hospitals with psychiatric diagnoses during the fiscal year 1997-98: after this group of 13,476 individuals had been followed for two and a half years, it was determined that the standardized mortality ratio was six times that of the general population (Health Canada 2002a). In Nova Scotia, researchers found that an additional one thousand persons with a mental illness die each year than would be expected if their mortality risk was the same as that for the general public (Kisely et al. 2005). It was also found from service records in Nova Scotia that persons with a mental illness had increased mortality for cancer, which could not be explained by differences in cancer incidence (Kisely et al. 2008b).

A number of factors may contribute to these higher mortality rates and poorer medical outcomes:

- Psychiatric medications, in particular antipsychotic drugs such as olanzapine, are known to cause weight gain and have been implicated in the development of "metabolic syndrome," a disorder with a cluster of symptoms that include obesity, high blood pressure, and high cholesterol levels (Chacon et al. 2011; Kisely et al. 2009).[1]
- Socio-economic circumstances clearly are significant, with poverty often relegating mentally ill persons to poorer diets and unsafe inner-city environments (Wilton 2003). The mentally ill are overrepresented among homeless populations, and homelessness is associated with poorer physical health (see Chapter 12).
- Concerning lifestyle factors, surveys have determined that the mentally ill have higher rates of smoking, alcohol consumption, and illicit drug use, which means an increased risk of associated illnesses, such as hepatitis and HIV (Gerber et al. 2003; Rush et al. 2008).
- Physical symptoms may be misattributed to mental illness by attending physicians, a phenomenon known as "diagnostic overshadowing" (Abbey et al. 2011).

Perhaps the most significant factor in understanding physical illness and mortality has to do with the mentally ill not connecting with the primary health care system. Lawrence, Kisely, and Pais (2010) note, for example, that higher cancer mortality rates among the mentally ill persist even after controlling for other physical health and lifestyle factors, suggesting that the mentally ill cohort is not receiving appropriate treatment, or at least not early enough to prevent more serious outcomes. These authors note that a number of studies have found that rates of procedural interventions are much lower among the mentally ill. An example comes from a US study that compares treatment rates for several physical illnesses using a sample drawn from the general public and another sample from persons diagnosed with schizophrenia (Vahia et al. 2008). The treatment rates for the general public/psychiatric cohort are as follows: high blood pressure: 93percent/ 75 percent; heart disease: 75 percent/38 percent; gastrointestinal ulcers: 100 percent/53 percent. This under-treatment could be a consequence of persons with mental illnesses not connecting with medical personnel in the first place, receiving indifferent care when they do (Dupuis 2008), or problems with respect to follow-up (Druss et al. 2001). On this matter, Lawrence, Kisely, and Pais (2010, 757) suggest that physicians may be "reluctant to offer some procedures because of the ensuing psychological stress, concerns about capacity or compliance with postoperative care, or the presence of contra-indications such as smoking."[2]

Other impacts of mental illness are covered in more depth in other chapters of this book and are briefly touched on here:

- The unemployment rate for persons with serious mental disorders is very high, a topic covered in more detail in Chapter 17. This means that in many cases these individuals will be living in impoverished circumstances. For example, persons who qualified for provincial disability incomes in Canada in 2010 in most cases received less than $1,000 per month, with basic welfare rates considerably less than that (National Council of Welfare 2011).[3]
- Not surprisingly, given their limited financial resources, persons disabled by mental illness are often in inadequate, unsafe housing. Surveys have determined that the mentally ill are overrepresented among homeless populations: about one in three of the nation's homeless have a serious mental disorder and consequently are at greater risk for illness, injury, and exploitation (Reid, Berman, and Forchuk 2005). Housing and homelessness is covered in Chapter 12.
- Caregiver burden, both in terms of emotional and financial resources, may be considerable when one is talking about serious mental illness, a subject addressed in Chapter 7. Concerning the situation of family members, a Health Canada (2002a, 20) report notes that "[they] face the anxiety of an uncertain future and the stress of what can be a severe and limiting disability. The heavy demands of care may lead to burnout. Families sometimes fear that they caused the illness. The cost of medication, time off work, and extra support can create a severe financial burden for families. Both the care requirements and the stigma attached to mental illness often lead to isolation of family members from the community and their social

support network and may even contribute to the suicide of a family member."

- The mentally ill are considerably overrepresented in the criminal justice system, leading observers to conclude that "prisons have become our new mental hospitals" (Torrey et al. 2010). This topic is covered in Chapter 13.
- Finally, the mentally ill and their supporters face stigma – ostracism and discrimination – which two Canadian researchers conclude is "the single most important factor undermining ... quality of life" (Stuart and Arboleda-Florez 2001, 251). Stigma is the subject of the next chapter.

The Aging Population

By the early twenty-first century, the number of seniors, particularly those over eighty, had grown dramatically in Canada relative to other age groups, and this trend is expected to continue as the baby-boomer cohort ages. It is estimated that by the year 2036, persons aged sixty-five and older will make up roughly one quarter of the population in Canada (Turcotte and Schellenberg 2007). Concerning persons over eighty, this group increased in numbers between 1981 and 2005 from 196,000 to 492,000, respectively, and this figure will continue to grow in relative and absolute terms, to an estimated 800,000 persons in 2021 and 2.5 million in 2056, when the over-eighties will make up about 6 percent of the Canadian population (Turcotte and Schellenberg 2007). Given this, rates of dementia are expected to increase since incidence is directly related to age: while it is estimated that about 5 percent of those over sixty-five will have severe dementia, this figure jumps to 20 to 40 percent for persons over eighty-five (Sadock and Sadock 2007), with a Canadian study determining that 34 percent of those over eighty-five suffer from some form of dementia and that, by the year 2031, over 750,000 Canadians will have Alzheimer's disease or a related dementia (Canadian Study of Health and Aging Working Group 1994).

Apart from dementia, there are a number of changes related to normal aging that can put seniors at increased risk for mental illness and diminished mental health, and these include physical (e.g., visual and hearing deficits, decreased mobility), cognitive (e.g., diminished memory and processing speed), and social factors (e.g., bereavement, care-giving, isolation, and relocation) (British Columbia Psychogeriatric Association 2012). Depression is not uncommon among the elderly, with one review finding a rate of depression of 15 percent among seniors in the community, reaching 44 percent among those in long-term care facilities (British Columbia Psychogeriatric Association 2012). In some cases (20 to 30 percent) depression coexists with dementia, and there is evidence that the onset of depressive symptoms in the year preceding the onset of Alzheimer's disease may represent the early symptoms of this dementia (Butters et al. 2004; Green et al. 2003). An onset of depression in later life may be influenced by the loss of friends and partners and by chronic medical conditions. It may also be exacerbated by alcohol use. An association has been found between depression and reduced cerebral blood flow, and it may be that the declining mood seen later in life is related to the higher rates of cerebrovascular disease evident in older persons (Ruo et al. 2003). Later-life depression may produce cognitive impairment, which can be confused with true dementia (Sadock and Sadock 2007). Canadian data show that elderly men are a significantly higher-risk group with respect to suicide (British Columbia Psychogeriatric Association 2012; Public Health Agency of Canada 2006). Suicide risk factors among the elderly include being isolated, living alone, anticipating admission to a nursing home, experiencing financial problems, having a psychiatric illness, and having a serious medical condition such as cancer (Quan and Arboleda-Florez 1999). Despite the losses and decline in physical health that older adults may experience, surveys of seniors living in non-institutional settings have found that scores for self-reported mental health (using criteria such as psychological distress, well-being, mastery, and stress),[4] particularly in the sixty-five to seventy-four age cohort, are in fact higher than other age groups (Blanchflower and Oswald 2008).

What are the implications of this? One concern is increased demands on the health care system, with workers having to care for increasing numbers of persons with complex care needs. Another implication is that mental health workers will increasingly be involved in investigating abuse and neglect cases among the elderly, in part because of evidence that persons with dementia are at higher risk for abuse (O'Connor, Hall, and Donnelly 2009) and also because provincial statutes now place a positive onus on health care workers to intervene in cases of suspected abuse or neglect of an older adult (Regehr and Kanani 2006). Concerning medical specialists, a 2006 report suggested that Canada needed at least four hundred more geriatricians and that this deficit would grow with time (Torrible et al. 2006). With care for the elderly being provided in most cases by family physicians, a resource that is already over-burdened (Condon 2006), it is notable that a 2007 survey found that 80 percent of family physicians in Canada considered the aging population to be a significant concern for their practice (College of Family Physicians of Canada 2007). It is estimated that students currently graduating from medical schools in Canada will spend as much as 50 percent of their time treating patients over the age of sixty-five (Shaw 2007).

Interventions
Prevention, as the term has been used in medicine, can be further broken down as follows (Brown and McGrath 2011):

- *Primary* prevention: the prevention of the onset of an illness, for example, immunizing children against polio. If primary prevention is successful, the incidence of an illness (number of new cases) should go down.
- *Secondary* prevention: when there has been an onset of illness, to modify its course by intervening early. Another medical example would be treating high blood pressure to prevent cardiovascular disease.
- *Tertiary* prevention: there is an established illness that is being managed, for example, by medication, to prevent worsening of symptoms.

Historically, psychiatric treatment programs have looked to prevent the worsening of a client's mental illness and to maintain that individual at his or her "baseline" (which may mean the presence of residual symptoms). Thus, they could be said to be engaging in tertiary prevention.

What about the secondary or primary prevention of a mental illness? Using schizophrenia as an example, this disorder is understood to be the result of an interaction between a genetic vulnerability and environmental stressors early in a child's development, in particular while the infant is in utero (King, St. Hilaire, and Heidkamp 2010). In the case of schizophrenia, the link with maternal illness has been established in large-sample studies that have looked at higher incidence in offspring when there has been maternal malnutrition (St. Clair et al. 2005) and maternal anemia (Sorensen et al. 2011). In the case of bipolar disorder, a link with maternal exposure to the flu has been established (Parboosing et al. 2013). Thus, it can and has been argued that population health (universal) strategies aimed at improving maternal health should lower the incidence of these disorders. The case for this is provided in more detail by Brown and Patterson (2011), and the reader is directed to this source for a fuller discussion of the statistical methods used. These authors review the evidence that eliminating several common infections among women who are pregnant would have an appreciable impact on reducing the number of schizophrenia cases and that incidence has, in fact, been lowered in countries (such as Finland) with widespread immunization programs. They argue that influenza vaccinations should thus be a mainstay for pregnant women and non-pregnant women of reproductive age.

Another potential area for intervention, corresponding to *secondary* prevention, is the identification of persons in the early stages of schizophrenia, often by targeting persons considered to be higher-risk. Early psychosis intervention programs exist in a number of centres in Canada, although in many cases these programs are working with individuals for whom there has been a clear breakthrough of symptoms, so they could be said to be involved in illness management or tertiary prevention. Can we identify schizophrenia in an individual before the disorder has fully merged? Currently, higher-risk status is based largely on family history, particularly if first-degree relatives have the illness. However, even when a parent has schizophrenia, the likelihood of an offspring developing it is only about 12 to 13 percent, so clearly history is not destiny (Asarnow 1988). Some illnesses can be identified through biomarkers – lab tests – but while research on this is ongoing, at present there is no way that schizophrenia can be identified on this basis (Lieberman 2011).

What about clinical signs and early symptoms of the illness? The challenge with schizophrenia is that illness onset is often insidious and gradual, with symptoms that are nonspecific; typically, it is only in hindsight that clinicians can point to a behaviour in the "prodrome" (the period prior to full expression of the illness) as suggestive of the full-blown illness. That said, research is under way on the identification of a "psychosis risk syndrome," a state reflective of illness but prior to full onset (Brown and McGrath 2011), and a potential target for "stop[ping] the disease before it has really begun" (Aviv 2010, 36). This concept is controversial, however; Aviv (2010, 37) notes that identifying a risk syndrome means identifying delusions "before the patient really believes in them":

> When does a strong idea take on a pathological flavour? How does a metaphysical crisis morph into a medical one? At what point does our interpretation of the world become so fixed that it no longer matters "what almost everyone else believes." Even William James admitted that he struggled to distinguish a schizophrenic break from a mystical experience.

While there have been some promising developments with respect to the risk syndrome (Brenner 2010), the challenges are both economic (given the potentially high rate of false positives) and ethical (given that early psychosis interventions potentially involve the introduction of pharmacological agents that may have significant side effects). (For a review of the research on the psychosis risk syndrome, see Brenner et al. [2010] as well as the section in Chapter 11 on early intervention programs.)

For economic arguments supporting early intervention in psychosis, see Knapp, McDaid, and Parsonage (2011), who use economic models to look at cost-benefit, which, in the case of early intervention – defined as assisting persons who have had a first psychotic episode – are based on reduced hospitalization for those receiving specialized services. The authors also make an argument for early detection, based on a model that assumes that transition from prodromal symptoms to full psychosis occurs for 35 percent of clients in standard care compared to just 20 percent of clients in specialized care, although the empirical basis for this assumption comes from just a single journal publication (Valmaggia et al. 2009).

In sum, regarding prevention in schizophrenia:

- Primary prevention is currently best addressed with universal health strategies that target maternal health and early childhood development; for examples of these, see World Health Organization (2002). Although the specific benefit of this with respect to schizophrenia is still uncertain, it seems difficult to argue with a strategy in which "there are potentially large public health gains available" (Kirkbride and Jones 2011, 262). Public education on mental illness is also important, especially initiatives targeting young persons since this is when mental disorders may start to emerge, when fears about stigma and not fitting in are felt most acutely, and when help-seeking would potentially achieve the greatest impact (Stuart 2006).
- "Selective" prevention strategies, ones that target persons considered to be higher-risk (Brenner et al. 2010), are problematic in the case of schizophrenia in that our ability to identify vulnerable individuals is still relatively poor (Brown and McGrath 2011). For example, research linking substance misuse to the manifestation of schizophrenia has led to the recommendation that marijuana use among vulnerable persons be discouraged, a recommendation difficult to achieve, given not only the challenge of identifying vulnerable persons but also the fact that marijuana-use is considered normative in a number of settings (Degenhardt and Hall 2006; Welch et al. 2011).
- Persons who have developed schizophrenia need to consider different protective strategies, including medication, adequate rest, adequate diet, limited substance use, avoidance of social isolation, and problem-solving and stress-management skills.

What about other mental disorders? Research on preventive interventions suggests outcomes may be better with depression (Beardsley, Chien, and Bell 2011), which may have to do with the different nature of the disability, vulnerability, and risk factors associated with that syndrome. Cuijpers and colleagues (2008) undertook a meta-analysis of randomized clinical trials that looked at the impact of psychological treatments – in most cases, CBT – on the incidence of depression, and they found a reduction in the incidence of depressive disorders of 22 percent compared to that found in control groups. Most of the studies targeted young persons (ages eleven through eighteen), while some targeted women who were in the perinatal period – both groups that would logically be included in prevention initiatives. The interventions being evaluated were for the most part not universal; that is, subjects recruited could be considered a higher-risk group. Risk was assessed in some instances by a screening instrument designed to elicit signs of a mental disorder short of meeting the full diagnostic criteria.[5] Significantly, the meta-analysis found that universal interventions were less effective; that is, they did not show appreciable differences in outcomes between treatment and control groups, suggesting that depression prevention programs need to be targeted. The authors also noted that more study was needed on the question of what types of psychological treatment are most effective. A position paper published in the *Canadian Medical Association Journal* concluded that "the lack of evidence about the benefits and harms of routinely screening for depression in adults" meant that routine screening in primary care settings could not be recommended (Canadian Task Force on Preventive Health Care 2013, 7).

Prevention and Health Promotion among the Elderly

There is a growing body of research on interventions intended to slow or prevent the onset of dementia, and these include diet and nutritional supplements, social contacts, leisure activities, physical exercise, and medication, although specific recommendations remain elusive, in part because of the quality of the research evidence (Coley et al. 2008). Prevention has been used in another sense with respect to dementia, referring to preventing unnecessary hospital visits and admissions since these have been found to be related to patient stress, risk of iatrogenic illness, and poorer health outcomes (Donnelly, McElhaney, and Carr 2011). An Ontario study of hospital admissions of long-term care residents concluded that about one-quarter could have been prevented if pre-existing conditions had been managed at an earlier stage. The authors found that, among this group, 62.4 percent were admitted and 23.6 percent died within thirty days of contact with the emergency department (Grunier et al. 2010). Recommendations included more regular monitoring by primary care physicians and care provider education. Concerning the prevention or mitigation of depression among the elderly, protective factors are similar to those for the general population and include exercise, sense of purpose, meaningful activity, and an active social network (British Columbia Psychogeriatric Association 2012). With respect to the high rate of depression seen in residential care facilities, there are implications here for organizational and environmental modifications, given that depression is related at least in part to opportunities for resident participation and control, social engagement, and emotional support (British Columbia Psychogeriatric Association 2012).

Workplace Mental Health

There is increasing attention being paid to prevention as it applies to mental illness in the workplace. The extent of the problem is reflected in the rising number of sick days taken due to illnesses like depression and anxiety, and the substantial proportion of short-term and long-term disability claims attributable to mental health and addiction issues, which have become the fastest growing category of claims (Conference Board of Canada 2008; Government of Canada 2007; Mental Health Commissions of Canada 2012; Shain 2008). Dewa and colleagues (2004) note that, in a thirty-day period, about 8.4 percent of the workforce in Ontario will experience a mood, anxiety, or substance-related disorder. In the 2006 Canadian Senate report on mental health reform, the authors speak about the need to implement "strategies designed principally to reduce the effects of stressful work situations by improving the ability of individuals to adapt to and to manage stress" (Standing Senate Committee on Social Affairs, Science and Technology 2006, 180), strategies that include disability management and employee assistance programs as well as workplace accommodations. Workplace stress may be reduced by reviewing workloads, promoting positive relationships, and clearly defining performance expectations, while worker resilience may be improved through support of healthier lifestyles and stress management techniques (Lau and Monro 2008). Toronto legal scholar Martin Shain (2008, 32) notes that the courts are now holding employers accountable for providing a "mentally safe" workplace; an environment that is fair, civil, and respectful; and a place "that does not permit harm to employee mental health in careless, negligent, reckless or intentional ways." To this end, the Mental Health Commission has developed a voluntary national standard on psychological health and safety in the workplace (Gilbert and Bilsker 2012).

Physical Health Interventions

As noted above, clients of mental health programs, particularly those being treated for psychotic conditions, have higher mortality rates and higher rates of theoretically preventable illnesses such as cardiovascular disease and type II diabetes (Hsu et al. 2011). It can be argued that mental health practitioners have an ethical imperative in these cases to intervene, particularly since the pharmacological treatments given contribute to the problem. Interventions can take the following forms:

- *Screening.* This can be regular "metabolic monitoring," that is, measurements of blood sugar, weight, waste circumference, body mass index, and blood pressure.

- *Referrals.* This could involve connecting the client with a general practitioner (GP) if he or she doesn't have one.
- *Outreach.* This refers to workers taking clients to labs, doctors, and hospitals, which is a vital function for those who are apparently unwilling or unable to make medical appointments, especially following surgery or other procedures.
- *Healthy lifestyle programs.* Clinical and rehab staff may run groups to address smoking cessation, healthy eating, and weight loss. This may take the form of walking, swimming, going to community centres, and going on grocery store tours. Mental health staff may also partner with dieticians or contract with other service providers, such as yoga instructors. A review of psycho-social treatment and rehabilitation programs concluded that interventions for weight management could be considered an evidence-based practice (Dixon et al. 2010).

In this author's experience, the implementation of these initiatives has been greeted with enthusiasm by mental health staff, who see them as obviously worthwhile. One potential area of concern has to do specifically with the role of the physician/psychiatrist at the mental health team and whether that person should be ordering tests or medication for conditions outside her or his scope of practice (something that is, in fact, usually discouraged by the professional licensing body). Obviously, the preferred option is for the client to get this done by her/his own GP; however, not uncommonly – particularly among the more disabled – the client's only doctor is the one she/he sees for psychiatric reasons. A possible solution to this problem is for mental health administrators to contract with GPs to provide service at the same site, which may happen in any case when the mental health team is located in a multi-program health centre. For stand-alone teams, this would neces-sitate creating a separate clinic room and information-keeping structure.

Challenges

A number of significant challenges exist concerning the implementation of a whole population approach to health care, as was noted in a 2002 Canadian Senate report. In the first place, the multiplicity of factors that influence health status means that it is extremely difficult to associate cause and effect, especially since the effects of a given intervention are often obvious only after many years. Because political horizons are often of a shorter-term nature, the long time frame for judging the impact of policy in this area can be a serious disincentive to the elaboration and implementation of population health strategies. Furthermore, it is very difficult to coordinate government activity across the diverse factors that influence health status. The structure of most governments does not easily lend itself to inter-ministerial responsibility for tackling complex problems. This difficulty is compounded several times over when various levels of government, together with many non-governmental players, are taken into account, as they must be if population health strategies are to be truly effective (Standing Senate Committee on Social Affairs, Science and Technology 2002, 252). Concerning mental health promotion in the workplace, Dewa, McDaid, and Ettner (2007) observe that, since the costs and potential benefits of this approach are distributed across several stakeholders, there may be less incentive for any single stakeholder to invest.

The cost-effectiveness argument for prevention, while intuitively appealing, still lacks a solid evidence base (Standing Senate Committee on Social Affairs, Science and Technology 2006). For effectiveness and efficiency, early interventions with mental illness need to be targeted at higher-risk individuals, and, as was noted in the case of schizophrenia, our ability to identify this disorder before a clear breakthrough of symptoms, is limited. In the case of depression, higher risk can be determined to some extent by pre-screening with a self-report instrument, which was the case for most of the studies included in the meta-analysis conducted by Cuijpers et al. (2008, see above). While the review did find some benefit with respect to the incidence of depression, conclusions about the effectiveness of the approach, based on the number needed to treat (NNT) statistic, were equivocal. The NNT is the number of patients that need to be treated in order to prevent one additional bad outcome, in this instance one person suffering from depression. A more effective treatment has a lower NNT, the best possible result being 1.0, which would mean that everyone improved with treatment and no one improved in the control condition. In the depression treatment meta-analysis the pooled NNT figure was twenty-two, which the authors concluded was "rather high" (Cuijpers et al. 2008, 1,278).[6]

If the evidence base for prevention in psychiatry is still developing, this would support undertaking more basic neuroscience research on the aetiology of illness and also more research on refining pharmacological and psychological treatments. Caregivers may be concerned that limited funds are being moved into an initiative with uncertain results when there are problems that need our attention "right here and now," such as insufficient treatment resources. However, universal public health approaches that focus on maternal and infant health, particularly among disadvantaged groups, would seem to offer a number of potential preventive benefits across a range of physical and mental health outcomes with no real "downside." Finally, prevention and promotion efforts are hindered by the stigma attached to mental illness, which negatively affects help-seeking for those in the early stages of illness. Stigma – its manifestations and possible initiatives to combat it – is discussed in the next chapter.

Notes

1 Chacon et al. (2011) note that the high prevalence of diabetes among persons with schizophrenia is a result of multiple factors, which include a vulnerability at the genetic level.
2 This author was involved with a client with schizophrenia who was refusing treatment for a detached retina. There were consultations with various parties, including ethicists, about whether the treatment could be imposed involuntarily under guardianship legislation. Ultimately, the decision to *not* force treatment hinged to a considerable extent on the reality that necessary post-operative care could not be ensured without the client's cooperation.
3 The source for this data, the National Council of Welfare, folded in 2012 when all federal funding was withdrawn.
4 It should be noted that the survey referred to was one targeting persons living in "private occupied dwellings," presumably excluding less independent and more disabled seniors.
5 Prevention initiatives may be *universal*, *selective* (targeting higher-risk groups such as single mothers living in poverty), or *indicated* (targeting persons who through preliminary screening show some signs of a mental disorder) (Brenner et al. 2010).
6 Although, as these authors also note, "there are no clear guidelines for what is a high NNT and what is not" (Cuijpers et al. 2008, 1278). For a discussion of the limitations of the NNT statistic, see McAlister (2008).

Other Resources

The Canadian Coalition for Seniors' Mental Health: http://www.ccsmh.ca/en/default.cfm.

Stigma

Stigma refers to the negative beliefs and attitudes held about mental illness, which can lead to public prejudice, stereotyping, and discriminatory behaviour (Charbonneau et al. 2010). A survey by the Canadian Mental Health Association found that the most common of these beliefs were that persons with mental disorders are dangerous or violent, lack intelligence, cannot be cured, cannot function or hold a job, are lazy and lack willpower, are unpredictable and cannot be trusted, and are to blame for their illness and should "shape up" (cited in British Columbia Partners for Mental Health and Addictions Information 2003c). In addition to the identified mentally ill person, stigma is often experienced by that individual's family and supporters.

Being diagnosed with a mental illness – a "traumatic death sentence" in the words of a recipient of psychiatric services (Capponi 2003, 110) and "social annihilation" in the words of a practitioner (Arboleda-Florez 2003, 635) – can be a devastating experience because of uncertain future prospects and the anticipated negative reaction by others. Two Canadian researchers observe that "schizophrenia sufferers and family members continue to experience social stigma as ... the single most important factor undermining their quality of life" (Stuart and Arboleda-Florez 2001, 251). In reviewing the literature on this subject, Corrigan and colleagues (2003, 1105) conclude that "a majority of [clients] perceive themselves as being stigmatized by others, expect to be treated poorly by the public because of this stigma, and suffer demoralization and low self-esteem due to the internalization of the stigma." Persons identified as mentally disordered can anticipate landlords not wanting to rent to them, employers not wanting to hire them, and potential friends and romantic partners not wanting to associate with them. All of this can create a "why-bother-even-trying" sort of hopelessness (Barkhimer 2003). A Canadian Mental Health Association publication sums up the devastating psychological impact of stigma: "Discrimination has an all-encompassing, corrosive effect on personhood and citizenship ... the social isolation that results from discrimination impedes recovery and, given that people with mental illnesses are members of the same culture that stigmatizes them, they often internalize negative stereotypes and convert them into self-loathing and self-blame, attitudes that further affect recovery, because people come to expect devaluation and rejection" (Everett et al. 2003, 13).

Stigma is one of the key reasons that persons with mental health problems may delay or avoid seeking treatment (Arboleda-Florez 2003; Canadian Alliance on Mental Illness and Mental Health 2007; Judge et al. 2008). For example, a Toronto study involving interviews with young adults following their first episode of psychosis found that stigma was the primary reason given for ignoring, denying, or hiding their experience (Boydell, Gladstone, and Volpe 2006, 57). "People don't want to hear it and when you do tell them, they don't want to be your friend anymore, 'cause they think you're crazy ... I didn't want to go to my family doctor because I was embarrassed about it." The Canadian Community Health Survey, a study involving thirty-seven thousand respondents from all provinces, found that 60 percent of those reporting symptoms of mood, anxiety, or substance-use disorders did not seek treatment (Statistics Canada 2003). Among this group, those who stated that they *needed* treatment were asked why they did not seek it; the most common reasons given were that they preferred to manage it themselves (31 percent), that they did not get around to it (19 percent), and that they were afraid to ask or were afraid of what others would think (18 percent) (subjects could choose more than one answer). Readers should note that this study did not include questions about psychotic conditions – such as schizophrenia – which are known to carry the most stigma (Dinos et al. 2004; Capponi 2003; Stuart 2008).

People may also choose not to disclose that they have a mental illness for fear of how this could affect their career. A survey commissioned by the Canadian Medical Association (2008) found that only 23 percent of those surveyed said they would feel comfortable talking to an employer about their mental illness. Similarly, a 2007 Ipsos Reid survey of the Canadian public found that most respondents considered depression to be a serious condition but one that you would not necessarily want to report to your employer: 79 percent said that a diagnosis of depression should be kept secret to avoid damaging future employment opportunities, and nearly half believed that someone missing work because of depression would be more likely "to get into trouble and maybe even fired" (Proudfoot 2007). Commenting on this a Canadian Mental Health Association official notes that supervisors and co-workers tend to see not an illness but, rather, difficult behaviour: "They see someone who may be irritable, withdrawn [and] not meeting deadlines" (quoted in Proudfoot 2007). Researchers studying the underreporting of mental health concerns among the Canadian military suggest that this "may in part be explained by the fact that in military populations, individuals may delay seeking treatment for fear that it may prematurely end their military career, especially before completing the number of years of service required for pension or retirement eligibility" (Fikretoglu et al. 2009, 365).

Fear of disclosure affects even those working in the medical and mental health fields (Barkhimer 2003). An illustration of this comes from a 2009 survey of students at the University of Michigan Medical School (Schwenk, Davis, and Wimsatt 2010). The study authors found that respondents reported somewhat higher rates of depression than for the general public (possibly related to training demands); however, among this group, a majority stated that disclosure of this condition would be risky and would be interpreted as the student having poor coping skills. Respondents suggested that revealing their depression would make them less competitive for residency training positions and future job placements.[1] In an interview the lead author of the study concluded that "students who are depressed feel highly stigmatized by their fellow students and faculty members" (quoted in Chavis 2010; see also Dupuis 2008). A Canadian Psychiatric Association position paper notes "the reluctance of physicians and mental health workers to accept and seek help for their [own] mental health problems," which is attributed to the deleterious effects of "the divide between 'us' and 'them'" (Abbey et al. 2011, 4). While disclosure may not necessarily help the individual disclosing, it may give hope to others affected by the same condition. A poignant example of this comes from a *New York Times* story about Marsha Linehan, a famous psychologist and the creator of dialectical behaviour therapy (described in Chapter 16). In a session a client noticed the scars on Linehan's arms – a cutting behaviour characteristic of borderline personality disorder – and asked if she was "one of us" since this would "give all of us so much hope" (quoted in Carey 2011). Linehan did then disclose her past experiences in the psychiatric system, saying in the *Times* article: "I owe[d] it to them."

Dealing with disclosure is an issue that frequently affects staff working with clients in mental health settings.[2] Practitioners, particularly in the rehab field, work with clients around writing resumes and applying for school and employment, and they must contend with how to report a "gap" in a person's employment history that is related to mental illness. Privacy is paramount to the point at which, even when sending letters to a client's residence, one must be mindful of the return address on the envelope: a street address is preferable to one that shows the name of a mental health program.

Stigma may be reinforced by the reduced circumstances in which mentally ill persons often find themselves. Wilton (2003, 151) notes how poverty contributes to the stigma of having a mental disorder: "Perceptions of 'bizarre behaviour' and 'poor social skills' may at the very least be exaggerated by poverty where a lack of resources forces consumers to wear old or unmatched clothing, and to do without personal care items. In this sense, the stigmatizing effects of poverty intersect with, and exacerbate, the stigma of mental illness."

Self-Stigma and Identity

Researchers distinguish public stigma – actual experiences of rejection – from *self*-stigma, a process of internalization whereby mentally ill persons apply negative stereotypes to themselves (Corrigan 2004; Dinos 2004).[3] Internalized stigma is associated with hopelessness and low self-esteem and, in turn, poorer recovery outcomes (Livingston and Boyd 2010; Yanos et al. 2008). A characteristic reaction among persons with low self-worth is avoidance and social withdrawal in *anticipation* of rejection, even if the rejection does not actually occur. As noted by Angell, Cooke, and Kovac (2005, 71), "in turn, these avoidance behaviors and the dampened self-esteem may be perceived by others as socially awkward, leading to a vicious cycle of withdrawal and rejection." In the case of schizophrenia, social awkwardness – such as lack of motivation and social withdrawal – may be classified under *negative symptoms*, and, while these have often been seen as a response to psychosis or as biologically based, Rector, Beck, and Stolar (2005, 247) suggest that they may also represent "a compensatory pattern of disengagement in response to ... anticipated failure in tasks and social activities." Concerning apathy and amotivation, in an account written by a service user, the author states that "giving up is a highly motivated and goal directed behavior ... [a way] of trying to protect the last fragile traces of our spirit and our selfhood from undergoing another crushing" (quoted in Davidson 2012, 7).

Persons struggling with the stigma associated with a psychiatric diagnosis may deal with this in different ways. The treating professional may be sympathetic and humane, but she or he is nevertheless asking the client to accept the identity of someone with a mental illness, to "have insight" into her/his condition and the need for treatment – a "club" that some people would rather not join. In some cases clients may lack the capacity to see the mental illness simply because it appears so real (Boydell, Gladstone, and Volpe 2006). Others may have some awareness but resort to denial or rationalization rather than confront the daunting prospect of having a mental disorder. These psychological defence mechanisms are ones that many of us adopt in difficult situations in order to allay anxiety and discomfort as well as to support our sense of identity. As Angell and colleagues (2005) note, a client's resistance to accepting a psychiatric diagnosis can be seen as being difficult or "non-compliant" by treating professionals, yet, at the same time, it may have healthy and self-preserving aspects. For example, these authors quote from a client's personal account, wherein he speaks about his resistance being necessary in order for him to retain his "power and self-confidence" (Angell et al. 2005, 72). In another personal account – subtitled "What I Didn't Know Helped Me" – the author speaks about the importance of downplaying an illness identity in order to maintain "motivation and focus" (Einhaus 2009, 145). Davidson (2012) suggests a more productive approach is for the practitioner to speak to practical issues, to how to make the client's life better, rather than to emphasize a buy-in to a diagnosis.

Resistance to diagnosis and treatment can obviously lead to poorer functional outcomes, but awareness of illness can also have harmful outcomes if that awareness is associated with hopelessness (Lysaker, Roe, and Yanos 2007). The significance of this becomes clear when one considers the findings showing a positive correlation between illness awareness and suicide risk among persons diagnosed with schizophrenia (Bourgeois et al. 2004). This association is a complicated one and is mediated by other factors, such as self-stigma, as was found in a study by Lysaker, Roe, and Yanos (2007). Using several different instruments, these authors assessed a group of seventy-five persons diagnosed with schizophrenia to establish degrees of illness awareness, self-stigma, hope, and self-esteem. A cluster analysis of the results produced three groups of roughly equal numbers: (a) lower self-stigma and lower awareness, (b) lower self-stigma and high awareness, and (c) higher self-stigma and high awareness. It was found that group "c," with higher self-stigma, indeed had the lowest levels of hope, while group "b" – aware of illness but with less internalized stigma – had significantly less impaired social function than those experiencing greater self-stigma, who tended to withdraw more. In the same vein, a conceptual analysis of how people respond to being identified as mentally ill is offered by University of Toronto professor Charmaine Williams (2008). In this conception, people may be differentially situated with respect to (a) internalized stigma and (b) identification as mentally ill. Some may be strongly affected by stigma and strongly resist the mental illness label; these individuals may be difficult to engage in treatment and consequently experience periodic crises and involuntary interventions, yet may have their self-esteem protected by this same resistance. A different group comprises those who are aware of the illness and identify as psychiatric clients but are also strongly affected by internalized stigma. These are people who may understand the need for treatment yet at the same time suffer from low self-esteem and feelings of hopelessness.

There are a number of practice implications here, particularly with respect to first experiences in the mental health system. First, we need to recognize that not everyone will respond to a diagnosis the same way. Some may lack any awareness of illness and never accept the identity conferred upon them. Some may find a diagnosis reassuring ("now I know what's wrong") and set about learning more and trying to achieve some mastery with respect to their disability. And there are those who have awareness of their illness but carry this as a great burden and struggle for a sense of purpose and hope in their lives. Practitioners need to explore what the illness identity means for the individual, which may necessitate a change in the approach or the way the problem is conceptualized or even a change in the treating personnel. Mental health programs need to consider interventions that increase mastery and decrease internalized stigma (Lysaker, Roe, and Yanos 2007; Sibitz et al. 2011). For many, the idea that that they are active agents in their own recovery is itself healing, and promoting this requires trust and hopefulness on the part of the clinician.

Public Attitudes

Public attitudes towards persons with mental illness may be inferred from actual behaviour and from self-report surveys. Each of these methods has its limitations in that discriminatory behaviour may be subtle and not always visible, and self-reports may be affected by what researchers call social desirability bias – that is, not wanting to appear reactionary or intolerant. One of the most blatant examples of prejudicial behaviour is the NIMBY phenomenon: "not in my back yard."[4] This refers to protests and demonstrations when the public finds out that a new psychiatric facility will be opened in their neighbourhood, protests that are based on perceptions about lowered property values and "dangerous" mentally ill persons being set loose in the area. The latter perception does not of course account for the fact that persons affected by mental illness are *already* in the neighbourhood, although usually in unsupported settings. It appears that in most cases NIMBY protesters are a minority group, albeit a vocal one (this has been the author's own experience). For example, a poll of 609 British Columbians conducted in 2008 found almost 84 percent agreeing with the statement "I would support a supportive housing project for people with mental illness or addiction issues in my community" and only 11.4 percent opposing it (Loy 2008). Interviewed about the survey, a non-profit agency director – who had been dealing with considerable opposition to the opening of a proposed thirty-unit facility in

Vancouver – noted that it may be different when responding to a hypothetical situation: "It's easy to respond to a poll when it's not actually happening ... how many of them are thinking, I'd welcome [supportive housing] in my neighbourhood – but not next door?" (quoted in Loy 2008, 4).

Health authorities planning new facilities may employ different strategies to notify and engage local residents and community groups in the process, in addition to the mandatory development permit hearings held by municipal governments. A US researcher came up with some interesting findings on this issue in a study that involved interviews with 169 administrators about their community engagement strategies (Zippay 2007). Federal anti-discrimination laws passed in that country now give mental health agencies the authority to forego notifying neighbours when new facilities are being planned, although many still do this "in the belief that outreach enhances community integration" (109). This belief was called into question when the study found that "reported levels of acceptance, indifference, and hostility [among neighbours] did not vary significantly among sites, regardless of whether initial opposition was present or whether neighbours were notified" (112). The author did find that agencies that implemented social activities with neighbours *after* move-in reported "very accepting" attitudes, such as citizens offering baked goods, helping shovel snow, and smoking outside with the facility residents. The study appears to support the view that, while possibly a minority, the views of persons hostile to a facility move-in are entrenched and not affected by early engagement strategies.

The association between mental disorder and violence is a particularly strong one in the perception of the public. This is illustrated by the results of a large-scale American survey involving 1,444 subjects who were given five vignettes, depicting: (1) a person with schizophrenia, (2) a person with depression, (3) a "troubled person," (4) a person with alcohol dependence, and (5) a person with drug dependence (Link et al. 1999). Respondents were asked how likely they felt it was that the person described in the vignette would do something violent towards others: one-third (33 percent) indicated that violence was somewhat or very likely in the case of the depressed person, with the figure for the person with schizophrenia being 61 percent, even though there was no mention of violence in any of the vignettes. The figures were somewhat higher for the drug user and alcohol user, and substantially lower for the "troubled person."

Public attitude surveys often use the concept of "social distance," based on the strength of agreement/disagreement with statements about associating with mentally ill persons (e.g., Angermeyer, Beck, and Matchinger 2003; Lauber et al. 2004). An example of this comes from a study of 1,653 randomly chosen residents of Calgary, in which, by means of a telephone survey, respondents were asked several questions about persons diagnosed with schizophrenia (Stuart and Arboleda-Florez 2001). As the authors note, social distance increased with the level of intimacy required in the relationship; while fewer than 7 percent of subjects said that they would "feel ashamed if people knew someone in [their] family was diagnosed with schizophrenia," one in five (18.1 percent) said that they would be unable to maintain a friendship with someone with this diagnosis, almost half (47 percent) said that they would feel "upset or disturbed" about having such a person as a roommate, and over three-quarters (75.2 perent) said that they would not marry a person diagnosed with schizophrenia. Studies of this type have found an expressed preference for greater distance from persons with schizophrenia than other psychiatric disorders, again showing it to be the most stigmatizing diagnosis. This was found, for example, in a survey of two hundred Ontario university students, with schizophrenia being associated with greater concern about socially inappropriate behaviour and danger (Norman et al. 2008).

In 2008, the Canadian Medical Association commissioned a Canada-wide public survey that contained a number of attitudinal questions concerning mental illness. Regarding the negative beliefs associated with mental illness, the report concludes that "this stigma persists among a significant proportion of the public" (Canadian Medical Association 2008, 4). Results from the study include the following:

- Seventy-one percent of respondents considered schizophrenia to be a *serious* mental illness, compared to 36 percent for depression, 26 percent for drug addiction, and 19 percent for panic and anxiety attacks.
- More Canadians agreed (46 percent) than disagreed (35 percent) that "some things described as mental illness offer an excuse for poor behaviour and personal failings" (Canadian Medical Association 2008, 26). Respondents here were apparently making a distinction between persons with a "real" mental illness and those using a "mental illness excuse" since 90 percent endorsed the view that mental illness was not something you could just "snap out of."
- Respondents were asked whether they would be "fearful being around someone who has a serious mental illness." Fifty percent replied in the negative, and only 27 percent in the affirmative, although the question was limited because it used neither diagnostic sub-types nor scenario descriptions.
- Respondents were asked whether they would socialize with a "friend" who had either a mental illness, a serious mental illness, clinical depression, drug addiction, or alcoholism. Just over half said they would socialize with a friend with clinical depression or a mental illness, while just under half

endorsed socializing with a friend with a *serious* mental illness. Interestingly, drug and alcohol addiction produced the greatest preference for social distance, with fewer than one-third of respondents willing to socialize with friends with these problems.

- As with other surveys, preferred social distance became greater when the relationship was intimate or required the mentally ill person to provide a service. Respondents were asked about the likelihood of interacting with a seriously mentally ill person in various types of relationship, with the following results: socializing with her/him as a work colleague: 35 percent; hiring her/him as a landscaper: 17 percent; marrying her/him: 10 percent; hiring her/him as a financial advisor: 8 percent; having her/him take care of my children: 10 percent; having her/him as a family doctor: 8 percent.
- Respondents stated they would be less likely to tell friends or co-workers about having a family member with a serious mental illness than about having one with a serious physical illness. Notably, the youngest cohort (age eighteen to thirty-four) was the least likely to endorse telling others, suggesting stigma is a particularly prominent concern for this group.

Concerning stigma, an important question is whether public attitudes are *changing*. Surely, one might think, with a more sophisticated understanding of mental illness, Western society would be more sympathetic to the plight of those who, in the words of one service provider (Rossi 2007, 9), have "lost the genetic lottery" and, through no fault of their own, struggle with a psychiatric disability. The data bearing on this question give a complicated and not altogether reassuring answer. There is evidence that attitudes about help-seeking are shifting, for example, from Canadian service-use patterns that show that the public is becoming more comfortable in approaching family doctors and getting pharmacological treatments for symptoms of depression (Slomp et al. 2009; Vasiliadis, H. et al. 2005; Watson et al. 2005). A US study on help-seeking, which compared results from general population surveys eleven years apart, found an increase of 35 to 41 percent in the number stating they would "definitely go" for professional help for mental health problems (Mojtabai 2007). There is also evidence that, at least in an abstract sense, the public is sympathetic to the needs of the seriously mentally ill. For example, the Canadian Medical Association (2008) study cited above found a clear majority of respondents agreeing that funding for mental health should be on a par with funding for physical health issues.

But what about where the "rubber hits the road": community acceptance and solidarity, and the befriending, housing, and employment of persons with mental illness? For instance, while acknowledging that the sample and survey instrument were somewhat different, it is nevertheless disconcerting to note that the percentage of survey respondents hypothetically willing to marry someone with a mental illness was *lower* in the 2008 CMA study (10 percent) than that of the Calgary study conducted by Stuart and Arboleda-Florez (25 percent) several years earlier. In fact, this example illustrates what researchers have found in a number of settings in North America and Europe: that public stigma towards the mentally ill has not been declining, that – in the words of Canadian stigma researcher Heather Stuart – "prejudices run deep" (Stuart 2010, 324). This has been all the more disappointing since it was assumed that, by publicizing neurobiological discoveries and getting the public to see mental illness as a *biological* condition, prejudicial attitudes would be diminished: "Stigma could be reduced, many believed, if people could be convinced that mental illnesses were 'real' brain disorders and not volitional behaviors for which people should be blamed and punished" (Pescosolido et al. 2010, 1321).

An American research team examined the historical trend in two major studies. The first one compared national US surveys conducted in 1950 and 1996 and found that, despite a better understanding of the causes of mental illness in the later cohort, stigmatizing beliefs had actually *increased* (Phelan et al. 2000). The second study, which is examined in more detail here, compared responses from national surveys conducted in 1996 and 2006 (Pescosolido et al. 2010). Results included the following:

- More respondents endorsed a neurobiological understanding of mental illness in 2006 than 1996; for example, 86 percent of the sample saw schizophrenia as a biological illness in 2006 compared with 76 percent in 1996.
- Social or moral conceptions of mental illness decreased across most indicators, with the exception of alcohol dependence, which 65 percent of respondents in 2006 saw as reflecting "bad character."
- There was an increase in support for medical treatment, with 85 percent in 2006 agreeing that someone with major depression should go to a psychiatrist, compared to 75 percent in 1996. Support for hospitalization for persons with schizophrenia increased from 53 to 66 percent.
- Significantly, measures of stigma – such as the belief that a person with schizophrenia would likely be violent – remained high in 2006, did not decrease in any category, and increased in some. For example, considerably *more* people in 2006 reported an unwillingness to have someone with schizophrenia as a neighbour than in 1996 (45 percent versus 34 percent).

- Researchers looked at the association of a neurobiological conception of illness with other variables. It was found that holding this conception increased the odds of endorsing medical treatment. However, endorsing a neurobiological conception was also associated with significantly greater preferred social distance as well as greater perceived dangerousness. This explanatory model effect on stigmatizing beliefs was stronger in the 2006 cohort than in the 1996 cohort.

Canadian research has produced similar results; that is, while mental health literacy and endorsement of a biological model by the public have increased over time, stigmatizing attitudes – as reflected in preferred social distance and perceptions of dangerousness – have not diminished (Stuart 2010). And, in the UK, Pinfold and Thornicroft (2006) note that public surveys there showed no reduction in stigmatizing beliefs between 1993 and 2000, with stigma measures actually increasing between 2000 and 2003.

How do we explain these findings? A couple of hypotheses are explored here, although currently answers to this question are speculative. In looking at public attitudes in the second half of the twentieth century, Phelan and colleagues (2000) found that the perception that the mentally ill are *dangerous* increased significantly, and certainly this would affect other stigmatizing beliefs, such as greater preferred social distance. This perception has likely been fuelled by media portrayals, both fictional and journalistic. As Stuart (2010, 321) notes, "violence and mental illness are a winning news combination." A number of sensational killings in North America and elsewhere have been attributed to mental illness. In 2011, for example, a twenty-two-year-old Arizona man shot eighteen people, including a federal politician, killing six, with the media later reporting that he suffered from schizophrenia (Lacey 2011). Later that same year, in Norway, the thirty-two-year-old man responsible for killing seventy-seven people in a series of shootings and bombings was later assessed as suffering from paranoid schizophrenia.[5] In 2012, twelve people were shot dead at a Colorado movie theatre by a man with a history of psychiatric treatment who at his trial raised the insanity defence. And, in 2009, the forty-year-old man who killed and decapitated a passenger on a Greyhound bus in Manitoba the previous year was found not criminally responsible due to a schizophrenic illness and was remanded to a forensic hospital (Pritchard 2011). Advocates argue that these cases, while capable of swaying public opinion, are not representative of the vast majority of persons diagnosed with a mental illness. American psychiatrist E. Fuller Torrey gives a dissenting opinion: in a short, provocative article entitled "Stigma and Violence: Isn't It Time to Connect the Dots?," Torrey (2011c) argues that increasing stigma in recent years is directly related to an *accurate* appraisal that homicides are disproportionately committed by persons with untreated mental illnesses, citing several older and more recent studies (see also Satel and Zdanowicz 2003). Torrey suggests that the "dots do not get connected" because acknowledging a connection between mental illness and violence is politically incorrect. His suggested solution is enforced psychiatric treatment on a more widespread basis (see also North Shore Schizophrenia Society [2012]). (The association between mental illness and violence is discussed further below.) Similarly, journalist Marvin Ross (2012) observes that the fact that the media focus on sensational stories should not be surprising: "There is nothing newsworthy, unfortunately, in the stories of the many people with treated mental illness who are coping and accomplishing." In this article Ross, like Torrey, suggests that the focus of attention should not be on reforming the media but, rather, on addressing the fact that so many seriously mentally ill (the presumed perpetrators) are not in treatment.

A different hypothesis comes from those suggesting that the problem of increasing stigma lies with the explanatory model. As noted above, neurobiological conceptions of mental illness have not helped diminish stigma, and some now suggest that this conception has actually made the problem worse. As reviewed by Watters (2010), a series of studies have found that persons "who adopted biomedical/genetic beliefs about mental disorders were the same people who wanted less contact with the mentally ill and thought of them as more dangerous and unpredictable." In other words, blamelessness does not apparently translate into greater social acceptance: you may feel sorry for the individual but still not want to associate with him or her. Researchers who have explored this further have found that biological or genetically based conditions are seen as more *intractable*: "The biomedical narrative about an illness like schizophrenia carries with it the subtle assumption that a brain made ill through biomedical or genetic abnormalities is more thoroughly broken and permanently abnormal than one made ill through life events" (Watters 2010). Rusch and colleagues (2010) found that the endorsement of a biogenetic model on the part of the public was associated with less blame (of mentally ill persons) but greater preferred social distance. The same study found that the endorsement of genetic models on the part of the mentally ill was associated with stronger guilt and fear. In their survey analysis Phelan, Yang, and Cruz-Rojas (2006, 386) found that a genetic attribution meant that the problem was seen as "more serious, lifelong and chronic," requiring "powerful forms of intervention" (medication and containment in hospital), but that this also led to "pessimism that even these powerful treatments will be effective in the long run."

Violence and Mental Illness

The relationship between mental illness and violence continues to be an area of controversy. As noted above, the perception that mentally ill persons are violent has strongly contributed to the stigma these individuals experience, in particular preferred social distance and public desire for "containment." Perceptions about violence, aided by media portrayals, have also been shown to significantly influence legal response through the implementation of community treatment orders (an involuntary outpatient status) in a number of jurisdictions, including Canada (Nielssen et al. 2011; Taylor 2008). An example of these is "Brian's Law," an Ontario statute named for the sportscaster killed in 1995 by an apparently mentally disordered man in a highly publicized case.

There is now enough accumulated evidence to conclude that mental illness is a risk factor, albeit small, for violent behaviour (Choe, Teplin, and Abram 2008; Corrigan and Watson 2005; Rueve and Welton 2008; Stuart 2010). This finding obviously needs to be put into context. First, there are other risk factors that are much stronger predictors, in particular, youth, maleness, and active substance misuse (Corrigan and Watson 2005; Rueve and Welton 2008; Steadman et al. 1998; Wallace, Mullen, and Burgess 2004). Second, concerning the public's fear of "stranger violence," violence by mentally disordered persons is most often directed at intimates, particularly family members, rather than at strangers – the same pattern seen in the general public (Arboleda-Florez 1998; Estroff et al. 1994; Lefley 1997; Wehring and Carpenter 2011). Third, persons with mental disorders are much more likely to be the *victims* of violent acts than the perpetrators (Choe, Teplin, and Abram 2008; Wehring and Carptenter 2011). Fourth, environmental factors are significant. Estroff and colleagues (1994, 670) conclude that "persons with persistent psychiatric disorders may be at increased risk for committing violence because of socioeconomic factors and because of how, where and with whom they live, rather than because of their psychiatric disorders." Persons with serious, persistent mental disorders are overrepresented among homeless populations and in skid-row settings, where day-to-day survival is a significant challenge and a premium is placed on toughness.

A final qualification, and arguably the one with the greatest policy relevance, is that it is a small number of individuals with *untreated psychosis* that accounts for a substantial proportion of violent behaviour (Torrey 2011).[6] This is supported by findings showing that violent acts often occur around the point of hospitalization, the violence in many cases precipitating the committal and detention of the untreated individual (Choe, Teplin, and Abram 2008; Rueve and Welton 2008). Further, the psychosis often takes on a particular form, which may include command hallucinations and/or a sense of deep suspicion and paranoia. The psychiatric literature refers to TCO symptoms – threat, control, override – which include perceptions of being controlled, followed, plotted against, and/or having thoughts inserted into one's mind (Norko and Baranoski 2005). In a review of studies on this topic, Taylor (2008) notes that TCO symptoms have been found to be useful in differentiating violent and non-violent individuals.

On the face of it, there are at least two positive corollaries here: first, that most mentally ill persons are not violent; second, that, with greater access to treatment, many of these unfortunate events could be prevented. Family members in particular have argued for some time that, with greater access to treatment (e.g., having the ability to get their ill relative into hospital), they would not have had to wait until it was "too late," until things had escalated to the point of requiring police intervention. However, there are a number of logistical and ethical problems in realizing this vision, apart from limited health care resources. First, some persons with a psychotic illness, even at a time of relative stability, will refuse medication and other treatments. The solution to this, according to Torrey (2011), is the more widespread use of involuntary interventions and laws that support "assisted outpatient treatment" (see also Inman 2011c). However, these interventions have been found to be oppressive by some clients and advocates, and to potentially *add* to stigma and worsen the therapeutic relationship (Dreezer and Dreezer Inc. 2005; Stainsby 2000).

A second challenge is the *early identification* of potentially violent persons. A study bearing on this issue consisted of a review of forty-two homicides from Australia, Canada, and Europe in which the perpetrator had a psychotic illness and the victim was a stranger (Nielssen et al. 2011). Researchers found that, in over half (64 percent) of these cases, the assailant had *never previously been treated* for psychosis. In other words, particularly when the individual lives a solitary existence, or when the family lacks knowledge about mental illness, he or she will be 'flying under the radar," unknown to authorities and not targeted for treatment. This appears to be the situation with the man (noted above) who killed the passenger on the Greyhound bus in Manitoba, for example. It may be that improved early intervention approaches would help, but our current ability to accurately identify and plan for at-risk individuals in the early stages of a psychotic illness is poor (Brown and McGrath 2011; Kirkbride and Jones 2011).

In sum, we know that most mentally ill persons are not violent but that the small number who are get disproportionate media attention (Pinfold and Thornicroft 2006). And, in working with these higher-risk individuals, we need to carefully balance public safety concerns with respect for dignity and autonomy, and the potential for actually increasing stigmatization: "As health care providers and researchers, we must be wary of policy directions that could result in greater restrictions on people who use mental health services, as opposed to providing them with better supports to live full and rewarding lives" (Morrow, Dagg and Pederson 2008, 1).

Stigma from Health Professionals

One of the most troubling accusations concerns the role that mental health practitioners themselves may play in contributing to stigma. This can occur in different ways, such as with the insensitive use of psychiatric jargon. An example of this is the term "chronic," which has been used in psychiatry as an adjective ("chronic mental illness," "the chronic wards") and, even worse, as a noun ("the chronics") (Lesage and Morissette 2002). The curriculum for psychiatric residents in Canada still includes a rotation in "chronic care."[7] Another example was the disparaging identification of persons considered to have personality disorders, as "Axis 2's," this being a reference to the *DSM* classification system in use at the time. (Because of the pejorative aspect of the multi-axial system, it was abandoned with the publication of the *DSM-5* in 2013.) A Canadian Mental Health Association (British Columbia Division 1999, 8) publication gives examples of other value-laden terms used by professionals, such as "low/high-functioning," "inappropriate," "non-compliant," and "treatment-resistant."

Practitioners may also convey stigma through an attitude of pessimism and lowered expectations (Krupa 2008). Canadian author Ron Carten (2006, 18) relates his experience of this in a memoir: the attending psychiatrist informs his family in a planning meeting that after hospitalization Ron would "likely not be able to do anything but very menial labour at best," a pronouncement the writer describes as "being sentenced to a life of marginalization" and one that left him "stunned [and feeling] that [he] had been robbed of all [his] strength and ... confidence." Notably, the doctor's comments were directed not at the patient but at the family, even though Carten was present in the room: "my first lesson in becoming an object."

A number of studies have found that, in the case of schizophrenia, psychiatrists may not actually share the diagnosis with clients. For example, one study found that only 30 percent of respondents had been informed of this diagnosis (Magliano et al. 2008). In another survey, this one involving psychiatrists, 43 percent of respondents stated that they "never" informed clients of the diagnosis, with 41 percent saying they did it on a "case-by-case" basis (Ucok et al. 2004).[8] Explanations for this included the idea that "communication of the diagnosis of schizophrenia could be frightening or demoralizing for patients and relatives" (Magliano et al. 2008, 795), that clients would not understand the term, or that this knowledge would cause clients to drop out of treatment. Concerning the latter belief, the opposite can also be argued: *not* telling "is likely to be perceived by patients as further evidence that schizophrenia is unavoidably a severe and untreatable disease, thus contributing to their withdrawal and skepticism toward treatments" (Magliano et al. 2008, 795). Davidson (2012, 3) notes the contradiction between using this approach and still hoping that the client will gain "insight" into the condition: "If we did not view people with mental illnesses as capable of digesting and using this information, and therefore did not educate them, how could we expect them to 'accept' their diagnoses?"

In truth, when handling a loaded term like "schizophrenia," practitioners must sometimes walk a very narrow line, dealing with, on the one side, the need to demystify mental disorder and be "up front" with the client about diagnosis and, on the other side, concerns about how psychiatric labels are perceived by others. Kirk and Kutchins (1992) note that, in this regard, clinicians may deliberately "under-diagnose" to avoid the worst effects of "labelling." A not uncommon strategy is for clinicians to speak more to the *symptoms* of the illness rather than to the diagnosis itself, which may be more effective in the case of a client who does not accept having a mental illness (Davidson 2012). A report by the Schizophrenia Commission (2012, 12) in the UK recommends that psychiatrists be "very cautious about making a diagnosis of schizophrenia, in particular after a first episode of psychosis [because] at that point making such a diagnosis may do more harm than good."

Some comment is necessary here on personality disorder diagnoses, particularly on borderline personality disorder. While any psychiatric diagnosis can be stigmatizing, the personality diagnoses are particularly so *within the practitioner community* because of the view held by many that the problems seen represent willfulness and a deliberate undermining of the clinician's treatment plans (Potter 2011; Woollaston and Hixenbaugh 2008). On this point, a Canadian woman diagnosed with BPD notes that practitioners may believe, wrongly, that people who fit this diagnosis "enjoy [their situation] and don't want to get well" (Williams 1998, 173). Similarly, Potter (2006, 139) concludes that practitioners conflate their moral and clinical appraisals in the way that they "routinely perceive BPD patients as manipulative and so have less empathy for them." Negative expectations can also arise because of the anticipation that persons diagnosed with BPD represent a lot of work as well as potential liability concerns. As Paris (2005, 1581) states: "Managing patients with BPD can be burdensome for clinicians because they may have to deal with repeated suicide threats and attempts over years." In considering the pejorative effect of the "personality" labels, suggestions from different authors include eliminating the word from diagnostic manuals altogether (Peele and Kadekar 2007) or viewing "the concepts under discussion ... as a process and not as a diagnostic label ... [that] can aid the clinician's understanding and management of such individuals" (Andrews et al. 2000, 628).

Persons with mental illnesses may also encounter discrimination in hospitals and other parts of the public health system. Clients with legitimate medical concerns may receive indifferent care from physicians, who may believe the physical complaints have a psychiatric basis or who who simply find this population difficult and unrewarding (Dupuis 2008).[9] There is also the frequent observation that persons in a psychiatric crisis are not well received – and, in fact, are subjected to further humiliation and trauma – when they come to hospital emergency wards (Picard 2008a). A position paper published by the Canadian Psychiatric Association (Charbonneau et al. 2010, 2) in fact identified "discrimination in the emergency department" as the top priority area in combating the stigma of mental illness. While some hospitals in larger cities may employ psychiatric triage personnel to help identify and direct mentally ill persons, in most cases clients will be seen by physicians and nurses whose orientation is medical, not psychiatric, and who make a distinction on that basis: in these situations psychological distress may not be seen as a "real" medical problem. This is all the more problematic when one considers that the answering machine messages for mental health agencies typically tell callers: "if you are in crisis, please go to your nearest hospital emergency department." In a survey by the Mood Disorders Society of Canada (2011b, 8), a significant proportion of the 3,125 respondents expressed dissatisfaction with the care they received at hospital emergencies: "Respondents reported using the emergency room as a last resort when they have suicidal thoughts. It is very concerning that, in these cases, individuals were left to wait extremely lengthy periods of time and in many cases were not treated with the sensitivity required." The survey included comments from respondents, as follows (Mood Disorders Society of Canada 2011, 9):

- "48 hours waiting, 10 min. rushed consultation."
- "I would never go back. They treated me with total lack of respect ... laughed about me to another staff and I am not being paranoid but you see the problem ... I cannot complain as they think I am 'paranoid.' Anyone else would be taken seriously."
- "When I've been suicidal, it's been excruciatingly painful to wait in the emergency room for hours."
- "It's very hard to go to an emergency room for [a] mental health emergency ... it's not easy to be turned away when you need help and feel you cannot stay alone because you are afraid of yourself and your actions."

- "Mental health care in the ER tends to leave me feeling even more crazy when I leave than when I arrived."

Finally, stigma is created *within disciplines* by devaluing the work of those who choose to specialize in mental health (Abbey et al. 2011). This subject is explored in a paper by occupational therapist and Queen's University professor Terry Krupa, who recalls a student saying, in a class on mental health practice: "But I didn't come into occupational therapy to work with these kinds of problems." Krupa (2008, 202) notes that the response was troubling "because the structures of specialization within our profession can oddly legitimize the notion that we have the right to control who will receive our help and that we can abdicate responsibility when people do not fit our vision." She goes on to describe the *associative stigma* felt by professionals who work with stigmatized populations:

> Over the course of my career I have received messages from within the profession suggesting a devaluation of mental health practice ... The messages imply, sometimes not so subtly, that the work lacks a definitive knowledge base, is limited in technical expertise, and is of limited value. As an educator I worry about how students will receive these messages, whether they will internalize them and whether they will influence their career choices. Mostly I worry about the extent to which they themselves will replicate the expression of these messages. (203)

One may encounter concern expressed about the devaluation of mental health work in other fields, such as nursing and medicine (Arbodelda-Florez 2003; Charbonneau et al. 2010; Whitaker 2010). A 2012 editorial in the British medical journal the *Lancet*, in commenting on the declining enrolment in psychiatry on the part of medical graduates in both the UK and US, quotes a British recruitment official as saying: "Common perceptions within the medical profession include the view that psychiatry is just not scientific enough, is too remote from the rest of medicine, is often viewed negatively by other medical professionals, and is a specialty too often characterized by difficult doctor–patient relationships and limited success rates of therapeutic interventions" (*Lancet* 2012, 1,274).

Anti-Stigma Initiatives
Tackling the problem of stigma has become a top priority for non-governmental organizations, health authorities, and the Mental Health Commission of Canada (MHCC). This cause has been taken up internationally,

with the World Psychiatric Association's "Open the Doors" campaign, launched in 1996 to fight discrimination resulting from the diagnosis of schizophrenia (Stuart 2008). An anti-stigma initiative was considered one of the most important mandates for the MHCC, which, in 2009, launched "Opening Minds," a multi-site and multi-partner project designed "to identify and evaluate existing anti-stigma programs to determine their effectiveness and potential to be rolled out nationally."[10] At this writing, as the previous quote suggests, the field is still an evolving one, with some promising developments but still a shortage of evaluative studies and no clear "best practice" approaches (Queensland Alliance for Mental Health 2010; Stuart 2008).

Coercion
Corrigan and Gelb (2006) suggest that there are three broad, overlapping approaches to anti-stigma: education, contact (with service users), and protest. To "protest" one could add anti-discrimination laws, both being approaches that rely on coercion ("sticks" versus "carrots") to correct what is seen as a moral injustice. An example of a protest approach is "Stigma-busters," created by the National Alliance on Mental Illness (NAMI) in the US. In this program, members of NAMI and the general public may send an "alert" about disrespectful media images, which advocates then respond to through written expressions of disapproval and, in some cases, boycotts. According to the NAMI website about twenty thousand alerts are sent in a month, nation-wide.

Does protest work? An American example is the case of "Psycho Donuts," a store that opened in Campbell, California, in 2009. The outlet featured specialty donuts with names like "Bipolar," "Manic Malt," "Cereal Killer," "Headbanger," "Psycho Panda," "Jekyll and Hyde," and "Kooky Monster," among others (see http://psycho-donuts.com/menu.pdf). The store décor included straitjackets and a padded room, with staff wearing lab coats and nurses' uniforms. As recounted in *Wikipedia*, this set off protests from advocacy organizations, including NAMI, who pointed out, for the sake of comparison, that making fun of cancer, or making gay persons or ethnic minorities the butt of jokes, would never be tolerated. Owners and supporters of the store denied malicious intent and also referred to the "right to free speech" – upheld in the First Amendment to the US Constitution – as entitling them to choose the name of their business and products.[11] Some also argued that advocates should worry about "larger issues" instead of going after a small business and that the controversy over the store would cause people to not take mental health issues seriously. The protests did result in some discussion at the city hall, a consciousness-raising workshop, and some changes to the décor and language used by the store's owner. Despite all of this, three years later, the store – with products named "psycho" and "crazy," and with its "nurse-on-duty" – was still in existence, and a second outlet had been opened.

Discrimination is also addressed through legislation in Canada under federal and provincial human rights codes and under the Charter of Rights and Freedoms, which, in section 15, prohibits discrimination on the basis of "mental disability." Proscribed areas include accommodation, goods and services, and employment. Proving discrimination is not always easy to do, and there is evidence from the US – in the implementation of that country's Americans with Disabilities Act – that protective legislation can be circumvented in particular cases by narrowed interpretation (Petrila 2009). In Canada, despite human rights codes prohibiting discriminatory employment practices, there is no evidence that human rights complaints are declining (Dranoff 2005).

One of the problems with coercive strategies is that they address behaviour but do not necessarily tap into underlying beliefs. Corrigan and Gelb (2006, 394) note that protest may actually have an adverse effect in that it "can produce psychological reactions – 'Don't tell me what to think' – and more negative attitudes" (which one can infer may have occurred with "Psycho Donuts"). Concerning anti-discrimination legislation, Stefan (2002, 1) concludes that "the law to a large extent follows political trends rather than shaping them; enforces consensus rather than creating it." Nonetheless, the law is important for its symbolic value, for defining injustice, and for providing a recourse – albeit a crude one – for addressing behaviour that is hurtful and harmful. We may draw from earlier examples, such as laws against racial segregation, which initially were neither enforced nor embraced by some but that were a necessary impetus to gradually shifting the *zeitgeist*. Pinfold and Thornicroft (2006) suggest that, for anti-stigma programs to be effective, "carrot" and "stick" strategies may both have to be adopted.

Contact

Anti-stigma approaches that involve actual contact with a member or members of the stigmatized group are usually compelling and may be the most effective way of shifting public attitudes (Pinfold and Thornicroft 2006). Stuart (2008, 186, emphasis added) suggests that "the approaches that have been most successful in improving knowledge and attitudes (*but not necessarily behaviours*) have combined active learning with positive contact with people who have a mental illness."

There are a number of "contact" initiatives to which one can point. For example, the Schizophrenia Society, which has chapters across Canada, makes presentations to community groups at which a staff member provides educational material and a service user describes her/his own experiences and illness trajectory. Some professional training programs now incorporate learning modules in which service users participate. Jamieson and colleagues (2006) describe a curriculum initiative for occupational therapy students at Queen's University in Ontario that involved students visiting disabled clients, with the clients acting as tutors, and the students writing in their journals about this experience. In evaluating this, the study authors concluded that the initiative had helped facilitate student empathy, which they argue is a crucial foundation for client-centred practice.

The advantage of education materials *plus* client contact over education alone comes from a study conducted at the Centre for Addiction and Mental Health in Toronto and in which a multimodal program aimed at destigmatizing mental disorder, called "Beyond the Cuckoo's Nest," was presented to high school students. The study sought to evaluate the impact of a video produced by staff and clients at the centre, which the authors describe as a "powerful and moving portrayal of the challenges facing individuals doubly burdened by mental illness and homelessness" (Tolomiczenko, Goering, and Durbin 2001, 254). It was found, however, that students who only saw the video subsequently expressed more negative attitudes towards mental illness and stronger feelings of danger associated with homeless persons than did a control group of students who attended the centre's program without seeing the video. By comparison, the video combined with an audience discussion that included one of the video's subjects was found to decrease stigmatizing attitudes, leading the authors to conclude: "These findings point toward a pernicious aspect of stigma attached to mental illness; namely, a tendency to ratchet in a negative direction when emotionally charged material is not grounded or interpreted in the context of either direct discussion or proximate relations [through a friend or family member] with a person or persons living with mental illness" (256). The counter-intuitive finding that a video (alone) produces negative effects has been observed in other settings in Canada and Europe (Arboleda-Florez 2003; Gaebel and Baumann 2003).

Direct contact with clients has been crucial, in this author's experience, with respect to staff buy-in on the issue of employing clients as peer workers in mental health settings, a practice that has only been in effect in Canadian health authorities since the late 1990s (see Chapter 17, which deals with "occupation"). Initially, the idea that mentally ill persons would be coming into agencies to work alongside practitioners was greeted with pessimism, trepidation, and, in some cases, outright hostility – another example of the stigma that exists within the mental health system itself. While not always publicly expressed, there was a view among a number of staff members that peer workers were unreliable, unprofessional, and potentially harmful to clients – this before they had even started. Thankfully, key agency players with courage and vision pushed through the implementation of peer services, which gradually achieved credibility among regular staff members simply by exposing them, first-hand, to the capabilities of peer workers.

Education and Mental Health Literacy
Mental health literacy (MHL) is a public education concept that refers to "the knowledge and beliefs about mental disorders which aid their recognition, management or prevention" (Queensland Alliance for Mental Health 2010, 14). The hope is that increased MHL will help people recognize signs of mental disorder in themselves, or among family, friends, or employees, and avoid delays in seeking help. While not specifically targeting stigma, there is an assumption that helping people view mental disorders as relatively common, treatable medical conditions, with no blame attached, will diminish public fear and discrimination. MHL programs have been particularly well developed in Australia (Queensland Alliance for Mental Health 2010).

A national survey on mental health literacy in Canada commissioned by the Canadian Alliance on Mental Illness and Mental Health (2007), which combined questionnaires and focus groups, found the following:

- Focus group respondents made a distinction between "mental illness" and "mental health problems," with depression and anxiety being examples of the latter, and schizophrenia being an example of the former. When asked to estimate prevalence rates, most questionnaire respondents agreed that almost anyone could suffer from "mental health problems," but they tended to underestimate the prevalence of mental illness. Most correctly identified depression as the most prevalent mental disorder.
- Focus group respondents tended not to see mental disorders as "health problems." When asked to identify the major health problems facing their age group, no mental disorder was mentioned, even though, as we noted in Chapter 3, depression is one of the leading causes of disease burden worldwide.
- Concerning recognition of symptoms, tested through a series of vignettes, a majority of questionnaire respondents were able to recognize the signs of depression, but accuracy was much lower for schizophrenia.
- When asked about causes, questionnaire respondents chose "environmental" factors (stress, trauma) as most significant for depression and anxiety. For schizophrenia, "biomedical" factors (genetics, brain disease, chemical imbalance) were considered most important – correctly – although by only 49 percent of respondents.

- Focus group respondents were found to have "a poor understanding of the roles and responsibilities of different mental health professionals," with, for example, few knowing the difference between psychiatrists and psychologists.
- Concerning perceptions of dangerousness, many focus group respondents agreed that "other people" tended to see mentally ill persons as "unpredictable" or "out of control."
- Finally, when asked why mentally ill persons might not seek help, "being ashamed or concerned about stigma" were the most common reasons given by questionnaire respondents.

Mental health literacy is addressed through public education programs such as Mental Health First Aid, a twelve-hour curriculum developed and sponsored by the Mental Health Commission of Canada and delivered through community agencies. At the website (http://www.mentalhealth firstaid.ca/EN/about/Pages/default.aspx), this approach is likened to "physical first aid," with interventions targeting persons who are developing a mental health problem or experiencing a crisis:

> The MHFA Canada program aims to improve mental health literacy, and provide the skills and knowledge to help people better manage potential or developing mental health problems in themselves, a family member, a friend or a colleague. The program does not teach people how to be therapists. It does teach people how to:
>
> - Recognize the signs and symptoms of mental health problems.
> - Provide initial help.
> - Guide a person towards appropriate professional help.
>
> MHFA shares the same overall purpose as traditional first aid – to save lives.

MHFA is also intended to "increase ... knowledge about treatment supports and services, increase willingness to proactively seek out professional services and build the capacity of carers to provide support" (Queensland Alliance for Mental Health 2010, 14). A review document concludes that, particularly in workplace settings, MHFA is a "promising practice" (Canadian Alliance on Mental Illness and Mental Health 2007).

Recommendations
Combating stigma is a complex matter when one considers that the targets for change are not just knowledge but also attitudes and behaviour. It has become apparent that information alone, presented in a decontextualized

and non-interactive fashion, is not sufficient for changing attitudes (Queensland Alliance for Mental Health 2010). In fact, there is concern that, when the issue is framed the wrong way, stigmatizing beliefs may actually be increased. This concern stems from the finding, noted earlier, that neurobiological conceptions of mental illness do not appear to diminish stigma:

> Many consumer and family organizations share an enthusiasm for promoting a medical understanding of the causes of mental ill-health based on a belief that this will help to lessen the perception of moral responsibility or character failings that are frequently associated with mental illness. The assumption is that if mental illnesses are attributed to factors outside of the individual's control, then they are not responsible for their own behaviour and the reactions of others will be less negative. Research evidence does not support the efficacy of this approach ... When the disease model is applied to the brain, the belief is that people are incapable of exerting judgment, control, or reason. The result is not greater acceptance but increased fear and a desire for social distance. The public is more pessimistic about recovery, holds an exaggerated perception of difference (them and us), and is more likely to dehumanize people with mental illness. (Queensland Alliance for Mental Health 2010, 20)

The "framing" issue appears to be most problematic with disorders that are perceived to be *serious*, schizophrenia in particular. Social distance surveys and help-seeking patterns indicate that there is less stigma attached to depression; the reason, apparently, is that depressed persons are viewed as "less different," with the Canadian mental health literacy survey finding that "the symptoms of depression are considered part of normal human experience but the symptoms of schizophrenia are not" (Canadian Alliance on Mental Illness and Mental Health 2007, 27). This suggests that public education about mental disorders should be framed "as part of our shared humanity" (Queensland Alliance for Mental Health 2010, 8) rather than by referencing genetic anomalies and broken brains. A Canadian Psychiatric Association (Abbey et al. 2011, 4) position paper on stigma suggests that "discriminatory behaviours become psychologically acceptable when the other is denied essential human characteristics through their placement of other or them as distinct from Us." It would also seem to make sense to target public anti-stigma programs specifically at schizophrenia, as is the case with the World Psychiatric Association's "Open the Doors" campaign.[12]

With regard to anti-stigma campaigns, a potential area of tension concerns the positions of family support organizations, which have tended to *endorse* the biogenetic framing of mental illness and have suggested that "shared humanity" approaches may have the effect of minimizing the seriousness of a disorder like schizophrenia. On this matter, a branch of the Canadian Schizophrenia Society talks about the need to have "open and frank" depictions of mental illness in public education initiatives and argues that downplaying the severity (differentness) is "in effect reinforcing stigma rather than combating it" (North Shore Schizophrenia Society 2012, 1).

In addition to considerations about framing, stigma researchers have concluded that education campaigns should be *targeted*, in particular towards young persons, health care professionals, emergency unit personnel, the police, social service agencies, and the media (Arboleda-Florez 2003; Corrigan 2004; Stuart 2008). Strategies and curricula would vary depending on the audience. For example:

- Stuart (2006, 647) notes that adolescence is a "strategically important time" to implement such programs since this is when mental disorders may start to emerge, when fears about stigma and not fitting in are felt most acutely, and when help-seeking would potentially achieve the greatest impact. She describes a program rolled out across eight Canadian high schools, which was found to increase knowledge and reduce measures of social distance.
- As noted, persons with mental disorders may encounter indifference and stigma from health care workers, including general practitioners and emergency room personnel. Initiatives that have been developed to address this include: (1) "Understanding the Impact of Stigma," a program for frontline health care workers created in Ontario and being rolled out to emergency room personnel in other parts of Canada;[13] (2) "The Mind Course," a requirement for all second-year University of Calgary medical students that combines lectures, hospital visits, and speakers who are managing a mental illness;[14] and (3) a continuing medical education web-based course on the stigma of mental illness developed by a partnership between the Mood Disorders Society of Canada and the Canadian Medical Association (Mood Disorders Society of Canada 2011c).
- Concerning the need to target the media, Pinfold and Thornicroft (2006, 151) suggest that, "when we consider ... evidence that has influenced public perceptions of mental illness, the press, and the tabloids in particular, are the main candidates for attention primarily because they reflect, and some would argue fuel, the public's preoccupation with the link between 'risk' or violence and mental health problems." Goering, Wasylenki, and Durbin (2000) note that, in Canada, when mental health issues are covered at all, the media tend to focus on negative topics such as homelessness and

violence. In her report on an anti-stigma intervention with newspaper personnel in Calgary, Stuart (2003) suggests that mental health programs make accurate background briefs available to the media, maintain a list of local experts for interviews, and keep up regular contact with key editorial staff.[15] To reference a website whose purpose is "to provide tools and information for ... journalists ... on ways to improve reporting on mental health issues," see http://depts.washington.edu/mhreport/.

It is also recommended that service users be involved with the planning, execution, and evaluation of anti-stigma initiatives. As noted, interventions that include client testimonials are usually more effective, particularly when dealing with the most stigmatizing disorders such as schizophrenia (Canadian Alliance on Mental Illness and Mental Health 2007). Success stories, showing recovery and participation in work, school, and social life, can be effective. Concerning the evaluation of these initiatives – are discriminatory behaviours really changing? – service users are in a unique position to identify the yardsticks used to measure change (Stuart 2008).

Stigma research also needs a stronger evidence base, which is difficult given the large scale and complexity of the evaluation designs necessary. Pinfold and Thornicroft (2006, 156) note that "research limitations ... include inadequate follow-up periods, social biasing within attitude measurements, few measures of behavioural change and overreliance on self-reporting rather than observational evidence."

Given that public education programs need to be ongoing to be effective (Joa et al. 2008), an enduring national vision, in which national programs are supported with activities at the local level, will be important (Pinfold and Thornicroft 2006; Queensland Alliance for Mental Health 2010). Thus, the "Opening Minds" initiative sponsored by the Mental Health Commission is promising, as would be the continued funding of that federal body.

As we have seen in this chapter, stigma may be conveyed through an attitude of pessimism and lowered expectations on the part of practitioners. Persons who have fought to overcome the effects of mental illness will later speak, in many cases, of the importance of having someone who believed in them, of someone who was positive and hopeful. The significance of this attitude among service providers and service recipients is explored in more detail in the next chapter.

Notes

1 Coincidentally, while writing this, the author was asked to complete a reference form for a physician applying to work at a mental health program in another (Canadian) health authority. The form required that respondents comment on whether the applicant had "suffered

from or received treatment for any drug or alcohol dependency problems" or had a "mental or other health condition which might adversely affect his/her skills, abilities or judgment." While one can understand an employer's liability concerns, the questions do appear to reinforce concerns about disclosure among mental health professionals.

2 See Corrigan (2005) for a discussion of this issue, especially how he draws parallels with "coming out" on the part of persons with different sexual orientations. He notes that a key benefit to disclosure is the reduction in stress as a result of no longer having to keep this secret.

3 There is a parallel here with the sociological concepts of primary deviance (label being applied) and secondary deviance (person identifying with label).

4 In 2006, an anonymous individual or group in the Vancouver area launched the website NIABY (not in anyone's back yard) (http://www.niaby.com). The website describes NIABY as "a virtual community of hard working, tax paying, concerned citizens" who are "monitoring proposed addiction and mental health community treatment solutions proposed for residential neighbourhoods." The site emphasizes that non-wealthy neighbourhoods are represented as well, an apparent reference to the historical tendency for mental health facilities to be located in poorer areas, this a consequence of community tolerance levels and housing prices.

5 See http://www.bbc.co.uk/news/world-15936276. In this report a journalist notes: "The shock [of the killings] is heightened by the media portrayal of Breivik as carefully planning his actions as a functioning member of society. He does not match the public's idea of a paranoid schizophrenic."

6 This is consistent with the author's own experience, which, in over twenty-five years of working directly with the seriously mentally ill, produced only two instances of a client-on-staff (minor) assault, and in both cases the assailant was psychotic, fearful, and misperceiving the presence of the staff person.

7 See: http://www.psychiatry.ubc.ca/teaching/PGE.htm. A particularly egregious use of language is given by Angell, Cooke, and Kovac (2005), citing an account of a hospital setting in which staff would abbreviate the diagnosis "schizophrenia, chronic undifferentiated type" and refer to patients as "scuts."

8 According to Davidson (2012, 3), the psychiatric community in Japan has eliminated the term "schizophrenia" altogether, "having found it stigmatizes and compounds complexities associated with diagnosing serious mental illnesses."

9 See also: http://www.medicalnewstoday.com/releases/74958.php.

10 See http://www.mentalhealthcommission.ca/English/Pages/OpeningMinds.aspx.

11 On this point, legal scholar Stanley Fish (1994) suggests that the concept of free speech has proven to be problematic in the US context, being appropriated in some cases to support bigotry.

12 While schizophrenia may be the most stigmatizing diagnosis among the general public, borderline personality disorder is – arguably – the one that produces the strongest negative reaction among mental health practitioners, so it could be targeted for professional education.

13 See http://www.mentalhealthcommission.ca/SiteCollectionDocuments/opening%20minds/OM_News_Release_Dec6_%20Eng.pdf.

14 See http://www.mentalhealthcommission.ca/SiteCollectionDocuments/News/News_release_Mind_Course_English_Final.pdf.

15 In Stuart's (2003, 654) intervention with Calgary newspaper staff, stories concerning mental illness were analyzed over an eight-month, pre-test baseline period and over a sixteen-month post-test. It was found that, while positive mental health stories increased in number and length during the post-test period, unfortunately, so did negative stories. In particular, stigmatizing stories about schizophrenia – involving public security concerns linked to people not in treatment – "increased at a faster pace than positive news," which speaks to the importance of ongoing re-evaluation of stigma initiatives.

Other Resources

To read more about the Mental Health Commission's anti-stigma campaign "Opening Minds," see http://www.mentalhealthcommission.ca/English/Pages/OpeningMinds.aspx.

The National Consortium on Stigma and Empowerment contains a number of resources on combating the stigma of mental illness: http://www.stigmaandempowerment.org.

Mental Health First Aid Canada: http://www.mentalhealthfirstaid.ca/EN/Pages/default.aspx.

The Recovery Vision

Recovery – as the term is now used in mental health – refers, tentatively, to a model of care. "Tentatively" is used here because, notwithstanding its prominence and a now considerable literature, there is still misunderstanding about what this term means. Further, despite its being referenced in agency mission statements, and despite recovery fidelity scales being published, it is unclear as to whether the model is being implemented and fully achieved. Indeed, one could argue that if people are still debating the operational definition(s), it is virtually impossible to evaluate implementation. For these reasons it may be better to talk about recovery as an orientation, or a vision, as the chapter title suggests. While the details may still need to be worked out, certainly the values underlying a recovery vision seem clear. This chapter addresses definitional issues, why this orientation is considered important, how one measures and evaluates recovery, debates about feasibility, and, despite a status approaching orthodoxy, whether there is buy-in from all stakeholders.

A relatively concise definition of the recovery vision is necessary at this point. Unlike a traditional medical definition of recovery, which focuses more narrowly on symptom remission, this conception of recovery

> may include, but *does not require*, symptom remission or a return to normal functioning ... recovery is seen [instead] as a process of personal growth and development, and involves overcoming the effects of being a mental health patient, with all its implications, to regain control and establish a personally fulfilling, meaningful life. (Schrank and Slade 2007, 321, emphasis added)

From this, one can see that, whatever a recovery orientation is, it is *not* what was referred to as a "medical model" in Chapter 1, or what some people would call "old school." From the recovery perspective the client is dealing

Figure 3

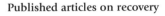

Published articles on recovery

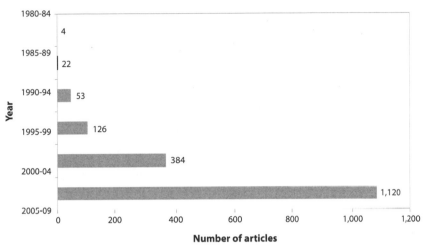

Number of articles

not just with symptoms but also other consequences of having a mental illness, such as stigma and social rejection. Recovery here is a process, rather than an outcome, in which self-management is emphasized and in which individuals strive for a good quality of life even in the presence of residual symptoms. The US Substance Abuse and Mental Health Services Administration (SAMHSA) (2012) gives an even more succinct definition of recovery, as follows: "A process of change through which individuals work to improve their own health and wellbeing, live a self-directed life, and strive to achieve their full potential." According to SAMHSA, this is achieved in part by managing symptoms of mental illness but also by addressing other determinants of health, such as having safe and stable housing, meaningful activity, a sense of purpose, and supportive relationships.[1]

The prominence of the recovery vision in mental health is reflected, partially, by the volume of literature written on the subject. Figure 3 represents a search, using Google Scholar, of peer-review publications that contained the phrases "recovery model" and "mental health" in the text. One can see the progression from virtually none prior to 1990 to a rate of four articles per week by the late 2000s. While the majority of these were authored by rehabilitation specialists and social scientists – as opposed to authors with a medical background – a professor of psychiatry at the University of Illinois suggests that "the concept of recovery ... has now entered mainstream psychiatry and is considered a legitimate area for academic focus and inquiry" (Weiden 2010).

Prominence is also established by the fact that the recovery vision has been adopted by the Mental Health Commission of Canada as a guiding principle. The Canadian Senate report that led to the creation of the commission concludes that "recovery must be at the centre of mental health reform," defining recovery as "a way of living a satisfying, hopeful, and productive life even with limitations caused by the illness" (Standing Senate Committee on Social Affairs, Science and Technology 2006, 42). In a later policy framework document, the Mental Health Commission (2009, 27) makes it clear that the definition of recovery being used is one that does not require symptom remission: "A person can *recover their life without recovering from their illness* ... This is the understanding of recovery used in this document" (emphasis added). Further, "a transformed mental health system must incorporate programs, treatments, services and supports that are not only geared to reducing the symptoms of mental health problems and illnesses, but [ones that] also promote the ability of people living with mental health problems and illnesses to attain the best possible mental health and well-being" (Mental Health Commission of Canada 2009, 26). Finally, the prominence of the recovery vision is reflected in the fact that it is now a standard used for the accreditation of Canadian community mental health programs.

In looking at the development of the recovery vision, one can point to a number of disparate influences and antecedents, some academic, some clinical, and some self-help:

- Grassroots initiatives developed by clients themselves, who were searching for support and social connections, and who found existing services to be either non-existent or overly medically focused. Examples include the Mental Patients Association, formed in Vancouver, BC, in the early 1970s, and "We Are Not Alone," a group of former psychiatric hospital patients from New York and an organization that paved the way for what became the clubhouse model. Some of these groups had an advocacy and civil-rights orientation and were more critical of psychiatry (Clark and Krupa 2002).
- "Labelling theory," a sociological perspective suggesting that the consequences of being diagnosed with a mental illness are more serious than the illness itself. This viewpoint differs markedly from biogenic explanations by focusing on *societal response* as a way of understanding how psychiatric disability is created. Authors in the labelling tradition included Canadian sociologist Erving Goffman, Thomas Scheff, and David Rosenhan. Goffman (1961), in his influential book *Asylums: Essays on the*

Social Situation of Mental Patients and Other Inmates, argues that it is institutionalization that fosters the regressive behaviours and symptoms seen among patients. Rosenhan (1973) is famous for a controversial study published as "On Being Sane in Insane Places," involving "pseudo-patients" (study confederates) posing as real patients in a psychiatric hospital, the conclusion being that that "once a person is designated abnormal, all of his [sic] other behaviors and characteristics are colored by that label" (253). Popular in the 1960s and 1970s, labelling theory has now faded from view, although some of its elements – the "stickiness" of psychiatric labels, the impact of stigma, and the idea that practice approaches may enhance dependency – are still relevant.

- Schools of psychotherapy emerging in the 1950s and 1960s that fell under the "humanist-existential" rubric – such as Rogerian therapy, or client-centred therapy – which were noteworthy more for underlying values such as egalitarianism and self-determination than for specific techniques.
- Practice schools that emphasize being client-centred and strengths-based (as opposed to being oriented towards deficits or disability, as medicine is presumed to be). Traditionally, social work and the rehabilitation disciplines have claimed this mantle, although in theory any practice discipline can adopt a strengths-based orientation. As noted in Chapter 1, there is a psychosocial rehabilitation (PSR) model recognized in Canada and other countries that is not discipline-specific; staff may attain certification in this model or, more generally, use it as a practice framework.
- Evidence from other areas of health care, for example, living with cancer, that quality of life and symptom profile are not as closely associated as we might assume (Waldron et al. 1999).

A number of the seminal professional publications on the recovery vision came from psychiatric rehabilitation specialists, notably Boston University professor William Anthony, whose 1993 paper "Recovery from Mental Illness" was very influential. In this article, recovery is conceptualized as follows:

- Recovery can refer to recovery from the disorder itself – that is, remission of symptoms – but is also possible even if some symptoms persist or return. Recovery, in other words, does not depend on the disorder being "cured."
- Recovery also refers to attempting to deal with and overcome the stigma associated with having a mental disorder, especially as it affects gaining access *to* education and employment.
- Recovery also means dealing with diminished confidence and self-esteem resulting from lengthy periods of unemployment and with feelings of loss

that result from seeing ambitions for career, family, and companionship go unfulfilled.

- Recovery is not a function of one's theory or theories about the causes of mental illness; that is, adopting a recovery vision does not commit a person to either side of the nature versus nurture aetiological debate.
- Recovery does not mean that the individual was not "really mentally ill"; that is, that their success was not a beacon of hope for others but, rather, an aberration or a fraud.
- Recovery usually requires having someone present who believes in you:

> People who are recovering talk about the people who believed in them when they did not even believe in themselves, who encouraged their recovery but did not force it, who tried to listen and understand when nothing seemed to be making sense. Recovery is a deeply human experience, facilitated by the deeply human responses of others. Recovery can be facilitated by any one person. Recovery can be everybody's business. (Anthony 1993, 18)

Recovery in this conception can mean dealing with debilitating aspects of the service system itself, which, even if unintended, may contribute to disability rather than diminish it. For example, a Canadian Mental Health Association publication suggests that, when clients are given no sense of personal responsibility by service providers, they reach a state of "learned helplessness and hopelessness," a state that practitioners contribute to by rewarding "easy to manage" clients – who do as they're told – and by defining "insight" as the client's capacity to accept a bleak prognosis (Everett et al. 2003). These authors also note the negative effects of being labelled and processed: "Access to needed mental health resources comes only through 'certification of impairment and disability' ... a process that in effect *creates* the social category of psychiatric disability" (12, emphasis added). Chamberlin (2010), in drawing from her own experiences as a "bad patient," suggests that "a 'good patient' is someone who has given up hope and who has internalized the staff's very limited vision of his or her potential."

Recovery, Rehabilitation, and Self-Management

Because of their similarities and areas of overlap, distinguishing a recovery-oriented approach from a rehabilitation-oriented approach is not easy. Corrigan (2003, 346), for example, suggests that "rehabilitation is synonymous with recovery: it means helping people get back to work and living on their own." In another instance, a Canadian report on best practices in psychosocial rehabilitation lists underlying principles that are very similar to those of the recovery model: client involvement, self-determination, personal choice, natural and peer supports, hope, and belonging (British Columbia Ministry of Health 2002f). One way to make a distinction is to see rehabilitation as more practitioner-driven and recovery as more client-driven. In this conception, people have to recover themselves – no one can do it for them (a perspective similar to that seen in the addictions field). Author Patricia Deegan (1988, 11), herself diagnosed with schizophrenia, writes that "it is important to understand that persons with a disability do not 'get rehabilitated' in the sense that cars get tuned up or televisions get repaired. They are not passive recipients of rehabilitation services. Rather, they experience themselves as recovering a new sense of self and of purpose within and beyond the limits of the disability." In distinguishing recovery from rehabilitation Deegan suggests that "rehabilitation refers to the services and technologies that are made available to disabled persons so that they may learn to adapt to their world. Recovery refers to the lived or real life experience of persons as they accept and overcome the challenge of the disability" (11). The Canadian Senate report *Out of the Shadows at Last* makes a distinction between recovery and rehabilitation by referring to a "psychosocial rehabilitation model" and an "empowerment model," the latter being more client-driven but still including resources and service provided by professionals (Standing Senate Committee on Social Affairs, Science and Technology 2006).

The idea of recovery as a client-driven process leads us to one of the most contentious elements of the recovery vision, articulated by William Anthony in his 1993 publication, that "professionals do not hold the key to recovery, consumers do" (18). In suggesting that there are "many pathways to recovery," Anthony raises the prospect that recovery can occur without professional intervention. Recovery probably does occur without professional intervention when one is considering transient states, or milder forms of depression, but the argument is less convincing when one includes persistent psychotic illnesses such as schizophrenia, particularly the early stages of these disorders. Recovery as a client-driven process is a theme that is carried through to the Mental Health Commission's 2012 strategy document: "To the greatest extent possible, [clients] control and maintain responsibility for their mental health and well-being, and they make their own choices about which services, treatments and supports may be best for them, informed by the advice of professionals, as well as families and peers" (Mental Health Commission of Canada 2012, 16).

Recovery and Hope
A critical component of the recovery vision is *hopefulness* and the role professionals play in enhancing or diminishing this. The importance of practitioners

instilling hope is apparent from a number of client surveys and testimonials, as Bachrach (1996, 31) summarizes: "The patient-authored literature reveals a number of relevant notions and ideas that are at best rarely given credence by professional program planners. Among these are the importance of hope to patients [and] their need for validation and encouragement." Similarly, in interviewing psychiatric service users, Borg and Rasmussen (2004, 493) found that "a central and greatly valued support from the professionals was finding ways to convey optimism ... and in general, keeping hope alive." Further, evaluations of outcomes in psychological treatments have found that "positive and hopeful expectations," apart from the particular method or technique, are a key determinant of success (Hubble, Duncan, and Miller 1999, 8).

Optimism may be crucial, but service user accounts suggest it is not typical. An example is the experience of Canadian author Ron Carten (2006, 18), who describes his first psychiatric hospitalization and the subsequent verdict rendered by the attending psychiatrist: that he would be "on medications the rest of his life ... [and] likely not be able to do anything but very menial labour at best." After "being sentenced to a life of marginalization," and "robbed of all [his] strength and ... confidence," Carten contemplates his future: "How could I tell anyone about it? How could I explain where I was and what had happened to me? Not a couple of years before this I had been a proud, strong free young man pursuing a dream, and now ... I was a freak, a loser" (18). (Carten went on to become the coordinator of a non-profit agency, a published author, and earned a degree in social work.) Similarly, Ellen Saks, a person with schizophrenia who went on to become a law professor at the University of Southern California, recounts an earlier experience with a doctor who told her the best she could hope for was "to work as a cashier making change" (Saks 2013). In another example, involving interviews conducted with thirty-two psychiatric clients, Killeen and O'Day (2004, 158-59) describe how low practitioner expectations – in this case, concerning returning to work – are "embedded in policies and programs":

> As we began to analyze the interviews ... we were struck by the degree to which their stories were saturated with negative messages and low expectations... Some had been told by a doctor or a nurse in their initial hospitalization that they would never work again. Others, with college educations or solid work histories were placed by well-intentioned vocational rehabilitation counselors into unskilled low-wage positions ... rather than risk relapse by going after more challenging work ... Often an individual's talents, abilities and interests are simply forgotten or unwittingly relegated to the background by the concerned and well-intentioned individuals.

The potential benefit of more hopeful attitudes can be seen when one considers the epidemiology of suicide on the part of persons with schizophrenia. Persons with this diagnosis have significantly higher rates of suicide than members of the general public (Palmer, Pankratz, and Bostwick 2005), and often this occurs not in response to symptoms, such as command hallucinations, but when the individual is seeing reality clearly and facing (apparently) a future of diminished prospects and social rejection (Lysaker, Roe, and Yanos 2007; Mourra 2013). Notably, researchers have found an association between suicide and "insight"; that is, persons with an understanding that they are mentally ill have higher suicide rates than those who lack this awareness or who engage in denial (Bourgeois et al. 2004).[2] Additionally, researchers have found that there is a spike in suicides around the initial onset of schizophrenia and initial contact with the treatment system, speaking to the need for practitioners to be positive and encouraging at this crucial early point in the trajectory of the illness (Palmer, Pankratz, and Bostwick 2005).

Pessimism about outcomes also affects the stigma and rejection experienced by people with mental illness. As we saw earlier, stigma researchers have found in "social distance" studies that members of the public who see a condition like schizophrenia as biologically "hard-wired," and thus persistent and intractable, are more likely to express a preference for greater social distance (Watters 2010).

Why the Pessimism?

Pessimism in psychiatry is influenced by several factors. In general, medical practitioners tend to be cautious and circumspect, partly because of concerns about liability – concerns that are shared by their employers in health authorities (more on this below). In the case of schizophrenia, pessimism comes as well from the fact that the disorder is considered serious and intractable *by definition*. Indeed, at an early point, schizophrenia was characterized as a condition with an inevitably downward or deteriorating course, initially by German psychiatrist Emil Kraepelin (1856-1926), when it was known as *dementia praecox*. Harding, Zubin, and Strauss (1992) note that, in Kraepelin's conception, a good outcome could only mean that the patient must have been misdiagnosed, a belief that is still with us today (and the basis for Anthony's [1993] plea that clinical recovery not be seen as evidence that the individual was "not really mentally ill").[3] Later on, the 1980 edition of the *DSM* included the statement that, in schizophrenia, "a return to premorbid levels of functioning ... is so rare as to cast doubt upon the accuracy of the diagnosis," an inclusion that psychiatrist Peter Weiden (2010) suggests helped to "reinforce an atmosphere of therapeutic nihilism." The statement on prognosis was softened somewhat a few years later, in a revision of the *DSM*, to "complete remission is probably not common" (American Psychiatric Association 2000, 309), although a companion text to that edition (Morrison 2006, 141) informs readers that, for a diagnosis of schizophrenia to be made, "functioning [must] be materially impaired," suggesting that "most people who have schizophrenia never marry, and either do not work at all or hold jobs that require a lower level of functioning."

Crucially, psychiatric pessimism is influenced by the simple fact that public mental health programs usually see only the most disabled clients. While this is arguably a good thing given limited resources, it does mean that practitioners are not witnessing success stories to any great extent (Kruger 2000). Persons who have symptoms of schizophrenia but are coping adequately may not come to the attention of the health authorities in the first place, and program clients who were coping poorly but are now doing well may move on – in fact are often *encouraged* to move on to make room for new referrals. Thus, the active caseload of the community clinician shows less variability in functioning and outcomes, but the evidence base – the population being captured – is more limited (Harding and Zahniser 1994). As a position paper on stigma from the Canadian Psychiatric Association concludes: "Psychiatrists may carry even more negative beliefs than the general public and be more pessimistic about prognosis and recovery perhaps as a result of often caring for patients at the more severe and treatment-resistant end of the spectrum" (Abbey et al. 2011, 3).

Clinical Recovery
One of the potentially confusing aspects of the discussion around recovery is that the "old" definition (recovery as sustained remission of symptoms) has been retained, in many instances, alongside the "new" definition (achieving full potential despite residual symptoms). For example, in its strategy document the Mental Health Commission of Canada (2012, 16, emphasis added) notes that "recovery does not always imply 'cure,' but it does acknowledge that the *full remission of symptoms is possible* for some." Why would *both* definitions – one requiring symptom remission, the other not – be incorporated in a recovery vision? The answer to this lies in the argument that conclusions about poor prognosis in schizophrenia come from a limited evidence base and a biased perspective, in particular, the concern is that researchers have not sufficiently examined the long-term course of the illness. If it can be established that clinical and functional recovery are possible in the longer term, then it could be said that, even by the *traditional* definition of recovery, the medical pessimists have got it wrong.

"Clinical recovery" is usually defined by symptom remission and restoration of function for a prescribed period of time. A cancer patient may be said to be in remission when the cancer is no longer present, and, while arbitrary, one convention is that the patient is considered recovered if cancer signs do not return for five years (Liberman and Kopelowicz 2005). Some mental disorders show promising rates of remission and clinical recovery. In the case of major depression, it is estimated that about 50 percent of the time the affected person will only experience a single episode, and even for those experiencing multiple episodes there is complete remission of symptoms between episodes in about 70 to 80 percent of cases (American Psychiatric Association 2000; Public Health Agency of Canada 2006).

What about schizophrenia?[4] In considering long-term outcome studies of persons diagnosed with this disorder, a number of methodological limitations need to be considered, which are mentioned here because these studies have been the source of disputes between different stakeholder groups. Briefly, persons critical of traditional psychiatric approaches have used positive findings from these studies to try to refute clinical pessimism and to support the recovery vision (Whitaker 2010), while others concerned about schizophrenia "not being taken seriously" have viewed the results with a more skeptical eye (Jaffe 2011). An example, and, because of its hopeful outcomes, one of the most cited follow-up studies is the Vermont Longitudinal Study conducted by Harding and colleagues (1987). In this study, 118 patients diagnosed with schizophrenia, and discharged from the state hospital between 1955 and 1960, were followed up from twenty-two to twenty-seven years later. The authors found that "outcome varied widely, but one-half to two-thirds of the sample had achieved considerable improvement or [had] recovered" (727). At the end of the study (by which time most subjects were in their sixties), 68 percent showed minimal or no symptoms and 61 percent were employed, although the criteria for employment were not reported. Significantly – and a finding that has not been duplicated elsewhere – participants diagnosed with schizophrenia did not fair appreciably worse than other subjects included in the study. In considering the study's limitations, a general concern of retrospective studies like this one is that it is harder to rule out confounding factors than it would be if a prospective design had been employed. Another concern common to follow-up studies is the drop-out over time: in the Vermont study, about 31 percent of the 118 subjects could not be found, refused to participate, or – mostly – were deceased by the end of the study. As Jaffe (2011) notes, the most disabled – those whose death is due to suicide or neglect, and those missing or homeless – are not commonly in the study at the end point, meaning the persons being assessed are the higher-functioning participants. And studies of this type may suffer from selection bias, which has to do with how participants are recruited. In the

Vermont study, there were two potential sources of selection bias, the first being that persons were recruited if they met the entry criteria for a new rehabilitation program, suggesting (again) that they were less disabled. The other concern – addressed by the authors – is that diagnostic systems change over time and that the first edition of the *DSM* used in the 1950s provided a broader definition of schizophrenia, which included persons with less functional impairment. This was dealt with by re-diagnosing participants according to newer standards (the original sample had been larger), although this was a retrospective, file-based process. Finally, it should be noted that the Vermont cohort benefitted from intensive outpatient services that did not exist in all jurisdictions.

While not discounting the methodological challenges in determining outcomes in schizophrenia, sufficient evidence has accumulated to make some tentative conclusions (Abdel-Baki et al. 2011; Davidson and Roe 2007; Harrow and Jobe 2007; Jeste, Wolkowitz, and Palmer 2011; Jobe and Harrow 2005; Picchioni and Murray 2007; Weiden 2010):

- Outcome is variable, but the more frequent course is stability or improvement, with only a small minority following a deteriorating course as per Kraepelin. Weiden (2010) suggests that schizophrenia is a neuro-developmental condition that, while serious, is not progressive, and he draws parallels with stroke victims who, in many cases, regain some or all of their functioning with the help of rehabilitation services (see also Andreasen et al. 2005).
- Clinical recovery following a first episode of psychosis is particularly promising, suggesting a subcategory of the syndrome.
- Many people show improvement at later stages of the illness. A review by Davidson and Roe (2007) suggests that up to 65 percent continue to show functional and symptomatic improvement over time. Canadian data show that frequency of hospitalization is greater in early adulthood, and then drops off considerably after individuals reach their mid-forties (Public Health Agency of Canada 2006).
- Some persons meeting the diagnostic criteria of schizophrenia recover without medication, although this is something clinicians are not able to predict.[5]
- Weiden (2010), using a more strict definition based on substantial remission of symptoms, suggests that 20 percent of persons with long-term schizophrenia achieve clinical recovery.

Finally, it is worth quoting from an article by Jeste, Wolkowitz, and Palmer (2011, 453, emphasis added), in which the authors note that a substantial number of persons with schizophrenia experience improved psychosocial functioning and lessened "illness impact" over time:

> [The study] participants described increasing their acceptance and self-management abilities as an active self-motivated process ... While they were not free of symptoms, they could now engage in strategies that diminished the impact of psychosis, consistent with skills taught in cognitive behavioral therapy. Thus, many older people with schizophrenia had *successfully adapted to the illness*, and, in addition, some had restructured their social networks to include peers and staff members to compensate for losses in original social networks. Other investigators have reported a stable or increased use of positive coping techniques in persons with schizophrenia over time, and this is associated with enhanced self-esteem and increased social support.

This passage is noteworthy since it validates the "new" definition of recovery – that is, successful adaptation and self-management even in the presence of residual symptoms, suggesting that the strict standard of complete remission is not the best benchmark for people with schizophrenia. Jobe and Harrow (2005, 896) note that clinicians sometimes "forget the importance of patient efforts and the importance of the patient's internal resources in his or her improvement and possible recovery" – internal resources that may be encouraged and developed by practitioners.

Definitional Confusion
Arriving at a definition of "recovery" that is meaningful yet relatively concise has been difficult, and the SAMHSA definition (above), which refers to self-direction and achieving potential, may come the closest. However, as this is being written, there is still confusion among service providers and service users as to what this term really means. Part of this comes from the fact that, as noted, a number of discussions about recovery include the older conception alongside the newer. This lack of clarity has made the evaluation of the concept more challenging (this is described in more detail in the next section). Davidson and Roe (2007) suggest that a possible strategy for lessening the confusion may be to distinguish between recovery *from* mental illness (the older conception) and recovery *in* mental illness. They note that the two constructs should not be seen "as hard and fast or as mutually exclusive, but as speaking to two different aspects of mental illness" (468). Indeed, seeing recovery not as a unitary construct but as encompassing different domains may have the greatest utility for practitioners in their work with clients.

Measuring and Evaluating Recovery

An ongoing challenge to the recovery vision is the question of how one operationalizes and measures this concept – how we know when or if recovery has been achieved. As noted above, there are two related but arguably distinct definitions of recovery, one referring to clinical or functional outcomes and the other referring to the newer conception of recovery: "a way of living a satisfying, hopeful and contributing life even with the limitations caused by mental illness" (Anthony 1993, 15). The problem with the newer definition is that recovery is *subjectively* determined: "Recovery is described as a deeply *personal, unique* process of changing one's attitudes, values, feelings, and goals, skills or roles" (15, emphasis added). This presents a challenge for service providers,[6] as Meehan and colleagues (2008, 178) note:

> Recovery is usually self-defined and each individual's experience of their recovery may be very different. Thus there is no clearly prescribed formula or defined set of service inputs for achieving recovery. Recovery principles and standards are available but these tend to focus on system level issues and provide limited guidance to practising clinicians. The subjective and personal nature of recovery makes it difficult for clinicians to comprehend and thus, operationalize at the service level.

While this may seem to be an insoluble paradox, a good starting point is for practitioners to be *client-centred* (or person-centred) in their approach to care; that is, to not assume that the clinician's priorities reflect those of the client (or at least to verify this), to ensure the client voice is heard, to respect autonomy, and to encourage participation in decision making. Person-centred care has been defined as "the experience (to the extent that the informed, individual patient desires it) of transparency, individualization, recognition, respect, dignity, and choice in all matters" (Whitley and Drake 2010, 1248).

In evaluating recovery, it makes some sense to separate clinical from other outcomes; this is similar to the logic used in the two-continua model described in Chapter 1 – separate axes for mental illness and mental health. Whitley and Drake (2010) take this approach in their description of five dimensions of recovery:

- *Clinical*: measures would include an individual's symptom severity and use of hospital and other crisis services.
- *Functional*: measures would include employment, education (starting and completing courses), and housing (obtaining and maintaining secure, independent housing).

- *Physical*: measures would include attendance at fitness and wellness programs, smoking cessation, weight loss, and participation in sporting events.
- *Social*: Indicators could be participation in activities, clubs, and groups, although here measures would be more subjectively determined since people may have varying definitions of a satisfying social life. Finding a supportive partner after a period of relative isolation would seem to be a reasonable success indicator.
- *Existential*: Outcomes here include a sense of hope, emotional and spiritual well-being, and a sense of self-efficacy, autonomy, and empowerment. These outcomes are less tangible, clearly, than an indicator such as "rehospitalization" and perhaps are best captured in the client's own narrative account. That being said, scales for quality of life – and now, recovery within mental illness – have been developed, although such instruments have not traditionally been widely used in clinical practice.

Burgess and colleagues (2010) note that the relationship between the different recovery dimensions is still uncertain at this point; for some, clinical improvement will be directly related to other domains of recovery, but for others, they may be independent.

Although the recovery vision is relatively new, and questions about operationalization remain, a considerable number of instruments designed to measure recovery have been developed. The reader is directed, for example, to two compendia published by the Human Services Research Institute in the United States: Ralph, Kidder, and Phillips (2000) and Campbell-Orde et al. (2005). These recovery scales fall into two clusters: those that are designed to measure the individual client's degree of recovery and those that are meant to assess the recovery orientation of the agency or service provider. The client outcome scales may be self-report, often in the form of a Likert-type questionnaire, while others have more open-ended questions and can be administered by staff. The instruments often incorporate several or all of the recovery dimensions noted above, for example, addressing symptom management but also including items such as "I have a purpose in life" and "I have goals I want to achieve" (strongly agree → strongly disagree). The scales designed to assess the recovery orientation of the agency include those to be completed by agency staff and others to be completed by clients. Generally, agencies are rated on the degree that services can be considered holistic in orientation. Scale items may refer to whether clients are placed in the agency in interview panels and decision-making committees, the range of choices in treatment, cultural sensitivity, collaboration between service providers and users, whether vocational rehabilitation is offered, whether hopeful messages are given, whether choice is respected, and other factors.

Concerning the evaluation of the instruments themselves, an Australian research group (Burgess et al. 2010) looked at thirty-three recovery scales – twenty-two designed to measure client recovery, and eleven the recovery orientation of the agency – on the basis of criteria such as being easy to use, yielding quantitative data, being published in a peer review journal, having at least some demonstrated psychometric properties, being created with service user input, and promoting dialogue between client and clinician. Eight scales met these criteria: for agency evaluation these were the Recovery Self-Assessment (RSA), the Recovery-Oriented Practices Index (ROPI), the Recovery Promotion Fidelity Scale (RPFS), and the Recovery Oriented Systems Indicators Measure (ROSI). For client recovery, these were the Recovery Assessment Scale (RAS), the Illness Management and Recovery Scale (IMR), the Recovery Process Inventory (RPI), and the Stages of Recovery Instrument (STORI). (Full versions of these are available in the Burgess et al. [2010] document.) While this research group was able to find several scales it considered acceptable, another group offers a dissenting view: citing problems with validity and service user acceptability, Drapalski and colleagues (2012, 49) conclude that "none [of the existing scales] has sufficient psychometric credentials to merit inclusion in a large trial on recovery or adoption by a public mental health system, and none has been widely accepted by the field."

Despite lacking clear benchmarks, accreditation standards used for Canadian community mental health settings now reflect a recovery orientation, as per the following guideline:

The concept of recovery is geared toward supporting individuals and families to establish a positive identity, build a meaningful life in the community of their choice, and feel in control of their illness and their life. Recovery must be accomplished using the individual's choice of services and supports. Principles of recovery orientation include harm reduction, fostering hope, enabling choice, encouraging responsibility, and promoting dignity and respect. (Accreditation Canada 2011, 3)

Accreditation Canada (2011, 22) also notes that assessments should be "completed using a holistic approach by assessing the individual's and family's physical, psychological, spiritual, and social needs." The service plan created by this assessment is similarly expected to be comprehensive.

An interesting example of a program applying a recovery orientation is the "Mental Health America Village" in Long Beach, California (http://www.mhavillage.org), a service that is publicly funded through contracts with the state government. The "Village" website contains a number of articles written by psychiatrist and founding member Mark Ragins, including the following, somewhat provocative "program inventory" designed to be a tool for evaluating the recovery orientation of other agencies (Ragins n.d.) (what follows is an abridged version):

- Do staff and consumers believe recovery with severe mental illnesses is possible? *Example:* Is there an expectation, mechanism for, and/or regular process of "positive graduation?"
- Do staff and consumers believe in empowerment and self-determination? *Example:* Are consumers included in advisory boards, planning and quality management committees, and research planning groups?
- Do staff and consumers believe in self-responsibility? *Example*: Are consumers "permitted to fail" or protected/rescued from failure?
- Do staff and consumers believe people with severe mental illnesses can contribute meaningfully to our world? *Example:* Are people with mental illnesses hired at all, in restricted consumer positions, and/or as fully equal staff?
- Are relationships between staff and consumers highly valued? *Example:* Are treatment assignments based on relationship fits?
- Do staff relate to consumers as people or do they relate to their illnesses? *Example:* Are subjective experiences explored or only objective symptom checklists?
- Are the barriers between staff and consumers minimized? *Examples:* Are there segregated bathrooms, lounges, telephones, work areas, eating areas, etc.? Are staff encouraged to share their personal experiences with consumers? Are staff encouraged to be emotionally expressive with consumers?
- Is treatment focused on improving lives or on treating illnesses? *Example:* Does goal setting reflect quality of life or clinical goals?
- Is treatment integrated? *Example:* Do staff act as overlapping "generalists" doing "whatever it takes," or are there substantial internal referrals because "that's not my job"?
- Does treatment build community supports and community integration? *Example:* Do staff focus on replacing themselves with "natural supports" in the community?

Some of these recommendations are more controversial than others. For example, the one concerning the "minimization of barriers," which flies in the face of what clinicians are taught about appropriate boundaries in the therapeutic relationship, could expect to be met with a fair degree of opposition from practitioners and some service users as well.[7] (It can be argued that sharing personal experiences and/or being "emotionally expressive" are approaches that still need to be purposeful, and that meet the needs of the client, not the practitioner.)

Readers are also directed to Rapp and Goscha's (2012) *The Strengths Model*, where, concerning the recovery orientation of service-providers, a number of "spirit-breaking" and "hope-inducing" behaviours are listed.

The Mental Health America Program has also created a scale, suggested as a way of tracking a client's progress in the journey towards recovery, with the following "milestones" (Mental Health America of Los Angeles 2005):

- at high risk and unengaged
- at high risk and engaged
- coping poorly and unengaged
- coping poorly and engaged
- coping, engaging in rehabilitation
- recovering, reconnecting
- advanced recovery.

At each stage the worker role and client goals would be different. Goals would shift from preserving safety to building the engagement between worker and client; increasing trust and hope; improving coping skills; shaping a personalized wellness plan; increasing participation in the larger community; and, finally, moving away from the mental health team. The potential benefit of such a scale, it is argued, would be not only in tracking client progress but also in identifying the sort of clientele an agency serves and the level and type of services needed. For example, a program with a crisis orientation (only) will likely do well with those urgent cases but do less well with respect to transitions to later recovery stages. This scale was used to give a snapshot of one of the Vancouver, British Columbia, adult mental health teams in 2011, teams mandated to assist persons with serious, persistent mental disorders.[8] The survey had a sample size of 457 clients, with the following findings:

- 23, about 5 percent, were high risk;
- 79, about 17 percent, were unengaged and coping poorly;
- 123, about 27 percent, were engaged but coping poorly;
- 142, about 31 percent, were coping and considered to be starting the recovery process;
- 70, about 15 percent, were further recovered and reconnecting with community;
- 20, about 4 percent, were considered to be in advanced recovery.

Thus, roughly half the caseload was "coping" and moving towards recovery, supporting the argument for a service delivery model that is not solely focused on stabilization and maintenance.

Concerns and Critique

Not surprisingly, concerns have been expressed by different stakeholders about the implications of moving to a recovery-oriented mental health system. With respect to the practitioner viewpoint, an article by Davidson and colleagues (2006a) outlines a number of these. Concerns identified in the article were drawn from a series of consultations and training sessions conducted with mental health personnel in the State of Connecticut, and they included the following:

- The argument that recovery is not new, and is something people are already doing.
- Concern about a potentially increased workload, and the need for more resources.
- Seeing recovery in clinical or symptom-based terms, which is believed by many staff to be impossible for most of the clients they see.
- Believing that recovery, if it occurs at all, can only happen later in the treatment process after a period of managing and stabilizing symptoms.
- Seeing recovery as a fad.
- Questions about the evidence base of recovery.[9]
- Concern that the role of the professional is devalued.
- Worry about the practitioner's increased exposure to risk and liability. "If recovery is the person's responsibility, then how come I get the blame when things go wrong?" (Davidson et al. 2006a, 642).

Some of these concerns are also addressed by Meehan and colleagues (2008, 180), who add the concern that recovery could become "a contemporary version of the 'anti-psychiatry' movement, discouraging people from accessing professional services that could benefit them."

Most of these concerns certainly resonate with this author, who was the manager of a Canadian mental health program undergoing a similar transition. Concerning the first item, that "we're already doing it," staff could become defensive when it was implied that their previous work was outmoded or "old school," or that perhaps they were lacking in compassion. "I have always tried to be holistic and client-centred in my practice approach" was a not uncommon response, which, if true, speaks to the importance of acknowledging previous good work on the part of staff. Another concern was identified through the use of a new, more holistic assessment tool, which asked clients about a range of psychosocial issues. While the tool was found to be effective in identifying previously unconsidered areas of need or interest, it also identified the fact that, in some cases, resources did not exist to address these needs (although the exercise is still a useful one for program planning).

As noted, the new definition of recovery is seen by some as unrealistic and not applicable to the most seriously mentally ill:

> The problem with the recovery vision is that it is a dangerously partial
> vision. It sets up unrealistic expectations for those who will never fully
> "recover," no matter how hard they try, because their illness is so severe.
> What's more, exclusive emphasis on recovery as a goal steers policymakers
> away from making changes vital to the needs of the most severely disabled.
> (Satel and Zdanowicz 2003)

This is an argument encountered previously in this book; that is, that emphasizing mental health rather than mental illness channels energy and resources away from those most in need. The idea that recovery is an unrealistic concept is echoed by *Globe and Mail* health journalist André Picard (2011) in his comment on a Mental Health Commission of Canada strategy document:

> There is far too much emphasis on the recovery model – the notion that
> everyone will get better with support – and not enough emphasis on brain
> science. It's a legitimate approach for those with mild to moderate mental
> health problems but not those with severe conditions such as schizophre-
> nia ... hope – and false hope – cannot be allowed to take the place of care.

Concerning the obligation of the practitioner, a psychiatrist speaks about the "fiduciary duty to be truthful that transcends the wish to please all" (Oyebode 2004, 49). In other words, there is an obligation to be realistically circumspect rather than unrealistically hopeful.

The new vision of recovery includes client risk-taking, and Davidson et al. (2006) found that liability was the number one concern among mental health staff. Supporting risk-taking is now seen as a desired trait for mental health practitioners: "Professionals must embrace the concept of the *dignity of risk*, and the right to failure if they are to be supportive of us" (Deegan, 1996, 95, emphasis added). An article on core mental health competencies reads as follows:

Providers should ... encourage independent thinking ... support consumers' freedom to make their own mistakes ... support risk-taking as leading to growth ... avoid controlling behaviors ... foster a sense of hope ... shift from a stance of demoralizing pessimism to rational optimism. (Coursey et al. 2000, 380-81)

The liability issue is potentially a major sticking point in the implementation of the recovery vision since it runs up against professional obligations such as duty of care as well as the fact that health authorities are by nature "risk averse"[10] (Davis 2008):

Most services for people with severe mental illness operate in a public environment where there is accountability to third parties (ultimately to the general public), whose priorities include individual and community safety and who are likely to have a low tolerance for adventurous services ... professionals will continue to err on the side of caution until they are assured the system will support them in times of crisis. (Meehan et al. 2008, 178, 180)

Some degree of risk-taking may be supported through careful assessment, the use of advance directives, and the more recent development of collaborative risk management instruments (see Burns-Lynch, Salzer, and Baron 2011). Nonetheless, there is always the danger that a bad outcome, while justified as an attempt to promote independence and autonomy, will be seen by others as negligence.

Another group that has been uncomfortable with aspects of the recovery vision are family members, who – not surprisingly – are nervous about the idea of risk-taking and, through support organizations, have expressed the need for assertive, proactive care in the case of seriously mentally ill persons, not necessarily greater independence.[11] One of the most contentious elements of the new vision, articulated by Anthony in his 1993 article, is the idea that there are many pathways to recovery and that it may occur without professional intervention. This notion was taken up by the Mental Health Commission of Canada in a 2011 draft strategy document: "Recovery cannot be done to, or on behalf of people ... [but] must be the result of individuals' own efforts and must be accomplished using their choice of services and supports" (Mental Health Commission of Canada 2011, 10). This assertion was harshly criticized by some family members and their representative organizations. In an interview, a family member, who was also president of the local Schizophrenia Society Chapter, is quoted as saying that the Mental

Health Commission had "stolen the word 'recovery'... [F]or the seriously ill, that's a small part of recovery that comes after the treatment for the illness itself, which is part of recovery, which requires a lot of not just support but structure, *provided by others*" (quoted in Brean 2011, emphasis added). Similarly, a psychiatrist-representative of the Treatment Advocacy Center in the US criticizes that country's federal mental health services administration (SAMHSA): "SAMHSA recently issued ten 'Guiding Principles of Recovery,' of which its first principle is 'Recovery is person-driven' with a foundation of 'self-determination and self-direction.' Although it doesn't actually take a medical degree to recognize that these are activities [that] are beyond the capacity of someone who has lost touch with reality, SAMHSA managed to overlook the connection between sanity and constructive self-direction" (quoted in Treatment Advocacy Center 2011).

In considering these comments, there is still evident confusion between clinical recovery and the other domains of recovery. It is reasonable to say that in the early, acute phase of a serious mental illness, clinical recovery – managing symptoms – should take priority. That said, once relative stability has been achieved, other approaches to healing and rehabilitation should be considered, which is really what the recovery vision is about. These can be provided by allied professionals at the same program, or they may be provided in other ways. Practitioners do have a tendency to be wary of "alternative" health strategies, and this wariness may be justifiable if the two approaches appear to be working at "cross purposes." However, the two may work well alongside each other: a survey of 311 clients of professional programs, half of whom also used self-help services, found that the use of these services was associated with *greater* satisfaction with the professional mental health programs, leading the authors to conclude that "self-help and traditional mental health services can function complementarily, rather than in competition with one another" (Hodges et al. 2003, 1161).

What do clients themselves say about recovery? We know from the Canadian Senate Report *Out of the Shadows at Last* (Standing Senate Committee on Social Affairs, Science and Technology 2006) that service users interviewed asked for more than just medical management, speaking to the importance of vocational services, adequate housing, and peer support. When service users have been asked more specifically about what recovery means to them, the answers have been complex but still show considerable deference to the "medical model." For example, a group of Quebec researchers (Piat, Sabetti, and Bloom 2009) interviewed sixty service users about recovery and found that:

- Twenty-four believed that recovery, as they saw it, was due mainly to medication.
- Twenty-two saw recovery as multi-determined, with medication part of the picture with other factors – such as positive relationships – being important as well.
- Twenty believed that you couldn't be recovered if you were still taking medication, and expressed the hope that one day it wouldn't be necessary.

The second group, the twenty-two who saw recovery as a multi-determined process, we would see as aligning more with the new vision of recovery, while the first group – making up 40 percent of the total – linked feeling well mainly to medical management. Interpreting the third group's responses proves somewhat difficult, but some at least would appear to be aligning with a medical conception – "recovery as cure." In another study, involving interviews with service users in Ontario and Quebec, the authors found that respondents viewed recovery "as both a medical and psychosocial concept ... [supporting the thesis] that different forms of recovery may co-exist in the relationship of individuals to mental illness, and at different times" (Piat et al. 2009, 205). The authors also found that respondents still aligned to a considerable degree with a traditional conception of recovery, *from* illness rather than *within* illness: "The prominence of the illness perspective was unexpected. Many looked for recovery outside of themselves: in a cure or in dreams of disappearing symptoms. Medication was viewed as important" (205).

That these researchers found the respondents' answers *unexpected* is significant for it raises the question: Who is driving the recovery model? This section of the chapter is entitled "concerns," and potentially the greatest concern of all is the prospect of a significant number of service users not actually endorsing the recovery vision. Certainly, there are service users (and academics) who speak eloquently to the need to form a new identity apart from illness, and the belief that recovery can occur in the presence of symptoms, but what is the obligation of practitioners if their clients do not appear to endorse this perspective? What are the ethical considerations? Again, a guiding principle involves being client-centred, noting that client preference needs to be actively solicited by the practitioner and that it should also be an *informed* preference.

One of the aspects of the recovery vision that may be very challenging has to do with "exiting" – that is, with the client's moving on and away from the formal mental health system. In some articulations of the recovery vision this is a necessary step in the recovery process, for example in Mark Ragins's (earlier noted) "program inventory": "Is there an expectation, mechanism for, and/or regular process of 'positive graduation?'" Moving towards this eventuality is facilitated by being purposeful and goal-directed, which may refer to the actions of the service user or the service provider. In focus groups and other discussions, this author has found some service users to be very concerned about being pushed out of the treatment team, and ambivalent about goal-tracking, recovery scales, and other instruments used to monitor client progress. Similarly, terms like "graduation" may be met with ambivalence. Clients may express the belief that, while they are seen as "high functioning" by the clinician – and thus no longer in need of the program's services – their stability is in fact tenuous and fragile. As well, there is the perception that, once you leave, it is hard to get back in. And, critically, there is the reality of very limited resources once the client leaves the mental health team. Typically, the approach taken is to pass on medical management to a GP, who may be hard to find and who usually will not have the time or training needed to deal with mental health concerns as effectively as a specialized program. Health authorities need to look closely at these transitions and consider ways of supporting a more graduated exit, whereby the client steps down to a less intense model of care, possibly through "alumni groups," which could be led by staff or peers. It is hoped that the recovery vision and its "expectation of graduation" will not have the effect of moving people on before they are ready.

Notes

1   The recovery concept has usually been applied to *adult* service users and, at first glance, would appear to have limited application to elderly persons, who may, for example, be dealing with a progressive dementia. However, one can argue that the same principles apply, such as engagement in meaningful activity and preserving a sense of personhood. A document on service guidelines for older adults prepared by the Mental Health Commission of Canada (MacCourt, Wilson, and Tourgny-Rivard 2011) concludes that elements of recovery such as choice, hope, respect, empowerment, and person-centred care are consistent with ideal dementia care.

2   Thus, a client's resistance to accepting a psychiatric diagnosis may have self-preserving aspects, even while this behaviour may be seen as being "difficult" by treating professionals (see Angell, Cooke, and Kovac 2005).

3   American psychiatrist Daniel Fisher, who went on to complete an MD and PhD after being diagnosed with schizophrenia, notes that the typical response to his own recovery was that people assumed that he must either have been misdiagnosed or, if "truly" schizophrenic, be incompetent to perform his professional duties (Fisher 1999; see also Saks 2013).

4   There has been some discussion about using *modified* standards to denote clinical recovery in schizophrenia, for example, allowing residual symptoms to be present, provided these are not painful, disabling, or overwhelming (Weiden 2010). A group of American researchers suggests a definition of remission based on at least six months during which symptoms are no more than "mild," this corresponding to a rating no higher than three on any item of

the PANSS (Positive and Negative Syndrome Scale) (Andreasen et al. 2005). However, previously published studies have used different outcome variables (usually including one or more of symptom severity, work history, conjugal status, and independent living) so that results are difficult to compare.

5 Journalist Robert Whitaker (2010) has advanced the controversial hypothesis that long-term treatment with antipsychotics is not only unnecessary in many cases but actually contributes to psychosis through altering neural pathways and creating a "supersensitivity effect," a phenomenon first described by psychiatric researchers in the 1970s. For a counterpoint, see Jaffe (2011).

6 Practitioners are often taught that, in order for client goals to be evaluated, they need to be "specific and measureable" as well as observable by a third party – a requirement made more difficult when success is subjectively defined.

7 To be accredited, mental health *clubhouse* programs do adhere to standards similar to those proposed in this section, although clubhouses are seen as programs *complementary* to – not replacing – the psychiatric treatment system (see Chapter 17).

8 This was an unpublished, in-house report.

9 In response to the question of whether recovery-oriented practices are evidence-based, Davidson et al. (2009) respond "not yet" because of the relative newness of the concept. These authors also note that, since recovery is individually and subjectively defined, pursuing one's own definition and pathway to recovery is perhaps more a question of human rights than of evidence. The question of the evidence base is discussed in more detail in Chapter 10.

10 For example, at the Vancouver Coastal Health Authority, staff members were required to fill out an "unusual occurrence form" after an adverse event such as a client's suicide attempt. The form (which is no longer used) contained the following questions: "Were the drugs prescribed by the mental health team? What actions were taken to rescue the client? Has this caused a change in treatment plan? Are there unsafe acts or procedures which contributed to the accident? What are the current mechanisms to prevent a similar accident? What corrective actions will be taken and when will follow-up occur on each?"

11 For example, see the bulletins of the North Shore Schizophrenia Society at http://www.northshoreschizophrenia.org/bulletin.htm.

Culture

In addition to having a recovery orientation, the Mental Health Commission of Canada in its 2009 framework document emphasized that mental health policies and treatments need to be culturally safe and culturally competent: "A transformed mental health system ... responds to the diverse individual and group needs – as well as to the disparities – that can arise from First Nations, Inuit or Métis identity; ethno-cultural background, experience of racism, and migration history" (Mental Health Commission of Canada 2009, 48). In the document the commission notes that, while progress has been made, there are still "significant barriers that keep people from seeking help, or from finding programs ... that both feel safe and are effective" (48). This chapter considers some of these barriers to help-seeking, in particular, different conceptual models and the differential impact of stigma. An introduction is given to the mental health concerns of the First Nations in Canada. Finally, some comments are made on how more culturally sensitive services could be achieved.

Demographics

Canada has seen a number of significant demographic shifts in relatively recent times and is increasingly a land of cultural and ethnic diversity. By the latter part of the twentieth century, the majority of immigrants were from Asia, the Middle East, Latin America, Africa, and the Caribbean, while the number of newcomers from "traditional" source countries in the United Kingdom and Continental Europe declined over this same period. In 2006, the main source countries for immigration were China, India, the Philippines, and Pakistan (K. Smith 2007). The new arrivals have predominately settled in the larger urban centres: figures from Statistics Canada showed that 70 percent of immigrants arriving between 2001 and 2006 settled in the Toronto, Montreal, and Vancouver metropolitan areas, with Calgary placing fourth

(Fitzpatrick 2007). On Census Day 2006, about 20 percent of the population were foreign-born, a proportion that grew much faster than the Canadian-born growth rate over the same period (K. Smith 2007). The 2006 census determined that the numbers of Aboriginal persons, particularly the Métis, had also grown at a rate much faster than the rest of the country over the preceding ten years.

In 2010, Statistics Canada published a report offering predictions of demographic patterns by 2031, based on recent data trends.[1] By 2031:

- About three in ten Canadians would be members of a visible minority, and these persons would be overrepresented in the younger age groups.
- South Asians and Chinese would comprise the largest visible minority group.
- At least 25 percent of the population would be foreign-born.
- Nearly one Canadian in two aged fifteen or older would be foreign-born or have at least one foreign-born parent.
- In the Toronto and Vancouver metropolitan areas, over 70 percent of residents would be either immigrants or the Canadian-born children of immigrants, and about three persons in five would belong to a visible minority group.

Meeting the mental health needs of minority groups has proven to be a challenge, given that our systems of enumerating and responding to mental disorder have an ethnocentric bias, one arguably reflected in our diagnostic manuals. On this point, Kirmayer, Tait, and Simpson (2009, 15, emphasis added) observe:

Psychiatric epidemiology faces many challenges in cross-cultural application because of *differences in how people experience and express distress.* Generally, the way to address these limitations is to begin with careful qualitative and ethnographic work in order to understand local models of illness and idioms of distress ... [which] can then be used to revise interviews, questionnaires and criteria in order to ensure that they make sense and capture the relevant dimensions of illness experience.[2]

These authors go on to note that estimates of the prevalence of psychiatric disorders among Aboriginal persons are often based on service-utilization records; however, "since many people never come for treatment [these records] are usually at best only a low-end estimate of the true prevalence of distress in the community" (15). Concerning assessment of need, there is the additional problem that minority groups have not always actively been included in clinical and epidemiological studies (Flores et al. 2002).

Culture and Mental Health

Culture influences the way a mental disorder is expressed by individuals, the coping styles employed, and the willingness to seek treatment (the latter term used here to denote Western-style psychiatric care) (McCabe and Priebe 2004).

Concerning treatment-seeking, cultural factors are important in understanding patterns of service utilization (Mok 2006). Previous studies have found that minority clients are either underrepresented among Canadian psychiatric treatment populations or that they drop out of treatment in disproportionate numbers (Deiser 2002; McCabe and Priebe 2004; Mojtabai and Olfson 2006). More recent studies suggest this still seems to be the case, with some qualifications. For example, a study using a large dataset from British Columbia, comparing recent Chinese immigrants with non-immigrants and longer-term immigrants, found that the newcomers were utilizing mental health services at rates ranging from 40 to 90 percent of the comparison groups (Chen et al. 2010). Similarly, a study in Montreal comparing service-use between immigrants and Canadian-born residents found that Vietnamese and Filipino newcomers were one-third as likely to use mental health services, a finding that could not be explained by socio-demographic factors, symptom profile, length of stay in the country, or use of alternative sources of help (Kirmayer et al. 2007). Similar findings have been made in the US when comparing white persons with Asians, Latinos, and African Americans (e.g., Alegria et al. 2008).

Understanding these findings is a complicated matter; it is possible, for example, that recent immigrants suffer lower rates of mental disorder in some cases (more on this below). More significantly, however, one must consider whether mental health services are accessible and relevant for minority groups, or if help-seeking patterns are similar, or whether idioms of distress are the same as in the dominant culture.

Cultures, and individuals, differ with respect to their *explanatory models* of illness, referring to the meaning someone imparts to their condition and the way they make sense of their subjective experience. As we noted in Chapter 1, the explanatory model includes beliefs about the cause, impact, and prognosis of a particular condition. Concerning the impact, stigma may be felt more acutely by ethnic minorities and can be a primary reason for their underrepresentation as service users. A number of studies have found stigma to be a particular problem in Chinese and South Asian communities (Li and Browne 2000), and, while there is some evidence that this may be shifting with acculturation, significant differences between Asian and white respondents remain (Fogel and Ford 2005). For example, Hsu and colleagues (2008) compared responses of fifty members of these two reference groups to several vignettes involving physical and mental illness. The response items were designed to reveal "stigma factors" such as fear, shame, social consensus, discrimination, and sanction. Stigma was higher in all five scenarios for the Chinese respondents, with examples of psychosis being especially stigmatizing. Interestingly, belief that depression was like a physical illness did not diminish the stigma attached to it. In looking at the underpinning of these beliefs, the importance of family becomes evident. A Vietnamese practitioner notes that "the notion of mental illness is quite dreadful to the Vietnamese people, who believe that there is a very remote chance of recovery. Along the way, the person also brings shame and disgrace to the family due to, as culturally believed, possible bad deeds in a past life – even though nothing was done wrong in the present" (Van Le 2000, 9). Similarly, in Chinese communities, the attitude may be that "family troubles stay in the house" (Li and Browne 2000, 150) since removing a mentally ill person from his or her family is often perceived as a failure or loss of control by the other members. A Canadian counsellor working with young persons suggests that the concept of "shared shame" applies to the South Asian culture – "that is, the shame of an individual becomes the shame of the family" (Rai 2006, 12). In addition, there may be concern about how an acknowledged mental illness will affect the marriage prospects of siblings (Macnaughton 2000; see also Pyke et al. 2001 regarding the Afro-Canadian experience). On this point, the author of a longitudinal survey of persons diagnosed with schizophrenia in India found that "in almost all cases, the fact that the bride suffered from mental illness was not disclosed to the groom or his family" (Thara 2004).

Explanatory models also influence whether a problem is seen as the manifestation of an illness or something else, such as routine sadness or disappointment (Watters 2010). As one reporter notes, traditional Chinese values "tend to emphasize suffering stoically, serving the hierarchy, blending harmoniously into the collective and accepting one's fate," with emotionally sensitive topics not talked about openly (Todd 2008). In this worldview, "depression" is not a meaningful concept and may, in fact, be seen "as a kind of weakness, and those who complain about it ... considered malingerers" (Scott 2007). Concerning psychological approaches to healing, observers of the traditional Chinese community note that self-scrutiny is not culturally encouraged and that emotional expressiveness can be seen as inappropriate and embarrassing (Mok 2006; Tolson 2006). From this perspective, turning to a doctor or therapist when depressed may not be a legitimate option.

Gaining access to outside services may also be discouraged in orthodox religious communities in which "mental illness" is seen more as "spiritual failure." In such settings, a psychiatric intervention may be seen as a threat to the moral authority and cohesion of the group. An instance of this comes from a study of the prevalence of depression among an American Amish community, which found relatively high levels of the disorder but concomitantly high levels of reluctance to seek treatment from mental health providers. The author concluded that "boundary maintenance was achieved through two social control mechanisms: religious-based stigmatization of depression, and the construction of mental health providers as illegitimate help agents" (Reiling 2002, 428). Seeing distress and suffering as a moral or religious problem has been associated with lower rates of service utilization among a number of ethnic minority groups (e.g., Whitley and Lawson 2010; Whitley, Kirmayer, and Groleau 2010).

Relative to persons from a Western orientation, ethnic minority groups may be more likely to express distress in terms of physical symptoms, requiring more careful interpretation by care providers. Mok (2006) notes that, among Chinese immigrants, psychological disorders may manifest as aches and pains, fatigue, weakness, headache, palpitations, dizziness, and bowel problems. Traditional Chinese medicine does not in fact separate emotions from physical functions. Chinese culture uses an "organ-oriented" concept of pathology, and the "language of distress" may refer to bodily organs such as the heart, liver, and kidneys. In a different cultural example, a study by Alegria and colleagues (2008) found, similarly, that under-utilization of treatment services for depression by Latin Americans was explained in part by their greater likelihood to somatize psychological distress, the signs of which could be missed by care providers. The study also found subjects expressing an "idiom of distress" known as *ataques de nervios*, signs of which include crying, trembling, heat rising in the chest, and a sense of being out of control. "Nervios" is an example of what is called a "culture-bound syndrome," in this case one more closely associated with the Hispanic culture (the 2000 edition of the American Psychiatric Association's *DSM* includes a number of these as an appendix).[3]

Culture also influences coping styles and the way individuals respond to problems. Here, one can point to a difference concerning the role of families: ethnic minorities may value to a greater extent the interconnectedness of families, a perspective that clashes with the North American ethos of individualism, which is reflected in practice approaches. Whitley and Lawson (2010, 510) observe that "family involvement is discouraged in [North American] delivery systems, which remain firmly individualistic in orientation." The practitioner's beliefs about treatment goals and procedures may not coincide with those of persons from other cultures, an example being the theory (taught to this author in university) that personal growth is contingent upon "individuation" and independence from the family of origin, with "enmeshment" being an expression of "family dysfunction" (see Inman 2010). For example, a Canadian practitioner working with the Hispanic community notes that parents contacted by the mental health system fear "that they themselves or their child-rearing practices will be blamed for the child's problem" and that "their parental authority could be undermined by a professional who does not understand the family cultural background" (Sanchez 2000, 10).

And there is the question of mistrust among persons from different cultural backgrounds. Practitioners need to be sensitive to the fact that many immigrants, persons of colour, and Aboriginal North Americans have had less than positive experiences with "the authorities" and with Western-oriented psychiatric services. Speaking about the African-American experience, Whitley and Lawson (2010, 509) conclude that this community "often does not perceive the mental health clinic as a service provider but rather as a place to be fearfully avoided," this stemming from a legacy of infamous practices, such as the Tuskegee syphilis trial,[4] and, more recently, the finding across a number of studies that black persons are more likely to receive involuntary commitment than their white counterparts. For some immigrants, based on experiences in their country of origin, maintaining a certain level of suspiciousness is normal and adaptive, whereas this may be interpreted as paranoia by practitioners in the new country (Ganesan 2000). Immigrants may also fear, not unrealistically, that their immigration status will be adversely affected by a mental health designation.

Cultural Formulation
An influential model for understanding cultural context in clinical practice comes from Harvard University psychiatrist Arthur Kleinman and colleagues (e.g., Kleinman and Benson 2006). The authors propose a *cultural formulation* with six components: (1) client ethnic identity, especially whether it matters to the client or is an important part of her/his sense of self; (2) determining what is at stake for the individual, in her/his own words; (3) reconstructing an "illness narrative" to understand the client's explanatory model for her/his problem (see below); (4) consideration of both social stresses and supports affecting the client; (5) self-reflection to consider the clinician's own cultural influences and to avoid stereotyping; and, finally, (6) determining whether a culturalist approach will actually *work* (or "do no harm"). Concerning the last point, the authors point out that focusing on culture or ethnicity may be interpreted by clients as being intrusive or may create a sense of being singled out and stigmatized; further, an "overemphasis on cultural difference can lead to the mistaken idea that if we can only identify

the cultural root of the problem, it can be resolved [when in fact] there is no easy resolution" (e294). The illness narrative is reconstructed through a series of questions:

- What do you call this problem?
- What do you believe is the cause of this problem?
- What course do you expect it to take?
- How serious is it?
- What do you think this problem does inside your body?
- How does it affect your body and your mind?
- What do you most fear about this condition?
- What do you most fear about this treatment?

The authors note that these questions should be used to *start* rather than to end a conversation. Generally, the clinician attitude should be one of curiosity and humility, and wanting to learn more about the client's experiences (Mok 2006).

At this point, we look in somewhat more detail at issues specific to immigrants to Canada and the Canadian Aboriginal population. The last part of the chapter is a discussion of how service delivery systems could be more culturally sensitive and relevant.

Immigration

The complexities of service utilization among immigrants have been explored in studies by McGill University psychiatrist Laurence Kirmayer and colleagues. In one study of newcomers from the Caribbean, Vietnam, and the Philippines, Kirmayer et al. (2007, 301) found lower rates of service-use to be associated with stigma, reliance on family, the idea that milder problems are dealt with through community or religious institutions, and "the conviction that clinicians would not understand salient cultural and linguistic issues." These authors found different levels of distress across groups, with the Vietnamese showing higher levels of somatic and psychological symptoms; however, different distress levels did not account for lower service-use, established after statistically controlling for this factor. In another study involving interviews with immigrants from the West Indies (Whitley, Kirmayer, and Groleau 2006, 205), reluctance to use mainstream services was found to be related to (1) beliefs in traditional folk medicine and religion, (2) a perceived over-willingness of doctors to rely on medication, and (3) "a dismissive attitude and lack of time from the physicians." (It is noteworthy that these last two factors, which result in the "perception that clinicians are not interested in the social context of suffering" [Kirmayer et al. 2007, 302], are no doubt relevant to understanding frustration among all service users, not just ethnic minorities.)

Interpreting service-use by immigrants is complicated by a phenomenon called the "healthy immigrant effect," whereby newcomers apparently manifest better physical and mental health than multi-generational residents across a number of indicators – such as depression and alcohol misuse (although these differences appear to diminish with time) (Greenfield et al. 2006; Hyman 2004; Kirmayer et al. 2011; Newbold 2009). From this perspective, lower service-use may then be a reflection of actual need, as opposed to discrimination on the part of the service user or provider. To attempt to assess the "true" prevalence of mental disorders, one needs to prospectively contact and assess individuals rather than rely on retrospective service records. This was done in a study by Tiwari and Wang (2006), which used data from the Canadian Community Health Survey, comparing white, Chinese, and "other Asian" populations. Among these groups, about 85 percent of the Chinese and Asian respondents were immigrants, compared to less than 10 percent for the whites. The study found that the Chinese participants had lower lifetime and twelve-month prevalence rates of mood, anxiety, and substance-use disorders than the other two groups and that the whites had higher lifetime prevalence rates than both comparison groups for these same conditions. There is an interesting qualification to these results, however. The survey also asked persons to *subjectively* rate their mental health and found that self-rated "fair to poor mental health" was actually *higher* among the Chinese than among the whites. This suggests the presence of mental health issues apparently not reaching the threshold of a diagnosable condition (although recall the reluctance of Chinese immigrants to use the term "depression").

There are several possible explanations for the healthy immigrant phenomenon, including screening by the receiving country and a self-selection effect so that newcomers are more healthy, wealthy, and determined than might otherwise be the case. However, vulnerability to mental disorder is not linear, and, in a systematic review of studies, Kirmayer and colleagues (2011) conclude that in general the prevalence of mental health problems among immigrants increases over time to become similar to that for the general population. An assessment of risk for mental disorder among immigrants needs to consider the *migration trajectory*; that is, pre-migration exposure, stresses during migration, and post-migration resettlement experiences (Kirmayer et al. 2011; MacPherson and Gushulak 2010). In some cases, these experiences may include placement in refugee camps or detention centres, which may aggravate mental health problems. After settlement, newcomers may experience a surge in hope and optimism, which in some cases may be followed by demoralization when expectations are not realized (Kirmayer et al. 2011). An example of this is immigrants who experience difficulties in having their credentials recognized. Given that the immigration experience may vary considerably from one group to another, readers need to be cautious in generalizing about the mental health of "immigrants." As MacPherson and Gushulak (2010, 295) observe, this term "as a single label for analysis and interpretation does not reflect their complexity and non-homogeneity."

The situation may be particularly difficult for persons escaping war-torn countries, and, in recent decades, Canada has seen refugees arriving from different source countries (from Asia and, more recently, from Europe) who have suffered considerable trauma and emotional upheaval. An example concerns the war in the Balkans in the late 1990s, with Canada having received fifty-five hundred Albanian Kosovar refugees fleeing this conflict. In a survey of health issues faced by the five hundred Kosovar refugees who settled in Hamilton, Ontario, participants reported difficulty in gaining access to medical, dental, and prescription services, in part because of language and cultural barriers (Redwood-Campbell et al. 2003, 2008). Researchers also found that respondents were significantly more likely to report poor health and lower satisfaction with health than the local population, and a screening instrument used to determine the presence of PTSD determined that about one-quarter met the diagnostic criteria, although rates among women were much higher, in some cases related to rape and other forms of sexual violence. Trauma-related conditions were found to sometimes take the form of somatic disorders.

Aboriginal Peoples

The Aboriginal peoples of Canada are made up of the First Nations (which includes status and non-status persons), the Métis, and the Inuit. According to the 2006 national census, 1.17 million persons self-identified as Aboriginal, with about 60 percent of this number First Nations, 33 percent Métis, and 4 percent Inuit. As noted earlier, the Aboriginal population experienced a much faster growth rate into the mid-2000s than that of the general population. There is considerable diversity within this population, with respect to language, dialect, and cultural traditions (Kirmayer, Tait, and Simpson 2009).

In Canada, persons of Aboriginal ancestry suffer from a range of health problems, and at higher rates than the rest of the population, this being particularly true for residents of more remote, sparsely populated areas (Canadian Institute for Health Information 2011a). Bearing in mind that survey data need to be updated, a review by Kirmayer and colleagues (2009) notes the following:

- Compared to the general population, life expectancy for both sexes was seven years shorter for the First Nations and at least ten years shorter for the Inuit.
- Aboriginal persons had much higher rates of tuberculosis, diabetes, heart disease, and hypertension.[5]
- Aboriginal persons had 6.5 times the national rate of death by injuries and poisonings.
- High rates of family violence and sexual abuse were self-reported.
- Rates of problem drinking and solvent use were significantly higher in some Aboriginal communities.
- Age-standardized rates of youth suicide were three to six times higher than the general population.

Among the Inuit, researchers have found much higher rates of premature birth, infant mortality, childhood malnutrition, and, even relative to other Aboriginal persons, higher suicide rates (Egaland et al. 2010; Luo et al. 2010).

In a number of cases, after statistically controlling for possible confounding factors, study data have revealed an "Aboriginal effect." For example, the higher risk for premature birth and infant mortality found by Luo and colleagues (above) still persisted after limiting the comparison to only other northern inhabitants. In another example, researchers in Vancouver found that, compared to other marginalized injection drug users, Aboriginal persons were significantly more likely to become HIV positive – by a ratio of 2:1 (Wood et al. 2008). A final example comes from a large-scale survey of Métis and First Nations persons in Saskatchewan conducted by Lemstra and colleagues (2009), which looks at the association between lifetime suicidal ideation and a number of predictor variables. The authors found that there was a significant association between suicidal ideation and household income and that controlling for the latter led to a result of lower rates of lifetime suicidal thinking for high-income Aboriginal persons, closer to the rates found for high-income Caucasians. However, as the authors note, there were two major qualifications: (1) poverty can be controlled for statistically but not in reality, with the Aboriginal members of the survey being much less affluent overall than the Caucasian comparison group; (2) even when controlling for all other significant covariates (household income, neighbourhood income, age, and life stress), Aboriginal persons were still 75 percent more likely to report suicidal ideation.

Concerning rates of diagnosable mental disorders, surveys have uncovered a higher prevalence of depression and low mood among Aboriginal persons than the general population – an example being a study of the Inuit that determined 26.5 percent of persons surveyed to be depressed (Haggarty et al. 2000) – although the reliability and specificity of the methods used in these studies have been questioned (Kirmayer, Tait, and Simpson 2009).

Suicidal Behaviour

Unquestionably, the reality of higher suicide rates must be seen as an indication of distress and poor mental health, and throughout the 1990s Canadians were given a series of grim reports about self-destructive behaviour in Aboriginal communities (Kirmayer, Boothroyd, and Hodgins 1998; McAndrew 1999). Davis Inlet, a government-made community built for the Innu people of Labrador-Quebec, was home to a number of horror stories, including televised images of young boys openly sniffing gasoline and talking to journalists about wanting to die. In reviewing records kept concerning the Innu of northern Labrador, Samson (2009) reports a suicide rate for Innu teenagers in the 1980s fifteen times higher than that for non-Native rates for the same area, and an estimate from the band council in Davis Inlet that one-third of all adults had attempted suicide in 1993. Concerning more recent events, a *Globe and Mail* story on the First Nations in rural BC communities (Hume 2007) reported a "suicide epidemic" in 2007 around the small community of Hazelton, with an average of over ten individuals a month being seen at the local hospital following suicide attempts. It was noted that these events followed other "outbreaks," one in 2007 and one in 2005, in small communities on Vancouver Island.

Concerning "epidemics," in an article entitled "Suicide as a Way of Belonging," McGill University anthropologist Ronald Niezen (2009, 180-81) uses the contagion metaphor in his analysis of "cluster suicides" in northern Manitoba:

> Suicide can be both an individual act – perhaps the ultimate expression of individual will and struggle with conscience – and a social phenomenon, influenced by common conditions and experiences and by shared values, beliefs, symbols and practices. [C]luster suicides seem to involve a central paradox that follows from the fact that those who commit or attempt suicide are often driven by profound loneliness ... or a sense of being unimportant and invisible, while, at the same time, this condition of loneliness becomes ... shared with others. There appears to be a perverse sociability at work in which self-destruction becomes a basis for linkage between individuals.

Understanding and responding to Aboriginal suicide is a major challenge (and the reader is directed to Kirmayer and Valaskakis [2009] for a more comprehensive analysis). While considering local and individual-level strategies, one must at the same time be aware of the historical context and *social origins of distress*, given that self-harming behaviour prior to European colonization was by all accounts "extremely limited" (Leenaars 2000, 58). Kirmayer, Tait, and Simpson (2009) review the postcolonial record:

- Early activity of European missionaries focused "on saving heathen souls through religious conversion" (7), leading to the suppression of indigenous spiritual beliefs and practices.
- Infectious disease and warfare, tantamount to genocide, decimated the Aboriginal population in many cases by the mid-1800s.
- Later in the colonial period, indigenous culture was further degraded through forced sedenterization, the creation of reserves, relocation to remote areas, and establishment of residential schools (see box). Crowding in the poor-quality housing provided increased the risk of infectious diseases like tuberculosis (a problem that still exists).
- To assimilate Aboriginal children, government policy dictated separation from their parents and, from 1879 to 1973, provision of a "civilizing" education in church-run boarding schools. It later became evident that many students had suffered physical, emotional, and sexual abuse from teachers and officials at these schools, a trauma that is still being re-lived by former students.

Theories of social cohesion – a cohesion torn asunder by the colonizers – have been used to explain suicide and self-destructive behaviour among indigenous peoples. For example, in his analysis of the Innu, Samson (2009) revives Durkheim's theory of anomic suicide, used in its original form to explain higher suicide rates in France at a time of industrialization and rapid social change ("anomie" is defined as a sense of dislocation or alienation).[6] Samson suggests that the circumstances described by Durkheim are similar to those affecting the Innu in more recent times: "a disturbance in the collective order, a breakdown of traditional authority, an attenuation of religion, and a rise in individualism" (121). A breakdown of social cohesion is also at the centre of a thesis explaining the phenomenon of drug addiction and destructive behaviour proposed by retired Canadian psychologist Bruce Alexander (2008). In his book, *The Globalization of Addiction: A Study in Poverty of the Spirit*, addiction is seen as an individual and social response to severe social, economic, or cultural dislocation. From this perspective, a need to belong, frustrated by alienation from both mainstream and traditional cultural values, is rechannelled into addiction and other self-destructive behaviours with similarly alienated individuals (Oslon 2007). Public surveys have found that Aboriginal persons are more likely than non-Aboriginals to identify environmental factors, such as racism and historical trauma, as causes of mental illness (Canadian Alliance on Mental Illness and Mental Health 2007), and the Mental Health Commission of Canada (2012, 98) concludes that, "in order to effect change, healing from this historical trauma must occur."

The connection between current mental health problems among indigenous persons and the colonial legacy has been made by a number of authors. Concerning approaches to healing, Leenars (2000, 59) notes that, in North

Residential Schools

Indian residential schools existed in Canada between 1863, when a school run by the Roman Catholic Church was set up in British Columbia, and 1996, when the last school was closed in the Northwest Territories (Chansonneuve 2005). In 1867, with the British North America Act, Indian education became a federal responsibility, and residential schools were operated from 1892 to 1969 as a partnership between the Government of Canada and the Catholic, Anglican, Presbyterian and United churches. The goal of these schools was to "civilize" and assimilate Native children into dominant society, in accordance with Euro-Canadian values. It was believed that residential schools – rather than day schools – would be more effective for this purpose since they would completely remove children from local influences and enable a more total indoctrination (Fournier and Crey 1997).

Since the closure of the residential schools, research into their effects has been undertaken, in particular the physical, sexual, and psychological abuse suffered by the students. In 1996 a Royal Commission report recommended that there be a public inquiry into the effects of residential schools on Aboriginal people, which led to the federal government's creation of a one-time, $350 million healing fund, designed to support community-based healing initiatives.

Canadian author Deborah Chansonneuve (2005) details the harms suffered by the residential school students, characterized as *ritual abuse*, which included isolation, monopolization of perception, degradation, and humiliation. She notes that assimilation by the schools can be seen as an example of *ethnocide* – the deliberate attempt to eradicate the culture or way of life of a people, and one that created historical trauma, "traumatic experiences that are cumulative across the life span of individuals, as well as across generations" (40).

America, colonization has had the effect of eliminating traditional practices that "offered Native peoples a complex and effective system of healing ... based on a holistic approach which attempted to balance the physical, mental, emotional and spiritual aspects of people." Concerning loss of identity, Kirmayer, Brass, and Tait (2000, 11) point to patterns of suicide among male Inuit and speak of the "greater disruption of traditional roles for males, resulting in profound problems of identity and self-esteem." Concerning paternalism and loss of responsibility, a study conducted in Nunavut (Harckham 2003, 74) involving interviews with Inuit residents of the community of Arviat found a number of them expressing the belief that "an individual cannot be mentally healthy without taking responsibility for their actions," leading the author to speculate that, over time, "colonialism [had] eroded a belief in self-sufficiency and encouraged a sense of dependency." Subjects in this study also suggested that, to have a healthier community, there should be more role models to look up to, which would represent proof of the "community's ability to foster and support healthy lifestyles and choices" (78).

Regarding loss of authority, researchers in British Columbia have posited an association between Aboriginal suicide rates and elements of "cultural continuity," which is defined as local control of human service organizations (police, fire, education, health, and child welfare), existence of local facilities for cultural activities, a degree of self-government, promotion of women into positions of leadership, and involvement in land claims (Chandler and Lalonde 2009). This research is based on a consistent empirical finding that must be seen as both curious and hopeful: that Aboriginal suicide rates in Canada vary widely from one community to the other, with some locales showing very high rates and others having few or no suicides at all. By way of example, Chandler and Lalonde (2009) point to a six-year period from 1987 to 1992 when more than half of BC's First Nations bands reported no youth suicides at all, with 90 percent of the suicides occurring in less than 10 percent of the bands. When these authors looked at why some bands were faring better than others, they found that the presence of an element of cultural continuity was predictive of suicide rates and that, when the data were grouped together across communities, suicide rates were inversely correlated with the number of elements present. The authors concluded that, among the BC bands studied, those scoring high on cultural continuity had no youth suicides and very low numbers of adult suicides.

Responses
Aboriginal persons dwell in urban areas and in smaller, more remote communities, and both situations present a challenge for service provision.

Generally, there are insufficient medical and mental health services in northern and more remote areas – a shortage of GPs let alone specialists, for example – and this disproportionately affects indigenous peoples (Hall 2001; Harckham 2003). Small communities present additional problems for service providers working in isolation, in particular a lack of anonymity for both the service user and provider, who may know each other socially or be related (Kirmayer, Brass, and Valaskakis 2009). The challenges facing remote communities was noted in a suicide action plan released by the Government of Nunavut, wherein the first recommendation was that northern residents should have access to "a wider range of mental health and addiction resources in their communities" (Working Group for a Nunavut Suicide Prevention Strategy 2011, 2). For city-dwellers, psychiatric services are often not culturally sensitive or relevant and, thus, are under-utilized; Kirmayer, Brass, and Tait (2000, 16) note that these services typically focus on the isolated individual, when "mental health services and promotion [should] be directed at both individual and community levels." Staying within the level of individual approaches, Aboriginal persons may be found ineligible for treatment programs because their problems do not fit the definition of a "serious, persistent mental illness," which is seen as a single syndrome typically manifesting with symptoms of psychosis and treatable pharmacologically. Persons with trauma histories often present with a range of symptoms in the anxiety and mood spectrum, to which practitioners may not know how to respond, other than by offering medication, so clearly there is a need for better training. Culturally specific mental health services may be available in some larger centres, but even when aware of their existence, traditionally oriented clinicians may be uncertain as to whether or how to combine Aboriginal healing practices with Western psychiatric approaches.

In the text *Healing Traditions* (Kirmayer and Valaskakis 2009), a number of authors describe holistic, traditional Aboriginal healing approaches directed at both the individual and the community. For example, among the Inuit, who see the individual as being connected to the land, an environmental or "land-based" psychology – in which the individual reconnects to the land through diet, activities, and values – is seen as promising (Kirmayer, Fletcher, and Watt 2009). Increasingly, stakeholders are making the case that mental health services for Aboriginal persons need to be holistic in orientation (e.g., Alberta Mental Health Board 2006), but as the authors of a provincial report for the BC Ministry of Children and Family Development note, if it is the case that "'ecological' approaches (i.e., intervening with families, schools, local governments, systems, and communities) hold greater promise than individual, clinic-based interventions," then clearly practitioners will require "a new and different set of skills" in the areas of community development and public education (Mussell, Cardiff, and White 2004, 32).

On a positive note, given the challenges in redesigning mental health services, there is evidence of benefit in *blending* Western and indigenous approaches. For example, Brass (2009) describes a treatment program in a correctional facility in Saskatchewan that combined standard methods of counselling with traditional Aboriginal healing practices, emphasizing pan-Indian spirituality, a "hybrid" approach that participants still found meaningful. The study notes the great diversity *within* the Aboriginal inmate population and, importantly, how one cannot assume a priori that an individual will identify more strongly with one orientation – Western or Aboriginal – rather than with another. Another hopeful finding, which is both interesting and, given past abuses, not a little ironic, is the number of indigenous persons in Canada who identify with and derive benefit from the Christian church, with a 2009 survey of eight hundred Aboriginal teens finding that one in two "valued" Christianity (Todd 2009). The same survey found, remarkably, that the proportion among this group who "trusted church leaders" was *higher* than the number for their non-Aboriginal counterparts. The key here again may have to do with the ability to blend practices – religious "syncretism" – something Aboriginal persons may be more comfortable with than are persons of European ancestry. In a report on this, Todd (2009) describes a "mixing of Christian devotion to Jesus Christ and the ritual of communion with customs such as the medicine wheel and sweetgrass ceremonies." The author notes that the Christian clergy may also have achieved more credibility in recent years with their activism and support of treaty claims.

Culturally Sensitive Services

Concerning the cultural context of mental health and mental illness, practitioners may make errors of both omission and commission. An error of commission would involve the worker's own preconceptions and stereotypes being applied clumsily or simplistically to clients. Kleinman and Benson (2006) give the example of a Mexican single-parent father, judged to be negligent in not connecting his HIV-positive son to the care system, which clinical staff attributed to a "different cultural understanding of HIV." In fact, after further investigation, it was found that the father had a relatively sophisticated understanding of HIV and that it was his *socio-economic* situation (working extra shifts at a low-paying job) that made it difficult for him to bring his son in for treatment.

Concerning errors of omission, this chapter offers a number of examples of how cultural aspects are missed or ignored in clinical practice, both individually and systemically. This ethnocentricity may not be accidental since the credibility of biological psychiatry rests to some extent on the idea of the universality of psychopathology; that is, "that cultural differences are a superficial 'mask' – a layer that must be peeled away to reveal the real, biological 'fact' underlying the disorder" (Hamid 2000a, 5). This perspective is reflected in practice documents, an example being an article on practitioner competencies in which it is noted that clinicians should be able to "separate cultural aspects from the person's psychopathology" (Coursey et al. 2000, 388).

One significant area of omission concerns language, the significance of which may still be underestimated by practitioners, despite the fact that language differences are a fundamental barrier to gaining access to and effectively utilizing mental health services. In an article on the role of professional interpreters in mental health, a McGill University researcher notes:

> Language is central to a person's cultural identity and is the most basic means through which people encode and express their emotions and their most complex thoughts, beliefs and values. Although it seems obvious that, in any clinical encounter, the ability to communicate effectively is essential, the under-utilization of interpreters by health professionals working with clients from ethnocultural communities with language barriers remains surprisingly common. Of concern is that most studies of immigrants in Canada find that one, if not the greatest, barrier to access to care is the lack of interpreters or of bilingual service providers. (Blake 2003, 21)

Blake (2003) observes that reluctance to use interpreters can come from the perception that the process will be too costly in terms of time and effort; it is also noted that there may be a misunderstanding of the role of the interpreter. The temptation to use untrained interpreters can lead to other difficulties with respect to accuracy and objectivity. Blake (2003, 22) suggests that "the use of informal interpreters represents a lack of recognition of the skills required to act as a competent interpreter. Mechanical word-for-word translation is often insufficient to convey meaning. Often, words cannot be literally translated from one language to another, owing to a lack of clear correspondence between the words of the two languages. Cultural 'idioms of distress' and the context or meaning of a symptom can be lost in attempts at literal translation." Professional interpreters also offer advantages with respect to impartiality, boundaries, and the handling of sensitive intra-family issues.

To attempt to remediate deficiencies in practice, health care organizations in Canada now strive for "cultural competence" among clinical staff

(Mental Health Commission of Canada 2012). In its *Framework for a Mental Health Strategy*, the Mental Health Commission of Canada (2009, 21) identifies responding to diversity as one of seven key goals:

> In a transformed mental health system, policies, programs, treatments, services, and supports are culturally safe and culturally competent. The system responds to the diverse individual and group needs – as well as to the disparities – that can arise from First Nations, Inuit, or Métis identity; ethno-cultural background, experience of racism, and migration history; stage of life; language spoken; sex, gender, and sexual orientation; geographical location; different abilities; socio-economic status; and spiritual or religious beliefs.

In its later strategy document, the commission recommends that the use of standards for cultural competency and safety be expanded through accreditation bodies and professional associations (Mental Health Commission of Canada 2012).

The term "cultural competency" refers to the ability of organizations to perform effectively in cross-cultural situations, and it is manifested in the values, attitudes, behaviours, policies, and practices of both individuals and systems. The assumption is that services sensitive to the needs of different cultural groups will be more inviting, will encourage minorities to get treatment, and will improve outcomes. A number of fidelity scales and self-assessment tools are now available for health care programs, and the National Center for Cultural Competence at Georgetown University is a good resource for these: http://nccc.georgetown.edu/. Accreditation Canada (2011) gives the following standard for community mental health services:

> The organization's acceptance of the diversity of the individuals and families it serves is evident in its policies and procedures. This may include having materials available in different languages and suitable for the hearing or sight impaired, access to interpretation services, and awareness programs and committees to understand different cultures and age groups.

In its strategy document, the Mental Health Commission (2012) recommends expanded use of standards for cultural competency and safety through accreditation bodies and professional associations.

The US Department of Health and Human Services (2007) has developed a more elaborate set of standards on culturally and linguistically appropriate services (CLAS),[7] which include the following:

- Health care organizations should ensure that patients/consumers receive from all staff members effective, understandable, and respectful care that is provided in a manner compatible with their cultural health beliefs and practices and preferred language.
- Health care organizations should implement strategies to recruit, retain, and promote at all levels of the organization a diverse staff and leadership that are representative of the demographic characteristics of the service area.
- Health care organizations should ensure that staff at all levels and across all disciplines receive ongoing education and training in culturally and linguistically appropriate service delivery.
- Health care organizations [should] offer and provide language assistance services, including bilingual staff and interpreter services, at no cost to each patient/consumer with limited English proficiency ... Family and friends should not be used to provide interpretation services (except on request by the patient/consumer).
- Health care organizations must make available easily understood patient-related materials and post signage in the languages of the commonly encountered groups and/or groups represented in the service area.
- Health care organizations should conduct initial and ongoing organizational self-assessments of CLAS-related activities and are encouraged to integrate cultural and linguistic competence-related measures into their internal audits, performance improvement programs, patient satisfaction assessments, and outcomes-based evaluations.
- Health care organizations should maintain a current demographic, cultural, and epidemiological profile of the community as well as a needs assessment to accurately plan for and implement services that respond to the cultural and linguistic characteristics of the service area.
- Health care organizations should ensure that data on the individual patient's/consumer's race, ethnicity, and spoken and written language are collected in health records, integrated into the organization's management information systems, and periodically updated.

Canadian organizations have been leaders in developing standards and curricula for working with Aboriginal persons as health care recipients and as research participants. For example, readers are directed to *Cultural Competency and Cultural Safety in Nursing Education* by the Aboriginal Nurses

Association of Canada (2009), and the Government of Canada's (2008) *Tri-Council Policy Statement* document on research involving Aboriginal peoples. An online curriculum is offered through the Indigenous Cultural Competency Training Program (http://www.culturalcompetency.ca).

Cultural competence can be seen as a continuum along which organizations and individuals can be placed. At the extreme ethnocentric end of the scale, approaches may be positively destructive, a historical example being the suppression of Aboriginal practices and beliefs by the early European colonists. While this example may be dismissed as outdated, Turbett (2000) notes that, even in the present era, there can be a tendency (perhaps unconscious) among clinicians to try to "convert" the client's worldview to one consistent with the medical model. Further along the cultural competence continuum is recognition but trivialization of cultural differences (tokeism). At the other end of the scale is an attitude of valuing and appreciating differences, along with possessing the skills to work effectively across cultures.

A first step for any practitioner is to examine her/his own attitudes and beliefs, which requires self-awareness and reflectivity. Sue, Arredondo, and McDavis (1992) suggest that culturally skilled counsellors are aware of how their own cultural background, experiences, and values influence psychological processes; are aware of their own communication style and of any stereotypes and negative emotional reactions held towards other ethnic groups; and are able to respect other, different belief systems and helping practices. This can be approached in a more structured fashion, through self-awareness exercises wherein clinicians answer questions about their own ethnic background and early life experiences, about the messages they received concerning racial differences, and about why people develop prejudices. Ideally, a budding practitioner should be someone who has both curiosity and humility. On this point, Tervalon and Murray-Garcia (1998, 117) suggest that *cultural humility* may indeed be "a more suitable goal" in clinical education than cultural competence (which implies that mastery can be achieved), one that "incorporates a lifelong commitment to self-evaluation and self-critique."

The next area of competence, after awareness, is knowledge: "The knowledge we use to inform our efforts should not be limited to the western biomedical model, but should include experiential knowledge gained from the person with the illness ... and also should include concepts of mental health or illness that come from different cultural traditions" (Macnaughton 2000, 14). To this end, practitioners need to actively seek out education and training experiences to enhance their understanding of the minority experience and worldview, which may in part be achieved by forging links with organizations representing these other communities. Practitioners also need to recognize the limits of their own expertise and seek consultation and/or make referrals as necessary. Knowledge may also refer to awareness of the limitations or bias of assessment and treatment procedures, especially those that have been "standardized": "Counsellors [should] proceed with caution when judging and interpreting the performance of minority group members and any other persons not represented in the group on which the evaluation and assessment instruments and procedures were standardized. They [should] recognize and take into account the potential effects of age, ethnicity, disability, culture, gender, religion, sexual orientation and socio-economic status on both the administration of, and the interpretation of data from, such instruments and procedures" (Canadian Counselling Association 2007, 12). As well, practitioners need to have knowledge of the socio-political context of minority clients, how discrimination may affect the manifestation of psychological disorders and help-seeking behaviour (perhaps within the practitioner's own agency), and how a "problem" personalized by the client may in fact stem from racism or bias. While it is impossible to come into a therapeutic relationship with a priori knowledge of all the cultural contingencies, an interested clinician can, it is hoped, gain some appreciation of these on an individual basis with clients, for example, by using a cultural formulation approach (described earlier) and constructing an illness narrative (see Lo and Fung [2003] for an articulation of a cultural analysis framework as a hypothesis-generating strategy for the practitioner).

A third area of competence refers to skills. This could include awareness of the different meanings of non-verbal communications such as gestures, silence, and eye contact; awareness of the limitations of a particular helping style; and an ability or willingness to engage in other "verbal/non-verbal helping responses" (Sue, Arredondo, and McDavis 1992, 48). The practitioner also needs to be careful about using psychological jargon and to be sure that the client understands the meanings of terms. Using the language requested by the client is desirable: there is evidence that bilingual counsellors are better able to retain clients in treatment and to obviate the use of crisis response teams (Ziguras et al. 2003), an assertion supported by a survey of seniors from the Chinese and Tamil communities in Toronto, which found that having access to an "ethnospecific," fully bilingual mental health service provider was clearly preferred by the subjects interviewed (Sadavoy, Meier, and Ong 2004). The unilingual practitioner should consider referral to, or consultation with, an interpreter or bilingual colleague and should also be open to consulting with traditional healers – such as those from the First Nations, who are establishing alternative treatment and healing programs in a number of mental health and institutional settings in Canada. Practitioners may also need to possess or develop advocacy skills for systems-level interventions when there is evidence that the client's "individual" concerns are a result of institutional barriers, biases, and gate-keeping arrangements.

In addition to consideration of practitioner competencies, mental health service providers need to look at how their programs are structured and delivered with respect to potential clients from minority groups. On this point, Humphrey and Townsend (2005, 5) note that "cultural competency is an add-on that program administrators find difficult to define, hard to implement, and often impossible to obtain reimbursement for, except in cases of programs that have been created to meet the needs of specific groups of consumers ... [which] sadly ... are few and far between." Taking cultural sensitivity seriously requires a conscious decision on the part of officials to make diversity and service equity "key issues for the agency to address" (Pyke et al. 2001, 182). Multicultural organizational change may be achieved through a number of approaches, including (1) recruitment and promotion of staff from diverse ethnic groups, (2) community outreach, (3) cultural events, (4) sensitivity training, and (5) developing partnerships that will facilitate improved attitudes between mainstream and other ethnic groups (Williams 2001).

Concerning service delivery, Kirmayer and colleagues (2003, 146) note that, historically, three main models have been developed to better meet the needs of minority clients: (1) the training of clinicians in generic approaches to cultural competency, (2) "ethnospecific" mental health services or clinics, and (3) the use of specially trained mental health translators and "culture brokers." Given fiscal restraints and the great diversity seen in Canadian urban centres, the development of ethnospecific clinics may be precluded, which "suggest[s] the potential value of a consultation-liaison model as a mechanism to address the impact of cultural diversity on mental health problems" (151). These cultural consultations may take three forms: (1) direct contact with the client by the consultant, usually with the referring person present; (2) a discussion with only the referring clinician, covering recommendations about treatment options and resources; and (3) education sessions or conferences with a number of representatives of the referring organization, who may present recurring problems, questions, and concerns. Kirmayer and colleagues (2003) describe the Cultural Consultation Service (CCS) established in Montreal in 1999 at the Jewish General Hospital. Personnel include part-time psychiatrists as well as psychologists, social workers, psychiatric nurses, and medical anthropologists. The authors found that referring sources most frequently made requests for help in clarifying the diagnosis or the meaning of specific symptoms (58 percent), for assistance in treatment planning (45 percent), and for information about or a link to resources related to a specific cultural group (25 percent). Issues raised in the consultations were most commonly as follows:

- variations in family systems, roles, and value systems (e.g., patriarchal families);
- identity issues related to age and gender roles (e.g., the importance of marriage and child-bearing);
- the impact of exposure to torture and war;
- the stressful impact of the refugee claimant process;
- the impact of immigration on intergenerational tensions;
- the effects of covert racism or biases in service provision;
- the prevalence of dissociative and somatoform symptoms that were initially misdiagnosed;
- previous experiences with healers in the country of origin;
- the importance of religious practices for coping and social support.

A preliminary evaluation of the program revealed positive outcomes as well as ongoing challenges. It was found that cultural consultation "often facilitated the therapeutic alliance between the referring person and the patient ... [particularly when] the consulting clinician was present during the clinical interview carried out by the culture broker" (Kirmayer et al. 2003, 150). On the other hand, it was found that, while having a culture broker from a similar background as the client could be positive, in some cases clients expressed concerns that being seen by someone from their own community compromised their privacy, a realistic concern for clients "from small cultural communities with high degrees of stigmatization of mental health problems" (150). Interested readers are directed to the CCS website at http://www.mcgill.ca/culturalconsultation.

Notes

1 Statistics Canada (2010).
2 This passage is taken from a text on Aboriginal mental health but applies to any minority culture.
3 "Nervios" is an interesting example of the difficulty in making a case for a culture-specific disorder, which, to be a valid construct, would need to show both differentiation from other psychiatric syndromes and association only with a particular ethnic group. This was tested in a study by Keough, Timpano, and Schmidt (2009), which consisted of a survey of members of three ethnic groups: Caucasian, Hispanic, and African-American. The question was whether *nervios* was simply another name for the most similar *DSM* category, panic attacks. The authors did find some measure of syndrome differentiation, supporting the claim that the two disorders are distinct; however, they did *not* find significant variation of rates of *nervios* across the three groups, suggesting that it is not culture-specific (see also Hamid 2000a).

4   A mid-twentieth-century study wherein black persons who tested positive for syphilis were given medical follow-up by the US Public Health Service but were never told they had the disease and were not given effective antibiotic treatments after the study started.

5   A 2008 Statistics Canada report found that 67 percent of Aboriginal women could be considered overweight and 41 percent obese, a difference from the general population that remained after controlling statistically for education and household income (Fitzpatrick 2008).

6   The validity and empirical basis for Durkheim's theory as it applied to France has been called into question (e.g., Kushner and Sterk [2005]).

7   Some of these standards are mandated, as per federal funding requirements, while others are suggested or recommended.

Other Resources

Laurence Kirmayer has been a leader in Canada in studying the cultural aspects of mental health. He and his colleagues are based at McGill University's Division of Social and Transcultural Psychiatry: http://www.mcgill.ca/tcpsych. Among other publications, Kirmayer has co-authored the Canadian Psychiatric Association position paper on guidelines for training in the practice of cultural psychiatry, available in the March 2012 issue of the *Canadian Journal of Psychiatry*.

Practitioners, Clients, and Family Members

7

In this chapter we take a closer look at the care providers and service users in the mental health system, their perspectives, and how these perspectives have shaped and are shaping the form that mental health services take. These parties are considered "stakeholders," which is a term that refers to individuals or groups who would expect to be consulted, or to have some input, regarding the development of public mental health policy. Historically, it has been the service providers themselves who have driven the policy agenda in Canada, with physicians having a particularly strong voice (Mulvale, Abelson, and Goering 2007). In more recent times, *service users* and *family members* have pushed for greater participation in the debate about mental health policy, even if fuller inclusion has not always been realized. Concerning service users, the slogan "nothing about us without us" has been adopted by disability rights groups to reflect the principle that no policy should be decided without the direct participation of persons affected by that policy (Charlton 1998; Morrison 2005).[1] Greater service user inclusion has also been driven by the idea of, and gradual move towards, a recovery-orientation in service delivery. Dickinson (2002, 381) suggests that, in Canada, there is "an increasingly explicit commitment to consumer empowerment and participation in the mental health field." Concerning families, support organizations such as the Schizophrenia Society have tried to make sure the family perspective is heard in discussions about access to treatment, as reflected in legislation and service planning (North Shore Schizophrenia Society 2011).

Support for greater inclusiveness has come from a number of sources. In 1993, the Canadian Mental Health Association published a report, *A New Framework for Support for People with Severe Mental Problems* (Trainor, Pomeroy, and Pape 1993, 1), which comments on the emergence of these "new stakeholders." The authors of the document address the need to include all stakeholders in the mental health planning process, challenge the idea of professional expertise as the only legitimate knowledge base, and emphasize the "undeniable importance of personal experience." This theme was taken up by Health Canada (1997, 112), whose report on best practices in mental health reform concludes that "the full range of stakeholders, including consumers and families, [should be] involved in the ongoing development and evolution of policy" and that "mental health policy [should be] supported by an explicit vision that the various stakeholders are aware of and in agreement with." And, more recently, the Mental Health Commission of Canada (2012, 41), as one of the "recommendations for action" in its strategy document, states that there is a need to "increase the active involvement of people living with mental health problems and illnesses and their families in governance, accreditation, monitoring, and advisory bodies in the service system."

While giving voice to persons not previously heard is almost certainly a positive development, this "new framework" has created some tensions and conflicts of interest. As Curtis and Hodge (1995, 45) note: "We are experiencing significant challenges to the assumptions underlying the balance of power in the service system." Indeed, a vision of client empowerment is not easily reconciled with a tradition of paternalism and hierarchical service delivery in which the practitioner role has been that of unchallenged authority/ expert. This vision is also challenged by, for example, the greater implementation in Canadian jurisdictions of community treatment orders (which permit involuntary outpatient treatment), a more coercive intervention whose introduction was partly the result of lobbying by family support groups – the *other* stakeholder. While program administrators have incorporated references to other stakeholder groups in their mission statements, it is not always apparent that the implications of this nominal commitment have been clearly thought through – that is, how, in practice, these concepts should be operationalized. As a professor of social work concludes in reference to client empowerment, professionals "have embraced this ideal, but it may be that we have not really examined the dilemmas that emerge and the choices to be made when a profession adopts empowerment as a mission" (Hartman 1994, 171).

This chapter reviews the behaviours and "vested interests" of three stakeholders – practitioners, clients, and family members – particularly in relation to a recovery orientation that sees client empowerment as an important goal. Attempts are made to bring into clearer focus areas where these stakeholder interests are complementary and areas where they may be conflicting. Before starting, a disclaimer is necessary: while it is useful to comment on themes that appear to be recurring, it is at the same time risky, and presumptuous, to generalize about stakeholders as having one shared voice or one particular agenda. Readers should bear in mind, then, that there is disagreement and great diversity of opinion *within* stakeholder groups, let alone between them (Carten 2006; Dickinson 2002; Everett 1994). It is also acknowledged that the three groups discussed here are not the only stakeholders in community mental health; other concerned parties, whose interests are addressed in other chapters, include government (Chapter 9), primary care physicians (Chapter 11), and the criminal justice system (Chapter 13).

To begin with, brief descriptions of the disciplines involved in mental health practice are offered. Following this, the relationship of these disciplines with other stakeholders is viewed from the perspective of professional duties and obligations, and from the perspective of self-interest. Finally, an attempt is made to explicate the interests of service users and family members, including the agendas of their advocacy organizations. This chapter focuses to some extent on psychiatry, which is in a particularly influential position in mental health settings because of the deference we give to physicians, their statutory authority to medicate and hospitalize, and the historical prominence of the medical model in service delivery. This is not intended in any way to devalue the role of allied professionals; indeed, it is this latter group that is responsible for delivering most of the other psychosocial treatment interventions. One other caveat: while speaking about separate occupations implies a distinctiveness of roles, in truth, many interventions, such as groups, are co-led by people of different disciplines, and there is a school of thought that mental health practitioners should in fact be generalists rather than specialists (Coursey et al 2000; see also Chapter 5).

Practitioners

A number of different professionals may be involved in the provision of services to mentally disordered persons. These include:

- *Family physicians.* While GPs are not considered mental health specialists, they are in fact the main contact point for many clients: surveys have found that a significant majority of Canadians requiring mental health care receive this care primarily or exclusively from their family physician and that the majority of prescriptions for psychotropic medications are written by GPs (Bilsker, Goldner, and Jones 2007; British Columbia Ministry of Health 2002e; Lavoie and Fleet 2002; Slomp et al. 2009; Vasiliadis et al. 2005; Watson et al. 2005). The available evidence suggests that, during the 1990s, the locus of treatment for depression shifted from the mental health specialty sector to the primary care sector – that is, family doctors (Harman, Edlund, and Fortney 2009). While this arrangement may be workable, GPs generally do not have the time, training, or fee incentive to counsel or case manage clients with mental health problems, so interventions tend to be based around medication (Hermann 2002). On the other hand, members of the public may experience a greater comfort level when dealing with their family doctor.

- *Psychiatrists.* Psychiatrists are physicians who complete an additional period of specialist training (a "residency") that lasts from three to five years. Psychiatrists may work in both public and private practice, tending to see fewer disabled persons in the latter. Psychiatrists (and physicians) are given special powers that consequently place them in a prominent position in the mental health system. First, they have the authority to arrange involuntary hospitalization, a procedure known as *certification* or *committal;* only in unusual circumstances can a non-physician be involved in this process (see Gray, Shone, and Liddle 2008). Second, they may prescribe medication, unlike most other mental health service providers (however, see box). The role of psychiatry is also distinguished by the fact that psychiatric services in both public and private practice are covered by provincial medical plans, meaning that they are effectively free to the client.[2] This is significant in that many persons with serious mental disorders are living in reduced financial circumstances and simply cannot afford private-pay arrangements. Gaining access to private psychiatrists in Canada has been found to be difficult, and there are often lengthy waiting lists. In a national survey, Canadian family physicians, when asked to rate access to psychiatrists on a scale from "excellent" to "poor," gave psychiatry the lowest access rating of any of the medical specialties, most often rating it "poor" (Goldner, Jones and Fang 2011).[3]
- *Psychologists.* For clinical psychologists, a PhD is the terminal degree and prerequisite for registration with provincial bodies. Psychologists have been prominent in the development and implementation of cognitive-behavioural therapies, an area of practice that is seen as being of increasing importance in the treatment of a range of mental disorders (described in Chapter 16). Psychologists may work in private and public practice, although they are not widely employed in community mental health settings in Canada and are used more in a consultative capacity, particularly to clarify diagnosis and treatment options through assessments and psychometric testing.
- *Educational* and *counselling* psychologists usually receive training through university faculties of education, with the MEd/MA or EdD/PhD being the qualifying degrees for practitioners. Persons with these credentials often (but not necessarily) work with families and younger clients.
- *Nurses.* Nurses are widely employed in the public mental health system, in hospital settings, and in the community as clinicians, case managers, and administrators. Their knowledge of medicine and pharmacology is

particularly valuable with respect to monitoring medication effects and side effects. Nurses working in mental health may be registered nurses (RNs) or registered psychiatric nurses (RPNs), with these two groups having separate professional associations. RPNs are trained, regulated, and employed only in the four western Canadian provinces (British Columbia, Alberta, Saskatchewan, and Manitoba).

- *Nurse practitioners.* Nurse practitioners (NPs) take additional training to at least a master's level, and are given many of the powers of physicians (i.e., to diagnose, prescribe, order tests, and refer to specialists).[4] This practice developed in Canada in the northern territories, presumably to compensate for a shortage of GPs, and legislation allowing full scope of practice has now been developed in most provinces. NPs are not yet widely employed in community mental health settings in Canada. In the US, advanced-practice psychiatric nurses (APPNs) are master's-level clinicians authorized to prescribe psychotropic medication in a majority of the states. As with the situation in the Canadian north, APPNs have been seen as a potentially important resource in rural locations (Hanrahan and Hartley 2008).

- *Occupational therapists.* Occupational therapy (OT) is a specialty that focuses on the rehabilitation needs of persons with both physical and psychiatric disabilities. In mental health, OTs may work in hospital and community settings, performing life-skill assessments and developing groups and programs that address social and vocational functioning. Training programs in occupational therapy are usually affiliated with university medical or health science faculties, with a master's degree now being the qualifying credential. Occupational therapy, with its emphasis on *function* as opposed to diagnosis and pathology, is well situated in a recovery-oriented system: Krupa and Clark (2004, 70) suggest that "the recovery framework is highly consistent with the profession's belief in our holistic understanding of the individual as an occupational being ... [and] with the profession's emphasis on client-centred and enabling practice" (see also Krupa et al. 2009).

- *Social workers.* Social workers are employed in hospitals, where historically they have played an important role in discharge planning, as well as in community settings, where they work as clinicians and administrators.[5] Training is at the baccalaureate or master's level, with most undergraduates receiving a "generalist" education. Most university social work programs make some reference to social justice, equity, or empowerment in their mission statements. One text notes that, with their ecological and systems perspective, "social workers have a unique perspective on the social and familial context of mental health problems, and are uniquely suited to advocate for and link with other systems in which clients are involved" (Sands and Angell 2002, 260). This orientation would appear to be a good fit with the recovery perspective: "Social work's distinct contribution may lie in the area of psychiatric recovery, especially those areas that link mental health with broader social issues, such as employment and education" (Shankar, Martin, and McDonald 2009, 28).

- *Recreation therapists.* A relatively new rehabilitation specialty, therapeutic recreation is provided to persons "who have physical, mental, social or emotional limitations which impact their ability to engage in meaningful leisure experiences" (Canadian Therapeutic Recreation Association 2003, 1). In recent years this discipline has moved towards being a licensed profession, with a clearer scope of practice and the ability to operate in a "sole charge" capacity. The qualifying credential, offered at several universities in Canada, is a baccalaureate degree.

Practitioner Duties

For practitioners, the relationship with other stakeholders can be seen in terms of a number of responsibilities, which can be examined by referring to codes of ethics and practice standards. It is noted that, in many instances, these responsibilities to different stakeholders (i.e., clients, families, and the public) are competing and not easily resolvable: a duty of care, concerns of relatives, and the obligation to consider safety and mitigate harm are not easily reconciled with a goal of client empowerment – a goal that is more

Prescription Privileges

The idea that physicians should have the exclusive right to prescribe psychotropic medication has been challenged in recent years, notably in two American jurisdictions. In 2002, the State of New Mexico passed legislation granting clinical psychologists qualified prescription privileges, which involves a two-year internship under the supervision of a psychiatrist as a prerequisite to independent prescribing. Similar legislation has been passed in Louisiana (Yates 2004). While these developments may seem surprising to some, they were justified on the basis of necessity: the New Mexico state government noted that few psychiatrists were available outside of the major metropolitan areas, that waiting lists were long, and that mental health needs were high, as evidenced by suicide rates among the populace in more remote areas.

In an article in the *Canadian Journal of Psychiatry,* Lavoie and Fleet (2002) review the reasons offered by proponents of prescription privileges for psychologists. One argument, consistent with the New Mexico example, is that this increases public access to treatment. The authors suggest that a shortage of psychiatrists has (in part) resulted in most prescriptions for psychotropic medication being issued by general practitioners, who have limited training in psychiatry and who may "frequently misdiagnose" their patients (445). A second argument is that treatment is more coherent and effective when both counselling and medication are offered by the same party. Finally, there is the "turf-guarding" view: that "psychologists do not and cannot function as independent professionals because the medical profession places many restrictions on their practice" (443). Counter-arguments include the position that prescribing would seem inconsistent with the mandate of psychology as well as the concern that non-physicians would be dealing with issues such as medication side effects, drug interactions, physical complications, and unrecognized organic causes of psychiatric symptoms (Scully 2004).

In Canada, the right to prescribe has been extended to two non-physician groups: nurse practitioners (as noted earlier) and, on a limited basis, pharmacists. Pharmacists in a number of locales have had the authority to dispense short refills of expired prescriptions, but in some jurisdictions these powers have been expanded. In British Columbia in 2001 pharmacists won the right to dispense contraceptive "morning-after" pills without medical authorization. The mixed feelings that this engendered were reflected by the fact that the move was opposed by the BC Medical Association but supported by the Society of Gynecologists and Obstetricians (O'Connor 2003). Then, in 2009, BC pharmacists were given the authority to renew prescriptions, alter dosages, and dispense substitute drugs without the oversight of a doctor. And, in 2008, a small group of pharmacists in Alberta, meeting new evaluation standards, were given the ultimate power: to write brand new prescriptions (exclusive of narcotics, steroids, and barbiturates) (Sinnema 2008). In an interview, an Alberta pharmacist suggested this initiative would "improve some of the efficiencies of the system" and noted that, given their education, simply dispensing drugs was "not really a good use of our training and expertise" (quoted in Sinnema 2008). Not surprisingly, representatives of the medical profession have opposed these changes. The Registrar of the BC College of Physicians and Surgeons went on record to say that the college was "not supportive of pharmacists adapting new prescriptions without prior collaboration with the physician" (VanAndel and Oetter 2008, 3). The chair of the Society of GPs in that province further detailed a number of concerns, including patient safety, privacy of information, liability, fragmentation of care, and a conflict of interest: the pharmacists would be dispensing/selling the same drugs they prescribe (Young 2008).

prominent now, in an era of recovery-oriented services. These competing interests have the potential to compromise the clinical relationship and to work against ethical ideals such as client autonomy. While mental health practitioners, individually and as a group, can be criticized for their failings, it can also be argued that the difficulty of the dilemmas they face is, if anything, under-appreciated by others.

Duty of Care
Practitioners face a considerable, sometimes daunting responsibility in providing care for their clients. In this they are guided by principles such as *beneficence*, which refers to "doing good" and preventing or removing harm, and *duty of care*, which is defined as acting with watchfulness, attention, caution, and prudence – and otherwise facing a possible charge of negligence. There is also the concept of "fiduciary duty," which is the obligation to act for someone else's benefit, as with a trustee, guardian, or parent. The relationship between physicians and patients has been seen as a fiduciary one (Chaimowitz, Milev, and Blackburn 2010), wherein "one person (a patient) entrusts his or her welfare to another (a physician)" (Gabbard and Nadelson 1995, 1,445). One could argue, then, that under these principles, which have the service recipient relinquishing power to the service provider, the doctor-patient relationship is, or at least has been, an inherently paternalistic one.

"Doing good" has become more complicated in an era of recovery-orientated services. Practitioners are now expected to "support consumers' freedom to make their own mistakes ... support risk-taking as leading to growth ... avoid controlling behaviors" (Coursey et al. 2000), and to "embrace the concept of the dignity of risk, and the right to failure if they are to be supportive of [service users]" (Deegan 1996). Reconciling these goals with a duty of care is not easy. Health authorities tend to be risk-averse and concerned about the issue of liability, which is reflected in, for example, risk-screening tools and audits after adverse events such as client suicide attempts. A US survey of mental health administrators found that the top concern about the potential impact of the recovery movement was that it would increase service providers' exposure to risk and liability (Davidson et al. 2006). Since they authorize treatment decisions, physicians in particular are concerned about looking bad, or being disciplined, or even being sued if a decision turns out poorly. Fear of litigation may be more a perception than reality-based – at least in the Canadian context[6] – but, to look at this another way, it can be argued that practitioners *should* be aspiring to high standards and to being accountable. At the same time, a natural consequence is that practitioner decisions tend to be cautious or conservative, which may have the effect of working against client autonomy and empowerment. So, for example, a psychiatrist may be reluctant to rescind a community treatment order – an involuntary reporting condition – because of the client's history of self-harming behaviour, even though the last incident occurred quite some time ago. Thus, the client is held at an involuntary status longer than is (arguably) necessary. While client autonomy *is* recognized in medical codes of ethics, it is stated as applying to *capable* individuals. For example, the Canadian Medical Association's Code of Ethics (2004, 2) includes respecting "the right of a *competent* patient to accept or reject any medical care recommended." Given that, historically, medical practice has been paternalistic, and given that the clients seen in public mental health programs are the most disabled, there is often a presumption of incompetence.

Among the stakeholders, families may have a different perspective than service users about risk-taking. Family support organizations, such as, in Canada, the Schizophrenia Society, have emphasized the need for proactive care and using involuntary interventions when necessary. They are uncomfortable with a model of care that promotes "consumers' freedom to make their own mistakes." Some family members have questioned whether the recovery-orientation can be applied at all to a serious disorder such as schizophrenia (Inman 2011b). For examples of this position, readers are directed to the advocacy bulletins of the North Shore Schizophrenia Society (http://www.northshoreschizophrenia.org/newsletter.htm). In sum, for many concerned relatives, the traditional notion of the practitioner as "watchful, attentive, cautious and prudent" is one they are very much congenial with, even if this is seen by others as "old school."

Mandated Treatment

For practitioners, achieving greater client autonomy and empowerment is limited when working in a mandated treatment setting. In some cases the relationship with the client is involuntary by definition; examples would be: employment in hospital settings with clients who have been certified under mental health legislation; in the field of forensic psychiatry, where client attendance is mandated by court order; or, increasingly, in outpatient settings, where involuntary treatment, not previously an issue, is now made possible with community treatment orders.

Confidentiality

Protecting client confidentiality is a key principle and responsibility for all mental health professionals (e.g., Canadian Medical Association 2004). A position paper from the Canadian Psychiatric Association (Beck 2000) notes:

Confidentiality is a prime condition in enabling the establishment of an effective therapeutic relationship. In no other medical specialty is so much private information required for establishing an accurate diagnosis and treatment plan. Breaches or potential breaches of confidentiality in the context of therapy seriously jeopardize the quality of the information communicated between patient and psychiatrist and also compromise the mutual trust and confidence necessary for therapy to occur.

While this seems uncontroversial, some tensions have arisen around how this principle is applied when working with family members of the mentally ill person and also around exceptions when safety concerns arise. With respect to family members, a Canadian Psychiatric Association publication states: "Be considerate of the patient's family and significant others and cooperate with them in the patient's interest. Psychiatrists recognize well the need to obtain the cooperation of relatives in providing collateral information and supporting treatment plans. They also recognize the need to assuage relative's anxiety about the care of their family member. However, ethical psychiatrists will recognize that *relatives' needs come second to the obligation to maintain confidentiality with the patient*" (Neilson 2002, 6, emphasis added). One can see that, in this reference, families are placed in a subordinate role, as "providers of information" and "supporters of treatment plans," and, in the case of competing interests, that family needs come second to the necessity of maintaining a therapeutic alliance with the client.[7] This stance has been criticized by family caregivers, who argue that being completely shut out of the treatment process is not helpful for the client/relative (North Shore Schizophrenia Society 2010). The subject of information-sharing with family caregivers is discussed in more detail later in this chapter.

Information can be shared without consent in certain circumstances, such as when reporting child abuse or responding to a court order. Since there is no blanket privilege given in law to clinician-client communications in Canada, practitioners should inform clients in advance that there is no absolute guarantee of confidentiality. In mental health settings, release without consent sometimes occurs in the context of client safety. For example, Ontario's Freedom of Information and Protection of Privacy Act permits release "in compelling circumstances affecting the health or safety of an individual." This leaves some question about how terms such as "safety" and "harm" are defined, and, unfortunately, other legal sources and precedents do not provide clear guidance in this respect (see Davis 2011; and Chapter 13). That being said, it has been argued that mental health service providers at times err too far on the side of privacy when safety is an issue. The Privacy

Commissioners of Ontario and British Columbia addressed this in a joint 2008 statement, following the tragic suicides of two university students who had been seen by the counselling services at their respective institutions (Loukidelis and Cavoukian 2008; see also O'Brian 2004). In their complaints to the universities, family members argued that if they had been told about their relatives' fragile mental states they could have provided support and possibly prevented the suicides. While predicting suicide is never an easy matter, the commissioners appeared to endorse the family position by concluding that "life trumps privacy, and our laws reflect that reality" (Loukidelis and Cavoukian 2008, 1).

Duty to Warn/Protect

While clinicians are generally comfortable with the idea of a duty of care, a more difficult role concerns the possible duty to protect others from the actions of a client. The discussion here flows logically from the previous section since warning any third party represents a breach of confidentiality, one that will almost certainly harm the therapeutic relationship. This aspect of practice achieved prominence in the US in the 1970s with the famous *Tarasoff* court decisions,[8] wherein a clinician was found liable for not warning/protecting the intended victim of/from his client.

With duty to protect becoming a more visible issue in Canada, a group representing Ontario physicians adopted the position that, where it was determined by the clinician, based on all the available evidence, a patient was more likely than not to carry out threats of serious violence, there was an obligation to notify the police or possibly the intended victim (Ferris et al. 1998). "More likely than not" is also referred to as the "balance of probabilities," which in law is a relatively low standard of certainty. The Supreme Court of Canada offered additional guidelines on this matter in the 1999 *Smith v. Jones* decision,[9] a case in which the client, "Jones," had revealed to a psychiatrist detailed plans for the torture and killing of young female prostitutes in a specified area of Vancouver. In this instance, the potential victims were identifiable and in imminent danger of serious bodily harm. In its ruling, the Court established a legal test, which, if all three criteria are satisfied, permits a breach of confidentiality on the basis of duty to warn:

- Is there a clear risk to an identifiable person or group of persons?
- Is there a risk of serious bodily harm or death?
- Is the danger imminent (i.e., close at hand or soon to actually happen)?

The standard of certainty here would appear to be higher than that proposed by the Ontario physician's panel, and it suggests that confidentiality should only be breached under extreme circumstances. Unfortunately, actual case scenarios are not usually as clear-cut as the *Jones* example since threats of violence by clients, if they arise, are often vague in nature. One legal analyst observes: "Inherent in the *Smith v. Jones* decision is the fact that many ethically challenging scenarios arise in which the law does not provide physicians with the appropriate or necessary legal directives. Absent specific legislative provisions, physicians are left to determine for themselves when disclosure will or will not result in a finding of professional misconduct and/or civil liability for negligence" (Tremayne-Lloyd 2003, 3). In discussing the dilemmas inherent in a duty to warn, in a position paper the Canadian Psychiatric Association notes that, in some cases, informing a third party may actually exacerbate risk and that "paranoid patients may have their persecutory beliefs reinforced by notification, and potential victims may be left with little protection beyond their newfound fear" (Chaimowitz and Glancy 2002, 4). The authors suggest that, if appropriate, hospitalizing the client might be a preferred alternative to breaching confidentiality. As with a duty of care towards a client, the obligation to mitigate harm to others will contribute to caution in clinical decision making and may compromise the goals of achieving trust and collaboration and of supporting autonomy in the therapeutic relationship.

Professional Imperialism?

While one way of viewing the actions of mental health practitioners is in terms of a number of obligations to clients and other stakeholders, a different, more skeptical view is to see their group behaviour as reflecting simple self-interest. Skeptics see professional activities in terms of turf-guarding or turf-expansion, examples from psychiatry being the resistance to extending prescription powers to non-physicians (see above) and the increasing number of conditions being defined as mental disorders – and therefore appropriate for psychiatric intervention – in successive revisions of diagnostic manuals such as the American Psychiatric Association's *Diagnostic and Statistical Manual* (Spiegel 2005; Wente 2009).

The idea that organizations act to further their own interests is not particularly remarkable; indeed, one of the key functions of any profession or labour union is to enhance the conditions of employment of its members. There are, however, several implications that flow from this, one being that professions act to maintain a competitive position in the "marketplace." In looking at the issue of which of these competitors is faring better in this respect, sociologists (e.g., Freidson 1994) point to several attributes that distinguish successful, or higher-status, professions and, in this case, psychiatry: (1) the ability to claim exclusive domain over an area of knowledge and skill; (2) the political power to control and organize their work, particularly the *content* of their work; and (3) the ability to be self-regulating. Licensure and self-regulation are promoted as the best means by which accountability is achieved and public safety protected. Canadian psychiatrist Jean Marie-Albert (2002, 919) observes that "the three major features of medical professionalism – the ethic of service, clinical autonomy, and self-regulation – benefit patients and society ... Individual psychiatrists should protect ... professionalism in psychiatry ... by contributing to the efforts of organized psychiatry and medicine to maintain and enhance the ethic of service, clinical autonomy, and self-regulation."

Psychiatry is particularly well situated in the Canadian mental health marketplace in that its practitioners carry with them the imprimatur of medical authority, the ability to admit persons to hospital, the licence to prescribe medication, and the ability to offer services that are covered (with some qualifications) by all provincial health care plans. Psychiatry's status is also linked to the pre-eminence of the biomedical model and its members' identification as physicians: in his revisionist history, journalist Robert Whitaker (2010) notes the decline of psychodynamic theories in the 1970s and a deliberate effort to "remedicalize" the profession in order to achieve greater credibility with the public. Psychiatrist and critic David Healy (2002, 217) suggests that the idea that mental disorders were produced by a chemical imbalance "set the stage for psychiatrists to become real doctors." Similarly, the advent of apparently effective psychopharmacological treatments, in the words of a former president of the Canadian Psychiatric Association, "confirmed and ratified the psychiatrist in his role of physician as a treater of severe mental disorders" (Marie-Albert 2002, 915).

Public funding gives psychiatry an advantage over other disciplines, such as psychology, whose practitioners generally are not eligible for payment through provincial health care plans – which means that persons on income assistance or the working poor are effectively excluded from this service. This supply-and-demand gap has become more apparent in recent years as the evidence base for psychological treatments – cognitive-behavioural therapy (CBT) in particular – has become stronger but has not been reflected in the skill sets of service providers (CBT is discussed in more detail in Chapter 16). This issue was raised in a 2009 position paper for the federal health minister authored by the executive director of the Canadian Psychological Association (2009, 2), with the following conclusion:

> Psychological services are not publicly funded by our jurisdictions' health care plans. With cuts to salaried resources and problems related to recruitment and retention in our public institutions (e.g. hospitals, schools,

correctional facilities), psychologists are increasingly practicing in communities where their services are not publicly funded and hence inaccessible to many in Canada. Although psychologists in private practice report ample work and demand for service within the private sector, individually and as a profession, we are very concerned that psychological services are not accessible to those without means to pay for them.

Concerning claims to "knowledge and skill," the skeptical viewpoint is to see the mental health professions – psychiatry in particular – overestimating in this regard, claiming broader tracts of psychic territory as a way of maintaining or expanding markets. On the tendency of professions to "overreach," Freidson (1994, 69) notes that "professional ideologies are inherently imperialistic, claiming more for the profession's knowledge and skill, and a broader jurisdiction, than can in fact be justified by demonstrable effectiveness. Such imperialism can of course be a function of crude self-interest, but it can as well be seen as a natural outcome of the deep commitment to the value of his [sic] work developed by the thoroughly socialized professional who has devoted his entire adult life to it."

Freidson's comments get at the complicated motivations of practitioners, who may want to do well for themselves but who also want to "do good" for their clients. "Doing well" in psychiatry has meant social status (although that may be arguable). It has also meant perks, benefits, and career advancement provided by an association with the pharmaceutical industry, a topic covered in more detail in Chapter 8. On this matter, the editor of the *Canadian Medical Association Journal* suggests that these "powerful pharmaceutical enticements have resulted in physicians believing that strong industry involvement is not only normal but also that they are entitled to receive the benefits. This culture of entitlement may be one of the most difficult obstacles to overcome" (Hebert 2008, 805). While benefits from the drug companies may speak to "doing well," psychiatry's reliance – and possible over-reliance (Ghaemi 2010) – on pharmaceuticals is also explained by the need to "do good." Clients are in distress, the clinician wants to help, and a prescription is at least *tangible*, an item the person can take away and evidence that the doctor is "doing something" (see also Doroshow 2007). The credibility of the intervention is enhanced by its being *medicine*, even if (as is detailed later) there is no compelling evidence that the new drugs are more effective in treating psychosis than products used fifty years ago.

Concerning treatment optimism being unfounded, Yale University psychiatrist Robert Rosenheck (2005) suggests that retaining faith in treatments, despite an equivocal evidence base, is due to "irrational exuberance." This author draws parallels between psychiatry and the stock market, arguing that, in both settings, "exuberant 'bubbles' occur when many voices reinforce one another, giving false credibility to wishful thinking" (Rosenheck 2005, 476). Similarly, a Canadian psychiatrist observes: "As physicians, we want to be helpful, but we often suffer individually and collectively from a pharmacological imperative: if we have a drug we feel compelled to prescribe it. We suffer from excessive therapeutic optimism" (quoted in Branham 2003). In considering the dramatic rise of psychopharmacology in the 1990s, Rosenheck (2005, 477) suggests that "drug company claims found a receptive audience among psychiatrists, whose profession was in the process of re-medicalizing itself ... partly in response to stiff competition from ... non-medical therapists ... A new generation of wonder drugs offered psychiatrists a unique niche among the crowded mental health professions as stewards of a valuable resource which they, alone, could prescribe."

Clients

While clients of the mental health system have for some years spoken and written about their experiences (Angell, Cooke, and Kovac 2005; Geller and Harris 1994; Morrison 2005), their opinions have frequently been overlooked, if not disqualified. Writing in the mid-1990s, sociologist Leona Bachrach (1996, 17) observed that "[clients] are, perforce, experts in the field of mental health program planning, and their products are often frank, articulate, and exceedingly sensitive. In fact, their writings contain important clues and information from which mental health program planners might take direction; yet surprisingly little note has been taken of the patient authored literature." Disqualification of the views of clients, particularly if these views are hostile to psychiatry, is made easier because their apparent "lack of insight" – which more recently has been given the medical term "anosognosia" – can be attributed to the disorder itself. As one client notes, "patients have had very little credibility when they do speak, because it's our minds that are in question" (cited in Brook 2003). A Health Canada (2002a, 2) report notes that having their agenda heard is made additionally difficult by the socio-economic status of many clients: "[clients may face] difficulties in mounting political lobbying efforts due to the poverty and disability of people affected by mental illness, and their consequent disadvantage in competing with other groups for limited health care services and supports." Health authorities, gradually, have been giving more of a voice to service users, although there is still a long way to go. Clients now sit on committees along with practitioners, and a numerically small but significant breakthrough was made in the author's own agency when a psychiatric service user became a decision-making member of the service's Policies and Procedures Committee.

It is difficult to talk about psychiatric clients as a "stakeholder group" in the sense of having one voice or having a consensus about how mental health services should be delivered. As a program manager, this author has been approached by service users who were critical and resentful of the role of psychiatry in their lives and others who were effusive in their praise for individual clinicians. Concerning the impact of the recovery model, one may read about the importance of system reform, client empowerment, and shared decision making while, at the same time, encountering – in this author's case through committees, focus groups, and interviews – a deferential attitude among some service users and a clear ambivalence about changing the status quo (see Gumpp 2009). An interesting example of this ambivalence concerns the preferences of service users regarding how they themselves are identified – that is, as "patient" (the oldest term), "client" (a somewhat newer term), "consumer" (one of the newest terms and the one seemingly preferred by people writing about and planning recovery-oriented services), or something else, such as "survivor." The significance of this is the symbolic value of the terminology: "Each of these words carries connotations regarding autonomy versus independence, illness versus health, fiduciary relationships, activity versus passivity, and so forth" (Covell et al. 2007; see also Essock and Rogers 2011; Morrison 2005; Torrey 2011a). If we are now in a more progressive era in mental health, we might suppose that service users would be happy with, for example, the more modern term "consumer." In fact, published surveys have found no clear consensus among service users regarding the preferred term (Covell 2007).[10] With these caveats in mind concerning the danger of over-generalizing, what follows is an attempt to identify some recurring themes that emerge in client critiques of the mental health system: (1) explanatory models, (2) use of coercion, (3) a focus by practitioners on symptom remission to the exclusion of other areas of need, and (4) a lack of "alternative" approaches to care.

To begin with, there may be disagreement over the fundamental question of the explanatory model: tension may exist between adherents of a biological concept of mental illness (typically practitioners) and those who attribute the disorder, or distress, to social factors, stress in particular (Pyne et al. 2006). For instance, in its mission statement, the National Empowerment Center, an advocacy organization staffed by current and former psychiatric service users, refers to helping those "with mental health issues, trauma, and extreme states" rather than using terms like "illness."[11] Finding common ground may be possible since these positions can be seen not as dichotomous but, rather, as representing different points on a continuum. However, if there is no common ground – if the client has a completely different interpretation of events – then working collaboratively or arriving at shared plans and goals is obviously very difficult. For example, a review article concludes that successful cognitive behavioural treatment of psychosis relies on the practitioner and client having "a shared understanding of the illness and its causes and consequences" (Somers 2007, 79), which is a problem in that a number of people affected by psychosis – and a majority in the acute phase – may not be able to meet this pre-condition. Davidson (2012, 5) suggests that finding common ground is helped by the practitioner staying "within the person's frame of reference as much as possible ... rather than asking him or her to take a leap of faith to believe in the utility of a diagnostic label that remains far from his or her experience base."

A second theme has to do with concern about the use of *coercion* in treatment, especially in the form of certification or, more recently, with the use of community treatment orders (Carten 2006; Morrison 2005; Sheehan and Burns 2011). In a review of the client-authored literature, Frese (1997, 18-19) concludes that, "while not all mentally ill persons are ... strident and ... unappreciative of services received, clearly a substantial segment of those who are willing to share their perspectives voice dissatisfaction, especially with mandated treatment." In a later review, this time of the professional literature, Newton-Howes and Mullen (2011, 465) conclude that "coercion was commonly felt by patients as dehumanizing." These authors also found that predicting who would be more likely to perceive an interaction this way was difficult, leading to the recommendation that "clinicians should routinely consider that all patients have the potential to experience an intervention as coercive" (465). Perceived coercion among clients has been found to be negatively associated with quality of life, sense of empowerment, and the working alliance with the caregiver (Tschopp, Berven, and Chan 2011). An example of a client perspective on the issue of enforced treatment comes from Canadian advocate Jill Stainsby (2000, 155):

> I believe that the therapeutic alliance which may be achieved between a patient and a physician or treatment team, which already has been eroded by involuntary committal in the first place, will be further weakened by the practice of [community treatment orders]. People will avoid the mental health system because of its focus on control over individuals with mental health diagnoses ... This approach to care is not a positive step for mental health: it is antagonistic, and it involves the use of threats – mandatory treatment, rehospitalization – in order to maintain individuals in the least expensive treatment regimen.

Among groups more explicitly critical of psychiatric practices, the slogan "If it isn't voluntary, it isn't treatment" has become a catchphrase (Morrison

2005). Coercion may extend to other domains, such as subsidized housing programs. In a study carried out by a group of Calgary service users (Schneider 2010, 77) the requirements concerning eligibility and ongoing tenancy were found to be onerous and demeaning, leading to the following recommendation for service providers: "Don't ask us for compliance. Work with us to help us make choices but do not tell us what we have to do. We do not want to be forced to live the way you think we should live."

Coercion, and the need to minimize coercive practices, is now on the "radar" of health authorities. Fidelity scales for recovery orientation refer to minimizing coercion, and instruments to help support shared decision making have been developed, significantly through the efforts of US advocate and author Patricia Deegan (e.g., Deegan 2007; Drake and Deegan 2009; Drake, Deegan, and Rapp 2010), although their implementation is not widespread. While shared decision making is intuitively appealing, it is notable that studies of service user preference have found ambivalence about this approach and a still-strong tendency to defer to professional expertise (Gumpp 2009). This subject was investigated by University of Toronto researchers through a large-scale ($n = 2,765$) survey in which participants were asked whether (1) seeking treatment information, (2) discussing treatment options, or (3) making the final decision should be patient-directed or physician-directed (the study referred to general medical care, not psychiatry specifically) (Levinson et al. 2005). The results showed that the vast majority (96 percent) preferred to be offered choices and asked their opinions but that a substantial number (44 percent) preferred to rely on physicians for medical knowledge rather than seeking it out themselves, and a substantial number (52 percent) preferred to leave the final decision to the physician. However, there were within-sample differences, in that women, better educated people, and – significantly – younger people were more likely to prefer an active role in decision making, suggesting, perhaps, that deferential attitudes are changing.

A third major area of critique concerns the mental health system's apparently narrow focus in responding to the needs of clients – that is, a preoccupation with symptom management to the exclusion of other important domains, such as housing, work, and social relationships. An illustration of this comes from a study that compared the responses of psychiatric service users and their care providers to questions about illness management (Pyne et al. 2006). Concerning "activities that maintain health," 65 percent of service users cited exercise, work, and hobbies as being important, compared to only 38 percent for the providers, who, by a wide margin, cited "taking medication" as the most important factor. Similarly, the service users were much more likely to choose "improved functioning" as a "sign of health," while the first choice in this category for providers was "decrease in symptoms." In another example, a survey comparing the priorities of practitioners, family members, and clients diagnosed with schizophrenia found that housing as an area of need was rated second in importance (out of seven outcome variables) by clients but only sixth by both practitioners and family members (Fischer, Shumway, and Owen 2002). Noting that clients "rarely" agreed with the other two stakeholder groups on the outcome variables, the authors found that practitioners tended to value "control of symptoms" and "medication management" more highly, whereas clients and family members rated social support, housing, and medical and dental services as more important (728). Finally, a study of 205 clients of a Canadian mental health service found statistically significant differences between the three stakeholder groups – clients, practitioners, and significant others – in seventeen of twenty-one outcome variables, which referred to "unmet rehabilitation needs" (Calsaferri and Jongbloed 1999). In this survey, the proportion of clients expressing an unmet need was compared to the proportion of significant others and practitioners who expressed the same unmet need as it applied, in their view, to that client. It was found, for example, that "job training or education" was seen as an unmet need by 43 percent of significant others, 37 percent of clients, but only 14 percent of practitioners; similarly, the percentages for "making friends" were 45, 32, and 14, respectively. One of the consequences of unmet (or unaddressed) needs is a potentially negative impact on the therapeutic alliance. This association was studied in a British survey of 160 clients and their care providers, which found a significant negative correlation; that is, the more unmet needs that were identified by the service user, the lower the score on a measure of the strength of the therapeutic relationship, from both the service user and provider's perspective (Junghan et al. 2007). A clear implication here is that an appraisal of client-chosen needs should be part of the engagement and ongoing discussion in the treatment process.

Concerning needs, Toronto advocate and author Pat Capponi (2003, xv) puts it quite simply: "The needs of members of the psychiatric community are not so different, really, from anyone else's needs – a home, a job, a friend." While some would worry that this sentence does not include "accessible and effective treatment," Capponi's words have been somewhat prophetic in that supported housing and supported employment have now become practices whose benefits have accumulated a solid evidence base (which is described in more detail in later chapters).

A fourth area of critique concerns access to alternative treatments and supports. "Alternative" is almost always defined as "non-pharmacological" and can refer to self-help and peer-support services as well as to treatment approaches not widely available in conventional public mental health programs. As an example of the latter, a Canadian advocate talks about the need to extend "medical coverage [to] non-drug medical support. Massage therapy, reflexology, counseling and 'talk therapy,' yoga and/or vitamin and herbal supplements to strengthen the nervous and immune system are all effective components of a health care regime that lowers stress and can protect any person from the debilitating effects of depression or psychosis" (Thor-Larsen 2002, 4). The reference here to "talk therapy" is significant in that clients have indeed expressed concern about over-reliance on medication (e.g., Gumpp 2009), which has helped fuel the development and wider implementation of psychological approaches such as cognitive behavioural therapy. Concerning peer support, a spokesperson for the psychiatric survivors' movement notes that, despite a lack of ideological unity, "the movement is held together by its common commitment to ... the development of self-help alternatives to professionally provided treatment" (cited in Dickinson 2002, 376). Access to client-run or self-help initiatives is limited by the finances of these groups: difficulties in attracting funding make their programming and viability more challenging – and tenuous. It is notable that peer support initiatives arose in many cases out of what was seen as *necessity*, to fill gaps that existed in the system, particularly around social support. For example, the successful and influential clubhouse program "Fountain House," based in New York City, was originally started by a group of ex-hospital patients who formed a mutual-aid organization called WANA (We Are Not Alone). In Vancouver, British Columbia, the Mental Patients Association (MPA) was formed in 1971 by a group of clients who first met at an outpatient treatment program and later created their own support network: "Their purpose was to establish a network of peer support, advocacy, self-help and empowerment at a time when only institutional care and support was available" (MPA Society 2011).

Agendas and Movements

As noted, it is difficult to talk about a common client perspective or agenda. Even on the most contentious issue, involuntary treatment, individual accounts and larger-scale surveys suggest that a substantial number of clients who have been certified will agree, in hindsight, that it was the right decision given their incapacity at the time (Priebe et al. 2010).[12] For example, an individual diagnosed with schizophrenia summarizes his own experiences as follows: "Although I recognize that some of my fellow mental health consumers are strongly opposed to the concept of forced treatment, I personally feel that I greatly benefited from being forced to accept treatment during periods in which I was incapable of understanding that I needed it. In fact, I sometimes wonder what would have become of me had someone not given me the treatment I so desperately needed but was so opposed to accepting" (Frese 1997, 17). Others, as noted, are much more critical of this practice, and when one speaks about a consumer "movement" in psychiatry it usually refers to people with this critical perspective. This may be contrasted with those with an anti-stigma agenda and who advocate for more resources (issues upon which all stakeholders can agree), but who stop short of open criticism of psychiatric practices.

Sociologist Linda Morrison (2005, ix) characterizes the "consumer/ survivor/ex-patient" (c/s/x) movement[13] as follows:

> Most members ... are people who have been diagnosed as mentally ill and are engaged in different forms of "talking back" to psychiatry and the mental health system ... Members of the c/s/x movement are not satisfied to settle into the ordinary sick role or accept the deviant "mental patient" identity assigned to them by their doctors and society. They work to take power in relation to their providers, and attempt to shape treatment to respond to their own needs or reject it altogether ... Instead of being passive objects of treatment, policy and social control they take an activist stance toward increased alternatives, informed choice, and human rights protection for people who find themselves within the power domain of psychiatric care.

While this passage suggests a coherence of purpose and vision, a somewhat different picture emerges in the following description of the "mental health movement" written by Canadian advocate Ron Carten (2006, 72-73, emphasis added):

> Many in the ... movement have grievances against the psychiatric systems in many countries. Some make shrill calls for the abolition of psychiatry. Others cry out for redress of abuses they and others have suffered at the hands of psychiatry ... There are yet others who feel they have, on balance, benefited from a psychiatric intervention. The shrill ones may object to the presence of the ones who feel less grievance than they. The legally-minded may object to the more pedestrian ones. The victims of abuse may resent those luckier ones who respond to their stories with skepticism and an apparent satisfaction with the status quo. In short, the mental health movement is *not a monolithic radical movement to abolish psychiatry*, nor is it a benign convocation of medicated ne'er-do-wells ... Being part of this

community breaks down the walls of isolation that surround so many who have been through the journey from asylum to community.

From this account the reader is given the impression that there is inclusiveness of different viewpoints and that mutual support is as important as the advancement of a political agenda. The contrast of the two passages supports the thesis of there being *two* consumer movements in mental health, one in which the aim is to achieve partnerships with mental health practitioners and a "survivor" movement in which the aim is to seek "complete liberation from psychiatry" (Everett 1994, 63). Dickinson (2002, 376) concludes, simply, that "the psychiatric survivors movement, at least as it has evolved in Canada since the 1970s, is not homogeneous in terms of either membership or ideologies."

Can there be reconciliation of different viewpoints? At the peripheries, this is difficult. As the above passage indicates, there is at times a tension between those clients critical of the system and those more or less satisfied with the services they have received. In her book on the c/s/x movement Morrison (2005, 5) speaks about "good patients" and "bad patients," the former someone who "continues to inhabit the sick role in a dependent or quasi-dependent state," and the latter someone who resists the sick role. Similarly, Capponi (2003, 30) contrasts "patients" ("[who] learn at an early age to trust professional experts, especially those with 'doctor' in front of their names") with "survivors" ("[who] have a jaundiced view of medical models, past and present"). While terms like "sick role" and "good patient" originally come from sociological, not consumer, literature, they have been adopted by the c/s/x community in a way that some would see as patronizing or arrogant when applied to other service users. Indeed, some take great exception to the implication that one group has a truer vision, while those who go along with the status quo are passive dupes. This issue is taken up by a service user in an editorial entitled "Client versus Client," wherein the author, who states that "treatment by professionals has saved my life" (Gibson-Leek 2003, 1101-2, emphasis added), criticizes current initiatives that have militant "super clients" being funded by public mental health dollars to act as advocates or peer-support workers:

> The *truly mentally ill* are bullied into silence. The "super clients" now speak on my behalf ... When I told one of these "leaders" that she did not speak for me and that I benefited from professional treatment, I was told "You have been brainwashed by the system" ... No client should ever be placed above another client or be paid to be a client. Funds that should be going

to treat the mentally ill are now squandered on extremists who constantly seek attention, awards, esteem, power and control over others ... I am sure that some people have not had good experiences. This does not mean they control my experiences. Many of these people *were never mentally ill.*

There are a number of interesting discussion points that flow from this passage. One is the perception that more strident, critical clients are not representative of the population of persons with mental disorders, not "truly mentally ill," and thus not entitled to speak on their behalf. This is all the more significant when one considers that, while voiced in this case by a client, these same sentiments have been expressed at times by practitioners (although not publicly), who may be used to dealing with individuals who are more quiet, compliant, and, for lack of a better expression, "seriously mentally ill."[14] Another author suggests that a distinction be made between persons who have and do not have schizophrenia: "It ... [is] impossible to know if people who claim the right to represent those with schizophrenia have ever actually been diagnosed with and had to learn to live with this disorder themselves" (Inman 2011b).

There may indeed be a "selection bias" in effect, in that service users who are more articulate, and less disabled, are more likely to attain committee and consumer advisory positions, but this should not be surprising. In fact, the selection bias is often exacerbated by practitioners, who will continue to load new assignments onto agreeable individuals (in some cases leading to their burnout). A problem only arises when the client in question is critical of the system, which, in this author's experience, is not usually the case: peer workers and client committee members appointed by the health authority, while capable of constructive criticism, tend not to be anti-psychiatry. Clients who are very critical of the system tend either to leave that system or keep a low profile within it. This makes life a bit easier for practitioners, but it also means that the population they are "capturing" – whether that means receiving treatment, participating in research, or being employed – is not a true cross-section of persons with mental health problems. One suspects that the confrontation described by Gibson-Leek above took place outside of a public mental treatment program; that is, at a non-profit society, a setting more controlled by clients. This speaks to the prospect of balkanization by program, meaning that "patients" and "survivors" – to use Capponi's terms – are less likely to cross paths.

One final point concerns the practitioner perspective, the idea that some clients – the passive ones, or the most disabled – are more representative and thus (perhaps) more sympathetic and deserving of service. There are several

concerns with this line of reasoning, one being that passivity and dependence are being encouraged (consciously or unconsciously) by the practitioner,
and self-reliance – which may be seen as non-compliance – discouraged. This
clearly conflicts with a recovery philosophy that sees people moving along
a path to greater self-reliance and self-management of their mental illness.
The idea that agency clients should all be at the same level of ability or disability seems to discount this prospect – that is, that some clients get better
and move on to greater independence. A more independent service user
comments on this bias, encountered when she was a speaker at forums and
conferences: "Despite a convincing collection of serious diagnoses, hospitalizations and treatments, we who get on with our lives and offer ourselves
as examples of recovery are dismissed as not really ill, as exceptions, as
misdiagnosed. Our experience is not valued" (Caras 1998, 763).

Families

Trying to support a family member with a serious mental disorder – a child,
sibling, or parent – can be an overwhelming task. In an article entitled "The
Family Experience of Mental Illness," Marsh and Johnson (1997) review the
challenges faced by families: these include dealing with grief and symbolic
loss because of expectations that have been dashed, chronic sorrow (never
reaching a stage of acceptance), the emotional roller coaster of not knowing
what to expect from one day to the next, the forced return to a parenting role
with an adult offspring, stigma, financial burden, self-neglect, frustrations
about dealing with the "system," a lack of support, and an apparent absence
of services. The burden of caregiving takes a toll in terms of physical and
mental health (Crowley-Cyr 2008; Dodge 2011). An illustration of this comes
from a US study that looked at the health of married fathers who were caregivers for adult children diagnosed with schizophrenia (Ghosh and Greenberg
2009). The ninety-five participants were administered structured scales
measuring depression, psychological well-being, physical health, and marital
satisfaction, and the results were compared with a random sample of fathers
from the same region who did not have children diagnosed with schizophrenia. Notably, the mean age of the caregiving fathers surveyed was just over
seventy, and the mean age of the children just over forty, showing how
caregiving can extend late into life. About one-third of the adult children
with the psychiatric diagnosis were still living at home with their parents.
The researchers found the caregiving fathers scored more poorly on all
measures of physical and mental health and marital satisfaction. A study of
the burden of care faced by caregivers in Australia found the following: "Some
of the possible long term effects of little or no respite on caregivers include[d]

exhaustion, bitterness, and even a sense of abandonment by the wider community. Such effects often strain family relationships and cohesion. Indeed, a fundamental question asked by many aging carers who are parents is 'when can I retire? And if I can't, what happens when I die?'" (Crowley-Cyr 2008, 384-85). Parents typically feel a sense of responsibility and guilt about the mentally ill child (Angell, Cooke, and Kovac 2005), which can be another source of tension between family members. A mother interviewed about this explains as follows: "You feel responsible for everything that happens in your son's life. So you have all the weight on your shoulders ... it's very hard because when he tried to kill himself my husband blamed me. 'Where were you?' he said. I said, 'What do you mean, where were you? Where were *you?*'"(quoted in McCann, Lubman, and Clark 2011, 384).

Concerning caregiver burden, a number of authors suggest that relying on families to provide care is a way for governments to offload costs and responsibilities (Crowley-Cyr 2008; Ross 2011a). An example is an Australian study on bipolar disorder that found 29 percent of families reporting serious economic hardship because of the care-giving burden (Dore and Romans 2001). A Canadian advocate argues that the organization created (in part) to promote caregiver concerns is failing in this regard: "The Mental Health Commission of Canada is not actively lobbying for reversing the trend to reduce the number of acute psychiatric beds nor is it advocating for the training of more psychiatrists. The responsibility for caring for people with untreated or inadequately treated schizophrenia will continue to reside with families" (Inman 2011b).

What is the experience of families when they interact with the mental health system in the shared care of their mentally ill relative? A large body of evidence, accumulated through surveys, family accounts, and the experiences of clinicians and administrators – including this author – suggests that the family-practitioner relationship has in many cases been a strained one and that families have not always been given the support they need (Calsaferri and Jongbloed 1999; Centre for Addiction and Mental Health 2004; Crowley-Cyr 2008; Dodge 2011; Gerson et al. 2009; Hall 2001; Inman 2011b; Perrault et al. 2011; Standing Senate Committee on Social Affairs, Science and Technology 2006). Often families do not know where to turn for help when their loved one has a first psychiatric episode, and, even after their son or daughter is "activated" with a mental health team, they may find that the team will not provide them with sufficient information, advice, or resources to help them in their caregiving role. Working with families, on the face of it, may seem to be an obvious role for community mental health programs. However, there are a number of institutional and philosophical factors that work against this. First and foremost is the fact that psychiatric treatment in English-speaking countries has a very *individualistic* orientation (Whitley and Lawson 2010). The argument goes that the person with the mental illness is the patient, not the family, and, further, that what goes on between doctor and patient cannot be shared with that family on ethical and legal grounds. (Expectations about the participation of families differ in other cultures. Kirmayer and colleagues [2011] suggest that, in these cases, "the cultural legitimacy of parental authority ... should be taken into account," and "interventions should be framed in ways that avoid alienating family members or aggravating intergenerational conflicts.")

A reflection of the individualistic orientation comes in the following response to a survey about family involvement given to staff at this author's agency:

> Is family involvement in medical treatment decisions a common experience for most adults? I don't think so. In the interest of wellness and a return to a normal pattern of living, I respect and value a client's autonomy in all aspects of their lives. Therefore, I am very judicious when I involve families. Bottom-line: is family involvement in my clients' best interest? This is a very strong value I have held in my 18 years of working.[15]

The respondent suggests here that, for any of us, it would seem odd to have an aging parent getting involved in treatment decisions that should be between you and your treatment provider. On the other hand, one could ask if the situation of someone *without* a serious mental illness is, for example, comparable to that of someone severely disabled by schizophrenia. The author of the quote also speaks about autonomy and a return to a normal pattern of living, which underlines the importance placed on individuation, of growing up and apart from the family of origin, and of not treating an adult like a child – in our philosophy of care.

Arguments in favour of greater family involvement include the fact that, in many cases, this is something families want: a study by researchers at Laval University in Quebec found that "collaboration with professionals" was the key determinant in predicting caregiver satisfaction with mental health services (Perrault et al. 2011). And there is the argument that inclusion of the family can be in the client's best interests. There is now a fairly large evidence base that indicates that family interventions work for clients; that is, that educating care providers in specific psychosocial and cognitive-behavioural approaches leads to fewer relapses and re-hospitalizations among clients, and reduced distress levels and enhanced coping among family members

(Bird et al. 2010; Dixon et al. 2001, 2010, 2011; Giron et al. 2010; Glyn et al. 2006; Hartocollis 2008; Jones 2005; Mottaghipour and Bickerton 2005; Pitschel-Walz et al. 2001).

The idea that families should be included as stakeholders is now reflected in policy documents. A best practices document published by the British Columbia Ministry of Health (2002c) made the following recommendations concerning family involvement:

- Families should be informed and aware of the treatment plan and discharge planning should focus not only on the individual's personal functioning, but also on the family's ability to care for the client.
- There should be provision of counselling for family members, which would include provision of information, support, skills teaching, and assistance in accessing services.
- There should be training opportunities and resources to support self-help.
- Support should include diversified respite care.
- Family members should have a role in the planning and evaluation of mental health services.

An appendix in this document contains a "Family Charter of Rights," developed by the Provincial Mental Health Family Advisory Council. The charter goes further than the recommendations contained in the main text, addressing attitudinal barriers encountered by family members. An excerpt is as follows:

Families have a right:

- To explicit information that families do not cause mental illness.
- To respect from professionals for the expertise of the family, as well as the sharing of power in the therapeutic process.
- To become appropriately assertive and to overcome traditional socialization that teaches families not to question authority (28).

At the national level, supporting families is one of the seven goals for transforming the mental health system articulated by the Mental Health Commission of Canada in its 2009 document *Toward Recovery and Well-Being:*

The unique role of families ... in promoting well-being, providing care and fostering recovery across the lifespan is recognized, as are the needs of families themselves. Families are engaged and helped through education and programs such as parenting and sibling support, financial assistance, peer support and respite care. Wherever possible, families become partners in the care and treatment of their loved ones and are integrated into decision-making in a way that respects consent and privacy. (Mental Health Commission of Canada 2009, 21)

And, at the agency level, an example of principles for working with family comes from the 2011 Family Involvement Policy of the community mental health programs of the Vancouver Coastal Health Authority:

- Staff will acknowledge the importance of family and endorse family participation, collaboration, and shared responsibility in the client treatment and recovery plan.
- Staff will actively involve families in the process of care and treatment of the client.
- Clients have a right to privacy while keeping in balance the need for family involvement and information sharing.
- When engaging families, staff will pay attention to the values and beliefs of all cultures.
- [The program manager will] ensure a welcoming environment for family members in the mental health teams/units, including engaging families from culturally and linguistically diverse backgrounds.

Realizing these principles and ideals has been difficult, however. Public mental health programs have not traditionally been involved in this area, apart from running some educational groups. Providing additional resources for families means fighting for limited funds within health authority budgets. The idea of "sharing power in the therapeutic process" is a bold one, but (truly) shared decision making is still in its infancy in working with clients, let alone with families. A role in planning and evaluation is starting to evolve, for example, through the establishment of family advisory committees at some agencies. And some changes in policy are emerging: a minor example from the author's health authority was to require that clinical staff ask clients about family involvement early in the engagement, including the use of a form that would identify a relative or ally with whom information could be shared. Currently, however, family involvement in a more systematic sense is lacking in many mental health programs. A chapter of the Schizophrenia Society of Canada, a family support organization, bluntly refers to the *"lip service* [that] is given to family involvement, sometimes tacked on in policy documents and clinical guidelines with bureaucratic rigour" (North Shore Schizophrenia Society 2010, emphasis added). One factor, limiting the wider implementation of family programs, is that relatively few practitioners have been trained in family work (Mottaghipour and Bickerton 2005). However, while staff training is important, there are barriers to working with families that are even more fundamental and are necessarily discussed here in greater detail. This discussion is broken into three sections: (1) family blaming, (2) information sharing, and (3) philosophy of care.

Family Blaming

It is unfortunately the case that the relationship between practitioners and family members is one that, historically, has been characterized by ambivalence, if not mistrust. To understand this one has to consider the legacy of aetiological theories that implicitly or explicitly blamed family members – the mother in particular – for contributing to the son's or daughter's mental disorder. To begin with, Freudian theory, which was very influential for a large part of the twentieth century, proposed that mental health problems often arose out of early life experiences, in particular with the family of origin. Scottish psychiatrist R.D. Laing, another influential figure, also implicated the family in the development of madness among the offspring. Concerning the genesis of schizophrenia, theories included the concept of the cold, rejecting "schizophrenogenic mother," the "double-bind" hypothesis (an investigation of contradictory messages from the parent), the role of marital "schism and skew" in the family of persons with schizophrenia, and an Italian group's findings based on a study of families in "schizophrenic transition" and their use of "paradoxical communications" (Davis 1987a). In the case of autism, this condition was said to be produced by "refrigerator mothers." This, according to child psychologist Bruno Bettelheim, who drew parallels between the demeanour of mothers with autistic children and guards at Nazi concentration camps – where Bettelheim himself had been imprisoned.

These older aetiological theories have now for the most part been discredited and abandoned (although this author can attest from his own university experience that a text published as recently as 1980 claims that the "double-bind hypothesis has grown into one of the most scientifically respectable theories of schizophrenia-producing family interaction" [Goldenberg and Goldenberg 1980, 87]).[16] Among other deficiencies, explanations of this sort face the problem of establishing the direction of cause and effect when studying communication patterns as well as the fact that apparently distorted interaction styles can also be found in "normal" families.

That being said, one area of study that continues to look at communication styles has to do with the concept of "expressed emotion," which predicts that, in social settings and families in which we find "emotional over-involvement" and excessive negative comments, relapse on the part of persons with schizophrenia is more likely (Raune, Kuipers, and Bebbington 2004). On the one hand, this hypothesis seems reasonable – it is, after all, consistent with the stress-vulnerability model of symptom breakthrough – but it remains somewhat controversial. Part of the criticism concerns the empirical basis of the hypothesis (e.g., Carslon 2011), with one treatment manual concluding that "there is little evidence that EE is associated with relapse in early psychosis patients or that family work designed to decrease expressed emotion reduces relapse" (Mental Health Evaluation and Community Consultation Unit 2002, 15). The other concern is the potential for finding fault, with social policy professor Phyllis Solomon suggesting that the conundrum concerning the direction of causality has still not been resolved and that the whole concept "continues to blame families" (Solomon 2001, 68; see also Inman 2011b). An online search in 2011 for articles on expressed emotion found that research in this area continues (and has in fact been extended to other syndromes), but in this author's experience expressed emotion is not being widely used to inform practice in Canadian settings.

Apart from aetiological models, there are traditions and principles within schools of therapy that have been seen as having the potential to blame families. An example of this comes from the memoir of Canadian author Susan Inman (2010), whose daughter was eventually diagnosed with schizoaffective disorder. Before the nature of the illness became clear the daughter was treated by a counselling psychologist whose orientation was to see mental disorder in familial, rather than in medical, terms and, after the daughter was finally hospitalized, advised staff at the inpatient unit that the family was "dysfunctional" and "shouldn't be around [the daughter] too much" (this according to the attending psychiatrist).[17] Later in the same admission the mother is chastised by staff for "not encouraging [the daughter's] independence" – this in the case of a fifteen-year-old girl certified to a psychiatric ward – a comment seemingly reflective of a therapeutic worldview that favours individuation and disfavours family "enmeshment" (see Sanchez 2000). Inman has continued to champion the cause of stigmatization of families, arguing that the most important way that practitioners can support the parents of people with schizophrenia is to "let them know that they did not cause this illness" (Inman 2011a). Inman and other family members have also made submissions to the Mental Health Commission of Canada on the subject, asking that the commission "openly acknowledge and address ... the destructive impact of unjustified blame for these disorders" and "advocate to raise the standards of programs training mental health professionals" since "professionals ... often still believe that families cause these mental illnesses" (quoted in Ross 2011a). These assertions will seem extreme to some, but they do capture the vulnerability family members with a disabled child often feel. It is also a reminder to practitioners to be more self-aware since there is still the chance that they may, even unintentionally, "send the message to struggling parents (whose sensitivity is already heightened to criticism) that they are failing as parents and that their failure is a primary cause of their child's problems" (Duncan 2004, 13).

Information Sharing

Sharing information with the family members of an adult client is a difficult ethical conundrum for the practitioner. *Sharing* information raises the concern of breaching confidentiality, while *not* sharing information may leave family members feeling shut out and abandoned, particularly in a situation in which a desperate parent or sibling does not know where their relative is living, under what circumstances, and whether they are safe and healthy.

There are, however, good reasons to protect client confidentiality. To not do so: (1) on the face of it violates professional ethics codes, (2) probably violates agency policy, and (3) may be unlawful, although legal guidelines in this area are neither clear cut nor well understood (more on this below). To deal with potential conflict between different policies from the same agency, principles need to be worded carefully to provide some flexibility: the agency policy statement (see above) that "clients have a right to privacy while keeping in balance the need for family involvement and information sharing" appears to do this, but in fact it gives no real guidance on particular cases.

Perhaps the most compelling reason for protecting confidentiality has to do with the therapeutic relationship: breaching confidentiality is often seen by the client as a betrayal of trust and, consequently, can grievously damage that relationship (Beck 2000). This is all the more significant when one considers that trust takes time and is not easily developed by psychiatric service users, in part due to symptoms of the illness and in part due to their experiences with the system (Gumpp 2009). Bogart and Solomon (1999, 1,322) conclude that requiring client consent to release information is vital to safeguard clients' trust, promote independence, and "communicate respect and validation of consumers' ability to make decisions in their own best interest." Family members may see references to "civil rights" and "trusting relationship" as a cop-out and argue that practitioners invoke confidentiality because they are frightened to deal with families, negligent, indifferent, or lazy.[18] While there are no doubt indifferent practitioners, there are also many who take the client-clinician relationship very seriously, meaning, unfortunately, that there is often no "middle ground."

Newcomers to the mental health field may wonder why more clients simply do not consent to having information shared. While some do, the fact remains that, in many cases, persons with serious mental disorders are estranged from their immediate family, particularly the parents, and when asked do not consent to share information (Perreault et al. 2005). For example, a 2010 survey of the Vancouver, BC, adult mental health teams found that over half of the roughly thirty-five hundred clients could be considered estranged, that is, that they had no regular contact with family and none at all in the previous year.

How does estrangement from family come about? In some cases it happens when parents misunderstand the nature of psychiatric disorders and interpret their child's behaviour as willfulness or laziness, leading to a falling out between them. A falling out may also occur when parents become involved in evicting the young person from the family home or, especially, in arranging an involuntary hospitalization, necessitated by the individual's refusal to get treatment. Lefley (1997, 9) describes the dilemma this situation creates for parents:

> Pragmatically and emotionally, family members view the involuntary intervention as an undesirable but essential safety net. Like mental health care consumers and all persons concerned with civil liberties, families would greatly prefer alternatives to involuntary interventions. They are humiliating and painful to all concerned. They not only have an adverse impact on the self-esteem and integrity of the individuals involved but also may generate resentment and alienation against family members faced with impossible choices.

Other sources of tension include situations in which children have been abused by their parents or claim abuse, situations in which they have the view that insufficient financial and material support has been offered to them by family and, in some cases, situations in which family members have become incorporated into a client's delusional system.

It can be argued that service providers could do more to promote and facilitate the connection between client and family member, particularly if it appears to be in the client's best interests. Families may be an important resource and support for clients, and they can also provide key information to the clinician, such as "early warning signs" of a worsening mental state. Clinicians may be reassured by the "need to know" principle in information sharing; that is, that parents do not need to know all the details – nor do they usually request this – and that more limited releases may still support the family connection. Sometimes there is no consent from the client simply because *the question has never been asked*. Agencies, as part of their intake process, should include a section in which the client can nominate a family member, friend, or other ally with whom information can be shared under certain conditions. This may be "in case of emergency," and, in fact, other forms used in mental health programs, such as crisis plans, may also include a reference to this. Forms can stipulate with whom the information may be shared, the nature of the information, and how long the consent lasts. Information sharing and crisis planning may also be covered in legal directives such as representation agreements. Consent can be seen as existing on a continuum rather than as a single decision at one point in time that is forever binding. It has also been suggested that the onus for initiating the consent process should be *on the practitioner*, not the consumer or family member, who may feel intimidated (Bogart and Solomon, 1999).

Information sharing without client consent can occur (1) when there are concerns about safety (as was noted earlier in the chapter), and (2) to support continuity of care of the client. The safety exceptions are contained in provincial freedom of information statutes, and family advocacy organizations have argued that practitioners appear to lack knowledge of the law in this area (see North Shore Schizophrenia Society 2010). "Continuity of care" applies between caregivers, such as a hospital that shares records with a GP concerning tests undergone by a patient. In BC's Freedom of Information and Protection of Privacy Act, for example this is contained in section 33, the "consistent use" provision, which, according to a provincial government publication, may allow sharing of information without consent with parents, if they are caregivers. The *Guide to the Mental Health Act* (BC Ministry of Health 2005, 121) provides the following example:

> An adult with schizophrenia is being discharged from a psychiatric unit. Although she does not have a close relationship with her family, they do take an active role in ensuring her day-to-day needs for food and shelter are met, and they also monitor her health status. The client is suspicious and distrustful of her family members, and asks her clinician not to share any information about her with them.

The *Guide* provides the following analysis:

> In deciding whether or not to disclose the client's personal information to
> the family, the health care provider should consider whether the family's
> "need to know" outweighs the client's wishes. If the provider believes it is
> in the best interests of the client to disclose personal information to the
> family so they can provide care to the client, the health care provider may
> do so [section 33.2(a)]. The provider should exercise caution to ensure only
> necessary information is released (B.C. Ministry of Health 2005, 121).

The balancing of interests is not easily achieved in this example; the parents
are clearly supporting the health of their daughter in the community, yet she
has explicitly requested that information not be shared.

Philosophy of Care and "Recovery"
A third area of tension that may arise in the family-practitioner relationship
has to do with approaches to care. Family members with a seriously ill relative, quite naturally, want care providers to err on the side of caution and to
be proactive in their approach – for example, hospitalizing the individual
sooner rather than later. In a 2009 family focus group facilitated by this
author, one of the participants described her unending anxiety concerning
her daughter: "There's a constant feeling of vigilance, especially when the
illness is more active. A feeling that if you let your guard down when they
are ill, they will commit suicide." The mother's perception is supported by
data showing that seriously mentally ill persons are indeed at higher risk for
suicide, financial and sexual exploitation, self-neglect, and premature death
from medical conditions. In short, in these cases families want care providers
to be *paternalistic*, for lack of a better word (e.g., Inman 2011c).

On the other hand, as we have discussed, we have entered an era of recovery-
informed practice. Clinicians are now expected to limit coercion and to
support risk-taking and self-determination. In short, they are expected *not*
to be paternalistic. Apart from a recovery-orientation, a clinician's decision
making about involuntary treatment is further complicated by (1) the need
to maintain trust with the client – a trust that may be broken when the client
is sent to hospital – and (2) the fact that, given the pressure on hospital beds,
the client will in many cases be discharged in just a few days. It can be argued
that involuntary hospitalization, while expedient, is a crude, all-or-nothing
approach that does not solve any longer-term issues. Clearly, clinicians must
at times err on the side of caution; the question is whether this stance must
be adopted indefinitely.

Service users have also taken issue with what is seen as a paternalistic approach endorsed by family members, the following personal account provides an example: "Authoritarian families curtail growth with coercive interventions ... accentuating the non-negotiable authority of the medical profession ... [P]erhaps the hardest, arguably the most important part of parenting is to trust the child enough to let go. Even children with disabilities deserve to be let go" (Caras 1998, 763-64).

In sum, families may be uneasy about any model of care that speaks about risk-taking and "alternatives" to conventional psychiatric interventions, which is something the recovery literature does. There is also the view that the concept of "recovery" simply does not apply to a serious illness like schizophrenia (Brean 2011; Inman 2011b). Concerns about this approach led to family members protesting the appointment of a professor from the University of Ottawa to the Mental Health Commission of Canada's Family Advisory Committee, given that individual's known support for alternative approaches and a recovery-orientation (Brean 2010). The apprehension about a new model may, in part, be a misunderstanding in that some analysis appears to conflate "recovery" with "anti-psychiatry" (which is made more likely given the lack of clarity and consensus about the former term). Nevertheless, a fuller implementation of recovery-oriented services will have to contend with potentially strong opposition from the family lobby.

Family Organizations and Agendas

The interests of families are advanced by family support organizations, examples being the Schizophrenia Society in Canada, the Schizophrenia Fellowship of New South Wales in Australia, and the National Alliance on Mentally Illness (NAMI) in the US (NAMI was formed as a grassroots movement in the late 1970s, initially to protest Freudian theory, which, as noted earlier, was seen as blaming mothers [Foulkes 2000].) The Schizophrenia Society provides direct services, such as information, referral, and educational programs, which include visits to classrooms and groups for families and friends such as Strengthening Families Together, a ten-session curriculum that is now available free online (see http://www.schizophrenia.on.ca/component/content/article/102.html).

Organizations like the Schizophrenia Society and NAMI also lobby on behalf of the mentally ill, raise systemic concerns, and provide advocacy support to individual families. In lobbying for more resources and launching anti-stigma campaigns, family organizations are supporting causes with which most other stakeholder groups are congenial. There are, however, agendas that have been polarizing (Caras 1998; Morrison 2005; Ross 2011a).

For one thing, family organizations support a medical conceptualization of mental disorder, a view that these are "severe brain disorders" that need appropriate pharmacological treatments (Reyers 2011; Whitaker 2010). Professional medical attention is seen as the only legitimate response, and alternative treatments are usually not endorsed. For example, in an interview, the president of a Canadian chapter of the Schizophrenia Society argues against the idea that recovery must be self-directed, stating that real recovery "requires a lot of not just support but structure, *provided by others*" (quoted in Brean 2011, emphasis added). Family organizations are supportive of medical research that looks for genetic factors and "biomarkers" as causal explanations.[19] On this point, there has been great interest in the concept of "anosognosia," which, if proven to be associated with schizophrenia, would help confirm the "hard-wired," intractable, and hence very serious character of the illness (and, further, its legitimacy). Conversely, there is some discomfort about talk of social determinants of health and the concept of prevention in psychiatry, for at least a couple of reasons. One is the concern that looking at trauma and early life experiences may have the potential, again, to blame families. The other concern involves resource allocation: Should funds be spent on population health strategies when we have, right here and now, very ill people who need treatment and research support? And family organizations very much favour "access to treatment," which, apart from sufficient resources, means committal laws that are not overly restrictive and the use of involuntary treatment (Goering, Wasylenki, and Durbin 2000; Hall 2000; North Shore Schizophrenia Society 2011). A more hardline approach to this issue is taken by the Treatment Advocacy Center in the US, whose mission includes "ensuring that individuals receive adequate psychiatric services and maintain medication compliance upon release from hospitals" and "educating policymakers and judges about the true nature of severe brain disorders, advanced treatments available for those illnesses, and the necessity of court-ordered treatment in some cases" (http://www.treatmentadvocacycenter.org/about-us).

Not surprisingly, this agenda is not supported by civil rights proponents and consumer-run advocacy and support organizations (referred to earlier in this chapter). Morrison (2005) describes at some length the "ongoing battle" in the US between consumer groups, on the one hand, and NAMI and the Treatment Advocacy Center, on the other. In a personal account disability rights advocate Sylvia Caras (1998, 763-64) takes issue with the "family lobby" – organized "to protect themselves from blame" – and which she sees as very much "engrossed" with "family image and misery," while the voice of the ill relative is suppressed or co-opted. Caras is referring here to families who, at public forums, describe their travails with the ill relative and, in so doing, "regularly breach privacy by telling their children's stories" and "sensationalize their children's antisocial activities." In some cases, unlike the author of this account, the ill family member will be part of, and go along with, the presentation. Morrison (2005, 149) refers to these individuals as "good, docile consumers."

In Canada, the "access to treatment" issue has led to clashes between consumer and family groups. For example, a dispute between practitioners and family organizations, on the one side, and civil rights advocates, on the other, dragged out the process of amending the British Columbia Mental Health Act by several years in the mid-1990s (Davis 1995b) (this statute governs the involuntary treatment and detention of mentally ill persons). In another example, the Schizophrenia Society of Ontario's appeal to legislators to support the implementation of community treatment orders (an involuntary outpatient condition) was strenuously opposed by clients' rights groups (Oakes 2003). More recently, as was discussed earlier, family advocates have expressed concern and disagreement with policy directions and appointments by the Mental Health Commission of Canada, which is seen as leaning too much towards a recovery-orientation and too far away from the medical model (Brean 2010; Ross 2011b). Significantly, the MHCC (2009) has explicitly named health promotion and prevention as one of its priorities for a reformed mental health system, which, as noted, is not seen as a priority by advocates speaking for families.

What about the relationship between family support groups and practitioners? Generally, if one is talking about clinicians working within a medical model, then the interests of the two groups would tend to align. If, however, one is talking about working within a recovery orientation that supports risk-taking and shared decision making (the latter apparently made dubious in the case of anosognosia), then, as we have discussed, there is the potential for friction. Even within a medical model, family members may be dissatisfied with the quantity and quality of follow-up offered to their relative, especially when the family member believes that the client is at risk and the clinician is not being sufficiently attentive or proactive. In these instances, organizations such as the Schizophrenia Society have supported family concerns by, for example, requesting and facilitating meetings between relatives and treatment personnel, and by drafting checklists of questions to assist relatives who may be uncertain about what to say in their dealings with professionals. This is arguably a reasonable approach, even though the clinician may feel uncomfortable about what appears to be second-guessing or challenging professional authority, since it is a means of ensuring accountability. This is especially so given our stated aim of greater inclusion of families, as reflected in recent policy documents. A more recent tactic used by some chapters of the Schizophrenia Society has been to articulate concerns about professional conduct in newsletters, internet bulletins, and news releases, naming the organization (although not the individual) and the client situation. For example, on the website of the North Shore Schizophrenia Society (http://www.northshoreschizophrenia.org), a BC chapter, in the "media centre" and "advocacy bulletin" a series of grievances against the local health authority are detailed, referring to negligent care, an unwillingness to certify people to hospital, hospitals discharging persons too soon, and doctors either not understanding statutory certification standards or applying them too narrowly.

Notes

1 "Nothing about us without us" can also be seen as a general principle underpinning person-centred care (e.g., one's relationship with a family doctor).

2 Provincial medical plans can limit the amount of time a psychiatrist may bill for an individual client.

3 There are no doubt a number of reasons for this finding, an apparent one being a mismatch between supply of and demand for psychiatric services. Also, if the treatment provided is long-term in nature (e.g., psychoanalysis), then there is limited client turnover. The article by Goldner and colleagues cited here reports on a survey of Vancouver-area psychiatrists, which found that only 24 percent – about one in four – of a sample of nearly three hundred were able to take on new clients, with the vast majority of the 24 percent not being able to commit to a date for the first appointment.

4 See the national website at: http://www.npcanada.ca/portal/index.php?option=com_frontpage&Itemid=1.

5 Based on local experience, this author's observation is that the role of social work in hospital discharge-planning has been diminished in recent years, with fewer social workers employed in secondary and tertiary care settings, and discharges being taken over by other individuals or specialized teams.

6 Litigation may be more of a reality in the US. For example, a 2008 survey of American psychiatrists found "threat of malpractice" to have had a "significant negative impact on career satisfaction" among respondents (DeMello and Deshpande 2011, 1013).

7 A later CMA (2004, 3) publication states that physicians should "be considerate of the patient's family and significant others and cooperate with them in the patient's interests," *without* elaborating on putting the patient first (although this document is directed at all MDs, not specifically psychiatrists).

8 *Tarasoff v. Regents of the University of California*, 188 Cal. Rptr. 129, 529 P2d 533, 1974.

9 *Smith v. Jones*, 169 D.L.R. (4th) 385 (S.C.C.), 1999.

10 The study by Covel and colleagues (2007) and other works cited in their article suggest a modest preference for "client," with "patient" second and "consumer" third. Writing in 2013, I have been told a number of times by service users on committees about their discomfort with the term "consumer." In a personal account, Hensley (2006) suggests that calling someone a "mental health consumer" is equivalent to calling a person with heart disease a "cardiology consumer," which means that the person is still identified by her/his illness ("schizophrenic"), albeit in a slightly different fashion.

11 See http://www.power2u.org/.

12　This has been referred to as the "thank you theory," proposed by Harvard academic Alan Stone in the 1970s.

13　While the terms "survivor" and "ex-patient" clearly have a challenging ring to them, "consumer," as noted, has been adopted by health authorities and practitioner-authors, and so its use is not necessarily reflective of an anti-psychiatry stance, despite the discomfort of some professionals (Torrey 2011a).

14　This claim is based on my own experience.

15　This quote comes from a 2010 survey of staff working at the Vancouver Community Mental Health Teams (Vancouver Coastal Health Authority).

16　Interestingly, a more recent article on the mental health of Aboriginal persons in Canada pulls the "double-bind" out of mothballs, at least in a metaphorical sense, as a way of understanding conflicting cultural pressures faced by the Innu of northern Quebec (Samson 2009; see also Chapter 6).

17　This anecdote, if accurate, also highlights a significant lack of discretion and professionalism on the part of the psychiatrist.

18　The contentious nature of client confidentiality is reflected in the newsletter of a chapter of the Schizophrenia Society of Canada, which refers to "the [clinician's] need to establish a relationship of trust with the patient" as "a faddish notion" (North Shore Schizophrenia Society 2009, 1). Concerning relationships with the mentally ill person, families may sometimes argue that if someone has to be the "bad cop" (making a decision with which the client is unhappy) then it should be the clinician, not the family member.

19　See Whitaker (2010) for a description of how NAMI and the American Psychiatric Association formally started collaborating in the 1980s to, among other things, lobby Congress to increase funding for biomedical and pharmacological research. See also Lieberman (2011) concerning research on "biomarkers."

Other Resources

For examples of groups representing service users that have a skeptical or critical view of the medical model, see the National Empowerment Center (http://www.power2u.org) and Mindfreedom (http://www.mindfreedom.org). For an example of an advocacy group that aligns itself closely with the medical model and involuntary treatment initiatives, see the Treatment Advocacy Center http://www.treatmentadvocacycenter.org and the writings of its founder, American psychiatrist E. Fuller Torrey.

The Family Association for Mental Health Everywhere (FAME) provides information for family members with a mentally ill relative: http://fameforfamilies.com.

Consumers' Health Awareness Network Newfoundland and Labrador (CHANNAL) is a provincial organization whose mandate is to build and strengthen a self-help network among individuals who live with mental illness: http://channal.ca.

The Drug Companies

8

This chapter deliberately follows a chapter that was concerned with stakeholders since, for better or worse, the pharmaceutical industry is an influential player in the mental health system, shaping public and practitioner perceptions about the nature of, and appropriate response to, mental disorders. Medication forms the cornerstone of the treatment offered in most Canadian community mental health settings, and, for many clients, it must be acknowledged that psychotropic drugs are an important component of their treatment. For example, a person suffering from delusions because of a schizophrenic illness will be less able to benefit from other rehabilitation approaches without first having those symptoms treated medically. Notwithstanding this, there is the argument that, with their considerable financial resources, the drug companies wield disproportionate influence with respect to mental health practice and policy – leading to what some see as an over-reliance on medication – and that the profit incentive inevitably results in a biased picture of pharmaceutical benefits. By partnering with and offering inducements to the medical community, the drug companies, it has been argued, help "manufacture consensus." As a professor at the University of Washington observes: "By subsidizing one research program instead of another, one conference or symposium, one journal, one publication, one learned society and so on, the pharmaceutical industry doesn't just make precious allies among the 'key opinion leaders' of the medical establishment, it also gains a very efficient means of steering the academic discussion toward the illnesses that interest it at any given moment" (Borch-Jacobson 2011). These concerns are addressed in this chapter.

Profits and Costs

Pharmaceuticals have historically been a very profitable industry (Angell 2004; Boodman 2012; Whitaker 2010). In Canada, spending on prescription drugs increased dramatically through the 1980s to the 2000s, reaching a figure of approximately $31 billion in 2010 (Canadian Institute for Health Information 2011b). The annual rate of increase declined later in the 2000s, to 4.8 percent in 2010, after having seen annual increases of about 9 percent in the first half of the decade (Canadian Institute for Health Information 2011b). During this period of increased spending, pharmaceuticals became the second largest component of the health care budget in Canada, next to hospitals, having exceeded the cost of physician expenses in the late 1990s, which put considerable budgetary pressure on Canada's pharmacare programs (Thomson 2003). It has been argued that more restrained drug spending would, for example, enable the hiring of more family physicians and other health care providers (Sernyak and Rosenheck 2004; Smith 2007a).

What was behind the surge in pharmaceutical spending seen in the 1980s and 1990s? Two important factors are patterns of use and product cost. Concerning the first factor, over this period more people were getting prescriptions, and more prescriptions per patient were being written (Pollack et al. 2009). As an illustration, in the US, the number of people who were prescribed an antidepressant grew from 13 million in 1996 to 27 million in 2005, with researchers additionally finding that over the decade more of this group were *also* being prescribed antipsychotics (Olfson and Marcus 2009; see also Fullerton et al. 2011). (Antipsychotic drugs are now being touted as an adjunctive treatment for mood disorders.) Antidepressant usage grew by a similar rate in Canada during this period (Branham 2003; Newman and Schopflocher 2008; Raymond, Morgan and Caetano 2007). In 2007, psychotropic drugs accounted for 12.5 percent of prescriptions dispensed by community pharmacies in Canada, second only to cardiovascular agents (Institute for Safe Medication Practices Canada 2012). Some of the increase seen in Canada and the US is the result of "off label" prescribing – ordering for conditions or populations, such as children, not specified within the product's monograph or licence. For example, in Canada there was a significant increase in prescriptions of antidepressant medication for persons under 18 from the 1990s to the 2000s (Branham 2004; Mitchell et al. 2008), and a 114 percent increase of antipsychotic drug prescriptions for this age group from 2005 to 2009, as treatments for conditions such as ADHD, conduct disorder, and behavioural problems (Kirkey 2013). In the US, off-label prescriptions of antipsychotic drugs doubled from 1995 to 2008 (Boodman 2012). It has also been argued that increased usage is due to more people being prescribed drugs who do not in fact meet the diagnostic threshold of the syndrome, depression in particular (Glenmullen 2000). In trying to understand this, researchers have found a greater comfort level about the use of psychotropic medication among family physicians and members of the public than was the case previously (Slomp et al. 2009; Vasiliadis et al. 2005; Watson et al.

2005). Concerning public attitudes, a survey of the US general population conducted by the National Opinion Research Center at the University of Chicago found that opinions about psychiatric medications became more favourable from the mid-1990s to the mid-2000s, with a substantial majority of respondents expressing that these drugs "helped to deal with day-to-day stresses," "made things easier in relations with family and friends," and "help[ed] people feel better about themselves" (Mojtabai 2009, 1015).

In addition to wider usage, increased spending on psychopharmacological products was due to the advent and successful promotion of "new generation" drugs in the 1980s and 1990s, agents that were *considerably* more expensive than their predecessors (Dewa et al. 2002). These drugs include the "atypical" antipsychotics, and the selective serotonin reuptake inhibitor (SSRI) class of antidepressants. The "atypicals" were advertised as a breakthrough in the treatment of schizophrenia, ameliorating a wider range of symptoms while producing fewer side effects. There was, as this author can attest, a feeling of increased optimism among clinicians at the time, although in the long run the drugs did not turn out to be that "atypical" and the hope of a breakthrough was not ultimately borne out. Enthusiasm may be related to "newness," in and of itself: there had seemingly been few advances in antipsychotic treatment since the advent of chlorpromazine decades earlier, so clinicians were ready to be optimistic. (The perception of "newness" may also be seen, for example, in public attitudes towards the drug lithium, still an effective treatment for bipolar disorder but regarded dubiously by some potential users simply because the product has been around for so long.)

The profitability of new drugs, like the atypicals and SSRIs, is ensured by patent protection, whereby governments legislatively limit the production of cheaper, generic equivalents by rival companies. As patents expire, particularly when several "blockbuster" drugs go off patent at the same time, companies may face a reversal of fortune. This was apparently the case in 2011, with one industry observer stating that it was "panic time" in that most companies realized "they don't have enough products in the pipeline or the portfolio, don't have enough revenue to sustain their research and development" (quoted in Wilson 2011; see also Jung 2012).

Patent laws are constrained by international trade agreements. In Canada, Bill C-22, enacted in 1987, weakened the licensing arrangement that permitted Canadian-made generic drugs to reach the market before brand-name patents had expired, a move that was purportedly made to gain US approval of the North American Free Trade Agreement (Fuller 1998). In 1993, Bill C-91 was enacted, giving twenty-year patent protection to brand-name medications, which a researcher at the Canadian Centre for Policy Alternatives characterized as a "deregulation of the drug industry [that] led to spectacular increases in the cost of drugs" (191). Currently, brand-name drugs have twenty years of patent protection in Canada (Jung 2012).

Drug patenting is a controversial issue. Lobbyists for the pharmaceutical industry speak about intellectual property rights, the importance of innovation, and thus the need to protect the research enterprise at these companies. It is also suggested that a healthy climate for research-based companies means more job creation and investment opportunities (Hadekel 2011). On the other side, critics of the drug companies argue that patents enable profiteering, result in First World/Third World inequities, and are not supportable by either the "cost of research" or the "innovation" claims. On profiteering, patent protection means there is no price competition. Goldacre (2008) provides the example of the drug loratidine, a "non-drowsy" antihistamine that initially dominated the market, and whose price was increased thirteen times in five years before the patent ran out. On inequities, drug companies resist supplying desperately needed medication (such as HIV drugs) to African countries too poor to afford the full cost because, so the story goes, the money from sales is needed to support research and development. While drug research may indeed be expensive, skeptics note that that the proportion of revenue spent by drug companies on research and development is still much less than that spent on "marketing and administration" (i.e., advertising) (Angell 2004). For example, a study by researchers at Toronto's York University determined that, in 2004, American drug companies spent $57.5 billion on promotional activities, 83 percent more than the $31.5 billion spent on research and development (Gagnon and Lexchin 2008). The importance of marketing in relation to research can also be seen by the difference in the number of staff working in these areas: American researchers found that between 1995 and 2000, there was a 59 percent increase in the number of marketing positions at pharmaceutical companies, while the number of research positions remained almost static (Pollack et al. 2009).

What about innovation? While drug companies may refer to newer products as "novel" or "atypical," in many cases they are merely slight variations on older agents, often with no new active ingredients and usually with no substantial therapeutic advantage over existing products. These are referred to as "me-too" drugs (Smith 2007b). British physician and author Ben Goldacre (2008, 185) notes that the number of "new molecular entities" being patented has dwindled since the 1990s, while the number of "me-too" drugs has increased:

> Me-too drugs are an inevitable function of the market: they are rough copies of drugs that already exist ... but are different enough for a manufacturer to be able to claim their own patent ... Sometimes they offer modest benefits

Figure 4

The chemical structures of paliperidone (Invega) and risperidone (Risperdal)

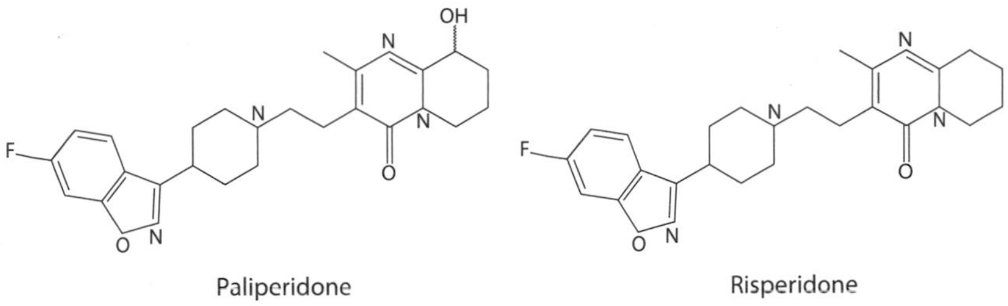

Paliperidone   Risperidone

(a more convenient dosing regime, for example), but for all the hard work they involve, they don't generally represent a significant breakthrough in human health. They are merely a breakthrough in making money.

(By way of example, in Figure 4, the newer antipsychotic paliperidone contrasted with the older drug risperidone – from which it is derived – and to which it is structurally identical except for the extra hydroxyl group.) A study in BC found that per person spending on prescription drugs more than doubled from 1996 to 2003 ($141 to $316) and that "me-too" drugs accounted for 80 percent of these rising costs (Smith 2007b).

Disease Mongering?

As noted, a wider range of people are being prescribed psychotropic medication than was the case thirty years ago – antidepressants in particular (Patten and Beck 2004; Smith 2011). Is this a good thing? It can be argued that, since depression has been historically under-reported – at least in part because of the stigma attached to psychiatric disorders – having more people in treatment is a positive development, albeit with some caveats. In general, medication is appropriate when (a) the person has a serious clinical condition and (b) the drug is effective in treating that condition (see Narrow et al. 2002).[1] Concerning point "b," we know that a majority of persons suffering from the positive symptoms of schizophrenia will benefit from antipsychotic medication. With depression, however, the picture is murkier: reviews of the available data suggest that a significant proportion of the benefit seen with antidepressants, especially for less serious forms of the disorder, is related to a placebo effect (which is still a benefit; this issue is discussed in greater detail in Chapter 15) (Begley 2010; Kirsch 2002; Kirsch et al. 2008; Vedantam 2002).

This then leads into point (a) above: whether it can be said that a particular experience constitutes a significant clinical condition – a pathology – warranting pharmaceutical treatment, particularly given the side effects that come with these products. For someone who is extremely ill, the cost-benefit equation would favour risking the side effects. On the other hand, should someone be given medication for a mild form of depression – something that will affect many of us – when we know that, with time, and "watchful waiting," there is a strong likelihood that it will go away on its own (Meredith et al. 2007)? Those responding "yes" would say, first, that if we have a tool available we should use it and, further, that in applying a medical treatment the practitioner is playing an important role in de-stigmatizing mental conditions – that is, having them seen as an illness rather than as a weakness or character flaw (Whitaker 2010). On the other hand, those replying "not necessarily" to the question would say that using a pharmacological treatment for milder forms of depression means going down a slippery slope, resulting in an increasingly wide range of human experiences in effect being labelled as abnormal and thus falling under the jurisdiction of the drug companies (Branham 2003; Peyser 2004). This process has been called by some "disease mongering," which is defined by Dictionary.com as "efforts by a pharmaceutical company to create or exaggerate a malady for the purpose of increasing sales of a medication." This may mean expanding the indications for drug treatment to cover less serious forms of an existing illness (Moncrieff 2009), or a wider age-range, or, in fact, to staking out new turf (i.e., a condition or experience not previously treated pharmacologically, such as "pre-diabetes" or "pre-hypertension") (Pollack et al. 2009; see also Kleiner 2011). For example, concerning the age-range, in 2011 the American Academy of Pediatrics revised its guidelines for attention deficit hyperactivity disorder (ADHD), lowering the age at which a diagnosis and pharmacological treatment could be applied from six to four. In response to this a prominent psychiatrist observed that "we have already experienced a vast expansion in the diagnosis and medication treatment of ADHD" and that this would lead to "a further feeding frenzy of aggressive marketing by drug companies" (quoted in Kirkey 2011). A physician defending the change argued that, by diagnosing and treating earlier, care providers were "trying to prevent kids from getting into situations where they are getting messages that make them think that they're bad kids" (quoted in Kirkey 2011).

Increasingly, there is evidence that drug company advertisements now promote medical conditions rather than just drugs, as Canadian academic Barbara Mintzes found in her PhD research: "To an unprecedented degree they portray the educational message of a pill for every ill – and increasingly an ill for every pill. It's a shift from a drug that's approved to treat people who are actually suffering from an illness to the idea that you just take a pill to deal with normal life situations" (quoted in Moynihan and Cassels 2005, 103). British physician Ben Goldacre (2008, 153) suggests that, "because they cannot find *new treatments* for the diseases we already have, the pill companies instead invent *new diseases* for the treatments" (emphasis in original). He uses as examples "female sexual dysfunction" (a new use for Viagra) and "night eating syndrome" (a new use for SSRI antidepressants),[2] and he observes that, while loss of libido may be a real problem, it is "not necessarily the stuff of pills, and perhaps best not conceived of in reductionist biomedical terms," adding that such an approach is "frankly disempowering" (153).

In their book *Selling Sickness,* Moynihan and Cassels (2005) use the examples of "premenstrual syndrome (PMS)," and the later variant "premenstrual dysphoric disorder (PMDD)," to illustrate disease mongering. The idea of PMS as a condition manifesting through irritability and moodiness first arose in the 1960s. Critics of this proposed syndrome pointed out, first, that the criteria were extremely vague and, second, that "women everywhere experience tension [and] irritability ... prior to monthly periods, [but] do not believe this is abnormal or feel any need for professional intervention" (Moynihan and Cassels 2005, 107). In response to this an attempt was made to distinguish a more severe form of mood disturbance, "serious enough in some women to be disabling and warrant treatment" (108), and "late luteal phase dysphoric disorder" (LLPDD) was proposed for inclusion in diagnostic manuals in the 1980s. More debate ensued, with proponents, ironically, using lack of knowledge about the new condition as a reason to add it to manuals to "facilitate more research on its causes and treatments" (109). As with PMS, critics expressed concern about labelling experiences of ordinary life as a mental disorder. The rebuttal to this was that the same arguments could be made about other conditions that exist on a continuum, such as depression, and that the appropriate course was to be careful in defining the boundary between normal and pathological. Despite the opposition, LLPDD was added as a provisional diagnosis (requiring further research) in the appendix of the 1987 revision of the American Psychiatric Association's *Diagnostic and Statistical Manual.* There continued to be lack of consensus about the validity of the proposed syndrome, but LLPDD, now renamed PMDD, was again included in the next (1994) revision of the *DSM* and, significantly, was now in the main body of the manual – non-provisional – as a variant of depression (depressive disorder not otherwise specified). With this inclusion, there was a clearer mandate for "doctors to prescribe drugs to treat the condition, and health insurers to fund them" (110). At this point, the drug companies enter the picture: Lilly, manufacturer of the highly profitable antidepressant Prozac, was about to lose a lot of money as this drug went off patent, with cheaper generics then becoming available. Lilly entered into discussions with psychiatrists pushing for the acceptance of PMDD, with the outcome that Prozac, under the new name "Sarafem" (now packaged in a lavender-coloured box with pictures of sunflowers), became approved by the US Food and Drug Administration as a treatment for PMDD, thus potentially extending the lifespan and profitability of Prozac – all this with still no consensus, even within the psychiatric community, about the validity of the syndrome.

Disease mongering may also occur in the context of drug company "illness awareness" campaigns – a potentially useful public service – in that the ostensible problem is almost always framed as a biological one that requires biological treatments. Pollack and colleagues (2009, 2) note that "pharmaceutical industry-funded disease awareness campaigns [are] more often designed to sell drugs than to illuminate, inform or educate about the prevention of illness or the maintenance of health." While direct-to-consumer ads for pharmaceutical products are restricted in Canada, drug companies may nonetheless run "awareness sites" on the internet such as Eli Lilly's "Depression Hurts": http://www.depressionhurts.ca/en/. A visitor to this site may assume it is a government-sponsored educational vehicle since nowhere is there a reference to any for-profit company until one clicks on the "terms of use" or "privacy statement" links at the bottom of the page. The "FAQ" section of the site includes the question "what causes depression?," then gives the answer: "One common theory is that depression is caused by an imbalance of naturally occurring substances called neurotransmitters in the brain and spinal cord." Nowhere in this section is there any reference to the psychosocial determinants of mood problems. Similarly, in the section "questions about treatment," all of the questions refer only to treatment with medication.

Product Promotion

As noted, the drug companies spend a lot of money marketing their products. A 2007 American study by health policy researchers, published in the *New England Journal of Medicine*, found that the largest proportion of this went to sales representatives visiting and providing free medication samples, gifts, and food for physicians;[3] 14 percent went to direct-to-consumer advertisements and only 2 percent to professional journal ads (Donohue, Cevasco, and Rosenthal 2007).[4] In 2005, it was estimated that there were over 100,000 drug sales representatives in the US, about one for every eight practising physicians (Pollack et al. 2009; Roslin 2008). In Canada, the number of sales reps increased by 30 percent – 3,990 to 5,190 – in the five-year period from

1998 to 2002, working out to about one rep for every eleven doctors (Roslin 2008). A survey by the British Columbia Medical Association found that two-thirds of physicians had a sales rep visit them at least once a month, with general practitioners experiencing the heaviest traffic: 42 percent of this group reported several visits a week. GP contact is significant since they are the major prescribers of psychotropic medication, antidepressants in particular (e.g., Slomp et al. 2009).

How influential are sales reps? When asked, doctors tend to say that promotion activities do not affect their prescribing practices (Pollack et al. 2009). This was found to be the case in a report by Canadian journalist Alex Roslin, who asked several physicians about attending drug company-sponsored educational evenings, where food and beverages were free. One respondent stated:

> I see drug reps every day, and I don't feel any pressure ... I would say by far the majority of reps are professional and we develop a relationship of trust ... I do appreciate hearing from pharmaceutical drug reps in a busy practice. It helps keep me up-to-date ... Yes, we go to dinners put on by companies, and I believe I'm representative of my colleagues. But are we swayed? Not on your life. I pick what's best for my patients. (quoted in Roslin 2008, 4)

Another respondent echoed: "Most physicians I've interacted with are comfortable accepting meals and don't think it influences them" (although adding that "that goes against all the literature, obviously") (quoted in Roslin 2008, 6). The comment about drug reps keeping the physician "up to date" is significant since there is considerable evidence that the information presented is biased to favour the salesperson's own product (more on this below). In reviewing the survey literature, Roslin concludes that "many doctors still rely on [sales reps] more than any other source for information about new drugs" (7).

The influence of sales rep promotion was investigated by McGill University psychiatry resident Ashley Wazana (2000), who reviewed twenty-nine published studies on the subject. The review found that physicians receiving free samples, research grants, free trips, and other honoraria were significantly more likely to prescribe the drug being promoted. This association appeared to be "dose-related" (no pun intended), in that doctors who went to free dinners on a frequent basis were more likely to request that the promoted drug be added to a hospital formulary than those who only went on an occasional basis. Similarly, a later survey of 473 US psychiatrists found a strong positive association between frequency of visits with sales reps and optimism about newer-generation psychotropic drugs (Arbuckle et al. 2008).[5]

In addition to physicians, since 1997 the marketing of pharmaceuticals has included "direct-to-consumer" (DTC) approaches in the United States.[6] The budget for DTC advertising increased substantially over the next ten years, both in dollar terms and as a percentage of all promotional spending, reaching a figure of about $5 billion annually (Alexander 2009). This form of advertising has proven effective in increasing sales (Pollack et al. 2009) but remains controversial. Proponents of DTC advertising suggest that it is a legitimate public health service, that it empowers clients, and that it addresses unmet needs with respect to persons who lack knowledge and who are suffering unnecessarily with an untreated condition (Alexander 2009; Gilbody, Wilson, and Watt 2004). The more widespread use of antidepressant medication is attributed in part to DTC advertising, which "both increased recognition of the symptoms of depression and diminished stigma associated with the disease, resulting in higher treatment rates" (Harman, Edlund, and Fortney 2009, 611). Opponents of DTC, on the other hand, argue that "ads entice patients to insist on unnecessary or ineffective drugs and to forego health lifestyle changes that might obviate the need for drugs in the first place" (Alexander 2009). Concerning the practitioner-client relationship, Hoffman and Wilkes (1999, 1,302) suggest that DTC advertising "unreasonably increases consumer expectations, forces doctors to spend time disabusing patients of misinformation, diminishes the doctor-patient relationship because a doctor refuses to prescribe an advertised drug, or results in poor practice if the doctor capitulates and prescribes an inappropriate agent." Finally, Canadian drug policy analyst Barbara Mintzes notes that "companies almost always advertise their newest and costliest products [when] usually very little is known about long-term risks" (quoted in Thomson 2010, 27).

To examine the influence of DTC advertising, a team of Canadian and American researchers surveyed a group of physicians in both countries, finding that "patient's requests. for medicines are a powerful driver of prescribing decisions" in that patients requesting a particular drug in the study were more likely to receive one, even though in about 45 percent of cases the doctor expressed ambivalence about the drug being requested (Mintzes et al. 2002, 279) ("ambivalence" was established by responses to the question "if you were treating another similar patient with the same condition, would you prescribe this drug?"). A later US study by public health researchers in Colorado looked at the same interaction – a patient asking his or her physician specifically about a new medication – and found that over half of the time the doctor acceded to the request, even though, in 62 percent of these cases, the requested medication was not the physician's first choice (Parnes et al. 2009). In another study conducted through the Centre for

Health Services and Policy Research at the University of British Columbia, researchers asked drug policy experts from Canada, New Zealand, and the United States about their perceptions of the impact of DTC advertising and found that the majority of respondents believed that the quality of information provided through DTC advertising was poor, that there were likely to be negative effects on the appropriateness of care, and that health care costs would increase (Mintzes et al. 2001).

While DTC advertising is not in theory allowed in Canada – despite overtures from the pharmaceutical industry (Smith 2003) – in reality it is a regular occurrence, given that most Canadians have easy access to American television channels, websites, and magazines. Journalist Pamela Fayerman (2013) notes that in their use of social media – Facebook, Twitter, YouTube, and sponsored blogs – drug companies are effectively circumventing DTC laws. Some restrictions on DTC have been relaxed in Canada: in 1996, Health Canada approved "help-seeking" ads that feature a medical condition without naming a brand of medication (as with "depression hurts," above), and in 2000 it allowed "branded reminder ads that state a product brand name without saying what it's for" (Thomson 2010, 27). Thomson (2010, 27) notes that, "of all the countries that have outlawed DTC, Canada is the only one that allows this level of advertising." The Canadian Medical Association is opposed to DTC and in a policy statement warns that "advertising may stimulate demand by exaggerating risks of certain diseases and generating unnecessary fear" (Thomson 2010, 27).

Evidence Base

Physicians base their decisions about using a particular medication, in part, on clinical experience; that is, on how the drug has benefited and been tolerated by patients in their practice. For newer products, as we have seen, they may also rely on promotional material provided by pharmaceutical sales reps. A better source of evidence is that which comes from studies published in peer-reviewed journals, usually based on randomized controlled trials (RCTs), which are considered the "gold standard" in the evidence hierarchy. Because drug trials are very expensive, about 90 percent of the RCTs conducted, and 70 percent of the trials reported in major medical journals, are sponsored by the drug companies themselves (Goldacre 2008) – and therein lies the problem. As Goldacre notes, "wherever you draw your own moral line, the upshot is that drug companies have a huge influence over what gets researched, how it is researched, how the results are reported, how they are analyzed, and how they are interpreted" (187). Concerning the interpretation of results, it is a robust finding that studies funded by a particular pharmaceutical company will be more likely to find a positive result for that company's product than independent studies or studies funded by a rival company (Goldacre 2008; Vedantam 2006). For example, a series of five studies sponsored by Eli Lilly, comparing its own antipsychotic drug Zyprexa to Janssen's rival product Risperdal, found Zyprexa to be superior in treating schizophrenia in all five reports. When Janssen sponsored the research, Risperdal came out ahead in three of four trials (Vedantam 2006).

What are the possible sources of misinformation in a drug trial?[7] One limitation of RCTs is their length of follow-up and the fact that some adverse effects may only materialize after several years. This, and the incentive/disincentive of drug patenting, creates what can be seen as a three-phase cycle for new products – such as the "atypical" antipsychotics. The first phase, lasting several years, is a period of initial optimism about the new treatment, during which time the longer-term adverse effects of the medication are not well understood by clinicians. In the second phase, also lasting several years, "anecdotal information" from clinical experience starts to accumulate about problems associated with the new product. Finally, in the third phase, case reports and more systematic research about adverse effects are published, the problems are now well established, and the initial optimism is a somewhat distant memory. And, around this time, the patent for the originators of the drug is expiring, meaning that the incentive lies in coming up with a new product rather than worrying about problems associated with the old one. In sum, study designs of short duration can miss "the big picture"; that is, how clients using the drug fare over the long term (Vedantam 2006). A key longer-term variable is *tolerability*, and it is notable that a major independent comparison of four newer antipsychotics with an old one found three of the four "atypicals" to be *less* well tolerated than the older medication (as measured by drop-out over an eighteen-month follow-up period) (Lieberman et al. 2005).

Another source of misinformation in RCTs is how – or whether – a new medication is compared to other drugs. Comparison with a placebo is necessary since it is well established that some people appear to derive a benefit from the treatment *process*, unrelated to the drug itself. A problem, however, is that manufacturers may get approval to market a new drug *just* by showing it to be more effective than a placebo rather than being more effective than an existing (and possibly much cheaper) medication (Thomson 2010). Goldacre (2008, 189) suggests that superiority to a placebo "proves nothing of clinical value: in the real world nobody cares if your drug is better than a sugar pill; they only care if it is better than the best currently available treatment." A better design, then, is to compare a new product against a placebo *and* an existing product. But the comparison must be fair. An unfair comparison is with a *non-optimal* dose of the existing drug – too low or too high – in the latter case resulting in more side effects. For example, early studies of newer-generation, "atypical" antipsychotic medications found them to have fewer movement disorder side effects, but critics noted that these results were based on comparisons with control groups that were given older drugs in disproportionately high doses, which exaggerated the differences between the two groups (Goldacre 2008; Whitaker 2010; see also Rosenheck et al. 2003).

Reporting side effects is also determined by how, or whether, the question is asked. Goldacre (2008) notes that the reported prevalence of anorgasmia, a side effect of SSRI antidepressant drugs, ranges from 2 to 73 percent, depending on whether the problem is addressed in a non-specific, open-ended question, or a more detailed inquiry. He also notes that some questionnaires given to participants may not even include sexual side effects as an option. In some cases, misinformation is due to the fact that negative findings are reinterpreted or suppressed altogether. A review of trials of SSRI antidepressants published in the *New England Journal of Medicine* found extensive evidence of suppression of results (Turner et al. 2008). This review looked at studies that had been registered with the US Food and Drug Administration and how the results were then reflected in the academic literature. There were seventy-four FDA-registered studies, with thirty-eight considered by the FDA to have positive results and thirty-six to have negative or "questionable" results. All but one of the positive studies were published in the journals. Of the other thirty-six, only three were published reflecting the negative findings; twenty-two were not published at all, and eleven were published "in a way that ... conveyed a positive outcome," for example by reinterpreting adverse events (Turner et al. 2008, 252). In fairness, the drug companies may not be entirely to blame in this situation: another factor is the importance placed on finding new, positive, or "interesting" results among researchers and journal editors, meaning that studies with negative results may be submitted but not published or not even submitted (Emery 2008).

The claim of publication bias has led to litigation in a number of cases: in 2004 the Office of the Attorney General in New York launched a lawsuit against GlaxoSmithKline (GSK), the manufacturer of the antidepressant paroxetine, accusing the company of fraud (*Lancet* 2004). This suit was based on the fact that, while GSK had conducted five studies on the drug's safety and efficacy with adolescent patients, four of them, which showed the product to have mixed or negative results, were suppressed and only one was published. There was also evidence that increased suicidal ideation among patients in the trials was recoded as "emotional lability." The suit alleged that, because the partial information provided by GSK caused doctors to have a biased picture of the drug, they were unable to assess risks and benefits and thus to properly advise their patients about its use. The manufacturers of the antipsychotic Risperdal, Johnson and Johnson, were found guilty of deceptive practices in three separate trials in the US in 2010, 2011, and 2012, with penalties totalling almost $1.7 billion (LaVeque 2012). Lawsuits have arisen in Canada as well over adverse effects caused by the newer-generation antipsychotic drugs, in particular, weight gain, high blood sugar levels, and eventually, diabetes. The claim in these cases, again, was based on suppression of negative findings, with plaintiffs producing internal Eli Lilly documents indicating that the risk of their antipsychotic drug Zyprexa was being downplayed down in communications with doctors (Berenson 2008). A lawsuit against Eli Lilly and Zyprexa was concluded in 2010, with the superior courts of Ontario, Quebec, and British Columbia approving a $17.6 million settlement. The legal counsel for the drug company in this class action denied wrongdoing and stated: "Lilly is taking this difficult step because we believe it is in the best interest of the company as well as the Canadian health care professionals who depend on this important medication" (quoted in Boyle 2010).

Suppression of negative findings is also achieved by requiring clinicians to sign multiyear "nondisclosure" contracts – what some have called "gag orders" – before participating in research sponsored by a drug company (see *Canadian Medical Association Journal* 2004). When one medical researcher affiliated with the University of Toronto, Dr. Nancy Olivieri, *did* attempt to publish results of a drug trial showing the product to have unexpected risks, the sponsoring company, Apotex, quickly terminated the trial and threatened Olivieri with legal action (Robinson 2001). Fearing the loss of grant money, other clinicians may be complicit in this process and may act to quell any dissent or portrayal of the pharmaceutical industry in a bad light. An example of this is the cautionary tale of Irish psychiatrist David Healy, as recounted by journalist Robert Whitaker (2010). In the year 2000, Healy accepted a position at the University of Toronto's Centre for Addiction and Mental Health. Around that time he presented a paper on the adverse effects of antidepressants – specifically, suicidal ideation – at a psychiatric conference. After his talk a prominent American psychiatrist warned him that his "career would be destroyed if [he] kept on showing results like the one [he'd] just shown, that [he] had no right to bring out hazards of the pills like these" (quoted in Whitaker 2010, 306). Just prior to his start date in Toronto, Healy presented at a colloquium at the university, again reviewing problems associated with the SSRI medications as well as antipsychotics. Shortly after this, Healy was contacted by the university, which rescinded the job offer. In an e-mail from the psychiatric director he was told: "While you are held in high regard as a scholar ... we do not feel your approach is compatible with the goals for the development of the academic and clinical resources that we have" (quoted in Whitaker 2010, 306). Clearly, physicians involved with drug company funding are in a conflicted position (Bekelman, Li, and Gross 2003).

Concerning drug companies and the evidence base, the last word is reserved for a former editor-in-chief of the *Canadian Medical Association Journal*:

> The evidence suggests that education sponsored by the pharmaceutical industry frequently distorts the topic selection, embellishes the positive elements of studies and downplays the adverse effects. In effect, the industry focuses primarily on treatments and treatment-related issues at the expense of the larger therapeutic picture, including quality of care and patient safety not involving drugs, determinants of health, prevention and health promotion and other modalities of treatment ... [T]here is no doubt that the current continuing education enterprise compromises the ethical underpinnings and the reputation of the medical profession. Physicians are seen as being aligned with the pharmaceutical industry and with its commercial priorities. We seem to have conveniently forgotten that the pharmaceutical industry is in business to make money, not to educate health professionals. (Hebert 2008, 805)

Responses

What can be done, or is being done, to address some of the concerns reviewed in this chapter? One step is to try to put greater distance between physicians and sales representatives. This can involve an appeal to a clinician's sense of ethics but has also taken the form of legislative intervention: Roslin (2008) reports on a motion by the Massachusetts legislature to ban any gifts from sales reps to doctors as well as initiatives in other states that limit the size of gifts or require drug companies to disclose all such transactions. Some Canadian health authorities have limited the visits that sales representatives can make to community mental health programs: in this author's own agency, once-frequent educational visits by sales reps to mental health teams, which included a breakfast for all medical and non-medical staff, have been curtailed by policy.

What about the issue of researchers who are sponsored by drug companies? Given the resources and infrastructure available through the pharmaceutical industry, it may be unrealistic to expect that clinicians researching new medications will have no attachment to a sponsoring company. That said, as much as possible there should be *transparency*, both with respect to affiliation and to the research enterprise itself. The affiliation issue has been addressed, at least to a limited extent, by medical journals requiring authors to declare any connection with a sponsor and to make publications and presentations as "transparent as possible" (Rae-Grant 2002, 513).

Concerning the research itself, which, as we have seen, can be manipulated or suppressed, a possible solution suggested by Goldacre (2008) is an enforced, open-access clinical trials register.[8] Drug companies would be required to publish research protocols visible to anyone before starting the trial, and if, subsequently, a registered study did not appear in the journals, then publication bias would be suspected since there would be an assumption that there was "something to hide" (204). Goldacre notes that this would also mean that changes in the protocol would become visible; he cites the example of an actual trial in which the outcome variables used were changed after the results were collected – "moving the goalposts."

On the question of the evidence base, clinicians need to consider using other, more independent sources of information on pharmaceuticals. A number of these are listed by Pollack and colleagues (2009), including the Cochrane Collaboration, an international initiative providing systematic reviews of the effects of healthcare interventions (http://www.cochrane. org). Two Canadian sources are the Common Drug Review (http://cadth. ca/en/products/cdr/) and the Therapeutics Initiative (http://www.ti.ubc.ca). The Common Drug Review, operated by the Canadian Agency for Drugs and Technologies in Health, conducts reviews of the clinical evidence and cost-effectiveness of new products, and it makes formulary recommendations (i.e., which drugs to include) to publicly funded drug plans in Canada. The Therapeutics Initiative (TI), operated through the University of British Columbia, states on its website that its mission is "to provide physicians and pharmacists with up-to-date, evidence-based, practical information on prescription drug therapy," adding: "We strongly believe in the need for independent assessments of evidence on drug therapy to balance the drug industry sponsored information sources." The TI also advises the provincial government through a working group about formulary inclusions, with its director noting that, prior to its creation, the "pharmacare program basically just approved every drug that came into the market" (quoted in Smith 2007b). In 2008, there was some concern about the future of TI after the provincial government considered "replacing" the program, based on the recommendations of a task force that included a top Canadian lobbyist for the pharmaceutical companies plus five other people with ties to the drug industry (Cassels 2008). These fears were realized in 2013, when the right-of-centre government suspended funding of TI amid specualtion that they had been pressured into this by the pharmaceutical lobby.

In dealing with escalating costs, provincial governments have instituted deductible, or "co-pay," arrangements that are borne by patients. There is some evidence that the introduction of these measures has led to a significant drop in the initiation of antidepressant treatment, the clinical consequences of which are unclear (Wang et al. 2008). Some have argued that, instead of increasing the costs borne by consumers, governments or their representative agencies should assume a more vigorous role in negotiating prices with the drug companies. A model that is held up in this regard is used by a Crown corporation in New Zealand called PHARMAC (Pharmaceutical Management Agency of New Zealand). The role of this model is to contain costs by holding tenders before buying drugs, applying reference pricing (wherein higher prices for new drugs must be justified by demonstration of substantial benefit), and negotiating lower prices in return for bulk purchases or longer-term contracts (Smith 2007a). Critics of this model suggest that it would potentially restrict treatment choices for patients and their doctors (Fayerman 2007). When asked about the New Zealand plan, a spokesman for the Canadian pharmaceutical industry said that "the capped budget on pharmaceutical products in New Zealand affects treatment options for patients and shifts costs to other areas of the health system, like hospitals" (quoted in Fayerman 2007, A2). Despite industry opposition, in 2010 the Canadian provincial premiers agreed to establish a medication purchasing alliance that, through the combined purchasing power of the different public plans, was intended to lower drug costs and increase access. This was followed in 2012 by provincial and territorial health ministers calling for the establishment of a value price initiative aimed at reducing the cost of generic drugs through a national competitive bidding process (Taylor 2012).

Notes

1 To these one could add a third criterion, that there are no alternatives such as psychological therapies. In the case of depression, there are, in fact, effective non-pharmacological treatments, a topic discussed in Chapter 16.

2 Goldacre also uses social anxiety disorder (SAD) as an example, although it has become increasingly accepted in the psychiatric community as a bona fide disorder. While anxiety can be a serious condition, Moynihan and Cassels (2005, 120) argue that SAD was a "little known and once-considered rare psychiatric condition" before the manufacturers of the antidepressant Paxil "helped transform it into a major epidemic ... affect[ing] one in eight Americans."

3 A smaller number of academic psychiatrists may receive larger amounts of money as "key opinion leaders," serving as speakers for and consultants to the drug companies. See Whitaker (2010).

4 In a review by Pollack et al. (2009, 4) the authors conclude that drug advertising in medical journals "has been found to not meet FDA advertising standards, to be of little educational value, and generally misleading."

5 Admittedly, the method used in these studies leaves open the question of direction of effect. While it would appear that exposure to sales reps results in greater use of and faith in the product being promoted, it may also be the case that physicians who by nature are more optimistic are also more likely to seek out new product information.

6 Some DTC advertising was allowed prior to 1997 but in a more restricted form, requiring detailed lists of potential side effects (Pollack et al. 2009).

7 The discussion that follows draws to a considerable extent from Goldacre (2008).

8 Goldacre notes that something approximating trial registers do exist but are inadequate. Concerning non-disclosure, applicants registering study proposals with the Research Ethics Board at the University of British Columbia are required to respond to the following: "Describe any restrictions regarding the disclosure of information to research subjects (during or at the end of the study) that the sponsor has placed on investigators, including those related to the publication of results."

Reforming Mental Health: Deinstitutionalization and Beyond

Prior to looking at current programs and practices in community mental health it is necessary to provide somewhat of a historical and political context, particularly since the legacy and perceived failure of the institutional era continues to haunt us today. With the influence of different stakeholder perspectives, the recovery vision, and the Mental Health Commission of Canada's (2009) principles for a transformed system, Canadian health authorities are striving to offer more responsive, coordinated, and effective care for mentally ill persons, reflected in agency reports and memoranda that refer to "reform," "renewal," "redesign," "moving forward," "transformation," and similar terms. There have, in fact, been significant tensions in moving from a hospital-based system to a vision of community care, in accommodating new stakeholder groups and care philosophies, in reconciling civil rights and duty of care, and in balancing budgets (Mulvale, Abelson and Goering 2007). A closer look at past practices and policies provides a necessary background for the chapters that are to follow, and, in this chapter, an overview is offered of the major historical trends seen in the delivery of mental health services in Canada.

The Asylums

Very broadly speaking, one can refer to three periods with respect to the care and containment of mentally disordered persons in Canada: (1) an early, pre-institutional era; (2) the period of the asylums, running from the mid-nineteenth to the mid-twentieth centuries; and (3) the post-institutional era, which encompasses the 1960s to the present day.[1] In Canada, the asylum movement started in the middle part of the nineteenth century, the first of these being built in New Brunswick in 1836 (Rochefort 1992). Provincial institutions were opened in Quebec, Ontario, Newfoundland, Nova Scotia, British Columbia, Prince Edward Island, and Manitoba during this period;

Ontario saw an expansion from one facility built in Toronto in 1850 to four provincial hospitals by 1891 (Mulvale, Abelson, and Goering 2007). In Saskatchewan and Alberta, psychiatric hospitals were opened in 1911 and 1914, respectively (Sussman 1998).

The word "asylum" now has a strong negative connotation, although part of this may be a reaction to the physical image: sprawling red-brick buildings with high ceilings, long hallways, and large dormitories. Readers should note, however, that the original intention (and meaning) behind the term had to do with the idea of respite, or sanctuary, of a place where patients could escape from the pressures and corrupting influences that were seen as endemic to life in the cities. By many accounts, the move to asylums represented a progressive shift, one that would "provide safe settings for physical and spiritual care and ... shield residents from the harm and peril that commonly befell people with mental illnesses in cities and towns" (Health Canada 2002b, 1; see also Chaimowitz 2012). Similarly, Sussman (1998, 260) notes that the policy of housing people in asylums in Canada "began with humane intentions as a part of a progressive and reformist movement, which attempted to overcome neglect and suffering in the community, jails and poorhouses." A survey in Halifax from the mid-1840s, for example, determined that "lunatics" made up 20 percent of the population housed in the city poorhouse (Rochefort 1992). The care philosophy in the early institutional era borrowed from ideas about "moral treatment" of the mentally ill first used in Europe, in particular minimizing coercion and restraint, and having a routine of work and leisure.

There were, of course, reasons other than good intentions for the longevity of the asylums, and the complexity of this is best captured in the title of a book on the subject by historian David Rothman: *Conscience and Convenience.* Reformers wanted to "do good" and care for the disabled (conscience), but the institutions could also serve other purposes (convenience). An interesting account of this as it applies to the institutional era in Ontario is given by Mulvale, Abelson, and Goering (2007, 371) who note, to begin with, that "the asylums 'took the problem away' from citizens in the community and relieved a major burden for family members." A key informant interviewed for their study recalls:

> The public were so fearful and rejecting of the fact that mental illness was a common illness that to the general public getting people out of the community was quite acceptable ... It was all part of the era, if you can't figure it out and you think it's a bit dangerous – remove it and send it somewhere else (quoted in Mulvale, Abelson, and Goering [2007], 371).

While removing the mentally ill person may have had the effect of decreasing the discomfort and stigma experienced by the family member (or member of the public), the experience was worse for the person being sent away. As a Canadian psychiatrist observes: "The custodial, institution-based model of care for those with mental illness contributed to their stigmatization by segregation" (Arboleda-Florez 2003, 646).

A second factor influencing the continuance of a hospital-based approach had to do with the payment structure and locus of policy making. Mulvale, Abelson, and Goering (2007, 369-70) note that, while governments managed the construction and operation of the asylums, policy-making decisions in Ontario psychiatric hospitals were largely left to the facility superintendents and medical directors "in isolation from the media ... and the political realm ... [A] resulting legacy was limited government capacity for internal strategic mental health policy-making and for many years the government relied heavily on external advice from the psychiatric profession." When medicare was introduced (in the late 1950s and 1960s) reimbursements from this source focused on hospital rather than community care and only covered hospital and physician services. Being thus in an advantaged position, "physicians were unlikely to support community-based services that could threaten their existing privileges" (Mulvale, Abelson, and Goering 2007, 379).

Finally, a factor that delayed the eventual downsizing and in some cases closure of the provincial hospitals was that they were a major source of employment, particularly in more remote settings that became, in effect, "company towns." Mulvale, Abelson, and Goering (2007) recount the reluctance of the Ontario government to downsize hospitals, in the 1980s and later, because of lobbying on the part of local communities and public service unions and fear of a political backlash should there be a significant impact on the local economy. Other stakeholders and lobbying groups, representing service users and families who supported a community care model, did not achieve any prominence until late in the institutional era.

Deinstitutionalization
The deinstitutionalization era started in Canada in the early 1960s. Regardless of good intentions, provincial mental hospitals had ultimately become overcrowded and understaffed facilities, which, in the absence of any effective methods of treating psychotic disorders, were vast warehouses providing "custodial care." Reports of physical abuse and cruelty by staff periodically surfaced (Reaume 1997; Regehr and Glancy 2010). Patients could be housed for months, or in some cases years, in a single admission.[2] At this time, for example, about four thousand persons were housed at the Essondale

(Riverview) Mental Hospital near Vancouver, British Columbia, while in Saskatchewan, thirty-five hundred persons were kept in two large institutions near Saskatoon and Regina, respectively (Livingston, Nicholls, and Brink 2011).

The 1960s saw a major shift in mental health policy, a shift fuelled by what an American sociologist describes as the "widespread belief that community-based care would be more humane and more therapeutic than hospital-based care" (Bachrach 1994, 24). American president John F. Kennedy, referring to new legislation that was to encourage the replacement of asylums by community clinics, proclaimed in a passage from a 1963 speech that "reliance on the cold mercy of custodial isolation will be supplanted by the open warmth of community concern and capability."[3] In Canada, starting in the 1960s and continuing through the 1970s and 1980s, there was a drastic downsizing of many of the old provincial psychiatric hospitals, a process referred to as *deinstitutionalization*, which Bachrach defines as "the replacement of long-stay psychiatric hospitals with smaller, less isolated community-based service alternatives for the care of individuals with schizophrenia and other major mental illnesses" (24). Bachrach (1994) notes that "deinstitutionalization, in theory, was to consist of three component processes: the release of patients residing in psychiatric hospitals to alternative facilities in the community; the diversion of potential new admissions into those alternative facilities; and the development of special community-based programs, combining psychiatric and support services, for the care of a non-institutionalized patient population" (24). By this definition "deinstitutionalization" refers more to a theoretical ideal than to what was actually accomplished, at least initially. What was accomplished was a considerable reduction in the in-patient census, done by increasing the number of discharges (opening the back door) and limiting new admissions (closing the front door), the latter being achieved in part by narrowing the legal criteria for certification (involuntary admission). Other legal changes provided for more procedural protections for individuals detained under provincial mental health acts and for shortening periods of mandatory detention.

From 1960 to 1976 there was a reduction in capacity in Canadian psychiatric hospitals from 47,633 to 15,011 beds, with general psychiatric hospital beds increasing from 844 to 5,836 over the same period (Goering, Wasylenki, and Durbin 2000). Regional examples include Greater Toronto, where the number of long-stay psychiatric beds fell from 3,857 to 761 between 1960 and 1994, and Saskatchewan, where the psychiatric hospital bed count dropped from 3,500 in the mid-1950s to about 200 in the year 2000 (Eberle 2001c). In British Columbia, the provincial psychiatric hospital reduced beds from four thousand to one thousand by the early 1990s, with a final closure taking place in 2012 (Livingston, Nicholls, and Brink 2011). Not all provinces downsized at the same pace, although the ultimate goal was the same. In surveying data from the different provinces, Sealey and Whitehead (2004, 249) conclude that there was "variation among the provinces in the timing and intensity of deinstitutionalization," with percentage decreases in provincial hospital bed capacity from 1965 to 1981 ranging from a low of 34 percent in Prince Edward Island to a high of 84 percent in Quebec. Despite these differences, a much greater proportion of persons with serious mental disorders were now, clearly, "in the community," particularly when one considered increases in the general population and the fact that people who previously would have been, in all likelihood, long-term residents of psychiatric hospitals were no longer being admitted.

Relative to a number of other jurisdictions, Canada has seen greater hospital downsizing. For example, data from 2005 show that per capita the number of mental health beds in Canada (both general hospital and psychiatric) was less than half that of New Zealand, Sweden, or the United Kingdom (Alberta Mental Health Board 2007).

It became evident in the aftermath of this wave of hospital bed closures that many problems still remained, notwithstanding optimistic beliefs about community care. Indeed, whether formerly institutionalized clients were achieving reintegration – were really "in the community" – seemed questionable. The situation is summarized in a Canadian Mental Health Association (2001, 5) document:

> By the mid-1970s, however, it was becoming clear that the realization of this vision (deinstitutionalization) was flawed. For many former hospital residents the new system meant either abandonment, demonstrated by the increasing numbers of homeless mentally ill people; "transinstitutionalization": living in grim institution-like conditions such as those found in the large psychiatric boarding homes; or a return to family who suddenly had to cope with an enormous burden of care but with very little support. In addition, fears and prejudices about mental illness, in part responsible for the long history of segregation in institutions, compounded the problems in the community. These attitudes increased the barriers to access to community life in areas such as employment, education and housing.

How did this state of affairs come about? In attempting to answer this question, one needs to look at the factors that originally influenced the deinstitutionalization movement, of which three are generally recognized as being significant: (1) new treatments, (2) changing ideologies and attitudes, and (3) economics.

New Medications

Concerning new treatments, the 1950s saw the first psychiatric use of two drugs that would radically alter mental health practice: chlorpromazine, used as a treatment for psychosis; and lithium, used for manic depression. Prior to the discovery of the antipsychotic properties of chlorpromazine, treatments for schizophrenia – which included electroconvulsive therapy (ECT), insulin coma, and psychosurgery – were found to be of questionable efficacy, if not harmful. Now, with the advent of an oral medication that patients would presumably take voluntarily, there was the promise that individuals would not require containment in hospitals but instead could be treated on an outpatient basis in community settings. Whether the community programs offering these new medications would be coordinated and accessible and whether all persons would agree to take these drugs were issues that would be struggled with subsequently. It soon became apparent, in the post-institutionalization era, that continuity of care would be a more pressing concern than the availability of medication (Eaton 2001).

Changing Attitudes

In the post-Second World War era a number of critiques, some popular, some academic, were levelled at the practice of "warehousing" huge numbers of patients in psychiatric hospitals. While many of these critiques came from the American context, they proved to be very influential among Canadian academics, policy makers, and the public. Examples include:

- *The Shame of the States*, a journalistic account of the living conditions in American psychiatric hospitals by Albert Deutsch (1948).
- *The Snake Pit* (1948), an Academy Award-nominated film that, while at least somewhat sympathetic towards psychiatry, led a number of American state governments to amend their legislation concerning the hospitalization of mentally disordered persons.
- *One Flew over the Cuckoo's Nest*, Ken Kesey's 1962 novel and, subsequently, an Academy Award-winning film (1975), wherein the protagonist is first given ECT, then lobotomized, in apparent efforts to quell his anti-authoritarian behaviour. To this day the term "cuckoo's nest" is used to refer to psychiatric hospitals. These vehicles made clear the role of mental health workers as social control agents.
- *Titicut's Follies*, a once-banned 1967 documentary film that is a genuinely horrifying account of life in a Massachusetts psychiatric hospital, in which patients are verbally abused, force-fed, and paraded about naked.

- *Asylums* (1961), an ethnography of life in a Washington, DC, psychiatric hospital by Canadian sociologist Erving Goffman. The thesis of this influential book is that institutionalism not only strips away individual dignity but actually fosters many of the regressive behaviours and symptoms seen among the patients.
- "On Being Sane in Insane Places," a controversial study by David Rosenhan (1973), published in the journal *Science*, which details the experiences of "fake" patients who had surreptitiously gained admission to psychiatric hospitals and who were never distinguished from the "real" patients by the professional staff. Among other things, Rosenhan looks at the *invisibility* and *depersonalization* experienced by institutionalized persons.

These critiques of the policy and effects of institutionalization coincided with a burgeoning civil rights movement that now incorporated the patients' rights agenda along with women's rights and minority rights. Based on the work of Goffman, Rosenhan, and others, it was now asserted that institutionalization not only did not help persons with mental disorders but also seemed to make them worse – that is, to exacerbate regressive behaviours – in a number of instances. The concept of "chronicity" as it was applied to mental disorders was attributed to the effects of institutionalization rather than to a disease process. Following from this, it seemed reasonable to suggest that being in the community, in and of itself, would have major therapeutic benefits for persons with mental disorders.

This, of course, was not enough. The provision of civil liberties – "negative" freedoms – did not obviate the need for positive care and support. We have also learned that some mental disorders can be long term by their very nature, apart from institutional arrangements. The over-optimism of the 1960s is summarized by Bachrach (1994, 26): "Early advocates were so completely certain of the curative powers of community based care that they sometimes elected to understate both the seriousness and chronicity that are part of long-term mental illness. Indeed, they were sometimes so expansive in their optimism that they chose to think [exclusively] in terms of mental health, and effectively to ignore the existence of mental illness." That said, while the social upheaval of the 1960s may seem somewhat distant and naïve now, this brief history shows that "ideas matter" and, as Mulvale, Abelson, and Goering (2007, 380) suggest, "changes in ideas may be sufficient motivation for incremental change to occur" with respect to the move towards enhancing community care. These authors point to, for example, the willingness of key public figures to talk about their own experiences with mental illness as helping shift the public *zeitgeist* and further lay the groundwork for reform.

Economic Factors

A more skeptical perspective on deinstitutionalization suggests that financial incentives and disincentives were the key drivers behind the process. One hypothesis is that the asylums were eventually closed to save money otherwise spent maintaining them since, by the 1960s, they were aging, outdated, and in poor repair. British sociologist Andrew Scull (1977), in attempting to explain what he referred to as the "decarceration" movement, argued that, by the 1970s, Western governments were facing a "fiscal crisis" and saw an opportunity to offload costs by closing hospital wards and discharging patients who, by the post-Second World War era, were eligible for new subsistence-level welfare and income assistance programs and new privatized services in the community. As summarized by Cohen (1985, 104), "money [could be] saved, and benevolent intentions proclaimed." Scull downplayed the belief that deinstitutionalization came about as a result of progressive reform and critiques of the asylums, arguing that similar critiques had been made in earlier historical periods. Similarly, according to this perspective, abstract references to "community care" and "family care" were smokescreens obscuring the reality that little or no care was in fact being provided.

Scull's thesis has been criticized on a number of points (Cohen 1985). It was noted, for example, that what appeared to be happening in North America was not necessarily applicable to other countries – for instance, Europe. Further, the time sequence seemed questionable: the census reduction in psychiatric hospitals had been well under way before the downturn in the North American economy of the 1970s. And there is in fact no compelling evidence that community-based services are cheaper when compared to long-stay psychiatric facilities, particularly given efficiencies associated with providing services at a single site and given that community programs are simultaneously running both inpatient and outpatient programs (Bachrach 1994; Latimer 1999). This leads to the question of whether the underfunding of community programs in the immediate post-deinstitutionalization period was, on the one hand, a matter of *intention* or negligence or, on the other hand, a matter of "unintended consequences" and over-optimism. In any case, it is clear that "the contraction of traditional institutional psychiatric care outpaced the expansion of community-based services and supports" (Livingston, Nicholls, and Brink 2011, 200).

While the conspiratorial aspect of Scull's argument is open to debate, one can nonetheless point to economic factors that facilitated the move away from the asylums and towards community care. Clearly, disability and income assistance payments available to individuals, starting in the post-Second World War period, made it more possible to survive on the "outside." On this point, journalist Robert Whitaker (2010) argues that the timing of the first wave of deinstitutionalization in the US is better explained by the initiation of these social security measures than by the advent of new medications. When in state hospitals psychiatric patients were the fiscal responsibility of the states, whereas new social security measures were federally funded, providing an incentive to discharge patients. In 1965, the US federal government excluded Medicaid payments for patients in state hospitals in order to encourage deinstitutionalization and to shift costs back to the states – which were seen as traditionally responsible for such care. This *disincentive* had the effect of patients being moved from state hospitals to community settings in which they would be eligible for Medicaid, which is funded at the federal level. In Canada, federal financial incentives also facilitated a move towards the community. In the 1960s, the federal government, through the Dominion Mental Health Grants Program, provided matching funding for provinces to move care from psychiatric hospitals to general hospital psychiatric units (Mulvale, Abelson, and Goering 2007). A key informant interviewed for this topic notes: "The Dominion Mental Health Grants started the shift away from the old asylums, but it wasn't done for therapeutic reasons, as much as for fiscal reasons ... [T]hese were 50 cent dollars. If you set up a psychiatric unit in a general hospital, you could get up to 50 percent of your cost paid" (quoted in Mulvale, Abelson, and Goering 2007, 373).

Aftermath

Through the 1970s and 1980s a number of problems associated with hospital downsizing became apparent. Former patients were found to be living in isolated, impoverished circumstances. The main housing "option" seemed to be private, unregulated, and often run-down boarding homes (Regehr and Glancy 2010). A number were winding up homeless or in the jail system. Notwithstanding earlier rhetoric referring to "the open warmth of community concern," the general public did not appear to be welcoming these former hospital patients, which was manifested as the NIMBY (not in my back yard) response. Ghettos arose in a number of Canadian cities, such as the Parkdale district of Toronto. And the treatment services provided were inadequate, with often a single outpatient clinic serving a large region. The treatment focus was narrowly medical, with rehabilitation services in short supply, these mainly taking the form of "sheltered workshops." Since the clients that

could reliably attend office appointments tended to be less disabled, it became evident that a number of those most in need were being overlooked.

To the present day people speak about the "failure of deinstitutionalization," and the perception of historical indifference or negligence has in some
quarters fuelled a cynical (if not nihilistic) attitude towards future reforms
in mental health services. Livingston, Nicholls, and Brink (2011, 201) suggest, however, that "these sentiments persist despite a burgeoning body of
evidence that careful implementation of deinstitutionalization policies may
thwart potential adverse consequences and may even foster favorable outcomes." In their own study these authors followed a cohort of clients discharged in one of the last waves – pre-closure, of a provincial psychiatric
hospital – comparing their outcomes to a cohort discharged in an earlier
period. They found that more careful planning along with a realignment
of tertiary services meant that this later group did not, to any significant
extent, encounter unintended consequences such as jail admission or frequent hospitalization. Characterizing deinstitutionalization as a failure now
needs some clarification. While it is true that a small number of the mentally
ill may need longer-term sanctuary, what some among the public appear to
be requesting is a more general return to the "containment" of a past era
(Howell 2008) – re-institutionalization – when in fact our current values
support interventions that are the least restrictive and invasive. For example,
in a 2012 op-ed piece in the *New York Times*, an American psychiatrist argues
that there is "too little institutionalizing of teenagers and young men (particularly men, more prone to violence) who have had a recent onset of
schizophrenia" (Steinberg 2012). Three Canadian authors comment on what
seems to be a nostalgia for the asylums:

> In the minds of many people, the focus of medical treatment, especially for
> those who are severely ill, is the hospital ... Hospitals provide a reassuring
> presence that is both highly visible and extremely tangible, and may for
> many epitomize care. It is hard then to understand that there are illnesses
> that may worsen in hospital, or may be severe and yet not require hospital
> care, as is often the case with mental illnesses ... When confronted with
> the sometimes unusual behaviour of a person with a mental illness, the
> immediate assumption made is that the individual concerned must need
> care in a hospital, and that their presence outside of the hospital is evidence
> of some kind of failure of delivery of health services ... The individual may
> in fact be involved in extensive community care, but their presence in
> public is often interpreted as a failure of the "hospital," which traditionally
> in many places in mental health care was the institution. (Morrow, Dagg,
> and Pederson 2008, 4)

Concerning the services available in community settings in Canada, progress has been made, and a broader range of services, more evidence-based vocational programs, and improved housing models – described in greater detail in later chapters – are now available for at least some of the seriously mentally ill. Deficiencies still persist, however, and these were referred to in two major Canadian Senate reports, published in 2004 and 2006, respectively (Standing Senate Committee on Social Affairs, Science and Technology 2004, 2006). The reports noted the following:

- Existing services and supports for individuals with mental illness were fragmented among many separate agencies and many access points.
- There was a need to better integrate the mental health system with the health care system and the addiction treatment system.
- Mental health services system still reflected an institutionally driven philosophy of care.
- The mental health services system was not comprehensive in terms of providing a continuum of services that persons could gain access to when and where needed.
- Mental health services were relatively under-funded.
- There were major human resource shortages in the mental health sector.
- There was a lack of measures of accountability in the mental health system, so that worker roles and responsibilities were not clearly set out and service effectiveness was not addressed.
- Stigma was a still a problem, not only among the general public but also within the health care system as a whole.

Service users interviewed spoke additionally about a lack of affordable housing, financial penalties for those on disability incomes able to work part-time, and a shortage of complementary, non-pharmacological treatment options.

Challenges and Responses

As noted, health authorities currently face a number of challenges with respect to service delivery, and these include fiscal realities, philosophy of care, and program coordination (Health Canada 2002b). On philosophy of care, service delivery in the post-deinstitutionalization era has been complicated by the recovery vision and the different and sometimes competing interests of stakeholder groups (discussed in more detail in Chapters 5 and 7). Client representatives have spoken to issues such as choice, empowerment, and civil liberties, while some clinicians, members of the public, and expedient politicians have sought stricter controls on mentally disordered persons deemed to be "non-compliant" and dangerous. At the same time, families have asked for greater support and greater input into the treatment process and may have concerns about aspects of the recovery model.

Concerning fiscal realities, health care consumes a very large and historically increasing proportion of provincial budgets in Canada (Regehr and Glancy 2010). The plight of the provinces has been made worse by cuts in transfer payments from the federal government: for example, from 1978 to 1998 the proportion of Medicare paid by the federal government shrank from 27 to 11 percent (Goering, Wasylenki, and Durbin 2000). *Cost containment* in health care is now viewed as a necessary and appropriate role for government and health authorities, something that is a relatively new development, with Goering, Wasylenki, and Durbin (2000, 347) observing that, historically, the provision of health care services in Canada has had "little accountability." One can landmark this shift by noting the references to "accountability" and "sustainability" in the 2002 report of the Commission on the Future of Health Care in Canada (known as the Romanow Report). References to "decreased use of more intrusive and/or more costly services" are also now seen in practice guidelines (BC Ministry of Health 2002e, 10).

To support greater accountability in the mental health system, Goering and colleagues (2000, 356-57) suggest that "there will be more attention paid to utilization review, measurement, and reporting of outcomes, and clearly defining roles and responsibilities between levels of care. [As well] the funding of hospital and community services is likely to be tied more explicitly to performance ... factors." Thus, one sees an increasing emphasis on *efficiency* and *effectiveness* in the delivery of mental health services.[4] Both of these rely on an evaluative approach, with quantifiable outcome measures and, where available, adherence to fidelity standards. Concerning efficiency, health care managers in Canada may receive training in the "Lean" model, a methodology originating with the Toyota automotive company (Womack and Jones 2003). "Lean" focuses on the elimination of waste or "non-value added" consumption of resources, and it looks at ways to avoid expenditures – of time, money, labour – that do not directly benefit the client. An example could be problems with the information (or lack of) available at transition points, such as when a client is discharged back to the community, resulting ultimately in delays for the client when it comes to accessing service. Waiting times are a commonly used success indicator in health care; this could refer to the wait for surgery or, in mental health, the length of time from referral to first appointment with a counsellor. Lengthy delays may mean that the person becomes ill again, possibly necessitating a return to hospital (Canadian Mental Health Association 2001). Evaluators may thus look at the ability of a mental health team to take on new clients, which is contingent at least to some extent on discharging "old" clients, which, in turn, requires some reliable means for determining level of function among clients. Efficiency has also been addressed in hospitals by moving to what is called "patient-focused funding" (also known as "pay-for-performance"), whereby revenues are related specifically to tasks performed (procedures, admissions) rather than block funding for an entire program (Mickelburgh 2011).

"Effectiveness" is a little more difficult to determine in mental health interventions and is a topic covered in more detail in the next chapter. Minimally, this would require periodic reassessment of illness and functioning (something that should but does not always occur), which can be promoted through the use of rating scales. An example is the Health of the Nation Outcome Scales (HoNOS), used in several Canadian jurisdictions and internationally (Kisely et al. 2008a; Spaeth-Rublee et al. 2010). The HoNOS is deficit-based, looking at problem areas across twelve scale items. The Outcome Rating Scale (Duncan, Miller, and Sparks 2004), used in some mental health and addiction settings, is a client self-report that gauges distress levels but also asks about subjective well-being.

Mental health programs have historically used hospitalization (length and frequency of) as an outcome indicator, although this is a measure fraught with problems given its multi-determined nature. Another way of considering effectiveness is the availability of "best practices" at a particular site (admittedly with the a priori assumption that a given client will benefit from them). For example, an intervention known as "supported employment" has been found through a number of evaluations to be successful in gaining competitive employment for clients and so is a recommended model for all community mental health programs.

Hospitals are a large cost driver in health care. In response to this, health authorities have in some cases privatized or "outsourced" hospital services such as housekeeping, laundry, food, and security, and have closed altogether some smaller general hospitals in more remote locales. In psychiatry, as elsewhere in acute care, there is usually great pressure on beds and, consequently, an emphasis on avoiding lengthy admissions, which is becoming even more challenging with an aging population. Limiting length of admission is ethically and fiscally defensible, given limited hospital resources, but it is a great source of tension for family members and community clinicians who may argue that clients are being discharged when still unwell, possibly into unstable housing arrangements. Groups representing caregivers have tended to argue for longer stays and more psychiatric beds (e.g. Buchanan 2011). The counter-argument is that it is wrong to tie up a bed when the client no longer needs acute care, but this may not account for the fact that there are no good alternatives (Davis 1996). This, then, points to the importance of having a *range* of services available in a community mental health system (see Chapter 11).

In addition to cost containment, better integration and coordination of services is now high on the agenda of health authorities, given past problems in this respect (Latimer 2005). Goering, Wasylenki, and Durbin (2000, 347) note that, "until very recently[,] the provision of mental health services in Canada has been characterized by fragmentation [and] lack of mechanisms to coordinate or integrate services." They go on to describe the "four solitudes" of the mental health system: provincial psychiatric hospitals, general hospital psychiatric units, "overburdened" community mental health programs, and private practitioners, each operating in relative isolation. For mentally ill persons this meant "negotiating a complex and fragmented set of services and supports," resulting in a deterioration of care (Durbin et al. 2006, 705).

In the Kirby Report (Standing Senate Committee on Social Affairs, Science and Technology 2006, 99), a transformed mental health system is seen as one that would provide an "integrated continuum of care" that would respect client choice, be comprehensive, "local and complex," and offer the least intrusive form of support. An integrated system is one "that provides a co-ordinated continuum of services to a defined population, and is held clinically and fiscally responsible for the health status of that population" (Durbin et al. 2006, 705). The benefits of such a system are outlined as follows:

> Duplication and inefficiency are reduced. Accountability is centralized so that clients are less likely to slip through the cracks. There is a full continuum of services to provide the right level of care in response to patient need. Access and movement within and across levels of care are easier. Care is more individualized, driven by client needs rather than program boundaries. As a result continuity of care is increased, with individuals more likely to receive needed services and supports and remain in care, especially during difficult transitions such as following hospital discharge. The ultimate expected benefit is improved clinical status and quality of life for the client. (Durbin et al. 2006, 705)

An important aspect of an integrated system involves bringing mental health and addictions treatment together under one portfolio, given the relatively large number of persons with these co-occurring disorders. Historically, persons with co-occurring disorders have in most instances had their concerns dealt with by separate programs, in separate locations, with different treatment philosophies, and under separate ministries. A report on the benefits of and barriers to integration notes that "bringing these two historically disjointed systems under one overarching administration/ management structure has been beneficial to the extent that there is clear evidence supporting stronger clinical outcomes for integrated treatment (Centre for Applied Research in Mental Health and Addiction 2007c, 6). And indeed, more health authorities in Canada are now combining mental health and addictions within a single administration. An example is Toronto's Centre for Addiction and Mental Health, created (in 1998) by the amalgamation of two addictions programs (the Addiction Research Foundation and the Donwood Institute) and two mental health programs (the Clarke Institute of Psychiatry and the Queen Street Mental Health Centre). It is my observation that, while these two historically separate services are now nominally combined in Canadian health authorities, true integration at the level of programs remains a challenge.

The approach used to achieve better integration of mental health in most Canadian jurisdictions has been *regionalization*; that is, the devolution of mental health services from provincial administration through the establishment of regional health authorities (Block et al. 2008), with these authorities now having "responsibility for the planning and operation of all health, including mental health, services for a defined population" (Goering, Wasylenki, and Durbin 2000, 347). Having a single regional health budget (as opposed to separate budgets for hospitals and the community) enables improved integration and comprehensiveness of services, it is suggested, "by discouraging cost shifting and by localizing, within one body, the full consequences of decision making" (Clarke Institute of Psychiatry 1997, 23). It is also hoped that, through regionalization, the system becomes more responsive to local needs (Wilson 2005).[5] On this point Dickinson (2002, 383) notes that "the anticipated advantages of decentralization and regionalization are twofold: It is hoped that they will enable the identification of location-specific service delivery needs, and that they will facilitate the creation of local commitment to the mobilization and reallocation of resources in the communities most directly affected. This last point is particularly important in light of the commitment to self-care and mutual aid as essential elements in the health promotion framework." Regionalization also means, ideally, that longer-stay beds, previously contained in the large, isolated psychiatric hospitals, will be dispersed to a number of smaller tertiary-care units that, by virtue of their size, privacy, and location, will be more homelike, normalizing, and integrated into local communities (Livingston, Nicholls, and Brink 2011). While regionalization holds significant potential, successful implementation is challenged by the different "solitudes" that exist within health care, in particular the historic lack of trust, and cultural differences, between the hospital and community sectors (British Columbia Ministry of Health 2002e).

How has regionalization played out? The Province of Alberta provides an interesting case study, one that has been followed by *Globe and Mail* journalist André Picard (2008b, 2009b). Alberta was the first province to adapt regionalization, in 1994, creating seventeen health regions, which were reduced to nine in 2003. According to Picard, regionalization did indeed work in Alberta – Calgary and Edmonton in particular – so that services became more responsive to local needs, creating one of the better health systems in Canada with innovative new programs and reduced wait list times. Picard notes in particular the efficiency of the Edmonton region, with among the lowest administrative costs in Canada. Then, in 2008, the provincial government announced a return to centralization: instead of regional boards there would be a single "health services board." Picard's account points to rivalries and tensions between the "powerful, independent health leaders" in the Calgary and Edmonton regions, and the premier, and the latter's desire to hold greater authority. In any event, it is a cautionary tale that shows that any new administrative structure will still be subject to political forces beyond its control. In Alberta researchers looked at an issue of some historical concern to mental health advocates in Canada; that is, the amount of funding for mental health relative to other health care expenses. This concern is based on evidence that mental health spending in Canada is low relative to other jurisdictions. For example, it is less than half the amount spent in Germany and the UK as a percentage of total health expenses (Alberta Mental Health Board 2007; Jacobs et al. 2008).[6] One of the hopes was that regionalization would bring this disparity into sharper focus and possibly increase the mental health portion of the budget. Alberta researchers examined this by comparing spending on mental health before and after budgets came under the regional health authorities, and they found, in fact, that there was no increase in the share for mental health (Block et al. 2008).

The Political Profile of Mental Health

As we have seen, the role of government has been to fund health programs and, more recently, to require accountability measures. However, when it comes to setting standards and shaping policy, mental health has not historically been given a high priority. In the drafting of legislation governing psychiatric treatment, political actions have been seen as expedient and reactive, influenced by media portrayals, as per the following overview by Goering, Wasylenki, and Durbin (2000, 354):

Public opinion has somewhat less direct influence on policy-making in a parliamentary system where special interest groups are not as powerful as in the United States ... Still, Canadian provincial and federal politicians are clearly influenced by the opinions of their constituency, and the media is the most common mode of communication ... Coverage of mental health issues tends to be centered on a few key topics with homelessness, suicide, and violence receiving the lion's share of attention. At times this coverage influences the development of mental health policy. For example, a number of recent threats and subway pushings by individuals with mental illness ... flamed public outrage and supported the efforts of the families of the mentally ill in advocating for a change in legislation to introduce community committal. Shortly afterward, the Ontario government announced its intention to pursue this course of action.

(Goering, Wasylenki, and Durbin refer here to community treatment orders, under which a person is subject to involuntary treatment even after leaving hospital – a law strongly opposed by patients' rights advocates.)

Concerning the low profile of mental health, a number of observers have suggested that government needs to do more in this respect; that is, to provide greater leadership with respect to mental health policy and standards (Smiderle 2003). This point is made in *Building on Values: The Future of Health Care in Canada* (Commission on the Future of Health Care in Canada 2002, 178) – the Romanow Report – in which the authors describe "mental health ... as one of the orphan children of medicare" and the need to "bring mental health into the mainstream of public health care."[7] Critics have pointed to the fact that research funding in Canada for psychiatric conditions is low relative to the funding for other disorders (Todd 2004) and that (until recently) Canada was the only G8 nation without a national action plan on mental health, the result being a "badly organized and under-funded" system, according to a 2004 Canadian Senate report (Kennedy 2004). It has also been suggested that the responsibilities for mental health be elevated to a deputy minister level within federal portfolios such as Health Canada and Human Resources and Skills Development (Mood Disorders Society of Canada 2011a). In its 2012 strategy document, the Mental Health Commission of Canada (2012) recommended an increase in the proportion of health spending devoted to mental health from 7 to 9 percent over the following ten years.

To present a stronger, more coherent voice, and to overcome what was seen as a disjointed effort among organizations advocating for reform (Smiderle 2003), several non-governmental organizations and professional associations formed a new umbrella organization in 1998 called the

Canadian Alliance on Mental Illness and Mental Health (CAMIMH). According to their website (http://camimh.ca/about-camimh) the mandate of CAMIMH is "to ensure that mental health is placed on the national agenda so that persons with a lived experience of mental illness and their families receive appropriate access to care and support." In referencing the considerable economic and personal cost of mental illness, CAMIMH states the following as a core principle: "Given the impact of mental health issues and mental illness (i.e. on the suffering of Canadians, on mortality, especially from suicide, on the economy, on social services such as health, education and criminal justice), Canadian governments and health planners must address mental health issues commensurate with the level of their burden on society."

The Kirby Report and the Mental Health Commission

The 2006 Canadian Senate report appeared to be a significant landmark in the history of mental health care in Canada since it provided the impetus to finally create a national action plan. The document, referred to as the "Kirby Report" after the chairman of the Standing Senate Committee on Social Affairs, Science and Technology, was entitled *Out of the Shadows at Last*, reflecting the marginalized status of mental illness in the political and social landscape. *Out of the Shadows* drew from a number of consultations with different stakeholders across Canada, including service users and family members. The report spoke about the inadequacy of mental health services and the lack of recognition of and support for caregivers. The authors pointed to the lack of a mental health strategy, which "symbolizes neglect of mental health issues by government" (Standing Senate Committee on Social Affairs, Science and Technology 2006, 429). However, the report also noted that, while there was a leadership role for the federal government, this body could not be the one developing and enforcing standards in mental health since, in Canada, under the constitutional division of powers, this is the responsibility of the provinces.[8]

A key recommendation to come out of the Kirby Report, and one that was acted upon, concerned the creation of a mental health commission – something that was supported by virtually all of the stakeholders. The establishment of the new Mental Health Commission of Canada (MHCC) was announced in 2007 by Prime Minister Stephen Harper, who stated that the commission would "seek to ensure that Canadians in every part of the country [would] have access to the best prevention, diagnostic, and treatment practices" (quoted in Fitzpatrick 2007). At this time the federal government committed to spending $10 million to start up the MHCC and $15 million annually for the operating budget. Shortly after this the MHCC announced that its three priorities were the development of a national mental health strategy, a stigma reduction campaign, and a knowledge exchange centre.

Concerning the mental health strategy, in 2009 the MHCC released a "framework" document, *Toward Recovery and Well-Being*, that articulated seven high-level goals. These included greater supports for families, recognition of diversity, using interventions that were evidence-based, reducing stigma, providing equitable and timely access to service, being client-centred and supporting individual choice, and addressing prevention and health promotion. The framework described was very much congruent with a recovery orientation. This was followed by the release of a draft "Mental Health Strategy for Canada" document in 2011, which set out a number of "priorities for action," building on the 2009 report. Again, the recovery orientation was emphasized, stressing the importance of involving clients in decision making and upholding their rights. And prevention and early intervention were emphasized, for example, the need to increase the capacity of families and schools "to promote mental health, reduce stigma [and] reduce mental illness and suicide" (Mental Health Commission of Canada 2011, 4). The full strategy document was released in 2012, articulating six strategic directions (referring to health promotion, the recovery vision, access to services, diversity, Aboriginal peoples, and leadership and collaboration), twenty-six priority areas, and 109 recommendations for action. Clearly, an ambitious agenda.

Not everyone was comfortable with the direction in which the MHCC appeared to be heading. The draft Mental Health Strategy document was criticized for being *too* "recovery-oriented" and even appearing to be anti-psychiatry, at least according to *Globe and Mail* health reporter André Picard (2011):

There is far too much emphasis on the "recovery model" – the notion that everyone will get better with support – and not enough emphasis on brain science. It's a legitimate approach for those with mild and moderate mental health problems but not those with severe conditions such as schizophrenia. In fact, reading the draft strategy, one is left with an unpleasant aftertaste: the distinct feeling that psychiatry and medications have no place in Canada's approach to tackling mental illness ... [T]he strategy gives too much credence to social science and not enough to neuroscience. It also pays far too much attention to the views of "psychiatric survivors" who hide their vehemently anti-treatment views in the promotion of "peer support" and the language of "rights."

Picard's comments were echoed by some family advocates who expressed concern that the emphasis on "upholding rights" would support treatment refusal by persons who, because of their psychosis, did not believe they had an illness (Inman 2011b). A more comprehensive critique of the strategy document came from CFACT, the Coalition for Appropriate Care and Treatment for Persons with Serious Mental Illnesses (http://www.cfact.ca). In a letter to the MHCC, a CFACT representative spoke about the commission's duty to protect the most severely mentally ill by maintaining access to hospital beds and medical treatment, and not potentially blocking this access by promoting more libertarian policies and statutes (Buchanan 2011). The writer also requested that there be no public funds made available to persons "promoting medication withdrawal," this an apparent reference to adherents of alternative, non-medical approaches to recovery. And the CFACT writer took issue with moving in the direction of health promotion and prevention, suggesting that "chronic brain diseases [such as schizophrenia] have a genetic predisposition and cannot be prevented."

The concerns expressed by Picard and others reflect a misunderstanding of what is meant by a recovery orientation, a topic covered in Chapter 5. Picard appears to be adhering to an older, symptom-based definition (recovery *from* mental illness), not a conception that sees the individual achieving her/his full potential across a number of existential domains (recovery *in* mental illness). The MHCC president addressed this in a 2011 letter "to all Canadians" (http://www.mentalhealthcommission.ca/ SiteCollectionDocuments/September_2011/MHCC_Open_Letter_ENG.pdf), which emphasized that the needs of persons with severe conditions would not be neglected while, at the same time, standing by the commitment to a broader recovery orientation. The final strategy document, published in 2012, addresses stakeholder criticisms, with more explicit references to illness, the need for basic science research, and access to hospital beds – albeit as part of a continuum of care rather than the predominant approach to care. It is noteworthy that, in the document, the Mental Health Commission (2012, 14, emphasis added) refers to "mental health *problems and illnesses*" (as a single term), noting that it is not attempting to draw a firm line between "problem" and "illness" but, rather, to be "respectful of a wide range of views," an acknowledgment that some are more comfortable with a biological conception. The exchange with advocates and other stakeholders nevertheless shows, again, how contentious the debate is around the issue of models of care as well as the difficult task the MHCC has set for itself in establishing a mental health plan that tries to accommodate all viewpoints and stakeholders.

Notes

1   The earliest human inhabitants of Canada were of course Aboriginal peoples, and the historical legacy with respect to their treatment is discussed in more detail in Chapter 6.

2   The possible iatrogenic effects of long-term hospitalization are now referred to in practice documents. For example, a Health Canada (2002a, 25) report suggests that, "although hospitalization provides important short term respite and care, prolonged periods in hospital remove individuals from their normal environment and can weaken social connections, making reintegration into community living more challenging."

3   Kennedy himself had a sister who spent most of her adult life in a psychiatric institution.

4   The first line in the job description of a mental health program manager in the Vancouver Coastal Health Authority reads: "The Manager is responsible for the delivery of effective and efficient community mental health programs."

5   Although this is challenged by the fact that "local regions" can still be very large geographically. For example, the Northern Health Authority in BC is over 600,000 square kilometres in size (although only about 300,000 in population).

6   Although by some "benchmarks" Canada meets the spending threshold (Lim, Jacobs, and Dewa 2008). On this subject, Lim, Jacobs, and Dewa suggest that "the benchmarking exercise should focus on similar countries that have achieved among the best health outcomes. However, even in countries with good mental health outcomes, the range of mental health spending may vary too widely for policy makers to decide on the optimal level" (30).

7   Ironically, mental health remained under-recognized in the Romano Report itself, which devoted only two of 357 pages to the topic, slotting it in as a subsection of a chapter on "homecare."

8   In section 8 of the Canada Health Act it is noted that health plans must be "administered and operated on a non-profit basis by a public authority, *responsible to the provincial/territorial governments* and subject to audits of their accounts and financial transactions" (emphasis added; see also Chapter 11). The federal government does, with some specific populations, have a responsibility for mental health care, and these would include the RCMP, the Canadian Armed Forces, Aboriginal persons, and federal prison inmates.

The Evidence Base and "Best Practices"

10

As we saw in the last chapter, funding bodies are increasingly emphasizing accountability and evidence of effectiveness in mental health services, which leads us to the question: How do we know "what works?" How do we know if the interventions used in psychiatric practice – for example, medication, cognitive behavioural therapy, or assertive community treatment – are effective? What evidence is used? These are important questions and are also more complex than they may seem at first glance. For example, how do we deconstruct and define a term like "effective," and *whose* evidence are we using in making these determinations? In exploring these questions, this chapter takes a critical look at the *evidence base* in mental health and at whether traditional methods and indicators need to be re-evaluated in light of a developing recovery orientation in service delivery.

To begin with, the fact that we are talking about evidence-based practices, despite all the difficulties and controversies associated with that term (e.g., Webb 2001), is almost certainly a good thing when one considers the alternatives. An example is the use of insulin-induced comas in the 1940s and 1950s as a treatment for schizophrenia, a practice followed despite a lack of scientific evidence or understanding of mechanism of action, and a treatment now considered to be ineffective and inhumane. In a historical account of "insulin therapy" Doroshow (2007, 243) notes that the practice persisted because of hopeful/wishful thinking on the part of the treating staff and also because it gave psychiatrists "something to do" and "made them feel like real doctors instead of just institutional attendants" (note that this was prior to the advent of antipsychotic medication). Clearly, this example shows that the desire to "do good" is not a sufficient basis for action. In looking at the history of psychiatry in Canada in the second half of the twentieth century, Paris (2000, 34) notes that, early on, the knowledge base was essentially "clinical inference," hunches that could be "unsystematic and open to bias." We have moved to an era in which we strive to be more systematic in our method of inquiry, and, while bias can never be completely eliminated in research, the scientific method, *at its best*, is transparent enough to allow possible biases to be identified.

In a Canadian Psychiatric Association position paper on this topic, the authors explain why evidence-based practice is an important concept:

> The most compelling reason to adopt an evidence-based approach is an ethical obligation to support patients and families in making informed choices about medical decisions. This is a central tenet of medical codes of ethics such as that of the Canadian Medical Association. It is reasonable for patients and families to expect the best available information about the efficacy of various treatments and their potential risks and side effects. Correspondingly, physicians have an obligation to provide high-quality information to their patients and to assist in summarizing and interpreting the research literature so that patients, incorporating their values and preferences, can make informed decisions ... Evidence-based information helps patients and families to counter popular misconceptions regarding diagnoses and treatments. Further, the level of credibility of the information that the physician provides may be a critical element in the subsequent acceptance of and compliance with treatment. (Goldner et al. 2000)

That clients now have greater access to information on mental health from sources such as the internet also underlines the importance of practitioners being current and conversant with the evidence base (Marie-Albert 2002). Finally, it may be noted that ongoing evaluation is one of the seven goals for a "transformed mental health system," as identified by the Mental Health Commission of Canada (2009, 22): "Mental health policies, programs, treatments, services, and supports are informed by the best evidence based on multiple sources of knowledge."

Developing an evidence base is also important from the viewpoint of funding bodies. Lim, Jacobs, and Dewa (2008, 31) note:

> To successfully draw funds to mental health, advocates must stress priority areas based on needs ... and needs in turn must be defined in tangible terms (such as being unable to live alone or work) ... [A]dvocates will be more effective if they can inform policy makers about evidence-based practices that support the effectiveness of various psychiatric treatments and find ways to translate the effectiveness of a particular treatment into tangible parameters, such as a decrease in hospitalization by two months, etc. ... [P]olicy and decision makers need to be convinced of the cost-effectiveness of the new interventions.

Using evidence-based practices may serve a number of purposes (British Columbia Ministry of Health 2002e; Hardiman, Theriot, and Hodges 2005):

- better outcomes for clients
- providing practitioners with tools for practice decisions
- informing policy and planning decisions
- improving fidelity (consistency) of services
- promoting accountability
- increasing cost-efficiency

Program fidelity is usually a desirable goal but is challenged by "individual practitioner, organizational and context-based factors" (Hardiman, Theriot and Hodges 2005, 108). An example is assertive community treatment, considered a best practice intervention but one in which full implementation is sometimes difficult to achieve because of resource issues or various local contingencies (McGrew, Pescosolido, and Wright 2003; Witheridge 1991; see also Chapter 11).

Evidence-based practices are seen as integrating (1) research evidence, (2) practitioner expertise, and (3) client values or preferences (British Columbia Ministy of Health 2002e; Hardiman, Theriot, and Hodges 2005). The second of these elements is an acknowledgment that applying research evidence still requires clinical judgment to account for client preferences and contextual factors, although doing so detracts from the goal of fidelity. Incorporating client values into the equation potentially creates another tension, with American researcher Boyd Tracy suggesting that this goal is necessarily compromised by an emphasis on research evidence and that service users should still have the option of "value-based services," defined as practices that have limited scientific evidence supporting their efficacy but high consumer satisfaction ratings (Tracy 2003, 1437). Similarly, Hardiman et al. (2005, 115) voice the concern that evidence-based practices will "lead to limited options and the defunding of programs that are quite effective, yet lacking scientific evidence to date." As we touched on in Chapter 5, recovery-oriented services present a challenge in this respect since outcomes in this model are more individually based and potentially harder to operationalize and measure. A rejoinder to this is to say that methods different from those traditionally used to evaluate outcomes can be applied or developed.

When considering the source of evidence for evidence-based practices, we start at the top of the traditional "hierarchy" seen in psychiatric research – the experimental design.

Evidence from Experimental Designs

While evidence may come from different sources, in medicine, and by extension psychiatry, the highest level of evidence – the gold standard – is seen as that produced by randomized controlled trials (RCTs) (Sackett et al. 2000). RCTs aspire to the true experimental design, considered to be the best method for making causal inferences and ruling out alternative explanations for the phenomena being observed. From this perspective other sources of evidence may have some utility but are considered second- (or third-) tier (see Figure 5). In the true experiment:

- Subjects are *randomly* assigned to treatment and control groups. Randomization is used to achieve initial group equivalency so that like is being compared with like. This achieves the ceteris paribus condition – "all other things being equal." Other methods of assigning subjects, such as volunteerism, increase the possibility that groups being compared are systematically different. Regarding control conditions, in the case of medication trials the new drug should be compared to a placebo *and* another – usually older – treatment to better establish benefits (Goldacre 2008; Rosenheck 2005).[1]
- The intervention (independent variable) is introduced by the researcher, as opposed to comparing groups after something has already occurred (the latter being called ex post facto research).
- Subjects do not know whether they are in the treatment or control group ("blind") and neither does the researcher ("double-blind"). The first condition theoretically deals with the *placebo effect*, the well-established phenomenon of people experiencing a positive effect from the *context* of receiving help, even if the treatment given – snake oil say, or a sugar pill – has no "active ingredient." The second condition concerns researcher expectancy, the tendency of the hopeful observer to read more into treatment response than may actually exist.
- The treatment environment is controlled so that other, external influences do not contaminate the results.

In RCTs, differences between groups are analyzed with inferential statistics and significant results highlighted. The strength of the evidence is increased when multiple trials produce similar results. These may be published in the form of systematic reviews, with meta-analyses sometimes used as a statistical method of calculating an average effect size across several previously completed studies on a particular topic.[2] A review is considered "systematic" on the basis of a stricter methodology (see Leucht 2006). The Cochrane Reviews

Figure 5

Example of an evidence hierarchy

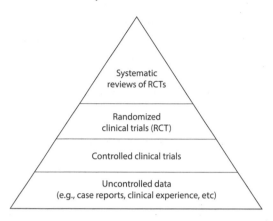

Source: From Ernst (1999).

is a database of systematic independent reviews and meta-analyses on medical subjects (see http://www.thecochranelibrary.com/view/0/index.html).

In psychiatry, the best example of the use of RCTs comes from medication trials. In these studies people are randomly assigned either to a treatment group or to one or more comparison groups. The effects of a new drug may be compared to an older one and also to a placebo, for example. Comparisons are made on the basis of quantifiable indicators, such as a symptom rating scale.

Limitations of RCTs

The apparent control and precision offered by medication studies may be somewhat illusory. In an article on antidepressant medication trials, Sparks and Duncan (2008) point out several possible flaws: (1) concerning "blindness," participants and clinicians may be able to tell who is getting what by virtue of the known side effects produced by the investigative medication; (2) clinician ratings of improvement may be at variance with clients' own measures; and (3) conclusions about effectiveness are limited by the fact that trial periods are short, typically twelve weeks, since medication/placebo differences often diminish with the passage of time. Concerning the first flaw, researchers may consider the use of an "active placebo," such as a substance that has side effects.

As well, medication trials are not necessarily a guide to action. Given that drug response is idiosyncratic, practitioners still need to use good clinical judgment when employing research evidence as a guide to choice of medications in individual cases (Vendantam 2006). Indeed, as noted by Kravitz, Duan, and Braslow (2004), the difficulty in applying global evidence – "average effects" – to individual clients is arguably one of the greatest challenges facing mental health practitioners (see also Davis and Leucht 2008).

Another limitation lies in the fact that the significance of RCT results is a function of sample size. Leucht (2006, S4) notes that "sample sizes in schizophrenia trials are usually too low to make statistically robust conclusions [and that] the quality of antipsychotic trials suffers substantially from high dropout rates." On the flip side, a very large sample may produce a result that is statistically, but not practically, significant. Statistical significance means that, by convention, we are prepared to conclude that a difference is not due to chance, even if the difference is not large, while *effect size* is the statistic that speaks to the "largeness" of the difference. For example, a study comparing newer- and older-generation antipsychotic medications, published in the *American Journal of Psychiatry*, found rates of relapse that "were *modestly but significantly* lower with the newer drugs" (Leucht et al. 2003, 1,209, emphasis added). Significance levels, then, must be placed in the context of effect sizes.

Finally, there is the possibility of bias when RCTs are sponsored by drug companies, who have an obvious incentive to demonstrate the superiority of a new product (Goldacre 2008; Rosenheck 2005). This bias can take different forms, such as the suppression of negative results (see below) or even, as some have claimed, the manipulation of the trial itself. For example, critics have argued that drug manufacturers' claims that newer-generation antipsychotic medications have fewer side effects were based on trial comparisons with control groups that were given older medications in disproportionately high, "non-optimized" doses, which spuriously made the new products better by comparison (Whitaker 2010; see also Rosenheck et al. 2003). Vedantam (2006) notes that rival pharmaceutical companies can "choose statistical techniques that show their drug in the best light," and that, since the trial goal is not to demonstrate cures but to measure symptom relief, this "allows more latitude in how the results are interpreted and marketed."[3]

Unpublished Research

The issue of unpublished research deserves at least some brief comment since there is evidence that it is not a random occurrence but, rather, is dictated by the commercial interests of drug companies, which do not want bad reports on a new product, or universities, which do not want to lose sponsors' contracts (Aleccia 2011; Bekelman, Li, and Gross 2003; *Canadian Medical Association Journal* 2004). Additionally, medical journals may prefer to publish exciting new findings rather than "boring, negative results" (Bekelman, Li, and Gross 2003, 463; see also McKnight 2007). Health Canada (2001a, 24) notes that the evidence-based approach relies "on a body of literature that is subject to pervasive publication bias."

An example of this concerns the unapproved use of antidepressant medication in children, particularly the class of drugs known as selective serotonin reuptake inhibitors. In 2003, regulatory bodies in Britain and Canada started issuing advisories to physicians concerning the use of these drugs with patients under eighteen since evidence of adverse effects appeared to outweigh evidence of therapeutic benefit. In looking at the evidence base to support the "off-label," or non-designated, prescribing of SSRIs, it was noted that fifteen clinical trials had been conducted with young people but only three published – because the results of the other trials showed that the medication did not work (Branham 2004). For example, an internal document obtained by the *Canadian Medical Association Journal* advised staff at the multinational drug company GlaxoSmithKline "to withhold clinical trial findings in 1998 that indicated the antidepressant paroxetine had no beneficial effect in treating adolescents" (Kondro and Sibbald 2004, 783). Similarly, a *New York Times* investigation of Eli Lilly found that the drug company at first withheld, then later reinterpreted, results of trials on the antipsychotic Zyprexa to make it appear that weight gain caused by the drug was less significant (Berenson 2006). In one final example, a review of seventy-four studies of antidepressant medication effectiveness published in the *New England Journal of Medicine* found that almost all studies with positive results (thirty-eight) were published; whereas in studies that did not show effectiveness (thirty-six) only three were published, while in another eleven results were reinterpreted (Turner et al. 2008).

In a report on the limitations of the clinical trial process for evaluating the efficacy of psychiatric medications, doctors interviewed by a Vancouver journalist expressed the need for an independent research body in Canada, akin to a national institute of health, and for the reporting of all trial data, positive and negative (Branham 2003). Similarly, in an editorial on this subject, the *Canadian Medical Association Journal* (2004, 437) concluded:

> The behaviour of industry, government and investigators must change. Investigators must demand access to all the data collected in clinical trials in which they participate and to suitably anonymized [sic] aggregate information from adverse drug reaction reports. Investigators should be at liberty and even encouraged to provide alternate analyses and interpretations of clinical trial results and adverse event reporting and to publish these. Physicians, research subjects and the public should demand no less.

Evidence from Research in the Field

Notwithstanding the limitations noted above, a well-designed RCT offers the potential for isolating and evaluating causal factors while ruling out alternative explanations. However, most research in community mental health is not carried out in laboratories and academic settings but in the "real world." This is a good thing, on the one hand, since it can be argued that findings from field research are more meaningful and generalizable. It is generally assumed that, compared to RCTs, field research is stronger with respect to *external validity* (generalizability) but weaker with respect to *internal validity* (ability to rule out confounding explanations). On the other hand, the standards and hence the advantages of experimental design are very difficult, often impossible, to achieve in research conducted in the field (Anthony, Rogers, and Farkas 2003). For example, in speaking about the difficulty of using experimental designs in the field of occupational therapy, University of Toronto professor Susan Rappolt (2003, 589) notes that, "even in the much larger, and relatively more quantifiable and controllable field of medical research, there is a shortage of coherent, consistent scientific evidence. How much more difficult is it, then, to produce research evidence on the effectiveness of occupational therapy practices, when occupational therapy focuses on the complexities of individuals in their occupational contexts rather than on their cells or biological subsystems?" Mental health researchers investigating non-pharmacological interventions – such as the benefits of assertive community treatment – must contend with issues such as not having a true control group, self-selection (volunteerism) of subjects, subject drop-out, inconsistent application of protocols and procedures ("low fidelity") between settings, and an absence of "discrete and controllable variables" ready-made for analysis (590). Concerning discrete variables, a problem with using trial designs to evaluate psychological therapies is that treatment models may be multifaceted and also have elements in common with other models, making the determination of "what works" more difficult. Duncan, Miller, and Sparks (2004, 40) argue that this finding means that the logic of the RCT cannot easily be applied to psychotherapy evaluations, noting that there are no unique factors and that "the common factors rule."

Studies that attempt to approach the rigour of RCTs in field settings are called "quasi-experiments," designs in which the investigator cannot control all extraneous influences and in which random assignment may not possible. Even in field research designs in which random assignment of subjects to intervention/non-intervention *has* been achieved, note that other requirements of the true experiment may not have been (i.e., "blindness" and a controlled environment).[4] For example, Lynch, Laws, and McKenna (2010,

10) suggest that the purported benefits of cognitive behavioural therapy are based on studies and reviews that lack true blinding as well as on "psychological placebos [control interventions] considered not to have specific therapeutic effects" and that, when more rigourous designs are used, the evidence base is much more equivocal. Another interesting example comes from a study of the effectiveness of peer-led mental health education programs (Cook et al. 2011) in which, because of an "anticipation effect," the investigators found positive outcomes not only for the treatment group but also for the control group. Despite these sorts of limitations, reasonable inferences may still be drawn if (1) limitations are recognized and made explicit, (2) alternative explanations are actively considered, and (3) design guidelines are conscientiously applied and, if possible, bolstered with the use of time-series designs. Anthony, Rogers, and Farkas (2003, 107) conclude that "correlational and quasi-experimental research are excellent sources of information for the development of evidence-based practices and can guide the development of appropriate studies of effectiveness."

Concerning the evidence base for community programs, an American panel of health professionals and researchers tasked with establishing standards for program effectiveness gave the following criteria (Kaplan 2004):

- evaluation with a randomized controlled trial
- statistically significant positive effect
- effect sustained for at least one year
- at least one external replication with RCT
- no known health-compromising side effects[5]

Programs that do not meet this standard may be considered:

- promising (RCT with positive effect but no replication)
- inconclusive
- ineffective (statistical significance not achieved) or
- harmful (negative main or side effects)

The logic of quasi-experimentation has extended to the realm of clinical practice, for example, with single-subject designs, which are approaches used to evaluate behavioural change in individual clients over time. Consistent with this approach, practitioners are taught when setting goals with clients to use the acronym SMART; that is, that outcomes should be:

- Specific: detailed enough that a third party would be able to tell when it had been achieved;

- Measurable: subject to client self-report, staff report, or third party objective appraisal;
- Attainable: within the capabilities of the client and staff (program) to achieve;
- Relevant: currently either a genuine need of or a challenge for the client; and
- Time-bound: achievable within a stipulated, finite period of time.

To measure change, clinical programs may use symptom rating and quality-of-life scales as well as other quantitative indicators, such as number of admissions to hospital, crisis units or emergency shelters, number of calls to the crisis line, number of missed appointments, time on and off the job, and so on.

Another method, widely used in the social sciences when RCTs are not possible, involves attempting to *statistically* control for confounding variables. This is achieved after loading a number of predictor variables into a regression equation, which, through a statistical software program, produces the strongest independent variable(s) after others have been held constant. For example, researchers in Saskatchewan studying suicide among the First Nations were interested in isolating Aboriginal status as a predictor variable after factors such as income were held constant (Lemstra et al. 2009), hypothesizing that poverty, apart from ethnic status, might be the stronger predictor of suicidal behavior (even after controlling for income they found that the prevalence of suicidal thinking was considerably higher among the First Nations). This is a useful research technique but one to be used with some caution. First, while helpful in narrowing to some degree the possible range of confounding factors, regression models cannot prove cause and effect. Second, the predictor variables used are often limited to those that can be most conveniently captured, so these studies may be weak with respect to content validity. Third, confounding associations between two or more variables can be controlled for statistically but not in the real world. In the example of the study (above) by Lemstra and colleagues, the authors found that poverty was much more widespread among Aboriginal participants.

Qualitative Research
Qualitative research (e.g., personal accounts or interviews and focus groups with stakeholders) has historically been placed lower down in the "evidence hierarchy." Qualitative researchers must contend with prejudice in the psychiatric community against the use of "anecdotal" sources of information, which may be applied in the case of the experiences of clients themselves (Uttal 2003). For instance, Boydell, Gladstone, and Crawford (2002, 21) note

that "experiential knowledge – the direct experience of a mental illness and the intimate knowledge of what it means in a human life – traditionally has been devalued in psychiatry." Even when written by practitioners, anecdotal accounts – case studies – have an inferior status in publications like the *Canadian Journal of Psychiatry,* being placed in the back end of the journal under "brief reports" rather than in the front under "original research."

This is unfortunate since it can be argued that the choice of method and evidence should be determined by the research question and that quantitative and qualitative approaches can be complementary rather than "two solitudes." Knowledge gained through personal accounts, clinical work, content analysis, and case studies – inductive methods – can form the hypotheses that are subsequently tested and analyzed through quantitative designs (e.g., see Hilty et al. 2003). Two British policy analysts support the need for a variety of methods as follows:

> Although many researchers and policy makers advocate a hierarchy of evidence, [we argue] that no one research method is automatically better than another. Instead, a research method is only helpful and appropriate if it fully answers the question that is being asked. Thus, if we want to test the effectiveness of a new drug, we may well wish to use a randomized controlled trial ... However, if we want to know how best to improve access to social care services, we might ask current workers (about possible barriers and what might help to make services more accessible) and ask previous service users (how it felt making contact with social services and how this process could be improved). (Glasby and Beresford 2006, 275)

Similarly, Hopper (2008, 711) asserts:

> There is a very good reason to embrace the call to expand use of qualitative research methods in mental health services: we can't understand what's actually going on without them. This isn't special pleading – it's a mundane fact. If we want to understand how it works (whatever "it" may messily turn out to be), what it means, and the enabling contingencies that seem to sustain it, we need to deploy such methods.

This situation may be changing. Boydell, Gladstone, and Crawford (2002, 22) suggest that "the experiential component has resurfaced in research with the burgeoning interest in the use of qualitative methods in tandem with the development of consumer/survivor initiatives and a growing consumer/survivor-authored literature."

Evaluation Research and Performance Indicators

Service utilization patterns are often employed by health authorities as indicators of success or failure. Historically, a commonly used outcome measure has been re-hospitalization, with number of psychiatric admissions, readmissions before a certain period of time, and hospital stays beyond a certain length all being counted as negative outcomes. For example, a document produced by the British Columbia Ministry of Health Services (2002b) proposes that a hospital admission for psychiatric reasons within thirty days of a previous discharge be counted, for evaluation purposes, as a negative outcome. Authorities may also assess system responsiveness through wait-times, for example, the length of time from a community referral to initial assessment or first face-to-face meeting with a clinician, with one government document suggesting that urgent community mental health referrals should be seen "within 72 hours, others within 10 days" (British Columbia Ministry of Health 2002e, 5). Wait-times as a performance indicator may also apply to inpatient services, with overcrowded emergency departments being a particular concern.

Using hospitalization as a success/failure indicator has been criticized from a number of perspectives. One concern is that the real agenda is cost savings, although being fiscally responsible with limited health care resources is an ethically defensible position.[6] Another concern is that if hospital admissions become too brief this can lead to negative outcomes, based on the claim that clients are being discharged prematurely while still in a fragile state. This argument has received empirical support, with surveys by the Canadian Institute for Health Information (2011a) finding an inverse correlation between length of admission and (subsequent) readmission rates. Because of this, "readmission within 30 days" is now used as a system indicator to qualify data on reduced length of stay.

For an overview of quantitative indicators used to evaluate mental health practice, the reader is directed to a document by McEwan and Goldner (2001). Performance across jurisdictions is assessed in the *accreditation* process, with standards specifically for mental health populations (see the Accreditation Canada website at http://www.accreditation.ca/en/default.aspx).

Evaluation efforts can – and should – be undertaken by clinical staff. Some practitioners may have lacked the training and encouragement to do so, while some disciplines (e.g., occupational therapy) have this aspect more clearly built into their practice and more routinely engage (for instance) in needs and outcome assessments. Concerning program evaluation, DePoy and Gilson (2008, vii) note that the schism between "those who do" (clinicians) and "those who scrutinize" (evaluators and planners) needs to be bridged, and they promote an "evaluation practice" approach that they define as the integration of systematic appraisal with professional thinking and action. A model for being outcome-informed when working with individual clients is presented by Duncan, Miller, and Sparks (2004) in their book *The Heroic Client*. Another model used in health care settings, more often by managers, is *root cause analysis*, which is a method for identifying how and why adverse events occur, with the goal of preventing recurrence. Rooney and Heuvel (2004) note that root causes should be those that can be reasonably identified, those over which management has control, and those for which effective recommendations can be generated. The Canadian Patient Safety Institute (2006) has produced a framework document on this subject.

Recovery-Oriented Research

The implementation of a recovery philosophy in mental health services has forced a re-evaluation of the concept of "evidence base." Looking at the evidence base through a recovery lens necessarily means addressing epistemological concerns, such as the limitations of quantitative approaches, as well as the need to actively seek input from the population being served.

Concerning the relationship between recovery and evidence-based practice, a useful discussion is provided by Davidson and colleagues (2009), who address three questions: (1) Is recovery evidence-based? (2) Are evidence-based practices recovery oriented? (3) Are recovery-oriented practices evidence-based? Concerning the first question, the answer depends on how one defines recovery. The authors make the distinction between the medical definition of recovery *from* mental illness and the newer definition of recovery *in* mental illness. On the first of these, they review longitudinal studies of persons with severe mental illness showing at least partial and in many cases full symptomatic remission over time. The second issue is more difficult to empirically investigate, given that recovery will be individually and subjectively defined, and, indeed, the authors argue that pursuing one's own definition and pathway to recovery is more a question of human rights than of evidence.

Are evidence-based practices recovery oriented? To answer this question one could look at current practices to see to what extent they could be considered to be client-centred, strengths-based, collaborative, and empowering. Supported employment and supported housing (described in more detail in Chapters 12 and 17) would score fairly high in this respect in that they both emphasize client choice as a central principle. On the other hand, assertive community treatment (ACT – described in Chapter 11) might produce a mixed evaluation: while scoring well on traditional indicators, such as re-hospitalization, the model's more coercive aspects would be considered less recovery-oriented. For example, a survey of ACT clients by Queen's University professor Terry Krupa and colleagues (2005, 23), while eliciting positive reviews, also found that staff could be perceived as authoritative and intrusive at times, especially "around choices regarding medication and the control of finances." Concerning the use of medication, a recovery orientation would be reflected more in the treatment *delivery* (e.g., using collaboration as much as possible) than in the treatment per se.

A different way of answering the question "are evidence-based practices recovery oriented?" is to look more closely at the evidence being used. Concerning the use of re-hospitalization figures as a measure of success/failure, William Anthony and colleagues observe that "simple dichotomous counts of ... hospitalization are an enormous conceptual distance from what might be described as recovery outcomes" (Anthony, Rogers, and Farkas 2003, 105). From a recovery perspective it is not always clear what such figures mean to the individual. While we may assume that, for most people, it is better to avoid hospitalization, the limitation is that the focus is on mental illness (symptom stabilization) rather than on mental health. Recalling the earlier discussion on the two-continua model (see Chapter 1), these two domains are not the same; and, indeed, for some people, taking risks to move ahead in their lives (e.g., through employment) may actually increase their level of symptoms in the short term. In sum, using *only* traditional psychiatric measures of success may actually work against achieving recovery goals (Davidson et al. 2009).

Finally, are recovery-oriented practices evidence-based? Davidson and colleagues (2009) ask, once again, whether the question is relevant since persons with a mental illness have the right to determine and choose their own individual pathways to recovery. That said, they note that, if one is talking about larger-scale, more systematic empirical support, the answer – in 2009 – is "not yet." This is because of the relative newness of the concept. While supported housing and supported employment may have a more solid evidence base, other promising developments (such as peer-run services) are still accumulating this evidence.

Participatory Research

A criticism of academic research is that the subjects – people – are used to suit the investigator's agenda and then, in effect, discarded. A different approach, typically employed with marginalized populations, involves a model called "participatory research," which differs not so much in the methods used as in having representatives of the population being studied identify the research question. Relevance of the question to the participant group and possible pay-offs to that group through the later exchange of knowledge are often the key criteria to consider. This is not to say that academic research never achieves any practical ends but, rather, that participatory research is more *explicitly* collaborative, praxis-oriented, and political. This discussion may be relevant in talking about research questions identified by service users of the psychiatric system since, according to Beresford (2006, 225), such research "tends to be associated with ... the empowerment of service users and the improvement of their lives, through both the process and purpose of research." The Mental Health Commission of Canada (2012, 115) concludes that a mental health research agenda should "enhance opportunities for people living with mental health problems and illnesses to ... participate meaningfully in all aspects of research including as lead researchers." With respect to the methods used, Canada's Kirby Report (Standing Senate Committee on Social Affairs, Science and Technology 2006) suggests that consumers and families favour "participatory action research and under-utilized ... qualitative methods" (244) as a means to "reclaim ones own story" (231).

An article by Griffiths and colleagues (2004) identifies both potential advantages and potential challenges concerning consumer participation in research:

- Advantages to the research enterprise itself include the inside experience and knowledge of service recipients; a potentially broader perspective on the research question; the greater likelihood that feasibility, relevance and client-sensitivity will be highlighted; insights into the interpretation of data – a phenomenological perspective; increased researcher accountability; and, greater appreciation for research by the consumers participating.
- Public health advantages include, hopefully, improved services and improved health outcomes.
- Advantages to clients of the psychiatric system include the acknowledgment of consumer expertise; providing clients with both a voice and a sense of ownership; providing an opportunity to contribute; and, diminishing stigma by making clients partners.
- *Challenges* to the research enterprise include the possibility of consumer-researchers becoming unwell and having to break off from the project; a lack of research knowledge and credentials among consumers; and, whether the consumers offering their inside experience and views of the mental health system can be considered representative. With respect to participants becoming unwell, a parallel concern is the added stress of the work causing symptoms of mental illness to worsen. Possible

challenges for the professional researcher include the additional time required to mentor consumer-colleagues, and the threat to a self-perception of "researcher as expert," this having to do with "a feeling of ownership regarding the intellectual quality of their research" (Griffiths et al. 2004, 52).[7]

Truly participatory, consumer-driven research, particularly as it applies to working in *teams*, is still an underdeveloped field, which is not to discount the exceptional personal narratives that have been written by persons receiving mental health services in Canada (e.g., Carten 2006). As reviewed by Schneider (2010), service user roles in research fall within a continuum:

- *Advisory*: clients are invited to be part of a board or committee to represent the "stakeholder" group.
- *Consultation*: service users are regarded as having knowledge that may be valuable, for example, in designing a survey, but control of the project is retained by the professionals.
- *Collaboration*: clients collaborate with professional researchers in all aspects of the project, including identifying the research question, study design, data gathering and analysis, and dissemination of results.
- *Control*: service users run the show, and if outside professionals are used at all this is at the request of the project team.

The fact that there are relatively few examples of the latter category may be because a collaborative approach is preferred by the parties involved but also clearly has to do with service users having limited resources in terms of finances and trained personnel. Academics and other professional researchers bring with them an infrastructure that includes, most critically, access to grant money. Client-only research teams are generally less eligible for grants, particularly those of any size, so collaborative projects may be the default option. These partnerships may be fruitful, and there are certainly progressive academics who want to honour the consumer voice, but there is always the danger of tokenism and co-option to guard against. Examples of enterprises that could be considered "consumer-controlled" are the Consumer Research Unit in Australia (http://cmhr.anu.edu.au/cru/index.php) and the National Empowerment Center in the US (http://www.power2u.org). In both of these centres, the program directors identify as being in recovery from mental illness.

In Canada, a number of collaborative projects have been undertaken by academics in partnership with service recipients, and one can point to the work of professors Geoff Nelson at Wilfrid Laurier University (http://info.

wlu.ca/~wwwpsych/gnelson/mainset.htm), Barbara Schneider at the University of Calgary (http://callhome.ucalgary.ca/), and Marina Morrow at Simon Fraser University (http://www.socialinequities.ca) as examples.

Knowledge Exchange[8]

Production of evidence is not sufficient: it needs to be put into practice (Straus, Tetroe, and Graham 2009). This may seem an obvious point, but the fact remains that, in many instances, mental health knowledge gained through research is not being implemented, and, hence, clients are not receiving what are considered to be best or better practices (Cook et al. 2009; Grol 2008; Marshall et al. 2008; Perkins et al. 2007; Waddell 2001). Not infrequently, for example, one reads accounts of parents with mentally ill children expressing frustration about the lack of availability of specific treatments for anxiety disorders (e.g., Barrett 2010; Inman 2010). In a different area, a study conducted by the Schizophrenia Patient Outcome Research Team in the US determined that fewer than one-quarter of clients of community programs received any vocational services at all, let alone "best practices" (Marshall et al. 2008).

There are a number of reasons for this state of affairs, many of them rather mundane. One, perhaps surprisingly, involves deficits in training at the undergraduate level (see Inman 2010). For instance, this author has been told in a number of discussions with colleagues that cognitive-behavioural therapy (CBT) and motivational interviewing are not subjects routinely offered to students in nursing, social work, and other helping professions. This may, in turn, be driven by faculty interest or disciplinary traditions that need to be revisited.

Another factor is cost, particularly with respect to physician time. Psychotherapy, CBT, and education sessions take longer than a brief visit during which the client "checks in" and has a prescription renewed. In a different example, there is now an evidence base supporting the efficacy of a behavioural treatment for autism (historically considered an intractable condition), but the expense of the treatment – around $60,000 a year – has been onerous for provincial governments and has led to some ugly disputes around cost containment (Greenberg 2007).

There is also the reality that professionals tend to stay within an orienting tradition or paradigm and to avoid incorporating new approaches, even if these are evidence-based (a seminal work in this respect is Thomas Kuhn's *The Structure of Scientific Revolutions*). For example, 2,607 psychotherapists in Canada and the US responded to a survey in which they were asked to "rate factors that influenced their clinical practice, including their adoption and sustained use of new treatments" (Cook et al. 2009, 671). It was found that their initial training, significant mentors, and informal discussions were the most significant and that "empirical evidence had little influence" on their practice. It was also found that they would be most likely to consider a new treatment if there was the "potential for integration with *the therapy they were already providing*" (Cook et al. 2009, 671, emphasis added).

There are other fairly mundane, self-serving justifications for practitioners not to adopt new practices. On this, Grol (2008, 275) observes that "most professionals, most of the time, [are influenced by] other drivers, such as practical problems, organizational barriers, patients' demands, avoiding unrest and conflict in their work setting, financial incentives, opinions of peers, and the wish to have a good time." Grol (2008) suggests that, before attempting to introduce changes, management needs to prepare carefully, to explore attitudes towards change and whether a culture of learning and collaboration exists, and to use complex change programs along with continuous evaluation. An example from my own experience involves the introduction of a new goals assessment tool among case managers – an instrument that had been positively evaluated in other settings – which was made difficult simply because of the additional demands with respect to time and recording requirements it placed on staff.

In addressing the challenge of knowledge exchange, Straus, Tetroe, and Graham (2009) note that knowledge dissemination (journal and conference papers) and even knowledge distillation (systematic reviews) are not enough. Concerning journal publications, a medical practitioner would have to read literally hundreds of titles a month to remain current. Further, most practitioners are not skilled in assessing and interpreting evidence since "until recently this skill-set has not been a traditional component of most educational curricula" (166).

To support knowledge exchange in medicine and psychiatry, *clinical practice guidelines* (CPGs) are published to "bridge the gap between producers of health care research and the providers" and to "reduce the variance between practice known to be effective according to the best evidence available and the actual practice taking place" (British Columbia Ministry of Health 2002e, 10). For example, a special issue (November 2005) of the *Canadian Journal of Psychiatry* provides guidelines for the treatment of schizophrenia, with reference to pharmacotherapy, psychosocial interventions, and systems of service delivery. In guidelines such as these, physicians may be given decision-trees ("algorithms") concerning the appropriate initial (first-line) medication, and alternatives should this treatment fail, such as augmentation with another drug or switching to an agent used with treatment-refractory presentations (such as clozapine in the case of schizophrenia). A first-line medication is so called presumably because of efficacy but also because of *tolerability* by the majority of persons receiving it. On this point, the clinician needs to be aware that people will respond differently and, indeed, "effective guidelines ... are flexible enough to allow both [clinicians and clients] some choices in individualizing care" (British Columbia Ministry of Health 2002e, 10). In reading CPGs, such as the ones for schizophrenia referred to above, it is notable that the "best evidence" being synthesized is not unequivocal and is not always clearly supported by RCTs or systematic reviews (i.e., CPGs may draw from evidence lower in the "hierarchy").

In larger community mental health settings staff education is supported by in-services and workshops, sometimes remedial in nature. The challenge for health authorities is not merely in presenting information in an engaging way but also in building an infrastructure that supports the maintenance and development of new skills (such as CBT) since, without practice, these skills are usually lost (Latimer 2005). Clinicians may be able to form peer-mentoring groups – "communities of practice" – to this end, something that should receive management support even if just in the form of the provision of space and time. This does, however, raise the question: Who is ultimately responsible for knowledge exchange and the maintenance of new skills? While clearly there is an onus on the individual practitioner, we have already spoken about the limited time individuals have to consume new information as well as the human tendency to resist change. Staff educators, present in larger organizations, presumably fulfill this role, although they may lack credibility since they are not practitioners and so may not be able to appreciate feasibility issues and the day-to-day struggles of staff trying to implement new initiatives – "talking the talk," but not "walking the walk," so to speak. This problem may be addressed by the employment of "knowledge brokers" or clinician-researchers who walk both sides of the line and can speak to the practical difficulties in implementing research findings in particular settings (Waddell 2001). This being the case, they cannot be as "easily dismissed as academics who do not understand what we do" (Yanos and Ziedonis 2006, 250). The challenge is not only in finding persons with both skill sets but also in gaining management support for this role. Yanos and Ziedonis (2006) suggest that, if anything, mental health settings have seen a decline in the number of clinician-researchers.

Mental health consumers themselves have a valuable role to play in knowledge exchange, and it is hoped that the practitioners working with them will engage in active listening to learn more about "what works." An evidence-based practice, after all, must rely on "practice-based evidence." Consumers may also demonstrate the potential of a new initiative more compellingly than would be the case if they had just read about it. An example from this author's own experience concerns consumers employed by health authorities as peer support workers. While there was research evidence supporting the value of this development (discussed in more detail in Chapter 17) there was also, in the author's work setting, trepidation expressed by staff about employing clients in the same workplace. However, once staff had seen peer workers *in action* greater buy-in soon followed. This does, of course, require managers with both courage and vision.

Best Practices Revisited

So, what can we conclude about "best practices" in mental health? To begin with, there is agreement that they must be evidence-based: "good intentions" are necessary but are not sufficient. With a weak evidence base, both the credibility of the practitioner and the buy-in of the client are diminished. However, as Glasby and Beresford (2006, 269) note, this still leaves us with a number of questions: "What constitutes valid evidence? Who decides? Do certain types of evidence seem to be treated as more legitimate than others? What happens when evidence is fragmented or even contradictory? How much evidence does there need to be before we can confidently develop and roll out a particular policy?"

We have suggested that "success" indicators need to include reduction in the symptoms of mental illness but should also address mental health or quality of life – in short, *both* of the two continua referred to in Chapter 1 need to be considered. Further, in evaluating new practices there is, increasingly, an expectation that these be *recovery-oriented*, indicators of which would include enhancing client choice, limiting coercion, and facilitating the self-management of mental illness (for more details on this, see Chapter 5). Community mental health programs have not traditionally used quality-of-life scales in clinical practice, but such scales have been developed (Keyes 2007; Lambert et al. 1996), including brief versions that can be used routinely in clinical practice (Duncan, Miller, and Sparks 2004). Such scales will not work for everyone, so a curious, flexible, and culturally respectful approach to understanding well-being will be needed.

Resource utilization data, which can be fairly reliably gathered, may still be a useful outcome measure. Hospitalization figures may reflect client dysfunction and may also point to gaps in other parts of the system. However, hospitalization rates as an outcome measure do not really tell us about quality of life and may just as well fuel the perception that the real issue is cost savings. On this point, Pollack and colleagues (2009, 5) note that best practices should not be seen as "a method for administrators to save costs."

As to the method by which evidence is produced, it was noted that in medical research the gold standard is the RCT, and, indeed, for certain research questions (such as psychiatric medication studies), RCTs offer the

Weighing the Evidence: Study Examples

The chapter concludes with examples of studies referred to in this book, in which conclusions reached must be qualified by limitations of the methodology used. It must be emphasized that *all study designs have limitations,* so, in a sense, the ones referred to below were arbitrarily chosen – although all address important areas of practice. The point of the exercise is to stress (1) that practitioners need to engage in critical thinking in their appraisal of the evidence base, and (2) that researchers need to transparently consider these limitations in drawing any conclusions.

Medication trials: experimental design (Chapters 8 and 15). While the randomized controlled trials used in pharmaceutical studies are considered the "gold standard," conclusions about the long-term benefits and costs associated with medication use must take into account the financial incentive for companies to favour their own products and to interpret or suppress findings accordingly. Medication trials may also suffer from follow-up periods that are too short as well as control agents that are "inactive" (in the case of placebos) or not optimally dosed (found to be the case with some studies of second-generation antipsychotics).

The Vermont Longitudinal Study: retrospective follow-up (Chapter 5). This now rather dated study is one of the most cited in support of the idea of functional and clinical recovery in the long term in schizophrenia (in a number of instances without treatment). The study, however, has a number of potential sources of bias: it is retrospective rather than prospective; diagnostic systems changed over the time period covered; some subjects could not be located ("drop-out") and likely had poorer outcomes; and there was possible selection bias in the way subjects were recruited.

Evaluating psychosocial interventions: quasi-experiments (Chapter 16). To establish that a practice is evidence-based researchers usually employ randomized controlled trials, but since these real-world studies lack the true control of laboratory settings they are referred to as "quasi-experimental." An example is the evaluation of WRAP, a peer-led curriculum in which participants design their own wellness recovery plan. Cook and colleagues (2011) randomly assigned 529 subjects either to WRAP or to control groups and, after six months, found the WRAP group to have statistically superior scores on scales measuring symptom profiles, hopefulness, and quality of life – although effect sizes were not large. One problem with field studies such as this one is that they cannot usually be "blind"; that is, subjects and researchers know who is and who is not getting the intervention, which means a placebo effect or researcher expectancy effect cannot be ruled out. In the WRAP study, subjects in the control group *also* improved across all three outcomes, possibly due to an "anticipation effect," as they had been promised an opportunity to receive WRAP at the end of the study. The problem is that this may have had the effect of *underestimating* the benefit of WRAP, and, in any case, differences between the groups were made more difficult to interpret. Another challenge in evaluating psychosocial interventions is the difficulty in isolating *specific* effects from *common* effects, getting inside the "black box" so to speak. Psychological treatments may have elements in common – such as relationship building and the expression of empathy – meaning that if clients find the intervention to be beneficial it may be difficult to say what is providing the benefit: a technique specific to that intervention or an element common to many?

Evaluating community treatment orders: various methods (Chapter 18). Community treatment orders (CTOs) are mandatory reporting provisions based in provincial mental health legislation that require clients to follow conditions set out by a treatment team. They are intended to prevent the "revolving door" of chronic re-hospitalization and to promote client and public safety. Conclusions that CTOs are effective have been criticized by those who say that they have rarely been evaluated using randomized controlled trials (RCTs). This, however, is an instance in which the use of RCTs would be ethically problematic since it would mean deliberately assigning persons who could benefit from an intervention to "no treatment" (a control group). There could also be liability considerations. Another example of this would involve using an RCT design to evaluate the benefit of a needle exchange program for injection drug users since control subjects would be deliberately exposed to health- if not life-threatening conditions. This conundrum is sometimes addressed using designs that employ waiting lists or "matching" (comparing in-treatment subjects to demographically similar persons). Studies of CTOs have tended to focus on re-hospitalization and arrest rates as outcome indicators and have not necessarily looked at the perceptions and buy-in of clients themselves, which, in a recovery-oriented system, would be important to consider. In some instances, when clients have been interviewed, this has been done with persons *still in the program* (i.e., in an involuntary status), meaning that they may have felt pressured to give positive feedback, making results harder to interpret.

most appropriate design. However, for other issues, particularly when exploring complex social processes, RCTs are usually neither feasible nor necessarily preferable. The safest conclusion is that a *range* of methods, both quantitative and qualitative, should be employed to create the evidence base in mental health practice (DePoy and Gilson 2008).

The most problematic question arising from the Beresford and Glasby quote at the start of this section is: "Who decides?" A provincial government document (British Columbia Ministry of Health 2002e), in defining best practices, lists several reference groups: clinicians, service users, family, and government. Reconciling what may be conflicting interests among these stakeholders is not an easy matter. For example, this author has, individually and in focus groups, had clients share with him their concern about implementing treatment practices that are time-limited and goal- or "graduation"-oriented, highlighting the tension between resource limitations and access to care. In other words, "graduation," however defined, can be seen as a good outcome by one individual but not by another. Families may be less interested in client self-determination (read: risk-taking) and more interested in practices that keep their loved one safe and in treatment – practices that may be coercive, unappealing to (at least some) clients and not what are called recovery-oriented (Inman 2010). Government action is driven by various factors that are not necessarily related to the interests of mental health consumers, cost containment being one and responding to public perceptions about safety and dangerous mentally ill persons being another (Goering, Wasylenki, and Durbin 2000). Here, there is a role for the conscientious clinician to attempt to balance interests. Practitioners need to be evidence-based with our interventions, using evidence from a variety of sources. Clinical guidelines may help us, but there is no "cookbook" method of practice (Pollack et al. 2009). Mental illness and safety should be our first targets, but we need to also include mental health in our scope and to understand the difference between those terms. And, since the knowledge base is being applied to *individuals* in clinical practice, we must take into account their values, choices, and expertise.

Notes

1   Rosenheck (2005) notes that, since this has not always been undertaken by the US Food and Drug Administration in trials of new psychotropic drugs (which were compared to placebos only), there has been a distortion of the evidence base.
2   Limitations of meta-analyses include the danger of skewed results due to the inclusion of methodologically weak studies with stronger ones and also due to the possibility of important studies being missed either by chance or because they were never published.
3   For a listing of "relatively unbiased sources on drugs and drug studies" see Pollack et al. (2009).

4 Concerning a controlled environment, see Cook and Campbell (1979) for a discussion of diffusion, imitation, compensatory rivalry, compensatory equalization, and resentful demoralization between comparison groups.

5 The requirement of "do no harm" is an important one since both pharmacological and psychosocial interventions can have unintended negative effects. Drug regulatory agencies may have a requirement of "non-inferiority" based·on a RCT (i.e., that the new product at least be no worse than the established treatment) (Leucht 2006).

6 A 2009 Vancouver Coastal Health internal document notes that "cost avoidance [e.g., through reduced length of hospital admissions] will help to improve access to meet pent-up demand."

7 Concerning these challenges, this author has been involved in a collaborative research group and indeed has struggled with the question of credentials asked for in the case of consumers: Should the purpose be to help train new researchers or to hire those at least minimally qualified to enable the research team to "hit the ground running?"

8 Similar terms used in this area are "knowledge transfer" and "knowledge translation."

Other Resources
The Mental Health Commission's Knowledge Exchange Centre provides a large number of tools, articles, and videos on a range of topics: https://kec.mentalhealthcommission.ca/mental_health_tools_and_resources.

The Continuum of Mental Health Services

What are the services considered essential to meet the needs of mentally ill persons living in the community? The Canadian Psychiatric Association (2005, 37S) addresses this question in its practice guidelines for the treatment of schizophrenia:

> All patients should have access to a comprehensive continuum of services
> that provides continuity of care, including physical care ... [T]he continuum
> of care should include 24 hour crisis services, acute inpatient care in a
> medical setting, nonmedical crisis stabilization, acute day hospital treat-
> ment, community-based rehabilitation, integrated addiction services,
> comprehensive services for early psychosis [and] assertive community
> treatment programs.

The passage above refers to the need for a *continuum* of services, which can be seen as ranging from less to more specialized/intense, depending on the needs of the client.[1] The Canadian Senate report *Out of the Shadows at Last* emphasizes that services should focus on supporting people in their local communities, be "close to home," and be delivered in the least intrusive way possible (Standing Senate Committee on Social Affairs, Science and Technology 2006). "Least intrusive" is a principle reflected in best practice guidelines, the recovery vision, codes of ethics, and legislation such as adult guardianship statutes. The Senate report also notes that, since specialized services (such as tertiary psychiatric inpatient care) are the "least available and most expensive resources[,] ... they must be reserved for those who truly need them and used only when ... [other] supports have failed to work for a given individual" (104). When intermediate resources are not available or accessible it becomes harder to "head off" psychiatric crises, with greater use of inpatient care being the result. At the other end of the continuum,

Figure 6

Continuum of mental health services

Increasing intensity →

First line	Specialized outpatient	Outreach	Residential care	Hospital care
Primary care (family doctor)	Early psychosis intervention	Intensive case management	Sub-acute facilities and crisis programs	General hospital psychiatry units
Crisis response	Programs for co-occurring disorders, eating disorders, and other conditions	Assertive community treatment	Residential recovery homes	Tertiary psychiatric units
Information, referral, and case management		Acute home-based treatment		Forensic hospital units
Community clinics	Telehealth			
Private counselors and psychiatrists	Forensic programs			
	Day hospitals			
Hospital emergency				

Cross-level services:
Peer services; housing; and social, educational, vocational, and recreational support.

Foundations of service:
Recovery-oriented, trauma-informed, and culturally sensitive.

first-line services, because they are located where most support is to be provided, "must be easily accessible to people no matter what their specific needs" (101).

Figure 6 is an (admittedly simplified) depiction of a mental health system as it might exist in a larger centre in Canada. Services listed in the diagram are described in more detail later in this chapter, and elsewhere in this book. Services can be seen as ranging from lesser to greater intensity, reflecting higher degrees of disability. "First line" indicates where most mental health contacts will occur. As will be seen, a majority of contacts are managed by family doctors alone; this is not necessarily a desirable situation, and it speaks to the importance of *shared care* initiatives, whereby family doctors receive support from specialized mental health services.

In a number of instances, contacts with the system will be crisis-oriented, with paramedics, police, or, in some cases, specialized mental health units responding. Some clients will *primarily* use hospital emergencies to deal with mental health concerns. While any system needs an adequate crisis response, clearly there is a problem if an individual's contacts are predominantly via crisis-oriented programs. This suggests that the person is not connecting or maintaining a connection with other services or that these services are absent. Continuity of care is better supported when there are information, referral, and way-finding services that are user-friendly and, for more disabled persons, case management programs that help coordinate care.

Persons being treated for a serious mental illness will in many instances be followed by public community clinics or teams and, in a smaller number of instances, "day hospitals." Access to other private treatment programs is often limited. Psychiatrists in private practice whose services are covered by provincial medicare plans may be difficult to gain access to or have long waiting lists (Goldner, Jones, and Fang 2011). Non-physician counsellors who do not work for a health authority, for example clinical psychologists, will in most cases not have their fees covered by provincial plans and hence offer services that are prohibitively expensive for low-income persons. Some centres will have public, community programs for specialized populations such as young persons first experiencing psychosis (early psychosis intervention), co-occurring disorders (usually referring to mental illness and substance misuse), eating disorders, and personality disorders. Forensic psychiatric programs, both outpatient and inpatient, operate under a very specific legal mandate and are described in Chapter 13.

Some seriously disabled clients will require, at least in the short term, more intense follow-up and outreach, which can be provided by intensive or assertive teams, the best known model being ACT (assertive community treatment). A different, shorter-term intensive model designed to manage acute crises outside of hospital is the acute home-based treatment program. When crises cannot be managed in the community, a staffed, sub-acute facility is an alternative, and when safety concerns become paramount hospitalization is the usual recourse. Most psychiatric hospitalizations in Canada are relatively short and occur in general hospital psychiatric units; smaller centres may, unfortunately, not have separate psychiatric units within their hospitals. When the clinical presentation is complex or very refractory to treatment, persons may be admitted to what are called *tertiary care* hospitals, where the length of stay is typically longer.

Using the example of a person with a psychotic disorder, and depending on the severity of illness, in a comprehensive system the client could (1) be seen at an outpatient team, (2) be followed by an intensive outreach program,

(3) be seen on a daily basis at home by doctors and nurses for home-based management of the illness, (4) be placed in a respite setting, (5) be hospitalized in acute care, or (6) be transferred to a tertiary care bed for a longer stay. In reality, many settings will not offer this range of services, and even where they exist, vacancies, allowing movement from one service to the other, may not open up in a timely fashion. Fortunately, the life-long trajectory of a mental illness will mean, in many cases, a later period of stabilization (Davidson and Roe 2007; Public Health Agency of Canada 2006) and less need for intense services.

Moving across the continuum of programs are *cross-level* services – housing (Chapter 12), peer support and rehabilitation programs (Chapter 17) – which, in a comprehensive system, should be available to all, regardless of level of care. And the mission of a comprehensive system should be to provide services that are recovery-oriented (Chapter 5), trauma-informed, and culturally sensitive (Chapter 6).

What follows is an overview of treatment services in Canada, moving across the continuum. Housing, peer support, rehabilitation, and forensic programs are addressed in later chapters. Readers should note that, while there is some consensus on what constitutes core services, the particular situation and manifestation of these services may differ from region to region, affected by "factors that are unique to the history and circumstances of each community" (Standing Senate Committee on Social Affairs, Science and Technology 2006, 105). In looking at inter-provincial differences in service provision, the federal government sets general guidelines, in particular through the Canada Health Act, but the delivery of health care remains a provincial jurisdiction, which accounts in part for the variation seen (see box). Because of these differences, the discussion here focuses on program *components*, which may be situated in various ways, depending on the locale.

Family Doctors and Shared Care

Before discussing *specialized* community mental health programs, a not unreasonable question to address is: Can mental health treatment needs be met by an individual's family doctor? Whether they can or not, it should be noted that in Canada most of physician care for persons with mental illness is in fact provided by GPs, not specialists (Alessi-Severini et al. 2012; Bilsker, Goldner, and Jones 2007; Lavoie and Fleet 2002; Picard 2008a; Slomp et al. 2009), with one report finding family doctors to be the sole caregivers in 80 percent of cases (Picard 2008a). Is this a good thing? While this arrangement may be workable, particularly for those with less disabling mental disorders, or for those who are in a later stage of recovery, the fact that such a large

Governance and Mandate of Health Care in Canada

The genesis of a national medicare system in Canada, following the lead of the Province of Saskatchewan, can be traced to 1965, when the Royal Commission on Health Services produced a report for the federal government that recommended a comprehensive and universal system of health care that would cover physician care and prescription drugs (Regehr and Glancy 2010). In 1966, the federal government passed the Medical Care Act, mandating federal funding for these services. Because health care in Canada is administrated by the provinces – a requirement dating back to the British North America Act of 1867 – individual cost-sharing negotiations had to be conducted with each province. In 1984, the federal Canada Health Act was passed, outlining five core principles that were to be followed by the provinces to qualify for federal funding:

1 *Public administration:* Health insurance plans must be administered and operated on a non-profit basis by a public authority, responsible to the provincial or territorial government.

2 *Comprehensiveness:* Health insurance plans must cover all health services provided by hospitals and medical practitioners. It should be noted that, while the Canada Health Act states that the provinces may fund additional health care services, at its narrowest, this section excludes mental health services that are not hospital-based or led by physicians. Thus, provincial medical service plans provide for a person who is seeing a private psychiatrist but not, in most cases, services provided by private, community-based therapists, such as psychologists.

3 *Universality:* All insured persons must be covered by the provincial health insurance plan. (The federal government has a separate responsibility to provide health care to certain populations, which include the Canadian military, the RCMP, and federal prison inmates.)

4 *Portability:* Canadian residents are to be covered by the plan when they move from one province to another. Initially the province of origin covers costs until care is transferred to the new province or territory of residence.

5 *Accessibility:* The health insurance plan must provide for "reasonable access" to services, unimpeded by charges (such as extra-billing) or other means (e.g., age, health status, or financial circumstances). The act allows for dollar-for-dollar withholding of transfer payments where extra-billing for insured services is allowed.

proportion of clients is not receiving specialized care is a cause for concern. That clients may not be receiving optimal mental health care in this arrangement is supported by findings that sessions with GPs "tend to be shorter in duration, less often include therapeutic listening, and more commonly result in prescription of medication" (Clarke Institute of Psychiatry 1997, 64). Conversely, there is evidence that, when psychotherapy can be provided concomitantly, reliance on, and possible overuse of, medication diminishes (Wiggins and Cummings 1998). Other studies have found that, compared to persons seen by GPs alone, persons seen by psychiatrists are seen more frequently (Slomp et al. 2009), are more likely to get counselling and optimal medication treatment (Young et al. 2001), and have lower drop-out rates (Olfson et al. 2009). There is also evidence that, when dealing with the initial onset of a psychotic disorder, involvement with a GP – rather than with a mental health specialist – may actually result in delays in receiving appropriate treatment (Birchwood and Brunet 2004). A 2011 online survey by the Mood Disorders Society of Canada (2011b) found that 52 percent of 844 respondents who identified as having a mental illness received treatment for this condition from their family doctor; of this number, less than half – 45 percent – reported being satisfied with care provided. Among those expressing dissatisfaction, the most commonly given reasons were lack of knowledge and the limited time available.

None of these findings should be particularly surprising, in that GPs in Canada generally see large volumes of patients in brief visits, do not have the same training as specialists, and – critically – lack the *fee incentive* to engage in longer, frequent counselling sessions (Branham 2003; Condon, 2006). Rather, they are paid on a per-person basis, regardless of how brief or how long and complicated the intervention is. Some accommodations are being made, an example being that, under the Medical Services Plan in BC, family doctors, up to eight times a year per patient, may provide and be compensated for a longer session to manage a psychiatric condition.[2] Financial compensation for GPs is less than that for specialists, with evidence that this gap has been widening in recent years (Condon 2006).

Family doctors also do not have the same access to resources: McEwan and Goldner (2001, 32) note that "many physicians work in isolation from community mental health providers who frequently are the gatekeepers to the array of services and supports required by those with serious mental disorders." GPs wishing to refer clients to specialist care may face various barriers, including (1) a lack of knowledge of these resources, (2) narrow admission criteria, (3) the fact that – particularly in remote areas – mental health specialists are relatively unavailable, and (4) the stigma associated with being referred to a mental health specialist (Ben Noun 1996), meaning that the client declines the referral even when it is offered. All of these may contribute to the fact that, as noted, many persons with depressive and anxiety disorders end up being treated by family physicians alone. GPs in private practice also lack access to educational in-services available to staff working at multidisciplinary clinics and hospitals.

Because of the potential difficulties associated with GPs working in isolation, there has been increasing interest in models of *shared care*, which has been defined as "collaborative activities between family physicians and psychiatric services designed to improve mental health care for clients" (British Columbia Ministry of Health 2002e, 48). One can note, for example, how important it is for GPs and specialists to be on the "same page" when working with a geriatric population, given the potential for problematic drug interactions and side effects. Shared care may involve GPs having telephone access to psychiatrists in order to discuss mental health issues, or psychiatrists and other mental health clinicians working, at least part time, at primary care clinics (Goering, Wasylenki, and Durbin 2000, 350). On this last point, a review in the *Canadian Journal of Psychiatry* concludes that *co-location* – having mental health staff on site – leads to better collaboration between service providers and better outcomes for clients (Craven and Bland 2006). An example of this approach comes from southern Alberta: in 1998 a shared mental health care model was implemented in the Calgary Health region, wherein mental health professionals provided consultation services right in the family physician's office. An evaluation of this found high satisfaction among all stakeholders, with GPs gaining greater knowledge on psychiatric issues and clients reporting improvement in their ability to manage problems (see the website http://www.sharedmentalhealthcare. ab.ca/home). Other examples of shared care include: making mental health intake processes more user-friendly; developing rapid access psychiatric consultation services; holding joint clinical or educational rounds; and designing educational programs for family doctors (BC Ministry of Health Services 2008). In its 2012 strategy document, the Mental Health Commission states: "As the role of primary health care in mental health expands, it will be important for all family physicians ... to work in new interdisciplinary ways and to possess core mental health competencies" (Mental Health Commission of Canada 2012, 58).

"Shared care" speaks to the problem of family doctors working in isolation, but there is also the reverse problem: mental health practitioners seeing clients who have no GP. It is unfortunately the case that persons with a serious mental illness are less likely to have access to a family doctor than the general public and to have poorer health outcomes as a consequence

(Bradford et al. 2008). There are different reasons for this, such as disorganization and insufficient advocacy and assertiveness skills on the part of the client as well as the more general difficulty – for anyone – of finding a GP willing to take on new patients. Gaining access to a GP can be supported through the mental health system by advocacy and outreach from case managers (see below) as well as by the co-location of family doctors at psychiatric (or multi-purpose) clinics.

Concerning the relatively poor physical health seen among persons with serious mental illnesses, a troubling ethical issue concerns the fact that some of these problems are the direct result of psychiatric treatments, in particular, the "metabolic syndrome" – weight gain and type II diabetes – attributed to second-generation antipsychotic drugs. American psychiatrist Benjamin Druss (2008, 833) suggests that "we are guilty both of sins of omission, through our failure to focus on our clients' physical health care needs, and commission, through the iatrogenic effects of psychotropic agents that we use." Increasingly in Canada, psychiatric programs are screening for these metabolic effects (i.e., checking weight, waist circumference, and cholesterol levels). However, there is still the conundrum of what to do when problems are identified, given the difficulty in gaining access to and maintaining care with a GP. This raises the question: Should psychiatrists themselves provide treatment for these conditions, which are not psychiatric? For example, should a psychiatrist order cholesterol-lowering drugs for a client who does not have a GP? While *practically* this may be inadvisable – doctors intervening outside their scope of practice – there nonetheless may be an *ethical* imperative here: a paper by Dixon and colleagues (2007, 600) on the "boundaries of responsibility" concludes that, in a decision-making hierarchy, "psychiatrists have the greatest responsibility for medical conditions that occur as a result of their own actions."

In 2010, a position paper on collaborative mental health care in Canada was jointly authored by the Canadian Psychiatric Association and the College of Family Physicians of Canada (Kates et al. 2010). The paper stressed the importance and effectiveness of shared care, pointing to studies showing improved health outcomes, the need to integrate physical and mental health care, and the need for "regional and provincial planners ... to look for opportunities to introduce collaborative projects into their service provision strategies" (1).

Gaining Access to Services: "No Wrong Door" and Centralized Intake
Gaining access to community mental health services can be a confusing ordeal for clients and loved ones, with the resultant delays in getting services

meaning that manageable problems may become crises (Hall 2001). Mental health workers will often hear, from clients and family members, about the trauma of an initial hospitalization and then the even more daunting challenges faced *after* discharge in trying to figure out where to turn to for help. For example, the mental health advocate of British Columbia reported in 2001 that the issue generating the most calls to her office (44 percent) was "difficulties with accessing the health care system" (Hall 2001, 18). A program model described below – ACT – was in fact developed to deal with the reality that people were not connecting with their communities after hospitalization.

In recent years, in recognition of the difficulties in gaining access to care, concepts such as "low threshold" and "no wrong door," and service models such as centralized intake, have begun to take hold in mental health, addictions, and housing. Concerning information and referral, service may be enhanced through the use of a centralized intake process – that is, a single contact point and phone number for all mental health services within a region. Such an arrangement is easier for clients to follow, and there is also evidence that accessibility and accountability are improved given that local responses to referrals can be idiosyncratic and inconsistent (British Columbia Ministry of Health 2002e). Centralized intake has been implemented in a number of British Commonwealth countries and is becoming more commonly used in Canadian jurisdictions. An example of a centralized information phone service is the "811" program available in a number of provinces, designed to provide "health information and medical advice and help navigate [the] health-care system," according to one media release. Callers may be transferred to speak with nurses or pharmacists. BC has also implemented a province-wide 1-800-SUICIDE line for persons thinking of harming themselves. In Calgary, according to its website, a single "Access Mental Health" line "streamlines the process for accessing mental health" and "matches callers to the right service" (http://www.albertahealthservices. ca/services.asp?pid=service&rid=2381). In Ottawa, the no-wrong-door principle is applied by having an agreement, and common assessment tool, among twenty hospitals and fifty-two service providers in mental health and addictions, the intent being to steer people to the right service regardless of which "door" they come to first.

Finally, the "low threshold" concept is meant to address the historical tendency, seen particularly in addiction and social housing programs, of requiring potential applicants to jump through a number of hoops (give up all illicit drugs, agree to a list of rules, be screened through mandatory interviews or orientation sessions) before getting into the program. These requirements have been seen as defensible since they get at the applicant's motivation, and without motivation and a desire to change, so the argument goes, success in addictions treatment (for example) is unlikely. (This author recalls a treatment program for clients with addictions and mental health issues, in his own health authority, that required applicants to attend no fewer than *ten* orientation sessions before becoming eligible for the treatment groups.) The counter-argument is that requiring clients to clear so many hurdles at the outset will mean many will simply give up and become further alienated and marginalized, with the result that a possible window of opportunity will have been closed.

Case Management
Assuming a client gets into the "right door," there remains, at least in the short term, the question of maintaining continuity and coordination of care with respect to mental health and other needs, such as housing and connection with a family physician. In brief, this is where *case management* comes in, a function that, according to one report, has "the most relevance to the creation of an integrated system of care" (Clarke Institute of Psychiatry 1997, 20). The importance of case management, recognized in documents such as the Romanow Report (Commission on the Future of Health Care in Canada 2002), becomes apparent when one considers the complaint, expressed by clients and family members, that negotiating "the system" is a difficult, bewildering ordeal, in which information does not seem to be readily available and in which, at every turn, the individual must deal with gatekeepers whose job seems to be finding reasons for not providing assistance.

While recognized as important, "case management" is not easily defined or conceptualized, with Health Canada (1997b, 4) concluding that there is "no standard definition" for this term.[3] That being said, there is some consensus that it refers to a role – rather than a particular professional background or discipline – in which the focus is on linkage with resources and coordination of care, not necessarily direct provision of services (Commission on the Future of Health Care in Canada 2002; Maguire 2002). For example, one publication on case management suggests that the term is synonymous with "service coordination" (Frankel and Gelman 2004, 3). These authors make the further point that service coordination becomes problematic when there are insufficient services: "Case management ... is not seen as a way to fix an inadequate or incomplete system of care" (5).

Who provides case management? Historically, clients would go to a community mental health team, or outpatient clinic, where they would be assigned a physician and case manager, and this still is a common approach. The case manager's role is to support medical management, make referrals, and investigate issues like housing and income assistance. This role, while important, has been seen by some as being too limited in that the case manager is not necessarily providing other interventions to persons who are further along in their recovery trajectory. Indeed, documents on staff competencies suggest that community mental health workers should be conversant with a range of possible client needs and interventions (Coursey et al. 2000), and treatment programs may emphasize more advanced clinical skills in potential hirees, such as the ability to run therapy groups or to conduct trauma counselling. That being said, it is important that the case management function not be lost in the redesigning of mental health systems. This could be achieved by within-team specialization but, it is hoped, would also be recognized as an area of practice within a profession, even if it may not be a profession in itself (Rossi 2003).

Case management, in this author's view, is neither esoteric nor arcane. Its "active ingredients" are knowledge of resources, an ability to provide a single point of accountability, and perseverance. Being accountable and a good advocate are qualities that can be encouraged but are not necessarily teachable, and it may be that some individuals are "naturally" better case managers.

There are variations within the case management approach that relate to the degree of direct service provision, staff specialization, and worker "assertiveness." One distinction that can be made is between a *brokerage* model, in which linkages are made but no direct services are provided, and a full support model, in which the client attends a program offering a range of services, such as medical management, counselling, and rehabilitation services. A second distinction is between generalist and specialist models (Maguire 2002). The generalist case manager is someone who in theory provides assistance in a wide range of goal areas (such as counselling around drug addiction, vocational planning, and facilitating healthier lifestyles), to be contrasted with the worker who focuses on medical management and otherwise refers (and defers) to team colleagues from other disciplines (such as occupational therapy). There is now greater recognition of the need for generalist knowledge among case managers. For example, findings that physical illness is under-recognized and under-treated in persons with serious mental disorders has placed a greater onus on practitioners to be knowledgeable about and alert to the medical conditions of their clients (as is discussed in Chapter 3). As noted, there is also a greater expectation that case managers will be familiar with a range of psychological interventions, such as cognitive-behavioural therapy (CBT) (Coursey et al. 2000). At the same time, it may be unrealistic to expect that an individual practitioner will possess the requisite knowledge, skills, and interest to be able to expertly perform all manner of duties. For example, registered nurses hired as case managers may not have been exposed to CBT in their training. In many cases the practitioner's role will fall somewhere between broker and generalist, with services being provided directly in some areas and referrals being made in others.

Finally, a distinction can be made between "regular" case management and assertive or intensive case management. Assertive case management, described in more detail below, differs from other approaches in that it targets the most disabled clients, is outreach-based, involves more frequent and prolonged contact with clients, has a lower client-to-staff ratio, and focuses on the "nitty-gritty" activities of daily living that are apparently causing difficulties for the client. A report submitted to the Ontario Ministry of Health estimated that about 25 percent of individuals with severe, persistent mental disorders require an "assertive" treatment approach (Goering et al. 1994).

One can encounter other case management "models" in the literature (Frankel and Gelman 2004). For example, a review article by Mueser and colleagues (1998) distinguishes five case management variations according to program philosophy, although the essential difference is, arguably, caseload size: the brokerage model has the highest ratio of clients to worker; the ACT model (see below) being the lowest; with the "clinical," "strengths," and "rehabilitation" models in between. The ACT model, with a client/staff ratio of about 10:1, is differentiated from the "intensive" model, with a client/staff ratio of about 20:1 (Ontario Ministry of Health and Long-Term Care 2005), and some authors have broken the intensive model down into further subtypes (Frankel and Gelman 2004). That being said, a study involving interviews with program experts found that differences tended to be overstated and that "intensive case management may not represent a distinct program model" (Schaedle et al. 2002, 208). In sum, the criteria distinguishing these models, to the extent that they exist, are poorly understood, and this author would agree with the authors of a literature review that "the differences between these models are difficult to establish ... [and] there appears to be little consensus around the best way to specify models of case management" (Centre for Applied Research in Mental Health and Addiction 2007a, 58). Frankel and Gelman (2004, 153) conclude that there is "too little data to suggest an optimal caseload size, particularly because of the many different settings in which case managers work." However, caseload size clearly dictates what can be achieved with clients: programs with significant caseloads will indeed provide less direct care and more brokerage and may predominantly be engaged in crisis management.

There are several assumptions underlying the presumed need for case management (Maguire 2002). One, as noted, is that coordination of care is required. A second is that services will be required for the long term. And a third is that, because of the degree of functional impairment, clients will need assistance in a number of areas, such as mental health, physical health, housing, finances, substance misuse, leisure, education, work, interpersonal relationships, and life skills. Although case management is potentially an effective model for assisting persons with mental disorders, it must be acknowledged that this approach comes from a tradition in which mental disorders are viewed as poor-prognosis illnesses (which could only be "managed" and not successfully treated) and is an approach that some clients may view as overly paternalistic and controlling (Davis 2002). Sullivan and Rapp (2002, 182) observe that "it is easy to see why some consumers and professionals find the term 'case manager' distasteful, and antithetical to empowerment and strengths models of practice." Practitioners should be aware of these concerns and, in their role as case managers, should carefully assess the level of functional impairment *as well as strengths* in their clients, work on areas of deficit, and build on client assets. This will require going beyond a narrowly defined "medical" role. Some clients will need support for the long haul, but we should not assume this to be the case for each new client.

Crisis Response
Care providers unfamiliar with the mental health system may unfortunately have to turn to 911, and police response, at a time of crisis. A survey conducted by the Canadian Mental Health Association (1998) found that, in 30 percent of cases, an initial psychiatric admission involved the individual's being brought to hospital by the police. The public may also be assisted by crisis lines, which are run by health authorities and non-profit societies. Community mental health programs that have a case management function should also be able to provide crisis response as part of that role.

A more specialized program involves the mobile crisis team, which generally provides a seven-day-a-week service with some after-hours capacity that provides brief crisis intervention through telephone contact or home visits. The staffing complement is made up of nurses or other clinicians with psychiatric experience and on-call physicians. These programs may be specialized by the age of the target group – that is, adults, older adults, and children and adolescents. Concerning the nature of the intervention, a manual on emergency mental health suggests that "the orientation of psychiatric emergency services should develop from an emphasis on triage to incorporate crisis resolution, based on thorough assessment of available patient coping resources and of environmental supports" (Mental Health Evaluation and Community Consultation Unit 2000, 16). In Vancouver, the local health authority runs an after-hours emergency service in partnership with the police (who in Canada have the statutory authority to take mentally disordered persons to hospital). In this program, nurses and plainclothes officers make after-hours home visits on an urgent basis.

Crisis response may also include residential crisis units (Howard et al. 2008). McCabe, Butterill, and Goering (2004) describe two Canadian examples, the Gerstein Centre in Toronto and Seneca House in Winnipeg, both notable for their principles of peer support and for employing clients as care providers. Such facilities provide an important intermediate option – between home and hospital – for persons in crisis. They have not been widely implemented in Canada, although a survey notes that crisis response systems – mobile crisis teams and free-standing crisis centres – have been particularly well developed in the Province of Manitoba (Goering, Wasylenki, and Durbin, 2000, 349).

Early Intervention Programs
It has been consistently observed that persons experiencing mental health problems for the first time will avoid or delay seeking treatment (Scholten et al. 2003). There are several reasons for this: (1) lack of knowledge of resources and/or problems with gaining access to the mental health system; (2) stigma; (3) social isolation – which is more common among persons with mental disorders – and hence a lack of concerned others who could contact treatment resources; (4) family members and care providers who lack knowledge concerning psychiatric disorders; (5) a perception by the individual and others that there is no problem – that the person's experiences are within the realm of normality – or an attribution to other causes such as recreational drug use; and (6) in some cases the onset of the disorder is insidious and hence more difficult to identify.

Another factor contributing to treatment delay is program mandates: until relatively recently, community treatment services have taken a "downstream" approach to mental health problems, with early detection and prevention not being high on the agenda. Using untreated psychotic disorders as an example, one can identify a number of harmful outcomes that may result from treatment delays following the first onset of symptoms:

- *Greater disruption of domestic relationships, parenting roles, schooling, employment, and career planning* given that the onset of psychotic disorders is typically in early adulthood. The finding that early social functioning is the best predictor of social functioning later in life provides a rationale, in the case of treating psychosis, for intervening at the earliest possible point (Birchwood, Todd, and Jackson 1998). A meta-analysis of early psychosis interventions concludes that "there is a critical period extending over the first two to five years following the onset of a psychotic disorder, during which treatment is likely to have the most significant impact on long-term outcome" (Harvey, Lepage, and Malla 2007, 471).

- *Risk of suicide.* Suicide rates for persons with schizophrenia are significantly higher than for the general population in any case, but, with respect to early intervention, it may be noted that the risk is even greater within the few years immediately following the first presentation and for young males with higher than average IQs (Palmer, Pankratz, and Bostwick 2005).

- *Poorer long-term clinical outcomes.* A number of studies have examined the association between duration of untreated psychosis (DUP) and clinical outcomes, and while there are inconsistencies and "unresolved methodological differences" (Scholten et al. 2003, 561), the preponderance of evidence appears to support a relationship between these two variables – that is, that "long durations of untreated psychosis have been associated with slower and less complete recovery, more biological abnormalities, more relapses, and poorer long-term outcomes" (Mental Health Evaluation and Community Consultation Unit 2002, 4). Subsequent relapses, in turn, are associated with "more social impairment, higher levels of secondary morbidity, and more residual symptomatology" (Mental Health Evaluation and Community Consultation Unit 2002, 16). Lines (2000, 5) notes the "growing evidence that untreated psychosis is 'toxic' – that left untreated, neurological damage progresses."

With concerns being expressed among stakeholders about mental health problems going unrecognized and untreated in the general population, health authorities are increasingly addressing the issues of prevention and health promotion, areas in which these bodies have not historically been prominent. In Canada, a mental health awareness week was launched in 1992, with the stated aims of de-stigmatizing mental illness, providing education, promoting public discussion and informed treatment decision making, and improving access to mental health services (Steiner and Amir 2003). This initiative has continued annually under the umbrella of the Canadian Alliance on Mental Illness and Mental Health and in many locations includes a depression screening day, which is held in venues such as shopping malls and community centres. In reporting on the depression screening day held in Montreal in 2002, Steiner and Amir (2003, 15) found that 5,639 citizens participated at twenty-seven sites and that, of those completing the screening instrument (the Harvard National Depression Screen), roughly half (442/879) had a score "consistent with a 95 percent sensitivity ... for a diagnosis of major depressive episode" – interpreted as being at risk for depression – and had not sought treatment for it. The authors note one of the dilemmas of this type of screening event: because of anonymity, there was no follow-up of individuals identified as at-risk.

Concerning the treatment of psychosis, early psychosis intervention (EPI) programs have been initiated in a number of Canadian centres (Tee and Hanson 2004). As reviewed by Lines (2000, 1), EPI "refers to current approaches to the treatment of psychosis that emphasize the importance of both the timing and types of intervention provided to persons experiencing a first episode of psychosis," with "early" being defined as "early as possible following the onset of psychotic symptoms." The aim of these programs is to "improve outcomes by promoting as full a recovery as possible, thereby reducing the long term disability and costs," with this being achieved by strategies "designed to limit the duration of the psychosis – prior to and during treatment – and prevent relapse" (2).

EPI programs contain elements that distinguish them from other psychiatric treatment programs, principally, early detection and phase-specific treatment (Marshall and Rathbone 2011). Lines (2000, 7) notes that treatment approaches targeting young persons need to be stage sensitive: "This population not only represents a unique developmental stage, but is naïve in terms of neuroleptic [medication] use and system exposure, and appears highly sensitive to the impacts of both." Concerning medication use, one can encounter different opinions about the treatment of psychosis in its early stages. One set of treatment guidelines emphasizes the need to start with lower doses that are increased only gradually because of the greater sensitivity of young persons to the effects of antipsychotic medication (Mental Health Evaluation and Community Consultation Unit 2002). Alternately, there is the view of Columbia University psychiatrist Jeffrey Lieberman, who in a newsletter of the National Alliance on Mental Illness is quoted as saying: "We need to throw the kitchen sink at this illness right from the start and we need to retain this person in treatment for a sustained period of time" (Reyers 2011). There is often, understandably, great ambivalence on the part of young clients about being on medication and, consequently, a dilemma for the clinician as to whether pharmacological treatment should be "intermittent" (discontinued once symptoms disappear) or continuous (lasting one to two years after a "first break"). For example, newer antipsychotic drugs, while not as likely to produce movement disorders, still have side effects such as weight gain, a problem particularly hard to deal with for a young person worried about self-image (Lester et al. 2011). While published practice guidelines emphasize the importance of medication and favour the use of longer-term maintenance regimens, there is the acknowledgment that "development of the therapeutic relationship may take precedence over treatment initiation in order to increase the probability of long-term success" (7).

Concerning "system exposure," receiving a diagnosis and being processed by the mental health system for the first time can be extremely traumatic for a young person, who has no frame of reference for this experience. Often an initial hospitalization is precipitated by a crisis in the family home, necessitating in some cases the involvement of the police and resulting in involuntary treatment and detention in a psychiatric ward. The experience is also traumatic because of the longer-term implications: What does this diagnosis/intervention mean for the individual's life and career plans?

The potentially traumatic experience of hospitalization speaks to the importance of early identification and treatment of psychotic disorders, thus – in theory – obviating the need for involuntary institutional care. Whether this can be achieved, however, is complicated by a number of factors. One is that, as noted, the individuals in question, as well as their significant others, may engage in denial and rationalization when presented with a mental health explanation for problem behaviours – which is, in many respects, an understandable response.

There is also the simple fact that psychiatric disorders, in their early stages, are not easily identified (Aviv 2010; Brown and McGrath 2011). Changes may not be abrupt; rather, there is typically a *prodromal* phase, within which are manifested the signs and symptoms seen before the development of a full-blown psychosis – symptoms that are often non-specific, such as depression, anxiety, and social withdrawal. Indeed, according to a document on EPI practice guidelines, the "prodrome" is by convention only diagnosed retrospectively, after the development of florid features of psychosis (Mental Health Evaluation and Community Consultation Unit 2002). The Canadian Psychiatric Association (2005, 43s) states that "not all behaviours and symptoms regarded as prodromal lead to psychosis, and hence the utility of this concept is limited." Attempts have been made to better identify incipient psychosis at the prodromal stage, and, more recently, researchers have spoken about an "ultra high-risk mental state" (Canadian Psychiatric Association 2005, 43s), which is identified by (1) symptoms suggesting psychosis, (2) a decline in functioning, and/or (3) a family history of psychosis among first-degree relatives, with some evidence that, by using these criteria, a transition to psychosis can be predicted in 30 to 40 percent of cases in the first year. This line of research has led to discussion about the possible inclusion of a "psychosis risk syndrome" in the American Psychiatric Association's *DSM* (Aviv 2010). However, in reviewing the evidence base, Kirkbride and Jones (2011) suggest that this risk-based approach is still problematic given our incomplete understanding of the aetiology of schizophrenia.

Given the difficulties in accurate prediction there are very real ethical dilemmas in treating persons at the prodromal stage, such as the negative effects of "labelling" and the use of antipsychotic medication before the presence of a disorder is clearly established (Ehmann, Yager, and Hanson 2004).[4] Further, the evidence base as this edition of *Community Mental Health in Canada* was being written is still lacking: a systematic review of EPI studies published in 2011 found that the evidence supporting early treatment was "inconclusive" (Marshall and Rathbone 2011). Authors with the Mental Health Evaluation and Community Consultation Unit (2002, 18) at the University of British Columbia conclude that "it is not possible to accurately predict if a person displaying features of a prodrome will make the transition to psychosis. For these reasons, and because little is known about how to prevent the onset of psychosis, psychosis-specific treatments (e.g., antipsychotic medications and education about psychosis) should not be implemented until a psychosis is definitely present." Rather, these authors recommend that clinicians address the presenting problems (e.g., depression, anxiety, insomnia), maintain a therapeutic alliance, monitor closely, and work on skills training to help the client deal with stressful events. Concerning the maintenance of a therapeutic connection, the separation of mental health programs into age divisions – child, adolescent, adult, and older adult – may in some instances be a barrier to care: some "childhood" mental health concerns may represent the prodromal phase of an adult mental disorder, pointing to the importance of integrated care and linkages to avoid the gap between termination of one program and initiation of another. Early identification, while a difficult task, is enhanced by public education programs, which would involve family doctors and other health care providers and, in particular, would include liaisoning with the school system.

Once a young person has been engaged in treatment, it is recommended that there be frequent reassessment, at least initially, because of the issue of diagnostic uncertainty and consequently the risk of applying inappropriate treatments and providing inaccurate information. Practice guidelines also emphasize the importance of professional involvement that is "ongoing and intensive" (Mental Health Evaluation and Community Consultation Unit 2002, 7).

Family involvement and education are key components of EPI. With the family being part of the therapeutic system, it is important that family members be given the resources, skills, and risk-reduction strategies to better support their loved one. Similarly, for the young client, education and skills training are crucial and will probably require the involvement of occupational therapists and other rehabilitation staff. While stigma and demoralization are important issues for psychiatric clients of any age, it is particularly crucial that they be addressed in programs for persons who have had a "first break." The rationale for this "enriched intervention" is that, as noted earlier, there is a critical period during which treatment impact is most significant, a hypothesis borne out in comparing EPI models with standard care in treating recent-onset psychosis (Harvey, Lepage, and Malla 2007).

In summary, as reviewed by Lines (2000), emerging best practices with respect to early psychosis intervention include:

- reduction of periods of untreated psychosis through public education;
- building a therapeutic alliance, which is so crucial at this first entry point into the mental health system;
- family engagement and support;
- comprehensive, phase-specific, individualized treatment, including low-dose medication, education, and psychosocial rehabilitation;
- prolonged engagement to sustain gains.

The evidence base for these practices is still limited. A 2011 systematic review conducted by university-based researchers in the UK concludes: "There is emerging ... evidence to suggest that people in the prodrome of psychosis can be helped by some interventions. There is some support for specialized early intervention services, but further trials would be desirable, and there is a question of whether gains are maintained. There is some support for phase-specific treatment focused on employment and family therapy, but again, this needs replicating with larger and longer trials" (Marshall and Rathbone 2011).

In Canada, clinical/research programs in EPI have been developed in a number of centres, including Calgary, Halifax, Toronto, Hamilton, Kingston, and London. London's Prevention and Early Intervention Program in Psychoses (PEPP), described on its website (http://www.pepp.ca), utilizes an assertive case management model wherein a case manager "walks the client through the mental health system, though whenever possible, relying on generic community services to reintegrate the young adult to his/her full potential over a two-year follow-up period." In a published description of the program, the authors note the importance of a flexible intake policy and quick response to referrals (twenty-four to forty-eight hours) in attempting to reduce treatment delays (Scholten et al. 2003). Concerning barriers to treatment, a mobile, home-based intervention program for early psychosis was introduced at the Centre for Addiction and Mental Health in Toronto in 2001 in an attempt to deal with the stigma that is attached to receiving treatment from a psychiatric clinic or hospital. Despite arguments in favour of separate EPI programs, some have contended that it would be more efficient to provide this service within a "generic" mental health program (on this point, see Malla and Pelosi [2010]).

Programs for Persons with Co-occurring Disorders

Persons suffering from mental disorders have higher rates of co-occurring substance use disorders than the general population. (The term "co-occurring," referring to mental disorder and substance abuse/dependency, has been used interchangeably in the literature with "concurrent disorders" and "dual diagnoses," although readers should be aware that the latter term has also been used to describe persons with mental disorders and intellectual handicaps.)[5] A report by the Canadian Centre on Substance Abuse (2010) found that 15 to 20 percent of those seeking help from mental health services were also living with an addiction, and over 50 percent of those seeking help for an addiction also have a mental illness. This same publication reported rates of illicit drug use among persons with schizophrenia six times that found among persons with no mental disorder. Other Canadian data come from studies conducted by University of Toronto professor Brian Rush and colleagues. In one analysis, co-occurrence rates were derived from a large-scale 2002 survey of the Canadian public, in which it was found that persons who had experienced a mental disorder in the preceding twelve months were twice as likely to have also experienced alcohol use problems in that time, and three times as likely to have experienced illicit drug problems, compared to persons who had not experienced a mental disorder (Rush et al. 2008). The twelve-month rate of co-occurring mental disorder and problematic substance use (combining drugs and alcohol) was 20.7 percent in this sample, with the rate of co-occurrence significantly higher for men than for women. In a separate study Rush and Koegl (2008) looked at rates of substance misuse among Ontario residents receiving psychiatric treatment, comparing inpatients who had more persistent, complex mental health problems with persons receiving treatment on an outpatient basis. The inpatient group had significantly higher rates of co-occurring substance misuse, 27 percent overall, showing that misuse was more likely for persons with more severe forms of mental disorder. The figure was higher still for men and for younger persons: rates of co-occurrence among inpatients in the 16 to 44-year-old age group ranged from 35 to 55 percent. Concerning diagnostic groups across the entire sample, Rush and Koegl (2008) found that co-morbidity was highest among persons diagnosed with personality disorders, followed by persons diagnosed with anxiety disorders.

The use of street drugs by a person with a condition such as schizophrenia is associated with a number of negative outcomes, such as an exacerbation of psychotic symptoms, greater risk of violence – both commission and victimization – increased risk of infectious disease, criminal involvement, high service utilization, and homelessness (Davis 1987b; Negrette 2003; Schwartz et al. 2006; Steadman et al. 1998). Substance misuse also makes diagnosing a mental disorder more difficult in that the effects of and withdrawal from the substance may mask other symptoms.

In trying to explain high rates of co-occurrence several hypotheses have been advanced:

- Use of alcohol and non-prescription drugs may be a form of self-medication (Swartz et al. 2006), a connection that Mueser (2006) suggests is strongest in the case of anxiety disorders.
- At a physiological level persons with a mental disorder such as schizophrenia may simultaneously be predisposed to substance use or to be "supersensitive" to the effects of substances (Negrette 2003; Mueser 2006).
- Cognitive impairment caused by the mental disorder may inhibit learning associated with adverse drug experiences, a hypothesis based on the conceptualization of an addictive disorder as "a faulty volitional process caused by a cognitive impairment that prevents the addict from making volitional decisions on the basis of all necessary memory" (Campbell 2003, 672).
- *Social* factors may be relevant, including (1) the reality that persons with serious mental disorders disproportionately live in poorer urban environments, where there is greater access to drugs and more environmental "triggers" (Phillips and Johnson 2001), and (2) the greater isolation experienced by persons with mental disorders and hence the use of drugs to facilitate interaction and socialization (unfortunately, clients may have to engage in drug use to be accepted as part of a group of peers).
- Persons with serious mental disorders typically have fewer coping resources, in part because of their socio-economic status and also because of skill acquisition being interrupted by the course of the disorder.

Despite their numbers and care needs, persons with co-occurring disorders have not typically been well served by the health care system or, in particular, by mental health practitioners. Several potential barriers to service can be identified. First, staff working in community mental health have not traditionally been trained in the assessment and treatment of persons with addictions, which has been seen as a separate specialty, with services being delivered in a separate location. As Latimer (2005, 568) notes, "people with severe mental illness and substance use disorder in Canada most often encounter separate services that often do not communicate with each other."

Second, there is the unfortunate fact that "helping professionals" can be quite judgmental when it comes to dealing with persons with drug addictions. This may have to do with the perception that drug addiction – unlike, for example, the manic state of a person with bipolar disorder – is a *volitional* condition, meaning that the individual is responsible for his or her own demise and is in some sense less deserving than other clients (Committee on Addictions of the Group for the Advancement of Psychiatry 2002). On this point, researchers who conducted focus group interviews with clients in three provinces as part of a Health Canada (2001a, 72, emphasis in original) report on co-occurring disorders found that "the strongest theme that emerged was the *additional and severe stigma* associated with having both substance use and mental health problems. The stigma expressed itself in various forms, including repeated and chronic self-harm experiences, self-deprecation, the fear of being judged, and the hurtful experience of judgmental attitudes."

A third barrier to service is the reality that co-occurring disorders may still be under-recognized, which at this point in time is probably inexcusable given the volume of available literature and discussion about high rates of co-morbidity (Castel et al. 2007). While underlying addictions may be missed among mentally ill persons, the opposite – seeing something as "only" an addiction – may also occur. Critically, with respect to the provision of care, this can happen at "entry points," such as intake by a mental health team or attempted admission to a hospital psychiatric unit, where incoming clients may be deflected or given short shrift if there is any sense that the psychotic symptoms seen are related to drug use.

While addiction issues may be addressed briefly at an initial assessment, there may be a lack of ongoing and systematic evaluation. To this end, Health Canada (2001a) describes several "Level 1" screening procedures, so called because they require little time and effort on the part of the clinician. These include (1) asking a few questions (although it is noted that clients may not be forthcoming about drug use before a trusting, non-judgmental relationship has been developed); (2) a brief screening instrument, such as the GAIN-SS (McDonell et al. 2009); or (3) use of an "index of suspicion," which is a checklist of indicators that include housing instability, difficulty budgeting, prostitution, sudden unexplained mood shifts, employment problems, suicidal behaviour, hygiene problems, weight loss (especially with stimulant use), and legal difficulties. "Level 2" procedures include instruments, validated with persons with mental health disorders, that take somewhat more time to incorporate into practice. These include the Dartmouth Assessment of Lifestyle Instrument (DALI), the Michigan Alcoholism Screening Test (MAST), the Drug Abuse Screening Test (DAST), and the Alcohol Use Disorders Identification Test (AUDIT) – all of which are in the public domain.

A fourth barrier has to do with psychiatric traditions that do not account for the reality of co-morbidity. An example here is the concept of the "primary diagnosis," which is usually defined as the condition that is the main focus of attention or treatment, a definition that is not particularly helpful when considering persons with two equally challenging sets of problems, each affecting the other.

A fifth barrier has to do with the lack of integration of services at either the governance or the program level. At the governance level, addiction and mental health programs have often been placed in different government ministries or departments, which usually do not communicate with one another. At the program level, these two services have not only operated in different physical locations but have also been influenced by different philosophical traditions, resulting at times in poorly coordinated treatment. Examples of these competing perspectives include:

- Differences in the educational backgrounds of mental health and addictions practitioners: the self-help emphasis and practice of hiring former addicts in some addictions programs may be contrasted with the "professional" model seen in mental health programs.
- Differences in the client's role. As noted by Minkoff (2001), some addictions services, such as traditional twelve-step programs, emphasize individual responsibility rather than disability and use confrontational methods in group meetings (generally considered inappropriate for persons with serious, persistent mental disorders), which may be contrasted with mental health case management approaches, in which care – versus confrontation – is emphasized and more is done "for" the client. This may be changing in mental health settings with a greater emphasis being placed on developing self-management skills and on recovery as a client-driven process.
- Different views about medication, with some addictions and residential treatment programs having a low tolerance for client use of prescribed psychotropic drugs (particularly anti-anxiety agents).
- Different views about abstinence. Some programs mandate abstinence from the drug of abuse as a precondition to participation. Critics have suggested that this approach discourages or prevents engagement in treatment (Minkoff 2001) and that abstinence should be considered a goal rather than a prerequisite. Harm-reduction approaches – in which ongoing substance use by the client is tolerated – have the potential to better maintain a therapeutic relationship but in some cases have produced discomfort among practitioners.

By contrast, in an integrated approach to treating persons with co-occurring disorders, efforts should be made "to ensure that the individual receives a consistent explanation of illness/problems and a coherent prescription for treatment rather than a contradictory set of messages from different providers" (Health Canada 2001a, vii).

In addressing the lack of integration in the provision of services to persons with co-occurring disorders, Minkoff (2001, 598) suggests "[the] adoption of a consensus mission statement incorporating a coherent set of principles on which system design will be based, embodying an integrated philosophy that is acceptable to both mental health care and substance use treatment providers." Minkoff outlines these principles as follows:

- Co-morbidity is an expectation, not an exception, necessitating a service delivery system that is welcoming and accessible.
- Admission criteria should be designed to promote acceptance of clients at all levels of motivation rather than preventing persons from receiving services.
- Both psychiatric and substance use disorders should be regarded as "primary," with each requiring specific and appropriate treatment.
- Both co-occurring disorders should be considered persistent, relapsing conditions, conceptualized by using a disease and recovery model, with parallel phases of treatment or recovery.
- Treatment should be phase-specific, corresponding to the stage that clients are in with respect to recovery from both conditions.
- Whenever possible, treatment should be provided by individuals, teams, or programs with expertise in both mental health and addictions.
- The system should promote a longitudinal perspective on the treatment of persons with co-occurring disorders, with service providers being available for the long term.
- The system should include interventions to engage the most detached or marginalized persons – for example, by providing outreach to the homeless.

Canadian jurisdictions are gradually seeing greater integration of mental health and addiction services. In British Columbia, for example, after years of "bureaucratic drift," Addiction Services was finally located administratively alongside other health and mental health programs with the creation of the regional health authorities in 2001 (prior to this it had been located within the Ministry for Children and Families, a department whose mandate was child protection and services for the mentally handicapped).

Health Canada (2001a) reviews a number of strategies to support integration at the program level, including the co-location of mental health and addictions treatment services, centralized intake and referral, shared data systems, shared training and education of staff, adding substance abuse specialists to mental health services (or vice versa), and creating "blended" teams. At the systems level, integration may be facilitated by the creation of inter-agency planning committees and networks, partnerships that could "go beyond joint planning exercises to the level of service agreements or potentially merged organizations" (85). Concerning the dissemination and transfer of knowledge, in 2001 Health Canada proposed the creation at the national level of a concurrent disorders resource centre and website. To this end the website of the Canadian Centre on Substance Abuse does publish reports on concurrent disorders.

Bearing in mind that local contingencies – attitudinal, fiscal, and bureaucratic – will influence how, or if, integration occurs at the level of individuals as opposed to teams or units of service, one can note that a number of different scenarios are possible. One approach is to broaden the skills of workers in existing programs. As noted earlier, one version of case management is a "generalist" model, according to which all mental health case managers are trained in techniques relevant to the treatment of addictive disorders. Examples of these are the concepts of staged treatment and motivational interviewing (Mueser 2004), approaches used in the field of addictions but more recently being taught to mental health specialists (staged treatment and motivational interviewing are described in more detail in Chapter 16). In this author's own jurisdiction, motivational interviewing is now considered a core competency for mental health practitioners. Clearly, notwithstanding traditions and individual preferences, it is hard to support a status quo in which mental health practitioners do not have at least a basic understanding of epidemiology and techniques in the area of co-occurring disorders. The idea that positive outcomes among persons with concurrent disorders can be achieved by mental health staff who are not addictions specialists is demonstrated by a study from the UK: clients randomly assigned to treatment from case managers who were later trained in managing substance misuse showed significant improvements in symptoms and level of needs met compared to those seen by case managers without such training, and at no additional cost (Craig et al. 2008).

Another approach to integrated treatment involves the inclusion of substance abuse specialists in mental health teams. This strategy has been most clearly developed in assertive community treatment program guidelines. For example, one overview of "indicators of high fidelity" in assertive community treatment (ACT) programs stipulates that there should be two or more full-time equivalent (FTE) staff with substance abuse training in each ACT program (Phillips et al. 2001, 774).

A different strategy for integrating treatment involves co-locating addictions and mental health programs (Carrigg 2004). The author of this book is located at a facility in which primary care, mental health, addictions, and other specialized services are offered under one roof. There is a recognition that, for this to work, at early stages, energy needs to be invested in forming relationships and establishing protocols with respect to information sharing and inter-agency cooperation.

Another strategy involves the development of programs specifically focusing on the treatment of persons with co-occurring disorders. As reviewed by Health Canada (2001b), a number of these specialized programs have been developed in Canada, although there is variation with respect to the range of services offered, with some focusing more on treatment (narrowly defined) and others also offering case management and outreach. Specialized co-occurring disorder programs represent an attempt to provide a more coherent approach to treatment and are a valuable resource not just for clients but also with respect to consultation and training of staff in other units of service. At the same time, there may be some danger of this model working against the goal of integrated services at the "macro" level: these stand-alone programs may become ghettoized within the larger system, with case managers on mental health teams routinely relegating clients with addictions to this other service without attempting to incorporate addictions treatment strategies in their own practice. It is almost certainly the case that no single stand-alone program can cope with the huge numbers of persons with co-occurring disorders (Carrigg 2002).

Acknowledging the historical attitudinal and bureaucratic barriers, Health Canada (2001a, 82) notes that achieving service integration in the field of co-occurring disorders is a difficult, "slow, evolutionary" process dependent on the leadership of individuals championing the cause and on the participation of stakeholders such as service users and family members.

Rural Mental Health and Telehealth
Canada is a vast country with many sparsely populated regions, and persons residing in more remote areas have had for the most part limited access to health care resources in general and specialized mental health care in particular. For example, Northern Ontario has an area of over 800,000 square kilometres, 90 percent of the total land area for the province, yet represents only 6 percent of the population. A 2004 survey found that the average number of practising psychiatrists was 13.1 per 100,000 population for Ontario, but only 3.3 per 100,000 for the northwest part of the province (Canadian Mental Health Association, Ontario, 2009). When psychiatrists and other specialists are available to remote communities this is usually "for a limited time, through temporary assignments, rotation programs ... or locums" (3). Further, staff turnover in mental health programs is typically

higher in rural areas, as much as 40 percent per year in some regions. Factors affecting staff shortages and turnover include large caseloads, the need to provide a wide range of treatments to diverse clients, a sense of isolation from colleagues, burnout from overwork, and a lack of resources (Brannen et al. 2012).

To compensate for the shortage of community-based services, residents will often rely on hospital emergency units. Staying with Ontario, it was found in 2004-05 that the use of emergency units for psychiatric reasons in the northern part of the province was more than twice the Ontario average (Canadian Mental Health Association, Ontario, 2009). Rural residents may rely on hospital emergencies for ongoing health care needs, such as medication renewal, and as the main point of entry into the mental health system.

What do we know about the health of Canadians living in more remote areas? While generally health outcomes are poorer (Kulig and Williams 2012; Monette 2012), there is also some evidence of a protective effect on mental health among young persons born and brought up in rural communities (Maggi et al. 2010).[6] Surveys have also found a stronger sense of community belonging among rural residents compared to their urban counterparts (DesMeules et al. 2012; Monette 2012). On the other hand, it has been determined that physical health outcomes are worse in rural areas in Canada, with higher mortality rates due to chronic illness, injury, and suicide, findings that need to be put in the context of a population with a poorer socio-economic status (DesMeules et al. 2012). A review by the Ontario chapter of the Canadian Mental Health Association (2009) notes that residents of Northern Ontario, compared to the provincial average, had higher self-reported rates of poor mental health and depression, a greater need for counselling, greater use of psychotropic medication, and a significantly higher rate of psychiatric hospitalization. Greater use of hospitals – as opposed to community-based agencies – may be due to a lack of alternatives but may also have to do with the help-seeking behaviour of persons living in rural areas: Brannen and colleagues (2012, 242) note that "norms and values associated with hardiness and self-reliance" may affect help-seeking, along with other factors (such as travel costs and the lack of anonymity that exists in small towns).

Telehealth

How can the mental health of rural residents be better supported? One response is through the greater use of *telehealth* or *telepsychiatry* initiatives, referring to the implementation of electronic communication and information technologies to support psychiatric care at a remote location. Such interventions have "evolved from a simple telephone service between clients and clinician into an ... information pathway involving the use of computers, videoconferences, and, in some cases, satellite communications" (Barranco-Mendoza and Persaud 2012, 181).

Telepsychiatry is designed to supplement, not replace, local treatment initiatives: a group with the University of Toronto Psychiatric Outreach Program (2002) notes that, for legal and practical reasons, consultation should be the primary model for telepsychiatry – that is, the local clinician should retain responsibility for ongoing care. Telepsychiatry can involve disciplines other than medicine, notably nursing (Hunkeler et al. 2000). While most episodes of telepsychiatry involve assessment, diagnostic clarification, and treatment recommendations, it is noted that applications are "theoretically limitless" (Hilty et al. 2003, 11) and can include case conferencing, psychological testing, student supervision, and continuing education. There has been some discussion about the use of telepsychiatry in emergency assessments, which might form the basis for involuntary hospitalization. Although video conferencing for the purposes of certifying clients under relevant mental health statutes has been sanctioned in Australia and New Zealand, the Canadian Psychiatric Association has no published position on this issue, and a survey of Canadian provincial mental health acts found that "all acts [were] either silent on whether assessments [had to] be conducted face to face, or their interpretations [were] ambiguous" (O'Reilly et al. 2003, 18).

Some concerns have been expressed about the ramifications of "virtual" interviewing – for example, how this affects rapport and whether the assessor can detect non-verbal cues, particularly when there are problems with the video transmission (Hilty et al. 2003). Calgary psychiatrist Doug Urness (2003, 21) notes that clients approaching videoconferencing for the first time may have different comfort levels, may wonder whether they will experience the "social presence" of the other person, and may ask themselves if they will be "treated as human beings or as depersonalized images on a television screen." It is thus noteworthy that a review of published evaluations of telepsychiatry found, notwithstanding expectations, generally high rates of client satisfaction with the process, concomitant with increased access to care (Hilty et al. 2003). In particular, reduced travel time, less absence from work, reduced waiting time, and more client choice and control were noted in the studies reviewed. Urness (2003, 25) suggests, with respect to concerns about new technologies, that therapist qualities are still more influential than the medium used (apologies to Marshall McLuhan) and that "the success of a telepsychiatry interview is more a function of traditional communication processes than of technology."

The expansion of telehealth initiatives is reviewed in a report by the Health Council of Canada (2012):

- At the time of the report the federal government had invested $108 million in telehealth projects, cost-shared with the provinces and territories.
- Telehealth was being used in collaborative initiatives with the First Nations and across provincial-territorial boundaries.
- In 2010, 5,710 telehealth sites were being used in over 1,175 communities.
- At the time of the report the use of telehealth had grown by 35 percent annually over five years.
- Mental health services accounted for over half of the consultations – 54 percent, far ahead of the next clinical service, internal medicine, at 15 percent.

Evaluations of the effectiveness of telepsychiatry, while variable in quality, have been "encouraging" (Halley, Roine and Ohinmaa 2008, 769). For example, Pignatiello and colleagues (2008) describe a successful Ontario program operated through the Hospital for Sick Children, which provides teleconsultation in both official languages to remote regions of the province and that has been favourably reviewed by the primary care physicians receiving the service. Along with user satisfaction, investment in telehealth is supported if the intervention can be seen as cost-effective, in particular through reduced travel costs, reduced hospitalizations, and improved health outcomes. On this point, a 2011 study determined that telehealth interventions had resulted in $55 million savings in cost avoidance for the Canadian health care system, a substantial part of this related to travel costs (Praxis Information Intelligence, Gartner, Inc. 2011). The study also concluded that telehomecare programs in Ontario, Quebec, New Brunswick, and British Columbia had averted almost $21 million in hospital costs over the study period.

The potential benefits of telepsychiatry are addressed both in the Canadian Senate report on mental health reform, *Out of the Shadows at Last,* and by the Mental Health Commission of Canada (2012, 58) in its strategy document, in which it is noted that "there are tremendous possibilities for new technology in promoting mental health and preventing mental health problems. Technology makes collaboration easier and can be a remarkable tool for supporting self-management, especially for younger people." In the strategy document the commission makes the use of technology to increase access to services one of its key "recommendations for action."

Staff Recruitment and Retention
Brannen and colleagues (2012, 254) note that, while technological solutions

such as telepsychiatry can increase access to services, they "should be viewed as supplements to rather than replacements for high-quality, community-based mental health services," and conclude that "the recruitment and retention of mental health professionals in rural and northern communities will undoubtedly require a broad, multi-level approach." Strategies here would include financial and housing incentives to attract mental health professionals, and professional development opportunities (continuing education) to reduce professional isolation (Canadian Mental Health Association, Ontario, 2009). In its strategy document, the Mental Health Commission of Canada (2012, 89) suggests that stakeholders should "enhance mental health training programs to match local people with local job opportunities in northern and remote communities." As well, the establishment of institutions of higher learning in rural areas may serve the dual purpose of providing local community service and the building of a professional "critical mass." Examples would include the Northern Ontario School of Medicine, near Sudbury, whose mandate is to support health care in rural communities, and the University of Northern British Columbia in Prince George, where the social work curriculum focuses on rural practice.

Day Hospitals

"Day hospitals" were one of the earliest forms of psychiatric community care, following the first wave of deinstitutionalization in the 1960s. Day hospitals were seen as an alternative to hospital admission, providing treatment and life skills training to persons who would attend during the week (Marshall 2003). In more recent years, day hospitals have fallen out of favour, in part because they were seen as old-fashioned and stigmatizing (attached to the psychiatric wards of hospitals in a number of cases), in part because of expense and in part because of the advent of community teams and other more intensive non-hospital services such as assertive community treatment, acute home-based treatment, and EPI (Marshall 2003). Day hospitals still exist in Canada, and while still described in a number of instances as an alternative to hospitalization (see, for example, the website of St. Joseph's Health Centre in Toronto, http://www.stjoe.on.ca/programs/mental/day.php), their role has shifted more to the provision of rehabilitation services (education and health promotion) as opposed to acute treatment, at least with younger adult clients. Day hospitals still play an important role in a number of centres for seniors suffering from depression and other mental illnesses; for example, the START Psychiatry Day Hospital Program in Edmonton provides treatment, including group therapy and pharmacotherapy, over a period of twenty weeks, with clients attending two days per week (http://www.albertahealthservices.ca/servicesasp?pid=saf&rid=1006094).

Assertive Community Treatment

The service delivery approach known as assertive community treatment (ACT) evolved in response to the recognition that, in the aftermath of deinstitutionalization, a number of clients in the community were not "connecting," either with treatment programs or with other community resources, and also appeared to lack the skills necessary to manage activities of daily living, skills that either had not been learned or practised or were not transferable from institutional to community settings. Unlike traditional, office-based case management, assertive community treatment is delivered in situ – on an outreach basis – and emphasizes the acquisition of life skills in addition to the clinical management function (Health Canada 1997, 5). The first version of ACT, and the model that has most strongly influenced subsequent programs, was the Training in Community Living Program, developed in the 1970s in Madison, Wisconsin, by Stein and Test (1980). As summarized by Drake and colleagues (2003, 45), in this program outreach teams were formed "to teach skills and provide supports in natural environments such as the client's home, neighborhood, or work setting. These approaches initially focused on teaching basic living skills, e.g., helping people learn the necessary skills for cooking, cleaning their apartments, and using public transportation, but they also began to focus on jobs, social relationships, housing and leisure activities." In addition to North America, ACT programs have been implemented in Europe and the British Commonwealth (Phillips et al. 2001). In Canada, ACT programs have become more widespread (although they do not exist in all regions) and in best practices documents are referred to as an integral part of a comprehensive mental health service (McEwan and Goldner 2001). In Ontario, for example, over seventy ACT teams were in operation by the year 2006 (Lurie, Kirsh, and Hodge 2007).

Given that ACT is a labour-intensive model of service delivery, some efforts have been made towards determining and delimiting the target population. One best-practices document concludes that clients of ACT programs should (1) have a serious, persistent mental illness; (2) exhibit functional impairment; and (3) be "intensive users of the system of care" (British Columbia Ministry of Health 2002a, 6). Examples of functional impairment would include poor hygiene, poor budgeting skills, inability to meet nutritional needs, transiency, poor problem-solving skills, and inability to develop or maintain a support system (British Columbia Ministry of Health 2002a). Given that most users of the public mental health system have a serious, persistent disorder and some functional deficits, the third criterion – "intensive system use" – often turns out to be the main distinguishing factor for potential ACT clients. While "system use" may refer to other community agencies or to the criminal justice system (McCoy et al 2004; Wilson, Tien, and Eaves

1995), for the most part, in the conceptualization and evaluation of ACT programs, it refers to the use of (costly) hospital resources. For example, a best-practices report (British Columbia Ministry of Health 2002a, 7) states that the first objective of assertive community treatment is "to reduce the need for hospitalization, and improve community tenure." "Need for hospitalization" in this context can mean: (1) frequent hospitalizations, which, while an arbitrary figure, is defined as two or more per year by one report (British Columbia Ministry of Health 2002e), (2) being at risk for re-hospitalization without additional supports, and (3) being detained as an inpatient when intensive outpatient services, if available, would make discharge a more viable option. Often re-hospitalization is the result of treatment non-compliance – that is, an inability or unwillingness to come in for appointments or to take medication. Thus, a core function of the ACT model is to address the "compliance" issue.

Unlike some of the case management models mentioned in the previous section, ACT has established guidelines, criteria, and fidelity standards, which are well described on the US Department of Health and Human Services website on ACT: http://mentalhealth.samhsa.gov/cmhs/CommunitySupport/ toolkits/community/. The following are considered to be key service components of an ACT program:

- A low client-to-staff ratio, typically around 10:1. This is necessary to sustain the frequent (several times per week) client contact characteristic of this type of program. Through frequent contact and more intimate knowledge of clients, the hope is that crises can be averted. Concerning staff attributes, there is some suggestion that "street smarts," pragmatism, initiative, and nonjudgmental attitudes among ACT workers are at least as important as formal credentials (Phillips et al. 2001).
- A shared caseload, meaning that clients are rotated among the different case managers. As reviewed by Rapp (1998, 366), the purported advantages of this are reduced worker burnout, better continuity of care, increased availability of someone who knows the client, and "more creative service planning." There are, on the other hand, a number of limitations to this team approach: (1) it goes against the "single point of accountability" tenet; (2) it can be confusing and frustrating for clients, who have to develop relationships with several workers or who may be getting the message that they are "so abnormal, bad or different that a whole team of people is needed to work with them" (Spindel and Nugent 1999, 7); and (3) it necessitates detailed information sharing among staff and frequent (daily) case management meetings to bring everyone "up to speed," all of which can be time-consuming.

- Assertive outreach. Most of the staff time in ACT programs is spent outside of the office, which is seen as "home base ... rather than a primary treatment site." "Providing services in the environment of the consumer's choice enables the team to assess the consumer's needs in the real world and to provide support and teaching in daily living skills. Assertive outreach is the key to engaging clients who do not connect with traditional office or institution-based approaches" (British Columbia Ministry of Health 2002a, 15).
- Continuous services. Working in conjunction with other services, ACT programs aim at providing comprehensive coverage, including during after-hours emergencies. Also key to this model is that, if necessary, service is indefinite, if necessary. This aspect is important when one considers that the target population is a group that others may have given up on, if not avoided, meaning that perseverance is important in order to establish trust and to make gains that are sometimes incremental. Workers may have to make repeated attempts to engage clients in the program, unlike a conventional service, which may close the file after a single failed appointment.
- Twenty-four hour coverage.
- A multi-disciplinary team, including a physician and a peer worker.

While closer adherence to ACT standards has been found to be associated with better outcomes (Latimer 1999; McGrew, Pescosolido, and Wright 2003), it should be noted that there are a number of "ACT-like" programs in existence that do not achieve complete adherence or fidelity to the model, and some question whether complete fidelity is necessary. Notably, a US survey of seventy-three ACT programs found that "several important ingredients [program components] appear to be *consistently* underimplemented" (McGrew, Pescosolido, and Wright 2003, 370, emphasis added). Sometimes standards may be compromised by practical considerations; for instance, having a psychiatrist on staff is made difficult by the shortage of these specialists, particularly in outlying areas (Latimer 1999; McGrew, Pescosolido, and Wright 2003). In another example, a survey of Ontario ACT programs found that not all were employing a peer-support worker, as stipulated by Ministry of Health guidelines. The reasons for this included a lack of enhanced funding, no guidelines concerning the role of peer-support workers, and "hesitancy to create the position because of worry of losing a clinical staff member to fund a peer support position" (White et al. 2003, 270). Exact replication of models may also be compromised by the fact that local contingencies will affect the implementation and eventual shape of any new program (Rapp 1998). This issue is addressed by the director of an ACT program in Chicago: "Although its inspiration came straight from Madison, the Chicago project took shape in a vastly different urban environment, under different agency auspices, with different funding circumstances, and with a different target population. Thus, a literal replication of the Madison model was not possible" (Witheridge 1991, 49). Finally, some differences in ACT-type programs may be deliberate. In defending their *time-limited* program, Bonsack and colleagues (2005) observe that this was motivated by: (1) limited resources and the need to create space for new clients, (2) getting clients to become more resourceful and less dependent on the program, and (3) getting clients to develop natural social support networks. While some ACT standards do speak to time-unlimited services, this is increasingly felt to be an inefficient use of resources.[7]

Does ACT "work"? ACT is now considered an evidence-based practice (Dixon et al. 2010), and evaluations of these programs have found them to be effective in reducing client re-hospitalization, maintaining housing stability, and retaining clients in treatment (Coldwell and Bender 2007; Dieterich et al. 2010; Health Canada 1997; Phillips et al. 2001). For example, in an Ontario study, investigators found that clients randomly assigned to an assertive outreach program spent only thirty-nine days in hospital during a follow-up period of one year, compared to 256 days for the control group, who were followed by a hospital outpatient program (Lafave, deSouza, and Gerber 1996). Canadian studies have found impacts in other areas, such as reducing suicidal ideation (Langley et al. 2009) and reducing jail recidivism (Wilson, Tien, and Eaves 1995). Impacts in other domains have been more limited: a review by the Toronto CMHA found that ACT involvement had the potential to improve vocational outcomes for clients, but to achieve this the employment of clients had to become as explicit a mandate as treatment and housing, and probably require a vocational specialist on the team, a position that, from their survey, they found was hard to fill (Lurie, Kirsh, and Hodge 2007).

Surveys of clients of ACT programs have also in many instances found user satisfaction to be high (Chue et al. 2004; Phillips et al. 2001), which may be related to the fact that clients gain access to more resources and services. When dissatisfaction with the ACT model has been expressed, it often relates to the more coercive, or intrusive, aspects of service delivery, the view that "assertive community treatment is paternalistic and has a tendency to overuse social and monetary behavioural controls, and to over-emphasize the role of medications" (McGrew, Wilson, and Bond 2002, 761; see also Davis 2002; Gomoroy 2001; Spindel and Nugent 1999). A Canadian user satisfaction survey by Gerber and Prince (1999, 549) found that substantial minorities of ACT clients expressed dissatisfaction with respect to "demands in treatment" (31 percent), "extent of clients' influence over treatment" (30 percent), and "whether their opinion was considered in treatment planning" (23 percent). Similarly, a survey of ACT clients by Queen's University Professor Terry Krupa and colleagues (2005, 23), while finding that "the participants, by and large, commended the services", also found that staff could be perceived as authoritative and intrusive at times, especially "around choices regarding medication and the control of finances."

While ACT programs are labour-intensive and have relatively small case-loads, this concentration of resources has been justified by the argument that, by preventing the re-hospitalization of a targeted, high-risk group, the intervention is still cost-effective (e.g. McCrone et al. 2009). Research has tended to support this hypothesis – that is, that ACT will be cost-effective if the comparison group, or target group, has had "extensive previous hospitalization" (Barry et al. 2003, 269) and thus can be considered at high risk for relapse (Essock, Frisman, and Kontos 1998). In a literature review by McGill University researcher Eric Latimer (1999, 443), the conclusion was that, using the costs of hospitalization in Quebec as a reference, ACT programs would need to enroll people with prior hospital use of about fifty days yearly, on average, to "break even." Given current hospital utilization patterns in Canadian community mental health programs (see below), a figure of fifty-plus inpatient days per year would be considered quite high, underlining again the need for ACT to be a carefully "targeted" program. Latimer (1999, 443) suggests that, since the fifty-day reference point will become increasingly difficult to achieve "as care systems evolve to reduce their reliance on hospitalization as a care modality with or without ACT," "the primary justification for implementing ACT services will then become their clinical benefits."

A variation of the ACT program is the Intensive Case Management (ICM) model. As noted above, the distinction between these two is not always clear in the available literature.[8] An Ontario government document on ICM standards specifies that, like ACT, ICM is community- not office-based, has a somewhat higher caseload at 20:1, and is not 24/7, i.e., it operates on weekdays (Ontario Ministry of Health and Long-Term Care 2005). In a review co-authored by Wilfrid Laurier University professor Geoff Nelson, it was found that, with housing stability as an outcome measure, the effect size for ACT interventions was greater than that for ICM (Nelson et al. 2007).

Acute Home-Based Treatment

Acute home treatment is defined as "acute care provided in the home for a limited period to treat acute psychiatric symptoms that would otherwise require inpatient admission" (British Columbia Ministry of Health 2002e, 40). The need for such a service is based on the view that many persons presenting and being admitted to acute care hospitals could in fact be treated at home by mental health clinicians and that, if available, this less intrusive intervention would have benefits with respect to both cost-effectiveness and client satisfaction. It is suggested that this approach would work best with "previously admitted patients with known patterns of decompensation" (42); that is, that one would not normally use home-based care as the first response to a crisis involving an unknown client. While this type of intervention appears similar in some respects to assertive community treatment, the latter is intended to be a long-term service, whereas home care might typically last only three to six weeks.

Acute home treatment has been relatively uncommon in Canadian and American settings, which may in part be related to the fact that, traditionally, unlike their British and European counterparts, North American psychiatrists rarely make home visits (Clarke Institute of Psychiatry 1997). Acute home treatment programs initially arose in Australia in the 1970s and have been implemented in Toronto in the mid-1990s and more recently in British Columbia. Acute home treatment is referred to in the federal government's Romanow Report, along with ACT, as one of the "two types of home care services that should be available for people with mental health problems" (Commission on the Future of Health Care in Canada 2002, 179). Research conducted in the UK has found acute home treatment to be preferred by clients and family (Knapp et al. 1998), to reduce hospitalization rates (Glover, Arts, and Babu 2006), and to be feasible for up to 80 percent of clients presenting for hospital admission (Smyth and Hoult 2000).

Wasylenki and colleagues (1997) describe an acute home treatment service, the Home Treatment Program for Acute Psychosis, established in Toronto. In this program, services were provided by nurses, homemakers, and social workers, with a psychiatrist available for back-up support. In urgent cases, services started immediately; otherwise, intensive support was initiated within forty-eight hours. Once the client was stabilized, he or she was referred back to the regular case manager at the Clarke Institute. The project was evaluated over an eighteen-month study period during which there were thirty-four episodes of home treatment averaging twenty-eight days in duration. It was found that there was a reduction in client symptoms, a reduction in the burden of family members, and that clients were satisfied with home treatment and preferred it to hospitalization. Home treatment was also found to be significantly less expensive than inpatient care at the Clarke Institute: $139.78 versus $637 per diem. In the Vancouver acute home treatment program, referred persons are seen within twenty-four hours, given a psychiatric assessment within seventy-two hours, and seen every day for about three weeks.

Hospital Programs

Hospital Utilization

As noted previously, from the mid-nineteenth to mid-twentieth centuries the treatment and containment of persons with serious mental disorders in Canada took place predominantly in "asylums." Now, with the downsizing and phasing out of provincial psychiatric hospitals, inpatient care takes place mainly in general hospital psychiatric units (GHPUs). For example, data from the period 2005-06 showed that 87 percent of hospital separations related to mental disorder were from GHPUs, while only 13 percent were from provincial psychiatric hospitals (Canadian Institute for Health Information 2010). (A "separation" is defined as a discharge or death, so a person being admitted and discharged on three separate occasions in a reporting period would be counted as three separations.) The smaller role played by psychiatric hospitals will presumably be a trend that will continue with their downsizing.

Lengths of hospital stay, both at GHPUs and provincial institutions, have grown shorter over the years. The average length of stay at a psychiatric hospital in Canada fell from 250 to one hundred days in just a ten-year period, from 1996 to 2006, while average admission length at GHPUs fell to sixteen days in this same time span (Canadian Institute for Health Information 2010). Length of stay may vary from one jurisdiction to the next and is affected by various factors, including the availability of community resources.

This trend towards briefer hospitalization is driven by both (1) cost containment and the relative scarcity of inpatient resources and (2) changing philosophies with respect to treatment, the role of the hospital, and the psychosocial impact of institutionalization. Concerning changing philosophies, different reports have concluded, for example, that "best practices in this area will contribute to reducing hospital average lengths of stay and hospital bed utilization rates" (British Columbia Ministry of Health 2002e, 17) and that "inpatient stays [should be] kept as short as possible without harming patient outcomes" (McEwan and Goldner 2001, 33). Long-stay hospitalization may, for example, place in jeopardy a client's housing arrangements in situations in which provincial income assistance policies do not permit continuing payment of rent when the individual remains in hospital. A best practices document describes the rationale behind hospitalization as follows: "The goal is to make 'sick' people less 'sick,' *not necessarily 'well.'* Once they can be managed in a less restrictive environment, they are discharged unless it can be demonstrated that remaining in hospital leads to a better clinical outcome" (British Columbia Ministry of Health 2002e, 17, emphasis added).[9]

In supporting shorter stays, hospital officials may refer to more effective patient flow and point out that patients with extended stays are blocking the admission of new persons needing care. There is also the argument that a significant proportion of those seeking and gaining hospital admission do not need inpatient care, with suggestions that 40 to 80 percent of those presenting for admission to hospital can be managed in alternative care settings, including step-down facilities and home-based treatment programs (Gordon 1997; Smyth and Hoult 2000). It has also been argued that, for some clinical presentations, hospitalization should be ruled out altogether (e.g., Dawson 1988).

While it is true that some persons in crisis can be adequately supported in less restrictive and less expensive transitional units, or by outreach workers (more on this below), in areas where these resources do not exist or are in short supply the community practitioner may be faced with an "all or nothing" decision (i.e., hospital or no intervention at all). Concerning possible benchmarks for appropriate bed levels in the mental health system, community clinicians, medical associations, family members, and first-responders such as the police have tended to argue for higher levels than those suggested by health authority planners (BC Medical Association 2008; Gordon 1997; Inman 2010; Lesage et al. 2003). In 2010, the Vancouver Police Department wrote a report critical of the short-stay emphasis at local psychiatric units (given that they were regularly responding to mental health calls in the community) and recommended that the health authority "establish sufficient mental health care capacity that can accommodate moderate to long term stays for individuals who are chronically mentally ill" (Thompson 2010, 27). Similarly, a 2012 position paper from the Canadian Psychiatric Association recommends that "there are sufficient psychiatric beds ... available for people with mental illness *for as long as they need them*" (Chaimowitz 2012, 6, emphasis added). A guideline suggested by University of Montreal psychiatrist Alain Lesage (2010) suggests that there be fifteen long-stay beds and twenty-five acute care beds available per 100,000 population.

Admission and Discharge-Planning

At present, hospitalization is primarily used when there are concerns about safety and security, although it may also be used when procedures such as ECT or initiation of clozapine treatment are being undertaken. In a Canadian Psychiatric Association document on the guidelines for the treatment of depression, it is noted that indications for hospitalization include "concern for the safety of others or the patients themselves, crisis intervention, diagnostic evaluation (especially with comorbid medical or psychiatric conditions), poor response to outpatient treatment, rapid deterioration or marked severity of depression (including hopelessness, suicidal ideation, or psychotic features), inability to function at home, and breakdown of social supports" (Reesal and Lam 2001, 25S).

The current emphasis on shorter admissions has at times created tensions between hospital and community-based practitioners, with the latter complaining about premature discharges and arguing for the benefits of longer inpatient stay. This position is supported by national survey data from the Canadian Institute for Health Information (2011a), which shows a significant correlation between shorter initial lengths of stay and higher risk of readmission. The thirty-day readmission rate for all mental disorders in this study was 11.4 percent, rising to 13.2 percent in the case of schizophrenia. Family advocacy groups have argued that this sort of data is proof that the premature discharge of a person – still presumably unstable – just exacerbates the "revolving door" of psychiatric care (Harnett 2008). This also means that any cost savings realized from shorter stays would be diminished by more frequent readmissions. Hospital readmission is a multi-determined event but, as noted by the Canadian Institute for Health Information (2011a), is related at least in part to suboptimal discharge planning and a lack of continuity of services. Consequently, thirty-day readmission rates are now used by health authorities as an indicator of coordination of care.[10]

Pressure on inpatient resources may also (unfortunately) influence decisions about whether to hospitalize a client in the first place: community practitioners may weigh the cost of certifying a client – in terms of damaged rapport with the individual – against the limited benefits that will be achieved, the assumption being, based on prior experience, that the client will be quickly discharged. However, practitioners need to be reflective and wary about this sort of cynicism in their decision making and should continue to advocate for the best care for their clients.

Following hospital admission, because the client is now dealing with (in most cases) a completely different treatment team, continuity and communication between the hospital and community become crucial. It is an obligation of both parties to transmit relevant documents so that, at point of admission, hospital staff have some history, background information, and a sense of the client's "baseline" functioning so that, at point of discharge, community staff get a review of what was done in hospital, whether there were changes in medication,[11] and how the client responded. It is unfortunately the case that, because of the pressure on hospital beds and staff time, clients may be discharged with little or no warning to the community and with insufficient supports in place. Hospital staff may in turn complain that they cannot get follow-up appointments from community programs in a timely fashion: for example, the Mental Health Advocate of British Columbia noted in her 2001 *Annual Report* that only 20 percent of community mental health clients had contacts for follow-up care within thirty days of being discharged from hospital (Hall 2001). (Concerning discharge-planning, the Canadian Schizophrenia Society has created and posted on its website a "discharge checklist" so that family members can see that issues such as medication, housing, and follow-up care have been addressed prior to discharge. See: http://www.bcss.org/2007/05/resources/family-friends/hospital -discharge-checklist.)

While these hospital-community tensions may not always be resolvable, face-to-face encounters between staff from the two areas are recommended, either in meetings, case conferences, ward rounds, or committees, as a way of understanding the vantage point of the "other." Having staff with cross-appointments – for example, physicians who work both in hospital and community settings – can be helpful with respect to bridging the disconnect between the two perspectives.

General Hospital Inpatient Programs
Most community hospitals will have only one psychiatric unit, and some hospitals, unfortunately, may lack even this. Inner-city hospitals typically have busy emergency departments and may at times be on "diversion," meaning that mental health clients being sent in ambulances are diverted to other, outlying hospitals. Clients with psychiatric crises may be backed up in the emergency department or may be held with paramedics in other waiting areas, including hallways, all of which can mean a more traumatic experience for the clients involved. While direct admission to psychiatric wards may be possible, often incoming certified patients have to be medically cleared first, which can take some time. Some jurisdictions may employ psychiatric triage nurses to work in emergency and help streamline admissions.

Larger centres, in addition to general psychiatric units, may have other, specialized programs. These include:

- A short-stay assessment unit, in which admissions are typically under fifteen days (Goering, Wasylenki, and Durbin 2000).
- A psychiatric intensive care unit, defined as a "secure unit for patients requiring the highest level of observation and containment" (British Columbia Ministry of Health 2002e, 20).
- A separate adolescent inpatient unit, based on the view that "adult ... inpatient units are not ideal for children and adolescents" and that each region should have a "residential assessment and treatment unit exclusive to adolescents and with programming specifically tailored to their developmental needs" (British Columbia Ministry of Health 2002e, 22). Adolescent

units may be located at general hospitals or specialized, children's facilities, although separate, smaller-scale residential settings may be preferable.

- Geriatric units. The admission criteria, clinical issues, and care needs are usually quite different with respect to the psycho-geriatric population, underlining the need for a separate unit with specialized staff. Best practices standards emphasize the importance of integrated care with an elderly population, meaning that continuity should be maintained with family, general practitioners, psychiatrists, mental health teams, and the community long-term care system while the individual is in hospital, which may be achieved in part with joint care rounds. Geriatric hospital units often include an outreach component.

Tertiary Care

"Tertiary care" usually refers to specialized inpatient programs for persons whose needs are not adequately addressed at a GHPU (Goering, Wasylenki, and Durbin 2000). Traditionally, persons admitted to a GHPU and found to have a more complex presentation could be transferred to a tertiary unit. This prospect may be diminished when there are significant bed pressures (i.e., it may not be possible for a GHPU to hold onto a patient awaiting a transfer).

Tertiary care can be contrasted with:

- *primary* care, which means care provided by a general practitioner or through a public health unit; and
- *secondary* care, which means specialized care provided either through a community mental health clinic or GHPU.

Examples of populations with specialized needs that may require tertiary resources include: persons with eating disorders, persons with treatment-resistant psychosis who may also demonstrate aggressive behaviours, persons with neurological complications, persons with co-occurring intellectual handicaps, persons with co-occurring substance misuse issues, elderly persons, and children and adolescents (British Columbia Ministry of Health 2002e). Apart from inpatient treatment, the goals of tertiary services may include consultation, education, outreach support, and research. Goering, Wasylenki, and Durbin (2000, 352) note that "the availability of tertiary care back-up often results in greater willingness among primary and secondary care providers to accept individuals with difficult conditions and behaviors." Tertiary units may be stand-alone or part of a larger hospital complex. Since assessing and managing treatment-resistant disorders can take more time, tertiary care can also refer to *longer-stay*, bearing in mind that extended hospital stays, once the norm for persons with complex, treatment-resistant conditions, are an increasingly unlikely outcome in the present era.

As with outpatient clinics, the idea that tertiary care should necessarily be associated with hospitals has been challenged, with the suggestion that services be provided in smaller, more homelike settings. One group of authors speaks about the "increasing interest in portable and community-based tertiary care models to delink delivery of tertiary care from particular settings or time frames" (Goering, Wasylenki, and Durbin 2000, 352). Concerning the evolution of tertiary care resources, a British Columbia report concludes that these services have developed "unsystematically" (British Columbia Ministry of Health 2002e, 45) and recommends that advisory boards be established at both the provincial and regional levels, with representatives from the primary and secondary care systems present to ensure that the needs of these stakeholders are addressed. This issue becomes more pressing given limited budgets and the need to avoid duplication of services, which can be the case in larger urban settings.

The Non-Profit Sector

The treatment programs referred to so far are generally provided under the auspices of provincial governments or health authorities. Complementing these programs are a number of services offered by non-governmental, not-for-profit agencies, which are funded by both government and private sources. In an overview, Latimer (2005, 565) notes that there are a large number of non-profit community mental health programs in Canada (at least four hundred in Quebec, for example) and that most have relatively small budgets and a "single vocation," which could include housing, vocational rehabilitation, family support, education, advocacy, and artistic expression. There are as well larger, multi-service agencies, such as the CMHA (see below) and, using an example from Vancouver, Coast Mental Health, which offers housing, drop-in services, employment, and management of trusts. While historically these agencies may have been given an inferior status by professionals working for government programs (Health Canada 2002b), there is now greater recognition that the services they offer are, for many clients and care providers, the ones that really "make a difference." Indeed, the evolution of these programs, a number of which were started by family members or clients themselves, was at least in part a result of the deficiencies or limited scope of existing government services.

While it is impossible to list all the various non-profit organizations, two are mentioned here because of their prominence and because they have both national and regional representation. One is the Canadian Mental Health Association (CMHA), founded in 1918, which has chapters in all provinces and territories. The CMHA provides direct services to clients, such as drop-ins and social/recreational programming, and also plays a major role in combating the stigma of mental disorders through systemic advocacy and public education. To this end, the CMHA sponsors workshops, seminars, and research projects and also issues pamphlets and newsletters. The CMHA has produced position papers for governments and bodies such as the Romanow Commission and has published influential policy documents – a number of them used as references for this book – such as *A New Framework for Support for People with Serious Mental Health Problems* (Trainor, Pomeroy, and Pape 1993), which highlights the importance of services and supports that have traditionally been outside the formal mental health service delivery system (Health Canada 2002b).

The other organization that has become an important voice for advocacy and public education is the Schizophrenia Society of Canada (SSC). While representing the interests of both clients and significant others, the SSC is especially known for its support groups and education programs for family members. For example, the website of the BC Schizophrenia Society (http://www.bcss.org) lists the following services, available free to the public:

- telephone support and referral information;
- online support groups, through which visitors can post and respond to questions about mental illness;
- links to informational articles and booklets;
- "Strengthening Families Together," a ten-session program designed to provide information and develop skill-building;
- "Kids in Control," an education and support group for children and teens that have a parent with a mental illness;
- "Reach Out," an interactive presentation on mental illness given to high school audiences.

Family support organizations like the SSC, and NAMI in the United States, align themselves with a biological conceptualization of mental illness and support "access to treatment" initiatives that may at times clash with a civil rights orientation, a topic that is covered in more detail in Chapter 7.

Notes

1 Although not widely used in Canada, scales have been developed with the intent of establishing a client care level, relating to need for more or less intense services. See Sowers and Benacci (2010).

2 Personal communication with Jackie Matsyk, MD.

3 In looking for definitions, Googling the term "case management" returns millions of hits, even after narrowing the search by including the term "mental health."

4 This author has been in discussions in which some client advocates depict early identification by genetic heritage as a form of eugenics, which speaks to the sensitivity of the issue.

5 Other terms have been used, which, as reviewed by Health Canada (2001a), include CAMI (chemically abusing – mentally ill), MICA (mentally ill – chemically abusing), and SAMI (substance abusing – mentally ill).

6 The study cited here involves children of sawmill workers in northern British Columbia.

7 A statement based on the author's own program planning experience in the Vancouver Coastal Health Authority.

8 For example, a review by Dieterich and colleagues (2010) concludes that ICM outcomes are better when the program has greater fidelity to ACT standards, suggesting the two models are on a continuum rather than being easily distinguishable.

9 In 2012, the Vancouver Coastal Health Authority announced the launch of "Home Is Best" in order to underpin the streamlining of patients away from inpatient care. The memo released to staff stated: "Home is Best isn't a project or service but, rather, a philosophy. It is the belief that home is the best place for people to live as long as they are safely able to do so, the best place for people to recover from an illness once they no longer require hospital care and the best place for patients and their family members to consider continuing care options, such as residential care."

10 Researchers have also found an association between hospital discharge and subsequent suicidal behaviour. For example, in a study of suicide attempts by clients of a Vancouver, BC, mental health program, it was found that, for those hospitalized within the year prior to the attempt, 40 percent (38/95) were discharged within one month of their subsequent suicide attempt (Davis 2000). See also Canadian Institute for Health Information (2011a).

11 Accreditation bodies recommend that a process of "medication reconciliation" be conducted periodically, and particularly at the point of hospital discharge, to make sure that the client and community clinician have a clear understanding of what has been included and excluded in the medication regimen. Errors and omissions at transfer points are not uncommon.

Other Resources

eMentalHealth.ca provides a directory of mental health services sorted by province and town: http://www.ementalhealth.ca.

The Canadian Centre for Substance Abuse: www.ccsa.ca.

Psychosis Sucks is a website providing information on early intervention in psychosis: http://www.psychosissucks.ca.

Housing

12

No discussion of a comprehensive mental health system and the ultimate goal of long-term client recovery is complete without addressing the issue of housing. Housing is unquestionably one of the key determinants of health (Dunn 2003; Health Canada 2002c; Standing Senate Committee on Social Affairs, Science and Technology 2006). As a Canadian mental health administrator (Thomas 2000, 5) puts it, there is a

> critical link between mental health and housing. A lack of safe, secure, affordable and appropriate housing is shown to have negative effects on both physical and mental health, resulting in increased need for and use of emergency, treatment, and support services. Research also points out that adequate, appropriate housing is often the essential ingredient needed to help people with mental illness move forward toward recovery. Having housing helps people better manage their illness, reduces the need for treatment and support services, increases stability, and generally improves quality of life.

Being homeless means more than just lacking shelter: it represents "absent or reduced social ties and the resources that these represent and a diminished sense of connectedness or belonging" (Vandermark 2007, 243).

It can be argued that housing is a fundamental right, one enshrined in the United Nations Declaration of Human Rights.[1] Unfortunately, for many mental health clients, the reality is that appropriate accommodation has been either unaffordable (in the case of independent market housing) or limited in range and quality (in the case of supported housing), with, historically, a "custodial" approach predominating. This chapter looks at the multi-determined association between mental disorder and homelessness as well as at developments in supported housing for clients that – on a more positive note – have led to better outcomes with respect to choice, satisfaction, and mental health.

Homelessness

Determining the number of homeless persons is a challenging task, given that this is a difficult group to reach and that different definitions are employed (Allen 2000; Canadian Institute for Health Information 2007). Definitions of "homelessness" may include:

- Absolute homelessness, referring to persons living on the streets;
- Persons staying in shelters;
- Persons "couch surfing" (temporarily staying with friends);
- Persons at risk of homelessness, which can be defined as spending more than 50% of total household income on rent;
- Persons in inadequate housing, or who lack security of tenure (Eberle 2001c, 22).

A definition of adequate housing provided by the United Nations includes five standards: (1) protection from the elements; (2) access to safe water and sanitation; (3) secure tenure and personal safety; (4) access to employment, education, and health care; and (5) affordability (Bryant 2003). By way of illustration, a skid-row hotel room may provide a roof and a mattress but not necessarily a toilet, and locks on doors are not always changed from one tenant to the next.

Prevalence

How many homeless persons are there in Canada? On this matter a federal government website concludes that "there are currently no reliable national statistics on the number of homeless individuals because of the methodological challenges surrounding counts of this population" (Human Resources and Skills Development Canada 2008). Researching this question is indeed difficult, mainly because of the various definitions used. A publication by the Canadian Institute for Health Information (2007), based on national census data, reports that at least ten thousand are homeless any given night, defining this as residing in a shelter. Other estimates, using broader definitions of homelessness, produce very large figures: one report puts the number of homeless persons in Canada at between 150,000 and 300,000 (Echenberg and Jensen 2008). Concerning those at risk of homelessness because of low income, it is worth noting that most of Canada's large cities have rental costs for two bedroom apartments averaging over $1,000 a month as well as relatively low vacancy rates (Canada Mortgage and Housing Corporation 2011).

Are the figures for homelessness increasing? Statistics bearing on this question are politically charged since they speak to the adequacy of response of the different levels of government to what is seen as a significant problem in Canada. Surveys from the early years of the 2000-09 decade *did* indicate an increase in the number of persons living in shelters and on the streets in larger centres such as Toronto (Irwin 2004) and Vancouver (Howell 2005). For example, it was reported that increasing numbers were being turned away from full shelters in Vancouver over this period of time (Centre for Applied Research in Mental Health and Addiction 2007a; Loy 2006). Since then, initiatives have been launched in these and other cities to provide more resources and support for persons who are homeless or inadequately housed (described in more detail below).[2] A survey released by the City of Toronto in 2010 reported a substantial drop in the number of "street homeless" in that city, with credit going to the resources provided through the new Streets to Homes Program (Jenkins 2010), although critics of the survey argued that it did not account for the "hidden homeless," such as couch-surfers (Shapcott 2010). In Greater Vancouver, homeless counts in 2008 and 2011 determined, similar to Toronto, that the number of street homeless had gone down while the number in shelters had gone up, although the total number stayed about the same (Lee 2011; Pablo 2008). Concerning the greater availability of shelters, a drop in the rate of property crime in Vancouver was attributed (at least in part) by the police to new, "low-barrier" shelter beds being opened in that city (Bellett 2010). A police spokesman concluded that "one of the key things is getting [the homeless] inside, getting them warm, getting them food so they are not outside having to do crime to survive" (quoted in Bellett 2010). This may represent a "good news-bad news" situation: while it is reassuring that fewer people are on the streets, the apparent shortage of permanent housing is still a concern.

Who are the homeless? Allen (2000) notes that the ranks of the "old" homeless – older, working-class males who resided in areas close to transient labour opportunities – have been swelled by the "new" homeless, who include women, young persons, and families. For example, in Toronto in 1998, shelter users aged fifteen to twenty-four comprised 21 percent of all persons using shelters that year, well above the 12 percent proportion of youth in the general population in Toronto (Canadian Housing and Renewal Association 2002). In its 2003 annual report, the Toronto Mayor's Task Force on Homelessness found that, of nearly thirty-two thousand persons staying in the city's hostels in 2002, 4,779 were children. In 2008, the City of Calgary opened a shelter just for families to cope with this problem. There is also now the phenomenon of the "working homeless," with studies in Calgary finding that as many as half of their shelter population already has jobs (Laird 2004). Refugees to Canada may face homelessness since, until their application process is completed (which takes a year or more), they are not eligible for settlement services or income assistance (Patterson 2007). And all available evidence indicates that members of the First Nations are over-represented among the homeless in Canada (Centre for Applied Research in Mental Health and Addiction 2007a).

Researchers also distinguish between episodic and "chronic" homeless-ness, the latter term describing persons whose status may persist for several years before stable housing materializes. It is estimated that the chronically homeless represent 15 to 25 percent of the cross-section of all homeless persons (Bula 2004).

What about persons with mental disorders? Estimating rates of home-lessness among this population is complicated by how one defines mental illness, in particular, whether substance misuse is included in the definition. In any event, it seems clear that a large proportion of the homeless popula-tion have mental health problems. Speaking of the American scene, psych-iatrist and author E. Fuller Torrey concludes that about 35 percent of the homeless population have a "severe mental illness," referring mainly to persons with psychotic disorders, bipolar disorder, and major depression. He adds that this figure increases to 75 percent if one includes alcohol and drug addictions as mental disorders (Torrey 1997). In Canada, reviews and surveys have arrived at similar numbers; that is, that about one-third of the homeless living on the streets or residing in shelters are persons with serious mental disorders (Allen 2000; Canadian Institute for Health Information 2007; Eberle 2001a; Golden et al. 1999; Stuart and Arboleda-Florez 2000).[3] There is evidence that these rates may be considerably higher if one is look-ing specifically at *chronic* homelessness (Todd 2004). Concerning particu-lar diagnostic categories among the homeless, studies have found between 6 and 11 percent reporting a diagnosis of schizophrenia, compared to life-time prevalence rates of roughly 1 percent for the general population (Can-adian Institute for Health Information 2007; Centre for Applied Research in Mental Health and Addiction 2007a) as well substantially higher rates of depression (Votta and Manion 2003). As noted, when substance misuse is included, either alone or as a co-occurring diagnosis, the numbers as a pro-portion of the homeless population are much higher still, with Canadian studies reporting rates of 40 to 68 percent (Canadian Institute for Health Information 2007). Finally, a Toronto survey of 904 residents of homeless shelters found that over half reported a previous traumatic brain injury, with 12 percent reporting "moderate to serious" injuries that left them unconscious for thirty minutes or longer (Hwang et al. 2008).

Impact

The effects of homelessness on the health of individuals and on the health care system itself are substantial. A Toronto task force on homelessness concluded in its report that "homeless people are at much higher risk for infectious disease, premature death, acute illness and chronic health problems than the rest of the population" (Golden et al. 1999, 103; see also Toneguzzi 2005). As reviewed by Eberle (2001a, 6-7), several factors negatively affect the health of homeless persons:

- Homelessness increases a person's exposure to infectious and communicable diseases, such as tuberculosis.
- Homelessness is a profoundly stressful experience, and severe stress can trigger genetic predispositions to diseases, such as hypertension.
- Long periods of malnutrition can cause chronic conditions such as anemia and degenerative bone disease.
- There is a higher likelihood of experiencing violence or trauma on the street or in a shelter.
- Difficult living conditions also result in poor hygiene, inadequate diet, exposure to the elements, lack of sleep, and physical injuries.

A Toronto study that involved interviewing 330 homeless persons found that suicidal thinking and attempts were common among this group (Eynan et al. 2002). In a study of young female "run-aways" in London, Ontario, Reid, Berman, and Forchuk (2005, 237) found that "most girls had fled from difficult, at times dangerous, situations at home to lives on the street that brought a new set of challenges, including a multitude of health problems and exposure to violence, chronic poverty, and discrimination." And a 2008 BC Coroner's report offers a grim depiction of the lives and premature deaths of homeless persons in that province (see Paulsen and Sandborn 2008). It was determined that fifty-six homeless persons died in 2006-07,[4] with the majority being under fifty years of age and only three making it into their sixties; two-thirds had been living on the street and one-third in shelters. Poisoning by drugs or alcohol was the leading cause of death, followed by blunt injuries (e.g., hit by a car), hangings, and stabbings, with nine deaths being undetermined. First Nations persons were overrepresented among the victims.

For persons who are homeless and have a mental disorder the situation, if anything, is worse, with one psychiatrist stating bluntly: "this kind of life is often a living hell" (Torrey 1997, 19). In the Calgary study by Stuart and Arboleda-Florez (2000) the authors found that homeless persons with mental disorders experienced more hardships on the streets, took greater public health risks, more often abused substances, were more often victimized, suffered greater negative economic and interpersonal life events, experienced greater dissatisfaction, and suffered more stress. Persons with mental disorders are particularly vulnerable to financial and sexual exploitation while on the streets, with a number of studies documenting an alarmingly high incidence of rape among female clients in this population (Torrey 1997).

Homeless persons also tend to use health care services in an inefficient and ineffective manner. A survey of homeless individuals in Toronto found that half did not have a family doctor, with most using hospital emergencies for routine care – half having gone to an emergency room in the past year (Golden et al. 1999). Similarly, data from an inner-city hospital in Vancouver showed that the number of patients with no fixed address seen at the hospital increased by about 300 percent from 1995 to 1999, while total admissions actually declined in this period (Eberle 2001b). A number of studies have concluded that costs borne by public agencies serving the homeless (such as ambulance, hospitals, the criminal justice system, and addiction services) are substantially reduced when these individuals are placed in secure, supported housing (Larimer et al. 2009; Mental Health Commission of Canada 2012; Thomas 2007), with the savings more than compensating for new housing costs (Centre for Applied Research in Mental Health and Addiction 2007).

Causes
While the association between mental illness and homelessness is empirically strong, teasing out cause-and-effect is complex. A number of overlapping factors contribute to homelessness among the mentally ill, and when arguments have arisen about how to respond to this problem, it has been when commentators have focused on one area, such as individual, as opposed to structural determinants. For example, American Author Edwin Fuller Torrey (1997) argues that homelessness is directly a result of the disorder itself – that is, an inability among this population to recognize the need for treatment or to have "insight" – in turn supporting the need for more coercive approaches to service provision, such as community treatment orders. On the other hand, there is the argument that homelessness is an issue of poverty and resource distribution and that focusing on individual factors, such as mental disorder, in effect blames and further stigmatizes the victim for government policies and cutbacks beyond his or her control. In an article entitled "How Psychiatric Status Contributes to Homelessness Policy," a policy analyst

suggests that a preoccupation with individual characteristics "removes from the level of discourse any indication of the macro-level changes that create and affect the day-to-day situation of homeless persons" (Lovell 1992, 256). Allen (2000, 18) points out that mental disorder or substance misuse can be a result of homelessness as well as a cause, noting that "the poorer an individual is, the more likely individual problems will precipitate homelessness, and it is arguable which is cause and which is effect."

In looking at *individual* factors, it is reasonable to assume that the manifestations of an untreated mental illness – psychosis, cognitive impairment, disorganization, and problem behaviours – will lead to decreased housing tenure if the person has no other supports. Drug and alcohol misuse, either co-morbid or on its own, is a particularly strong predictor of decreased housing tenure and eviction (Davis 1987b; O'Connell, Kasprow, and Rosenheck 2008). Concerning the direction of effect, Didenko and Pankratz (2007, 9) conclude that substance misuse is *both* a "pathway to homelessness" and a way of adapting to street life. In their review of the literature these authors conclude that about two-thirds of homeless persons cite alcohol and/or drug addiction as a major or primary reason for becoming homeless.

Homelessness may also result from family disruption. For example, a Toronto study found that 70 percent of young persons leaving home for the streets did so because of physical and/or sexual abuse (Eberle 2001a) and, similarly, analysis of data from an Ontario community survey, involving 3,760 females, found that physical and sexual abuse as well as parental psychiatric illness were strong predictors of running away from home (Andres-Lemay, Jamieson, and MacMillan 2005). A report on homelessness among young women in Canada concludes that "the predominant reason for homelessness among young women is family breakdown in all its manifestations" (Canadian Housing and Renewal Association 2002, 53).

Among the mentally ill, homelessness may also be linked to hospitalization. This is a complicated issue, with some persons simultaneously becoming ill, being hospitalized, and being evicted from their previous residence for behaviour related to the relapse of their psychiatric condition. Alternately, persons kept hospitalized in a psychiatric unit for an extended period of time may lose their housing because the provincial income assistance ministry will refuse to pay rent when the person is not residing there. However, the latter situation is increasingly rare since most psychiatric admissions in the present era are relatively brief, but this, in turn, leads to a problem: the hospital stay is so short it does not give hospital staff (usually social workers) enough time to line up appropriate housing, with the result that persons who came into the hospital homeless may be discharged back to the streets or to shelters. For example, an older survey by this author (Davis 1987b) of

232 mentally ill persons residing in Vancouver emergency shelters found that about one in five had just been discharged from a hospital psychiatric ward with no fixed address.[5] While in some of these cases hospital staff and the client would agree about the need for supported housing, the waiting lists for this type of accommodation were too long to allow the client to continue taking up a bed in the hospital. A more recent study in London, Ontario, found that, in the year 2002, on 194 occasions, persons were discharged from psychiatric units to shelters or the streets (Forchuk et al. 2006). The study's principal author, University of Western Ontario professor Cheryl Forchuk, followed this up with an intervention designed specifically to address this issue. In evaluating this, it was found that at-risk persons randomized to a group given immediate assistance in gaining access to housing (a "housing first" approach – see below) were still in housing six months later, whereas all but one of the comparison group remained homeless (Forchuk et al. 2008).

Homelessness is also affected by income assistance levels and policies. A striking example of this was documented in a study out of BC by the Canadian Centre for Policy Alternatives (CCPA) (Wallace, Klein, and Reitsma-Street 2006). Since the mid-1990s, the number of people on basic income assistance in that province had been declining,[6] which the right-leaning government attributed to people gaining employment in a recovering economy. However, the CCPA was able to gain access to data that showed more people were also being *denied* welfare, blocked at the "front door," by policies brought in in 2002 that made qualifying more difficult. Significantly, as acceptance rates dropped from about 90 percent in 2001 to slightly over 50 percent in 2004, the number of street homeless not on *any* income assistance rose, from 15 percent in 2001 to 75 percent in 2005. In a different example, single mothers on income assistance, if their child is apprehended, may have their shelter allowance cut, leading to unsuitable accommodation for the mother, which, in turn, means the child will stay longer in foster care (Pablo 2010).

In looking at structural factors leading to homelessness, a number of researchers point to unemployment and the increasing unaffordability of rental housing (Bula 2004).[7] A five-year study of homeless persons in New York found that the strongest predictor of homelessness was the lack of affordable housing, rather than individual traits or characteristics, and that "subsidized housing succeeds in curing homelessness among families, regardless of behavioral disorders and other conditions" (Shinn et al. 1998, 1651). In an interview on this subject, University of Toronto urban economics professor William Strange concludes:

> Some observers argue – often based on personal observation – that
> because many of the homeless are substance abusers or are mentally ill,
> that homelessness is not a housing problem ... [W]hile it is no doubt true
> that homelessness has some of its roots outside the operation of housing
> markets, it is demonstrably false to claim that homelessness arises independ-
> ently from the housing market ... [A]lthough the deinstitutionalization of
> the mentally ill occurred simultaneously in many places, the rise in home-
> lessness did not. Instead, increases in homelessness accompanied increases
> in income inequality. (quoted in Bula and Skelton 2004)

Interviewed for the same report, David Hulchanski, a University of Toronto
professor and authority on housing, notes the impact of government programs for housing and income assistance: "There are so many people on the
edge, it just takes small cuts to any of those [programs] to push people over
the edge" (quoted in Bula 2004).

In Canada, one can note a number of social and economic factors that
contributed to the rise of homelessness in the 1990s. At the federal level, the
national housing program, mandated to fund social housing projects, was
eliminated in 1993. At the provincial level, social programs were cut and
more restrictive welfare policies implemented in a number of jurisdictions
(Wallace, Klein, and Reitsma-Street 2006). A number of neighbourhoods
underwent "gentrification," whereby rental units were renovated or demol-
ished to make way for office buildings and condominiums. In some cases
cheap single-room occupancy (SRO) hotels were converted to daily rental
units or "backpacker hostels" (student dormitories) (Carrigg 2003). All this,
combined with high rents and low vacancy rates – around 1 percent in most
of the larger cities – has made life difficult for low-income renters in Canada.
Libby Davies (2000, 38), member of Parliament and New Democratic Party
spokesperson for Social Policy and Housing, argues that the housing crisis
is a direct result of these federal and provincial government cutbacks: "The
[federal government] solution is to institutionalize shelters, and that is no
solution at all. What they should be doing is admitting that the federal decision to retreat from social housing was not only shortsighted, it was shame-
ful ... We need the government to commit to a national housing strategy, a
strategy that calls for ... a federal investment of an additional one percent of
overall spending on housing, or two billion dollars annually; and an approach that is national in scope and in vision."

Apart from humanitarian concerns, the provision of decent, affordable
housing to marginalized persons can be supported on pragmatic and fiscal
grounds, with the National Housing and Homelessness Network (2001)
suggesting that federal and provincial investment in housing would produce

social and economic benefits, including direct and spin-off employment, income tax revenues, neighbourhood stability, and empowerment. Based on the finding that homeless individuals tend to use more costly emergency type services, a number of studies from Canada and the US have concluded that subsidized, supported housing for transient persons would be less expensive for the taxpayer than a disjointed response consisting of shelters, ambulances, and jails (Culhane, Metraux, and Hadley 2002; Larimer et al. 2009). For example, a report authored by David Hulchanski at the University of Toronto found that it cost $40,000 annually to provide shelter as well as social, criminal justice, and health services for a homeless person, compared to $28,000 if that individual was given permanent housing (cited in Irwin 2004). A later study by researchers at Simon Fraser University concluded, similarly, that annual costs of about $55,000 per person spent on homeless individuals in BC could be reduced to $37,000 per year with the provision of supported housing and that, even factoring in capital costs (spread over several years), the savings would be about $33 million annually (Centre for Applied Research in Mental Health and Addiction 2007a).

"Housing First"

What do clients themselves say about housing preferences? While there is no single answer to this, generally there is an emphasis on greater independence and privacy, hardly surprising in that few of us, given the choice, would relish sharing a bedroom with a stranger (Davis 1987b). In reviewing the literature, two McMaster University researchers found that choice in selection, privacy, the ability to exercise control in the residential environment, and safety were all salient concerns among persons surveyed (Edge and Wilton 2009). Another review concludes that "most people with [serious mental illness] desire to live independently in the community, not in congregate housing" (Centre for Applied Research in Mental Health and Addiction 2007a, 10). A Montreal survey of 315 clients living in seven different types of housing found that a majority would have preferred housing that offered them more autonomy than the housing in which they were currently living, although interestingly this was a preference their case managers – who were also surveyed – did not necessarily support (Piat et al. 2008). And a study from London, Ontario, concluded that clients wanted housing without "strings attached": persons interviewed stated a preference for independent housing in which supports would be available as needed, as opposed to "having to choose between the housing they wanted and the supports they needed, since supports were often contingent upon living in a less desirable housing situation" (Forchuk, Nelson, and Hall 2006, 42). Notably, this study was entitled "It's Important to Be Proud of the Place You Live In."

Historically, client preference for independence has not been realized in Canada: persons discharged from psychiatric hospitals and needing support could expect to be placed in congregate housing such as group homes and boarding homes. This author recalls a landscape in the early 1980s in which the typical "choice" for people with respect to supported accommodation was seedy, run-for-profit boarding houses with rules, fixed mealtimes, curfews, and shared bedrooms. The assumption was that these clients did not have, and apparently would never acquire, the skills to look after themselves, and the question of their own housing preferences was not usually raised at all. Gradually other options, such as self-contained suites, were introduced, but apart from insufficient supply there was also an attitudinal barrier that some clients had to face: they had to "prove" themselves by working their way from settings of lesser independence to more independence rather than simply being placed in self-contained housing in the first place. Further, to qualify for greater independence there were still rules to follow, such as agreeing to be seen by a particular psychiatric treatment program (which would be able to provide back-up should something "go wrong").

While some clients benefit from more structured congregate housing, we now know that there are those that simply will not tolerate the rules and institutional feel of this type of dwelling and, consequently or coincidentally, that this includes persons in the persistently homeless category (Greater Vancouver Shelter Strategy 2007; Pearson et al. 2007). In responding to this, a strategy called "housing first" has been developed and implemented in a number of settings. Definitions of this term vary slightly, but the key features are:

- direct placement into permanent housing, without any preconditions placed on tenancy and regardless of past behaviours (Remund 2007);
- while mental health and addiction services are offered, the program does not require participation in these to remain in the housing (Pearson et al. 2007);
- staff support is in the form of outreach rather than being based at the building;
- other aspects of the program may include greater tolerance of substance misuse and an effort to hold housing for clients even if they leave the program for short periods.

Following developments in the US, such as the Pathways to Housing model located in New York City (Tsemberis, Gulcur, and Nakae 2004), "housing first" projects have been initiated in a number of Canadian cities, including Edmonton, Calgary, and Toronto. As well, in 2009, the Mental Health Commission of Canada embarked on an ambitious, multi-city study of the housing first model by providing supported housing for 2,285 homeless mentally ill persons in Moncton, Montreal, Toronto, Winnipeg, and Vancouver. Health outcomes for persons provided with subsidized housing and outreach support were compared with a group screened and found eligible but assigned to a quasi-control group receiving "care as usual" (readers are referred to the commission's website: http://www.mentalhealthcommission. ca/English/Pages/homelessness.aspx). Evaluations of "housing first" programs have found, despite not requiring addictions treatment for tenants, that persons with co-occurring disorders can remain stably housed without increasing substance use (Tsemberis, Gulcur, and Nakae 2004). A preliminary analysis of the Mental Health Commission supported housing study found that, after one year, participants had been stably housed 70 percent of the time compared to 20 percent for the control group and that the rate of emergency department visits had significantly declined (Vancouver At Home Research Team 2012). A review by Simon Fraser University researchers concludes that "housing first ... may be effective with hard-to-house individuals" and that, in any case, "housing with supports *in any form* is an effective intervention for individuals with serious mental illness" (Centre for Applied Research in Mental Health and Addiction 2007a, 9, emphasis in original).

Mental Health Housing Models
Many clients will manage quite well in independent housing, although for those on income assistance the cost of appropriate market accommodation may be prohibitive. If support is needed, this can be provided on an outreach basis, assuming sufficient staff resources. Other clients, who are more disabled, may need on-site support. This can take the form of meals, medication support, and "gate-keeping," the latter term referring to the need to screen out predatory visitors such as drug dealers. Broadly speaking, then, one can talk about three models of mental health housing:

- Residential housing, defined as housing services that are provided "to enable individuals who cannot live independently at this time and/or who choose to acquire skills and confidence in a group setting to maximize their independence" (British Columbia Ministry of Health 2002d, 22).
- Supported housing, which refers to dwellings that offer greater independence and privacy (through self-contained suites) and where support services

are offered on an "as-needed" basis (9). "Housing first" would fall into this category.

- Emergency housing, which is provided for clients "who have no other housing or who require intensive stabilization (but not hospitalization) to return to adequate housing" (31). In some cases this will be in the form of specialized mental health facilities, but in many other cases this (unfortunately) will be in the form of shelters or hostels. As noted earlier, emergency shelters have become a necessary evil in Canada partly due to deficiencies in other areas of the social service and health care systems.

These three categories of housing are discussed in more detail below.

Residential Housing

Group homes and boarding homes represent one of the earliest approaches to mental health housing; indeed, this type of accommodation predominated in Canada for a number of years following the initial wave of psychiatric hospital downsizing. These facilities were usually large, older buildings with shared bedrooms that were run for profit by private operators. Parkinson, Nelson, and Horgan (1999) note that the approach tended to be custodial: client autonomy was limited, there was an emphasis on rules (regarding smoking, drinking, visitors, curfews, set meal times, etc.), and residents had little or no decision-making input. Older-style residential homes may have provided the basic necessities, but they tended to foster dependency by not involving clients in activities, chores, or rehabilitation and by "focusing on deficits, rather than strengths" (147; see also Browne and Courtney 2004). While it could be argued that the most severely disabled clients required this degree of structure and supervision, a problem for practitioners working in the 1960s and 1970s was that there did not appear to be any alternatives for clients to this "one-size-fits-all" approach. (Toronto author Pat Capponi [1992] gives a moving account of life in a custodial boarding home in Toronto – which housed as many as seventy other people – in her biography *Upstairs in the Crazy House*.) On the question of independence, a survey by this author (Davis 1987b) of clients referred to residential housing in Vancouver found that, of those who refused placement, most did so because of a wish for independence and an unwillingness to accommodate the rules and regulations of residential housing – even though at the time of referral they were homeless and residing in emergency shelters. (The survey was conducted at a time when the main placement options were older-style boarding homes.) An early example of residential housing that aimed for greater tenant empowerment – and, not surprisingly, that came out of the self-help sector – was the group home program of Vancouver's Mental Patients Association,[8] founded in 1971. In these homes the expectation was that residents would clean their own rooms, make their own meals, and look after their own health care and medications. This was one of very few programs that allowed residents some say in who their housemates would be by requiring that prospective tenants be "ratified" by the other members.

Later guidelines for residential housing suggested that these facilities should be small and homelike, offer more privacy, have more of a rehabilitation focus, and be run by non-profit societies (Parkinson, Nelson, and Horgan 1999). On this last point, a government document provides the example of a housing society whose land is owned by the province but whose services are contracted with care providers on the basis of proposal calls. With services separated from property ownership, residents do not lose their housing if contractors change (either voluntarily or as a result of not meeting standards) (British Columbia Ministry of Health 2002b). Concerning privacy, this same document recommends that, either by policy or regulation, a standard of one person per room be established in licensed facilities.

Residential housing is "segregated" in the sense that all tenants of a particular facility are mental health clients, which critics argue promotes stigmatization and social isolation (Aubrey and Myner 1996). To overcome these drawbacks, different authors have suggested that these facilities should be located within easy access to services and amenities, and be indistinguishable from other houses in the neighbourhood, and that residents should be encouraged and empowered to develop networks for peer support, family contact, and social support (Dixon et al. 1998).

There are several potential systemic barriers with respect to developing residential housing that meets best-practice standards and that is accessible to clients who need it. One, unfortunately, is lack of community acceptance, more commonly known as the NIMBY (not in my back yard) syndrome. A concern sometimes voiced is that social housing will lower property values in the area, although research conducted on the issue contradicts this claim (Hamid 2000b). Local opponents of residential housing may not appreciate that mental health clients will be living among them in any case – the days of the asylum are long gone, after all – but (potentially) as marginalized, unsupported citizens, a situation that benefits neither the clients themselves nor the other residents of the area. In attempting to overcome the NIMBY problem, a general strategy is to enhance public education about mental disorder. Particular projects may also require that project leaders make contacts with local officials: in describing the opposition to a group home in a small town in British Columbia, author Sarah Hamid (2000b, 28) describes how the mayor, city council, and police chief were invited for dinners at which clients attended and made presentations. These officials were "surprised to see people ... that they knew from other contexts ... [and] by the time the mayor and council left ... were in full support of this project." Another barrier to residential placement concerns client access to income and adequate support funding. In some jurisdictions a client's income assistance is suspended when that person goes into a residential facility, with the facility then receiving direct payment from government sources and the client receiving a small amount of money for personal expenses. In British Columbia, at the time of writing, the "comfort allowance" given to clients was about ninety-five dollars per month. While practitioners can attempt to persuade the client that he or she is getting a good deal in some respects – housing, meals, and other services are being provided – the small amount left over as "cash in hand" can make it a very tough sell when discussing residential placement. A recommendation here, in keeping with principles of client autonomy, is that clients receive income assistance directly and pay shelter and food costs out of this (British Columbia Ministry of Health 2002d). Another barrier concerns restricted access to housing across health region boundaries, an issue that has come up with the move in many jurisdictions to region-based funding of mental health programs. This policy may restrict the ability of clients to make choices about where they wish to live and may effectively block access to specialized programs that are only available in other regions. The recommendation is that "health authorities be required to establish policies and procedures that will maintain and support consumer choice in housing across boundaries" (British Columbia Ministry of Health 2002d, 30).

Supported Housing

The move to supported housing in mental health reflects an increased emphasis on the principles of recovery and empowerment and in particular the importance of client choice. As reviewed by Browne and Courtney (2004, 37), more recent surveys "indicate that, for people with a mental illness, boarding homes are the least desirable type of community accommodation and that living in their own homes is the most desirable." A survey of three hundred mental health clients in London, Ontario, for example, found that almost 80 percent stated a preference for living in their own apartment or house (Nelson, Hall, and Forchuk 2003).

Supported housing also represents a move towards greater physical integration – that is, dwellings that are "located in ordinary residential areas and widely dispersed in the community, rather than segregated" (British Columbia Ministry of Health 2002d, 15; see also Parkinson, Nelson, and Horgan 1999). Supported housing can take different forms, such as block apartments with self-contained suites, supported hotels, and satellite apartments, which are subsidized units in regular apartment buildings. In this model, particularly in the case of satellite apartments, the aim is to "de-link" services from the building, with clients then utilizing outreach support and/or office-based programs in the community.

As noted earlier, there was a view that saw more independent, supported housing programs as something clients could "work towards" after successfully completing a placement in residential housing. Currently, the emphasis is placement in supported housing as the *first consideration*, to be ruled out only if the degree of client disability and potential risk are so high as to necessitate using other options. This is based on the finding that supported housing is associated with increased client satisfaction, greater community integration, and increased residential stability as well as with favourable outcomes in clinical domains such as hospitalization rates and symptom reduction (Boydell and Everett 1992; Brown et al. 1991; Canadian Housing and Renewal Association 2002; Dixon et al. 1994; Kirsh, Gewurtz, and Bakewell 2011).

It is acknowledged that, compared to residential housing, there can be a greater risk of social isolation in supported housing. Different approaches to addressing this problem include the provision of outreach support as well as communal kitchens and shared activity groups in the block apartments. Another potential problem area concerns medication assistance: supported housing models do not normally make provision for supervising clients' medication, consistent with principles of autonomy and self-determination. In the worst-case scenario, this can lead to re-hospitalization and loss of housing. Client independence with respect to health care would normally be assessed prior to placement; additionally, options such as injectable forms of medication, medication delivery, outreach support, coaching, and use of blister packs and dosette containers may be considered to assist clients.

Major barriers to client access to supported housing include the supply and affordability of these units. Lack of timely access to housing means either that persons must spend extended periods in more costly housing or that eventual transition to supported housing is more difficult due to persons becoming acclimatized to supervised residential settings. A best-practices document recommends that provincial governments and health authorities should "aim to provide housing services for a minimum of 30 percent of persons identified as having a serious and persistent mental illness" (British Columbia Ministry of Health 2002d, 20). Access to apartment-style housing is also limited by high rents and inadequate income assistance for mental health clients. The result is that clients may be forced into inadequate, unsafe housing, a stressor that, in turn, may lead to greater clinical instability and greater use of hospitals and crisis shelters. A Canadian professor of geography observes that "a person's home may root them to a point in the landscape that exposes them to things that are unhealthy such as pollution, crime, vandalism, violence, discrimination, exclusion, social isolation, and a lack of services. In this way, people can easily become 'prisoners of space,' especially if they are poor and cannot afford to move and live elsewhere" (Dunn 2000, 4). It is consequently recommended that supported housing programs come with rent subsidies, which would be portable should the individual wish to relocate to another health region.

Emergency Housing

The discussion here considers two types of emergency housing: shelter/hostel accommodations and short-stay crisis units. Concerning the need for emergency shelters, it is noted that, "while emergency housing programs must exist to provide services to the homeless and must engage in best practices, they are clearly a stop-gap solution. Emergency shelters should be viewed as symptomatic of the lack of affordable, appropriate, safe and secure housing and as a reflection of an inadequate and inappropriate response to housing needs" (British Columbia Ministry of Health 2002d, 34).

Housing mental health clients in shelters or hostels is problematic in a number of respects. Shelters usually provide services to a wide range of individuals, with the potential that mentally disordered clients may be marginalized within the shelter setting or exploited by others. Shelters are often located in inner-city or skid-row areas, meaning a greater probability that vulnerable mentally disordered persons will be exposed to unsafe situations and activities, such as drug use. As a former shelter worker notes: "Large shelters tend to be dangerous places, especially for those who lack the social skills of getting by and surviving in a desperate milieu" (Allen 2000, 25). Shelters also tend to get clients with the greatest needs or who are the hardest to house – for example, persons with multiple diagnoses, such as mental disorder, intellectual impairment, and substance misuse – despite having limited resources to assist these people. Operating with minimal funding and staffing makes it difficult for shelters to intervene effectively in the lives of clients prior to discharge. Mental health clients face additional challenges with respect to emergency housing: transition houses for battered women may not take persons with mental illness even if they have been battered (MacPhee 2002), and older-style "men only" shelters (sometimes run under religious auspices) may force clients out of the building during the day, even though the individual may be fragile and in need of respite. Daly (1996, 157) describes these older shelters: "These practices [of the shelter] include placing a large number of residents in a dormitory-like setting; inappropriate short-term limitations on length of stay (which tend to induce transience);

night use only (residents are forced to leave early in the morning); minimal staff-to-resident ratios (which makes it difficult to provide a secure environment); staff members who adopt a controlling or punitive approach to residents; limited resident involvement in the planning of the shelter or its operations; and only tenuous connections to supportive community."

Given the above, it is perhaps not surprising that homeless clients may simply refuse placement in a shelter, despite the best efforts of mental health workers. This question was examined in a survey of thirty-four persons experiencing homelessness in the Greater Vancouver area, with participants being asked: "Why do some people prefer to sleep outside than in a shelter?" (Greater Vancouver Shelter Strategy 2007). The ten most commonly cited reasons were:

- the rules and institutional feeling of shelters;
- lack of safety and security (which most often referred to theft but could also mean sexual harassment);
- unsuitability of shelter hours;
- lack of privacy (which could refer to filling out forms and people "asking too many questions");
- pride, shame, and guilt, with participants feeling stigma and embarrassment;
- health concerns (e.g., bed bug infestations);
- noise;
- lack of available beds (the experience of being turned away was unpleasant);
- lack of storage;
- barriers to access (which could mean no accommodations for the disabled but could also refer to policies around not being let in without ID).

A document produced by the Canada Mortgage and Housing Corporation (1999) makes several recommendations concerning emergency shelters: (1) that staff have a nonjudgmental manner, offer support respectfully, and empower and encourage clients to accomplish the goals they have set for themselves; (2) that safety and security be emphasized; and (3) that services be provided flexibly, particularly that length of stay be negotiable and based on client needs with a view to longer-term stability. Some shelter organizations have ancillary services, such as an outreach program whose workers help clients to locate housing and make other linkages that support long-term tenancy. In Toronto, the Shared Care Clinical Outreach Service, an initiative of the Centre for Addiction and Mental Health, provides outreach workers, nurses, and part-time physicians to city hostels so that clients in need of health care services can be identified, given immediate assistance, and linked up with a doctor (Lechky 1999).[9] At the same time, while it is probably true that shelters could "do more" and provide more services on-site, one has to question whether concentrating services in a large, inner-city facility is the best solution.

Crisis units are programs for persons who need short-term stabilization but not hospitalization (ideally, a stay in such a program will obviate the need for hospital care). These facilities offer a safe environment with twenty-four-hour staffing, although they vary in terms of staff composition and the treatment model applied. In some cases the approach is medically focused, with the staff consisting of nurses and sessional doctors (e.g., Venture House in Vancouver). In other cases a non-medical, self-help model is used, an example being Toronto's Gerstein Centre, which provides crisis intervention to adults experiencing mental health problems. The Gerstein Centre offers telephone support and a mobile crisis team, in addition to the centre itself, which is a ten-bed facility in which the average length of stay is three days (see description at http://www.gersteincentre.org). A program that uses a peer-support model is Seneca House in Winnipeg, which provides crisis support and respite for adults and in which persons may stay up to five days up to eight times a year. Peer counsellors help clients to make linkages and assist them with problem solving and goal setting. The Seneca House website (http://www.senecahouse.ca) notes that "guests maintain their autonomy and freedom of movement." In settings in which twenty-four-hour assertive community treatment is offered, crises may be managed in the client's own residence, a "least restrictive" alternative that clients may prefer (Knapp et al. 1998). Alternately, some clients may prefer the safety and security of a staffed facility. Unfortunately, particularly in more remote settings, neither option may be available. The best-practices guidelines for crisis housing are similar to those for residential housing (see above). In particular, it is recommended that these facilities be small and homelike, be indistinguishable from other houses in the neighbourhood, be located within easy access of services and amenities, and offer single-occupancy bedrooms (British Columbia Ministry of Health 2002d).

There are several systemic problems with respect to the effective operation of emergency housing resources. As with residential housing, there is the question of community acceptance, with residents of suburban areas not uncommonly objecting to emergency shelters being built in their neighbourhoods. While these objections should be considered, citizens and practitioners must be aware of the problems associated with locating shelters only in inner-city areas, particularly the vulnerability of mentally disordered persons to drug use, assault, and financial and sexual exploitation.

Emergency housing resources also face the problem of increasing acuity in the cases presented to them, which is related to diminishing resources in other areas, particularly the relative unavailability of hospital beds. Because clients refused admission to a hospital emergency department are in many cases sent to a shelter, these facilities become de facto hospital wards (Forchuk et al. 2006; Torrey 1997). Some of these clients may be elderly or medically compromised, in addition to having mental health problems.

Finally, staff at emergency facilities may find it difficult – practically, clinically, and ethically speaking – to discharge persons due to a "lack of safe, affordable, secure and appropriate resources" (British Columbia Ministry of Health 2002d, 40). This author recalls the situation of a man with dementia being placed in a sub-acute facility because he was at risk living in his own apartment. The facility, which normally housed people for only about a week, had to hold onto this individual for two months while staff scrambled to arrange priority placement in a nursing home. Having persons wait for a long time in a shelter or crisis unit decreases access to the resources by other persons, who may also be in dire need, while discharging persons into unsuitable housing may only fuel the cycle of transience, instability, and shelter use. That shelter costs in many cases are higher than the costs of supported housing again speaks to the need for better housing options for mental health clients.

A form of temporary housing that exists in some centres is respite accommodation. Respite is primarily for clients who are living with or receiving care from a friend, partner, or family member who may be away, ill, or temporarily unable to provide care. In some cases, respite is provided to clients who are living independently but who need a brief reprieve in a setting in which some support and meals are provided. Respite options have been established for some time for persons looking after an older relative with a dementing illness such as Alzheimer's but are relatively new in the case of younger adults with other mental disorders. In Canada, family support groups such as the Schizophrenia Society have been instrumental in organizing respite services.

Notes

1 See article 25 of this document at http://www.un.org/en/documents/udhr/index.shtml#a25.
2 See also http://www.calgaryhomeless.com/.
3 The Mental Health Commission of Canada (2012, 72) cites rates ranging from 23 to 74 percent of homeless persons in Canada reporting having a "mental health problem or illness."
4 Critics of the report argued that this was an underestimate since it did not include formerly homeless persons who died in hospital from "natural/expected" deaths (e.g., from hepatitis C or HIV).

5 Eight percent of this group had just been released from jail.
6 It should be noted that, during this same period, more people had provincial disability status (PWD), which provides more money and benefits.
7 The Canada Mortgage and Housing Corporation gives regular updates on rental market trends. See http://www.cmhc-schl.gc.ca/en/hoficlincl/homain/index.cfm.
8 Whose name has since been changed to the "Motivation, Power and Achievement Society."
9 See the CAMH website: http://www.camh.net/About_CAMH/Guide_to_CAMH/Mental_Health_Programs/Schizophrenia_Program/guide_shared_care.html.

Other Resources

For descriptions and evaluations of the Mental Health Commission of Canada's homelessness initiative, "At Home/Chez Soi," see http://www.mentalhealthcommission.ca/English/Pages/homelessness.aspx.

The Interface with the Criminal Justice System

Apart from the mental health system, another large, publicly funded institution provides for the care and containment of persons with mental disorders: the criminal justice system. This chapter addresses the unfortunate fact that persons with serious mental disorders are overrepresented in the criminal courts and corrections systems. Hypotheses are advanced concerning what some have termed a "criminalization" process, and, in particular, the role of the police and the courts is examined. Programs facilitating the *diversion* of mentally ill persons are described. The chapter concludes by looking at a specialized branch of the mental health system: forensic psychiatry.

Criminalization

A number of studies show that the prevalence of serious, persistent mental disorder in jail, remand, and prison populations far exceeds that seen in the general population (Correctional Investigator of Canada 2009; Torrey et al. 2010). For example, a large-scale survey of the US states conducted by Torrey and colleagues (2010) showed the following findings: (1) At least 16 percent of jail and prison inmates have a serious mental illness, defined as schizophrenia or bipolar spectrum disorders and major depression; (2) 40 percent of persons with a serious mental illness have been in jail and prison at some time in their lives; (3) there are now three times as many seriously mentally ill persons in correctional facilities in the US as in hospitals, leading the authors to conclude that "jails and prisons have become our new mental hospitals" and that, consequently, the country had "returned to the conditions of the 1840s" (1). The survey also found that mentally disordered inmates, compared to the rest of the inmate population, had higher rates of recidivism, cost more (because of extra staffing requirements), and, on average, stayed longer, this likely due to inadequate supports post-discharge.

What about Canada? While it is tempting to think that with universal medicare and more generous social supports the situation would be better here, it is notable that the corresponding numbers are similar. For instance, a report on provincial system inmates in BC found that about 15 percent had a serious mental illness, a figure very close to the 16 percent cited for the US (Hall 2001). A more recent report on Canadian federal prison inmates (persons charged with more serious crimes and sentenced to more than two years detention) found that about 15 percent of the male, and *30 percent* of the female inmate populations had previously been hospitalized for psychiatric reasons (Public Safety Canada 2008). The same report found that 21 percent of inmates were being prescribed psychotropic medication at the time of admission. The lack of resources in the prison system to deal with these challenges, which included an "alarming" number of self-harm incidents, constitutes an area of "key concern" according to the Correctional Investigator of Canada (2009). Regarding particular diagnostic categories, a number of Canadian studies have found that 7 to 8 percent of inmates in remand, jail, and prison settings suffer from a psychotic illness, a figure much higher than that for the general population (Brink, Doherty, and Boer 2001; Gingell 1991; Hart and Hemphill 1989; Hodgins and Cote 1990).

Life in prison is not easy for anyone but is especially difficult for those with a psychiatric diagnosis. Such individuals, referred to as "bugs" in prison jargon, are low down on the inmate hierarchy and are often victimized and physically or sexually exploited by others (Blitz, Wolff, and Shi 2008). These inmates are sometimes punished for symptoms of the disorder itself, such as being noisy, disruptive, refusing orders, or even self-mutilation. A common response is to put such persons in isolation – "administrative segregation" – which may be for their own protection but which can actually have the effect of exacerbating psychotic symptoms (Quan 2011). The organization Human Rights Watch (2003, 2) describes prisoners "who, because of their illness, rant and rave, babble incoherently, or huddle silently in their cells. They talk to invisible companions, living in worlds constructed of hallucinations. They lash out without provocation, beat their heads against cell walls, cover themselves with feces, mutilate themselves until their bodies are covered with scars, and attempt suicide." In examining the administrative response to mentally disordered persons, Hodgins and Cote (1991, 181) surveyed inmates of Quebec penitentiaries who had been transferred either to "special handling units" or to "long-term segregation units," finding persons with schizophrenia and bipolar disorder to be overrepresented relative to the total inmate population in both of these special units. The same did not apply to those suffering from depression, leading the investigators to conclude that "withdrawn mentally disordered inmates are left within the general penitentiary population, while the troublesome ones are sent to isolation."

In considering the plight of mental health clients who, in disproportionate numbers, are ending up in criminal justice settings, the remaining questions are "how did this come about?" and "what – if anything – can be done about it?" With respect to the first question, this state of affairs has usually been seen as another failure of deinstitutionalization (Chaimowitz 2012). Like homelessness, the incarceration of the mentally disordered has been linked to the larger numbers of these persons now present in the community because of psychiatric hospital downsizing and to the fact that community treatment and support services are insufficient and/or unresponsive. The phenomenon has in fact been given a name, "criminalization," which refers to the hypothesis that troublesome behaviour on the part of mentally disordered persons that would presumably have been dealt with previously by the mental health system – usually by hospital detention – is now, post-deinstitutionalization, being dealt with by the criminal justice system. What kind of "troublesome behaviours" are we talking about? As Canadian forensic psychologist Stephen Hart (2006, 4) details:

> Symptoms of mental illness increase the risk for a wide range of inter-personal conflict that results in the police being called. In rare instances mental illness causes violent ... behaviour – people act in direct response to symptoms they are experiencing, such as delusions ... often in an attempt to protect themselves from perceived danger. Much more common, however, are situations in which members of the public misinterpret the behaviour ... as aggressive or threatening and call the police for assistance. In many of these cases, the only violation that has been committed ... is a violation of social norms – talking too loudly, self-neglect, incoherent speech, mannerisms and so forth.

One must add to this the possibility that a behaviour such as theft may simply be a rational act taken by someone who is short of food.

While the criminalization hypothesis is supported by the large number of mentally disordered persons seen in correctional settings, this does not rule out the possibility that these numbers have always been high but were previously under-reported. The problem with making historical comparisons is that archival information may be inadequate and incomplete, not to mention the change of diagnostic systems over time. That said, there is at least one piece of systematic research bearing on this subject from an earlier part of the twentieth century: in 1939, a British researcher named Penrose published a paper based on a survey of service utilization data from eighteen European countries, which proposed that the size of psychiatric hospital populations was inversely proportional to prison populations and that a dynamic relationship existed between the two. This thesis is not that far out of line with the conclusion of Torrey and colleagues (2010) that "prisons have become our new mental hospitals" (see above).

Are there any data showing that the proportion of mentally ill persons in jails and prisons is *increasing*, which would also support the criminalization hypothesis? Torrey and colleagues (2010) compared results from two major US studies, one conducted in the mid-1980s in Chicago with a sample of 728 jail inmates, and one conducted about twenty years later in New York and Maryland with a sample size of 822. Prevalence of serious mental illness had increased from 6.4 percent in the earlier study to 16 percent in the later study. While these come from different settings and times, a conclusion that this represents a notable increase is strengthened by the studies' sample size and methodological rigour. What about Canada? Data from the federal prison system in our country also appear to show a significant increase in mentally disordered inmates in recent years. A report from Public Safety Canada (2008) found that, for the period 1998 to 2008, there was a steady increase in the proportion of inmates at admission (1) with a psychiatric diagnosis and (2) on psychiatric medication. While it is possible that these figures could reflect better screening and more widespread use of psychiatric medication in the general public, it is nevertheless significant that, in his annual report, Canada's Correctional Investigator (2009, 12) stated that "the plight of offenders with mental disorders in prisons has become a major focus and priority of my Office."

In evaluating the criminalization hypothesis, a considerable amount of attention has been given to the role of the police since they represent the key "entry point" to the criminal justice system and since they can exercise a degree of discretion in how they respond to community disturbances involving persons who are apparently mentally disordered (Teplin and Pruett 1992). It is to this subject that we now turn our attention.

The Role of the Police

Police involvement with mentally disordered persons is, by all accounts, a relatively frequent occurrence. Indeed, research on this subject has found that the mentally ill are more likely than the general population to have contact with the police through street checks and complaints from the public (Brink et al. 2011; Crocker, Hartford, and Heslop 2009). A comprehensive literature review of publications written in English determined that two in five people with mental illness have been arrested in their lifetime and that about 5 percent of police dispatches or encounters involve people with mental health problems (Brink et al. 2011). Individual studies have found numbers considerably higher than the 5 percent figure. For example, in 2008 the Vancouver Police Department undertook a survey, based on calls received over a sixteen-day period, to determine the proportion of responses for which it was believed "that the mental health of an involved person was a factor in police attendance" (Wilson-Bates 2008, 1). Out of 1,154 calls, it was found that 31 percent involved at least one mentally ill person (averaging to over twenty-two calls a day) and, further, that, in some areas of the city, this figure approached 50 percent.[1]

The police may also be the "entry point" into the mental health system for persons experiencing their first mental health crisis: interviews of 107 clients and family members by the Canadian Mental Health Association (1998) found that in 30 percent of cases an initial psychiatric admission involved being brought to hospital by the police, making that experience even more traumatic (this figure is similar to that found in studies from other jurisdictions [Brink et al. 2011]). A survey of 244 mental health clients in BC found that 66 percent – two in three – had experienced a mental health crisis resulting in police contact at some point in their lives (Brink et al. 2011).

Concerning police decision making, it can said that, generally, depending on contingencies, police officers may take no action, may informally intervene (such as removing a person from the scene), may attempt to use another resource (such as taking a person on a voluntary basis to a shelter, hospital, or detox), or may invoke statutory powers, either under mental health legislation (which authorizes initiating involuntary hospitalization) or under the Criminal Code (whereby the person is arrested). Police discretion is limited by the nature of the disturbance, with more serious incidents being more likely to lead to arrest. So how is police discretion used in the case of mentally disordered persons?

Dating back to the 1960s – the early stages of post-deinstitutionalization – a number of American studies found that persons with mental disorders were being arrested at a higher rate than members of the general public (Mulvey, Blumstein, and Cohen 1986). The interpretation of this, however, was unclear. Did it mean, for example, that "dangerous" ex-hospital patients were now running amok in the community? To better examine the police decision-making process, American sociologist Linda Teplin and colleagues conducted a number of participant-observation studies in the 1980s, which involved "ride-alongs" with Chicago police officers (Teplin 1984; Teplin and Pruett 1992). Based on a large number of documented encounters with persons who were apparently mentally disordered, Teplin (1984, 794) concluded that these individuals were "indeed being criminalized" – that is, that all things being equal (the seriousness of the charges being constant) they were more likely to be arrested than members of the general public. Why was this happening? Teplin found that the mentally disordered subjects were not committing more serious offences but that other factors were in operation. In some cases, the mental disorder was not recognized by the police. Second, there was the "visibility factor" – that is, the disturbance was public, or the persons in question lacked social skills and might have been disrespectful, or they were more easily caught, or the behaviours/symptoms were disconcerting to other citizens, resulting in demands (implicit or explicit) that the police officer "do something." (The visibility of these incidents is made more likely by the fact that mental health clients are disproportionately homeless.) Finally, and most significant, other options were blocked for bureaucratic reasons. For example, in the case of someone with a drug addiction and a mental disorder, police would find that a detox centre refused to admit the individual because of symptoms of psychosis. Hospital admission, which one might think would be the most appropriate intervention, was relatively unavailable because of a shortage of beds, because the involuntary admission criteria were (or were interpreted to be) very narrow, and, in general, because of the "red tape" and amount of time needed to attempt this intervention. Teplin (1984) found that the police officers were all too familiar with the statutory criteria for hospital admission, thus persons ended up being arrested "by default."

More recent data show a persistence of higher arrest rates among the mentally ill. A large-scale study in Massachusetts found users of a public mental health program to have significantly higher numbers of arrests compared to members of the general public, matching for age and gender (Fisher et al. 2011), although the categories showing the largest differences were "misdemeanor crimes against persons and property and ... crimes against public decency" (67). The literature review by Brink and colleagues (2011, 6) concluded that "overall, people with mental illness who are suspected of committing a criminal offence are more likely to be arrested compared with those without mental illness."

In Canada, data from police records and other published studies have also found that the police have a higher rate of contact with mentally disordered persons than with the general public (Brink et al. 2011; Hoch et al. 2009; Wilson-Bates 2008). For example, a survey involving 304 participants in Vancouver found 24 percent, almost one in four, reporting twenty-five or more contacts with the police in their lifetime (Brink et al. 2011). A study in London, Ontario, took a more detailed look at this phenomenon and at what happened to persons after the initial police contact (Hoch et al. 2009). In this study the authors reviewed police data for one calendar year and compared dispositions for persons considered to be, and not considered to be, mentally ill (the reader is warned that the data analysis is somewhat complex). They found the mentally ill group was *more* likely to be arrested but not charged and *less* likely to be charged but not arrested. What does this mean? Since an arrest is the physical apprehension and removal of an individual, the priority of the police was apparently to "do something" and remove the perpetrator from the scene but not necessarily to pursue criminal charges at court. According to the authors, the disproportionate use of arrests with the mentally ill "may indicate a lack of options available to the police when citizens file complaints," that "the officers may have exhausted other options, such as attempting to access hospitalization or support services,[2] and may arrest and hold the person in custody to prevent the reoccurrence or continuation of an offending behaviour such as trespassing" (Hoch et al. 2009, 60; see also Howell 2007).[3] In short, these findings are similar to those reached earlier by Teplin in Chicago. It could be argued that, if charges are not pursued, the person is not really being "criminalized," which is probably small consolation to people being repeatedly approached by the police. But in fact the London study found that, when charges *were* pursued, mentally ill individuals were convicted and also jailed at a higher rate, a result that apparently could not be accounted for by differences in the type of offences. The data sources did not allow the authors to explain this finding, although it may have been related to a lack of community resources and poorer representation: Hart (2006, 4) notes that "people with mental illnesses are more likely to have problems getting good legal representation – especially given cutbacks in legal aid – and more likely to be convicted ... [M]ental illness can make it difficult to get a fair trial."

Criminal Record Checks

One unfortunate fact relating to police involvement with mentally ill persons concerns the way that information may be recorded and used later. As we know, sometimes persons may be taken involuntarily to hospital by the police. While not charged with a crime, they may nonetheless be flagged for future reference as having had involvement with the police, which may then turn up as a positive criminal record check when that person is applying for a job or dealing with border officials while entering another country (Teotonio 2011). Even though the reference may be to a different category of involvement than "charged with a crime," it may nonetheless be highly stigmatizing and damaging, for example in the case of a prior attempted suicide that becomes known to a potential employer. Some police forces have adopted policies to prevent the release of this sort of information, such as Saskatchewan in 2009 and Ontario in 2011 (with the Ontario Association of Chiefs of Police issuing guidelines requesting that non-criminal contact with police not subsequently appear during police record checks).[4] In its

2012 strategy document, the Mental Health Commission of Canada included as one of its "recommendations for action" that disclosure in police record checks of apprehension under mental health acts should be stopped.

Police Use of Force

Concerning interactions with the police, an area of great concern is the use of force – sometimes deadly force – with mentally disordered persons, who are overrepresented in these kinds of incidents (Brink 2011). For example, according to one published report, at least six mentally disordered persons (all with psychiatric histories, at least three with diagnoses of schizophrenia) were shot by Vancouver-area police from 1996 to 2000, four of them fatally (Wittek 2001). Another report identifies thirteen such incidents across Canada between 1992 and 2002 (Bryan 2004). In some of these cases police officers were faulted, with witnesses arguing that lethal force was unwarranted given the proximity of the parties to one another, the lack of imminent threat, and the availability of alternatives (such as mental health personnel, who were present but ordered to back off).

How do these unfortunate situations occur? For one thing, symptoms of mania and psychosis impair the affected person's ability to perceive, process, and respond appropriately to commands from law enforcement personnel. To the police officer, manifestations of mental illness may appear more dramatic and threatening, and, in such situations, officers may feel they have little choice given the apparent unpredictability of the individual, especially if that person is wielding a weapon.

Concerning the police officer's "hand being forced," it is hypothesized that the victims in some of these situations are deliberately provoking the response, a phenomenon referred to as "suicide by cop." Support for this claim comes from research conducted by Richard Parent (1996), a former Vancouver-area police officer who went back to university to complete a master's thesis. Parent reviewed fifty-eight incidents, spanning the period from 1980 to 1994, in which BC police officers were confronted by a "potentially lethal threat." Of the twenty-eight cases in which officers shot and killed the persons confronting them, Parent concluded that roughly 50 percent could be considered "victim-precipitated homicide." Parent later expanded his research in a PhD dissertation, analyzing 409 police shootings across Canada between 1980 and 2002 and 434 others in the United States during this same period. He concluded that 273 of these incidents – roughly one-third – could be considered victim-precipitated (Bisetty 2004; Parent 2004). One problem is that a characterization of "suicide by cop" does not appear to distinguish persons acting on the basis of a mental illness from persons who are in a highly agitated state of mind but who may not otherwise be considered mentally ill.

Regarding use of force, police use of the *Taser* has given rise to considerable controversy across Canada in recent years. The Taser is a device that immobilizes suspects with a jolt of electricity and was introduced specifically as a "non-lethal" alternative for dealing with mentally unstable persons. However, a number of deaths in Canada in Taser-related incidents have forced authorities to review policies and practices concerning this technology. In a five-week period in the fall of 2007, three persons died after being tasered by police, in Nova Scotia, Montreal, and Vancouver. The latter incident, involving the death of Polish immigrant Robert Dziekanski, was videotaped by a witness at the Vancouver airport, and the media airing of the video helped fuel a firestorm of criticism, including formal protests from the Polish government. Much of the criticism had to do with the view that police resorted to the Taser too quickly, and that the victim, agitated but unarmed, could have been talked down using basic non-violent crisis intervention techniques (Pablo 2007). The incident in Nova Scotia occurred when Howard Hyde was being booked into jail in Dartmouth. A struggle ensued, the suspect was tasered, then later died in hospital. A spokesman for the manufacturer argued that too much time had elapsed to attribute the cause of death to the Taser, but Hyde's death was especially poignant given that he suffered from schizophrenia, and this incident was seen by some as another example of the mentally ill being victimized in the criminal justice system (Mandel and Meaney 2007). A similar incident occurred in 2010 in Collingwood, Ontario, when Aron Firman, a twenty-seven-year-old man diagnosed with schizophrenia, never regained consciousness and died after being tasered by provincial police. What was interesting about this case was that the investigating pathologist, while acknowledging that there may have been other contributing factors, said for the record that the taser was "the most immediate factor" in the death (Mehta 2013).

Following these high-profile incidents, and subsequent reviews, it is noteworthy that Taser use by the RCMP declined in almost all Canadian jurisdictions, dropping by more than half from 2008 to 2009 (Ling 2010).[5] However, data from the RCMP also found that "mental health cases" were more likely to result in the deployment of the Taser once it was drawn – in almost 50 percent of cases, compared to 39 percent of "non-mental health" situations, which could include robbery, assault, or domestic dispute (Ling 2010). This result is worrying but is perhaps understandable if one assumes that the "mental health cases" represent persons who are less accessible. Interestingly, in the context of police use-of-force, a term has now been coined – "excited delirium" – to describe persons who are "combative and irrational" (Doskoch 2007). The term is controversial, not widely endorsed by the medical community (despite sounding "clinical"), and, according to one Canadian expert, is being used by the manufacturers of Tasers as an excuse for the over-utilization of that technology (Hall 2008). Despite the pendulum apparently swinging away from Taser use, a jury in a 2010 coroner's inquest into the death of a mentally ill man still endorsed them as a viable response to agitated mentally disordered persons (Olivier 2010).

Police Attitudes

Despite the difficult realities of police work, officers are not necessarily unsympathetic when it comes to attitudes towards mentally disordered persons, and, indeed, there are personal accounts written by clients that describe compassion on the part of officers who chose not to charge mentally disordered persons who had committed crimes such as theft (Sterle 2006). On the issue of police compassion, Ontario psychologist Dorothy Cotton surveyed 150 officers in Ontario and British Columbia using a questionnaire that measured four attitudinal dimensions (authoritarian, socially benevolent, socially restrictive, and oriented towards community integration) as well as their perception of the role of police in working with mentally ill people (Dorrance 2003). When the results were compared with those from the same survey given to the general public, it was found that the police officers were relatively more benevolent and less authoritarian: 80 percent of respondents believed the mentally ill to be "far less dangerous than most people suppose," 94 percent believed society should adopt more tolerant attitudes, and 93 percent believed the mentally ill should not be denied their individual rights. The study's author noted that "most police officers in fact have a great deal of trouble arresting individuals with mental illnesses and are much more interested in linking them to appropriate services" (quoted in Dorrance 2003, 8). An American survey of 382 police officers found that persons diagnosed with schizophrenia, all things being equal, were considered to be "more dangerous" but that – similar to the Canadian study's findings – individuals with this diagnosis were "less responsible for their situation" and "more worthy of help" (Watson, Corrigan, and Ottati 2004, 49).

System Responses

The Canadian Mental Health Association has written a number of documents on the question of police involvement with the mentally ill and on ways the mental health and policing systems could provide a better coordinated response (Canadian Mental Health Association, BC Division, 2003; Hall and Weaver 2008). Barriers to effective interventions identified in these reports include: (1) inadequate advance information – that is, information on mental health concerns not being passed on by dispatchers; (2) inadequate information systems, which could potentially identify mental health clients in advance and provide information about successful prior interventions; and (3) lack of access to consultation from mental health workers at the scene. A 2008 report by the Vancouver Police Department similarly spoke about "a profound absence of information sharing between mental health resources" as contributing to "excessive police interactions" with the mentally ill (Wilson-Bates 2008, 2). While there are legitimate concerns about privacy and stigmatization when one talks about information systems that flag persons as "psychiatric cases," it is interesting to note that a recent Canadian study found a majority of the sixty mental health clients interviewed *supporting* police access to background information "before arriving on the scene" (Brink 2011, 79).

Concerning police response, critics have questioned the adequacy of recruit training in mental health issues (which may be compounded in the field by staff turnover and rotation of assignments) (Olivier 2010). Training has become a contentious issue in some instances, with police spokespersons suggesting that education is in fact adequate (Howell 2007) and that the deficiencies lie elsewhere (i.e., if the mental health system was sufficiently resourced, the problems we have been describing would not arise in the first place). This was definitely the message in a report by the Vancouver Police Department subtitled *How a Lack of Capacity in the Mental Health System Is Failing Vancouver's Mentally Ill and Draining Police Resources* (Wilson-Bates 2008). On the other hand, clients with direct experience have themselves suggested that police training is critical and insufficient: possible topics for training suggested by participants in a Mental Health Commission-sponsored survey included communication, understanding mental illness, compassion and respect, and emphasizing non-violent approaches (Brink et al 2011). These and similar findings led the commission to include improved training of law enforcement personnel as a "recommendation for action" in its 2012 strategy report.

System integration has been successful in the case of crisis teams – police/ mental health partnerships – which exist in several urban settings in Canada. An example is the partnership between the Toronto Police Service and St. Michael's Hospital, piloted in 2000, in which plainclothes police team up with mental health nurses to respond to emergency calls involving mentally disordered persons. This program is designed to "better improve the police's response to dealing with people with emotional disturbances" and to "both reduce costly policing delays and move people with mental illness from the court system into the health care system" (Centre for Addiction and Mental

Health 2001, 2). Concerning partnerships, the Canadian Association of Chiefs of Police sponsors a website (http://www.pmhl.ca/Index.html) whose aim, in part, is to provide resources, reports, and examples for persons planning "joint response initiatives" between mental health and the police.

Diversion

The term "diversion" has been defined different ways, but generally it refers to the suspension of criminal charges and redirection of the individual away from the criminal justice system and towards the mental health system.[6] It can be argued that, rather than convicting and sentencing mentally disordered persons for minor offences, it is more appropriate, humane, and effective to divert these individuals. Indeed, prosecutors in Canada, when considering the approval of police charges, are supposed to consider whether the prosecution will be "in the public interest." Diversion is based on the assumptions that the offending behaviour is a result of the mental disorder (which sometimes may be open to debate) and that the appropriate type of resources to ameliorate this problem are available.

Diversion may occur at different points in the criminal justice process, starting, as we have seen, with the use of police discretion. Often diversion decisions are made post-arrest and pre-trial. Diversion can occur informally,[7] or under the guidelines of specialized court services, a subject discussed in more detail below. In its 2012 strategy document, the Mental Health Commission of Canada included as one of its "recommendations for action" the suggestion that diversion programs, including mental health courts, should be more widely available.

Fitness to Stand Trial

Once a police officer makes the decision to charge and arrest an accused person, that person is taken into custody at a remand centre and subsequently appears before a judge. A key decision to be made early in this sequence is whether the individual, if mentally disordered, is *fit to stand trial* – that is, whether he or she can competently participate in an adversarial criminal proceeding.[8] The accused's lawyer, for example, may point out to the judge that he or she is unable to communicate effectively with the client because that person is psychotic. The judge may then order a fitness assessment, which is usually carried out by a forensic psychiatrist, sometimes at the remand centre and sometimes following a transfer to a forensic facility. To assist persons doing fitness assessments, clinicians have developed structured guidelines, such as, in Canada, the Fitness Interview Test (Viljoen, Roesch, and Zapf 2002).

Studies of this process have found that most accused persons are found fit following the assessment (e.g., Davis 1995b; Ohayan et al. 1998), which may seem counter-intuitive and is possibly the result of the courts applying a low standard of fitness since a finding of unfitness results in further delays and deprivation of the accused's liberty. The fitness standard may indeed be lower than the certification standard (the legal criteria used for involuntary psychiatric hospitalization), and this author has seen cases in which a mentally ill person is certified but still found fit for court. Some have observed that the fitness threshold may be too low and judicial decisions too idiosyncratic, despite the criteria available in the Criminal Code. For example, interviews conducted by this author as part of a research project on the fitness process turned up the following quotation from a forensic psychiatrist: "Different judges can have much broader or narrower conceptualizations of fitness. I've been in court when the accused is so psychotic he doesn't even know where he is, let alone what the 'role of the prosecutor is,' and yet the judge will declare him fit" (Davis 1994, 115). This speaks to the possibility that an accused person's impaired mental state may be underestimated – or not recognized at all – during the remand process. One of the reasons for this is that provincial courts in larger urban centres deal with a huge volume of cases, meaning that persons with serious mental disorders may simply get swept along with the mass of other unfortunates entering the criminal justice system – which speaks to the need for adequate screening for mental disorder at the point of remand.

Bail and Probation

Persons found fit are, in most cases, released with bail conditions, requiring them to report to a bail supervisor and to return for further court appearances. This can be a problem for some mentally disordered persons: disorganization and cognitive impairment caused by the disorder, and a lack of community supports, may mean that he or she fails to make these appointments, which may lead to further charges since "failure to appear" is itself an offence (see Skeem and Louden 2006).

Persons on probation (a sentencing option for individuals convicted of an offence) face other difficulties: as with persons on bail, individuals who are more disabled may fail to make appointments or have a more difficult time following conditions such as geographical restrictions. Some persons given probation may be ordered to receive psychiatric treatment as a condition of their probation order, which in most cases means that they will be seen within the forensic psychiatric system. Non-forensic mental health services have historically been reluctant to accept these sorts of cases

(1) because they are a "voluntary" service (although, with the increasing use of community treatment orders, this is a debatable assertion) and (2) because of discomfort in dealing with clients who carry the "criminal" or "offender" label. As an editorial in the *Canadian Journal of Psychiatry* notes: "Most psychiatrists, like most physicians ... prefer not to deal with the often unpleasant characters with which forensic psychiatrists inevitably must deal" (Hucker 1998, 456). In this way mental health programs make a distinction between the "mad" and the "bad," with the latter group sometimes being turned away, despite being diagnosed with serious mental disorders. One of the problems with this response is that it becomes a self-fulfilling prophecy: the denial of services to "mentally disordered offenders" (as they are referred to in the forensic literature) may mean further deterioration of their mental state, resulting in more charges and subsequent reinforcement of the "bad" label.

Skeem and Louden (2006) note that mentally ill persons on probation or parole are twice as likely to fail on supervision – to be pulled back to court for a technical violation or new offence. From their literature review they point to five aspects of supervision programs that may lead to better outcomes with mentally ill clients, based on a "small but growing body of research" (333) that includes some randomized controlled trials. These are (1) exclusive mental health caseloads, (2) smaller caseloads, (3) sustained staff training, (4) integration of service provision (i.e., probation officers working closely with other care providers), and (5) use of "problem-solving strategies" (i.e., meaningfully engaging with clients to explore their problems rather than simply laying down the law). Their conclusion was that specialized supervision programs with these characteristics were more effective at linking clients with treatment services, improving their well-being, and reducing risk of probation violation.

Court Programs

Apart from informal diversion, reliant upon prosecutorial and judicial discretion, two related court-based approaches have been developed with respect to mentally ill persons charged with a crime: (1) formal diversion programs administered through the courts and (2) mental health courts that are exclusively mandated to work with this population (Canadian Institute for Health Information 2008a). Mental health courts are a largely American phenomenon, and, as reviewed by Watson and colleagues (2001), their development was influenced by the earlier establishment of drug courts in that country, a therapeutic jurisprudence model that identified substance misuse as a public health (not simply criminal justice) problem and that emphasized immediate intervention, a non-adversarial process, a team approach, and having clear rules and goals.[9] Therapeutic jurisprudence conveys the idea that "the law has therapeutic qualities and, if properly administered, [can] be used as a therapeutic agent to improve the lives of mentally disordered accused" (Schneider, Bloom, and Heerema 2007, 43). In Canada, drug courts operate in six cities: Toronto (the first, in 1998), Vancouver, Edmonton, Winnipeg, Ottawa, and Regina.

In Canada, the only full-time mental health court, opened in 1998, is in Toronto. Mental health court programs exist in other cities, such as Sudbury, Ontario, and Saint John, New Brunswick (Canadian Institute for Health Information 2008b). Objectives of these programs include:

- diversion away from the criminal justice system;
- expedition of the assessment of the accused person's fitness to stand trial;
- treatment of the mental disorder;
- reduction of recidivism (re-offending) among this population (Canadian Institute for Health Information 2008a).

Evaluations (mostly American) of mental health court programs, while limited in number and quality, have generally found them (1) to be effective in linking program participants to treatment and services and (2) to have achieved a high degree of self-reported satisfaction among participants (Schneider, Bloom, and Heerema 2007). In summarizing the evaluation literature, Schneider, Bloom, and Heerema (2007, 192) refer to perceived "high levels of fairness, low levels of coercion, and increased confidence in the administration of justice." A more recent study by Hiday and Ray (2010) found a significant reduction in recidivism among persons enrolled in the court program, although the study did not use a randomized controlled design. In Canada, an evaluation of the program in Saint John similarly found a benefit with respect to connecting clients with treatment services (Canadian Institute for Health Information 2008a). The study also found that the 76 percent of clients successfully completing the program either had charges dropped or were given non-custodial sentences, whereas those in the control group were, in all cases, convicted and in 64 percent of cases, incarcerated.

Diversion programs run within "regular" courts have been established and formalized in a number of Canadian cities, including Calgary, London, and Thunder Bay. These programs typically include appointment of counsel, mental health assessment, consultation with victims, and a review of the charges. Suspension of the charges is contingent on the client's agreeing to enter treatment (Canadian Institute for Health Information 2008a). The

Thunder Bay program, a partnership formed in 1994 between the Ministry of the Attorney General and the Canadian Mental Health Association, is "designed to give a more suitable response to mentally disordered offenders, both adults and young offenders, who find themselves in conflict with the criminal justice system because of their mental illness ... [and] to gain the necessary treatment and support they need to prevent future criminal activity" (Canadian Mental Health Association, Thunder Bay Branch 2001). Diversion is decided by the judge on a case-by-case basis, with diverted persons being referred either to a hospital, to a mental health professional, or to the Canadian Mental Health Association to seek treatment. A well-articulated example of a diversion program is the Provincial Diversion Program of Alberta (see website at http://www.amhb.ab.ca/Publications/reports/provincialDiversion/Pages/default.aspx). As described in one of their documents, eligibility for the program depends on (1) the nature of the incident, with low-risk, minor offences given priority; (2) the situation of the individual, which includes motivation to change; and (3) community resources – both formal and informal – which must be sufficient to support the accused person (Provincial Diversion Program Working Committee 2003). This program, successfully piloted in Calgary, is being expanded to other centres.

Evaluations of court diversion programs in Canada, while limited in number, have shown some promising results. Research on the Calgary program, referred to above, found a decrease in complaints, charges, court appearances, time at hospital, and per-client costs (Canadian Institute for Health Information 2008a). An evaluation of two programs in southwestern Ontario found that recidivism – defined as a re-arrest for any charge within the year following the initiation of the diversion agreement – was low in both locales: 2 to 3 percent, which the authors note compares favourably to rates of comparison groups taken from the literature (Swaminath et al. 2002). Authors of the Ontario study pointed out that the positive results were influenced by selection bias, given that cases were screened out when adequate community support services were unavailable or if the accused person had a more serious criminal record (but this was of course an *intentional* bias coming from the program's eligibility criteria). While the courts have a right and a duty to screen out higher-risk clients from diversion programs, application of overly restrictive eligibility criteria may at the same time result in the exclusion of the very persons that these types of programs were set up for in the first place. As well, the problem of appropriate treatment services not always being available speaks to the importance of community resources since diverted persons, after all, have to be diverted "to" somewhere.

The Forensic System

Mental health clients entering the criminal court process may become involved with the forensic psychiatric system, which provides assessment and treatment mandated by the courts and special provisions in the Criminal Code. Involvement with the forensic system can come about in several different ways:

- Pretrial assessment of an accused person can be requested to determine that person's fitness to stand trial, referring to his or her mental state while at court, or to determine criminal responsibility, referring to the mental state of the accused at the time of the offence and whether mental disorder negated the *mens rea* (the "guilty mind," or criminal intent) required to secure a conviction. In most cases these assessments are undertaken by psychiatrists with a forensic specialty. Assessments may be conducted at a remand centre, at a secure forensic hospital, or on an outpatient basis.
- Persons who are deemed either unfit to stand trial or not criminally responsible on account of mental disorder (NCRMD) may be detained in custody or given a conditional discharge, as determined by a board of review (or in some cases by the Court itself). In these cases, ongoing treatment and supervision of the review board order is provided by forensic practitioners, either in secure hospitals or in outpatient clinics in cases of conditional discharge. Persons found NCRMD and initially held in custody will in most cases graduate to conditional and then absolute discharge status. Persons found unfit to stand trial will return to court once deemed fit. The conditions attached to conditional discharges are in some respects similar to probation conditions, with references, for example, to abstention from alcohol, having no contact with certain individuals, and "no-gos" to certain areas, in addition to the requirement that the accused accept treatment as directed. Applications for discharge are made at review board hearings, when there are submissions from both the accused's representatives and forensic clinical staff.[10]
- In some cases persons may be required to report for psychiatric treatment as a condition of bail or probation, which is usually provided at a forensic psychiatric outpatient clinic. Enforcement of these orders can be a cumbersome process: if a client "breaches" an order by not showing up for treatment, no immediate action is necessarily taken; rather, the individual may be required to make another court appearance at some future date.
- Forensic clinicians may also become involved in the criminal process at the point of sentencing. After a defendant is convicted, the Court may ask for a pre-sentence report, wherein material is gathered and opinions

offered on the likelihood of reoffending – in particular under which conditions – and on the question of treatability. This typically happens in cases in which there has been repetitive violent behaviour and in particular sexual offending.[11] (It should be pointed out that, while conditions such as pedophilia are included in the American Psychiatric Association's *DSM*, sexual deviations are not usually included in the "serious, persistent" category of mental disorders, and there is considerable debate among practitioners as to whether they should be considered mental disorders at all.) Whether mental health practitioners should be in the business of predicting future violence is a very controversial issue, with opponents arguing that accurate prediction is impossible and that attempting to engage in it is therefore unethical. A counter-argument is that, like it or not, practitioners are, on a routine basis, forced to make risk assessments and that, in the forensic context, this process can be improved by the application of structured guidelines that incorporate clinical, actuarial, and environmental factors (Monahan 2003).

- Treatment for sex offenders is provided by forensic clinicians, either at correctional facilities or on an outpatient basis. A range of therapeutic approaches may be tried, including (1) drugs that reduce testosterone levels; (2) behavioural techniques such as aversion therapy, covert sensitization, and masturbatory satiation; (3) cognitive techniques that look at the rationalizations that support deviant behaviour; (4) social skills training, which may include anger management and sex education; and (5) relapse prevention, a process that attempts to interrupt the "crime cycle" by identifying behavioural precursors to sexual offending. For a description of a Canadian comprehensive treatment program, see the report by the John Howard Society of Alberta (2002).

Some built-in limitations arise with court-ordered treatment. To begin with, there is the fact that the client-practitioner relationship in this situation is by definition involuntary and may be perceived as more adversarial given that the "control agent" function is emphasized and that clinicians report to the courts, probation officers, and review boards. Of course, non-forensic practitioners may also have an involuntary relationship with clients, and in either case there is the potential for a skilful, compassionate clinician to make therapeutic gains. Court-ordered treatment is also time-limited, meaning that investment and commitment, on the part of either client or practitioner, can be compromised. As well, court orders are a clumsy, cumbersome means of enforcing treatment given the postponements and delays endemic to the court system and the unfamiliarity of court officers with mental health issues. Finally, because of mandate, philosophy, or fiscal restraint, forensic psychiatric services tend to be more narrowly focused and may not have the important ancillary and rehabilitation services offered in other mental health programs.

Forensic psychiatric programs have historically been separate from other mental health services with respect to location, governance, and organizational culture, although with the move to regionalization in Canada some forensic programs have come under the umbrella of local health authorities. As with mental health and addictions, an argument can be made for better integration of forensic and non-forensic programs, bearing in mind that this is complicated by different legal mandates, with forensic staff dealing with orders from the courts and review boards that operate under the Criminal Code. There is room for improvement with respect to linkages between forensic/correctional and non-forensic programs, particularly how clients leaving forensic treatment are received by the other system given the tendency to discriminate between the "bad" and the "mad." There is no necessary reason for mentally ill persons under probation orders to only be seen in the forensic system. Non-forensic clinicians may assume, incorrectly, that forensic staff have "special techniques" for working with, for example, a person with schizophrenia who gets into conflict with the law, when in fact the clinical approaches are much the same. It may be that comfort level is the main characteristic that distinguishes staff from the two programs.

Notes

1 This survey has been criticized on methodological grounds in that there were no independent raters or databases used to confirm the presence of mental illness in persons encountered (see Brink et al. 2011). Concerning the ability of the police to determine the presence of mental illness, the report states that, in these cases, "the symptoms [were] readily apparent and would likely be obvious to any layperson," although it might be noted, inter alia, that a drug-induced psychosis is indistinguishable from a "true" psychosis. There was a perception that the police had an axe to grind, given (for example) that the report was subtitled "How a Lack of Capacity in the Mental Health System Is Failing Vancouver's Mentally Ill and Draining Police Resources."

2 Readers should note that, while police have the legal authority to take mentally ill persons to a hospital, *admission* to the facility still requires the consent of the receiving doctor. Also, in some Canadian jurisdictions the statutory criteria for police apprehension are narrower – with references to "danger," for example – than those applying to physician certifications. Indeed, on this second point, this author has encountered situations involving the police and the possible transport of a client to hospital in which the officers in question were nervous about overstepping their authority.

3 Concerning access to hospital, a report by the Vancouver Police Department expressed frustration about the police being tied up for, on average, an hour and a quarter at local hospitals before a handover of the mentally ill person could be made (Thompson 2010).

4 See the OACP guidelines at: http://www.mentalhealthpolicerecords.ca/docs/guides/OACP_Guideline.pdf.

5 In 2012, a legislative committee was told by a senior RCMP official that officers of that force were "scared to use their Tasers because of public criticism" (Shaw 2012).

6 Some have defined the term more broadly, to include dispositions that address treatment even if the person is convicted (e.g., specialized probation and in-custody programs).

7 In British Columbia, persons charged with minor offences, detained, and subsequently certified under the Mental Health Act were, until the 1980s, in many cases channelled directly from the pretrial centre to the provincial psychiatric hospital, all of which ended because of policy changes and, more specifically, the downsizing and closure of many of the wards at that facility. There are problems, however, when diversion occurs informally – that is, without explicit guidelines and protocols. For example, is the consent/non-consent of the accused person taken into account? Also, without guidelines, diversion decisions may be idiosyncratic and biased.

8 The adversarial basis of the Anglo-American system may be contrasted with the "inquisitorial" approach used in some European countries, wherein the judge takes a more activist role. Interestingly, this approach is now taken in specialized mental health courts in North America.

9 Drug courts have been opened in Toronto and Vancouver, with an evaluation of the Vancouver program finding that participants had greater reductions in offending than a matched comparison group (Somers et al. 2011).

10 Historically, persons found "not guilty by reason of insanity" could expect to be detained in-custody for lengthy periods, so defence lawyers in Canada tended to avoid this plea, except in the case of very serious charges (often murder). This changed following a series of court decisions and Criminal Code amendments in the 1990s so that there was an onus on review boards to come up with "least restrictive" dispositions and for persons found NCRMD to be granted absolute discharges unless there was evidence that the individual was a "significant threat" to public safety (Verdun-Jones 2000). However, the picture changed again in 2013 when the federal government introduced legislation that shifted the emphasis away from "least restrictive" dispositions toward public safety as the paramount consideration (see Chapter 18).

11 The Canadian Criminal Code contains "dangerous offender" provisions, referring to persons who have committed a "serious personal injury offence" – in practice, usually a sexual offence. The application of these provisions must be supported by psychiatric testimony, and convicted persons given this special status may be detained in custody indefinitely.

Assessment and Diagnosis

An assessment provides the basis for a *planned* intervention, whether the intervention is medical or involves some other life domain. Practitioners can get locked into a routine so should be mindful about the importance of planning and *re*-assessing what they are doing with clients, given that needs and goals will change over time. While assessment is a structured process, it is not simply a mechanical recitation but, rather, one that is dependent on the assessor's ability to skilfully conduct an interview and, in particular, to be empathetic and engender trust. This chapter looks at different aspects of assessment and concludes with an introduction to diagnostic systems, in particular, the *DSM* – the *Diagnostic and Statistical Manual* of the American Psychiatric Association – which is used in almost all mental health settings in Canada.

Clinical Assessment

The clinical assessment is a multifaceted, ongoing process, one that involves interviews, gathering collateral information, and sometimes using scales and self-report instruments. Without collateral and historical information, a psychiatric diagnosis based on a single interview is necessarily tentative.

While sometimes seen as separate parts of the therapeutic endeavour, assessment and treatment can in fact inform each other and be conceptualized as one process (Mental Health Evaluation and Community Consultation Unit 2002). In particular, since the early phase of any intervention often involves the client's describing and setting goals, the assessment is an opportunity to engage the individual and motivate him or her to participate in the recovery process (Kopelowicz and Liberman 2003).

An initial assessment usually begins with the "chief complaint" or presenting problem (e.g., "So, what brings you here?"). Even if the client's version of events does not coincide with other sources, the practitioner should be respectful and serious in considering this information. The assessor may then ask about personal and family history, and previous encounters with the psychiatric system (not always possible in one session and usually involves material from elsewhere). Assessors need to be alert to the possibility of past or current physical/sexual/emotional abuse or neglect, and also of substance misuse, all of these known to be present at higher rates among mental health clients and to have considerable significance for treatment planning. An initial assessment may occur at a time of crisis for the client, so assessors must be tuned to the possibility of suicidal thoughts or intentions (more on this below).

Mental Status Exam

As part of the assessment procedure, and as a way of getting a snapshot of someone at a point in time, assessors routinely perform what is called a mental status exam (MSE). This may be done in full in an initial assessment, but can also be done on an "as needed" basis, particularly in times of crisis or distress. Thoughts and behaviours identified in the MSE are not necessarily syndrome-specific but do provide important clues. Components of the MSE are as follows:

- APPEARANCE: This can refer to dress, grooming, alertness, and facial expression.
- BEHAVIOUR: This can refer to eye contact, movements, and psychomotor activity.
- SPEECH: Assessors often look for rate of speech (e.g., is it so rapid it is "pressured?"). There may also be poverty of speech, or a delay in response called "latency." Latency may be seen in persons with schizophrenia, when their line of thinking gets sidetracked.
- MOOD: *Type*: euthymic (mood not excessively high or low); dysphoric (depressed, irritable, angry); euphoric (elevated, elated); anxious. Euphoria may be associated with mania. *Range*: full (normal) versus restricted, blunted, or flat. Persons with schizophrenia may suffer from flat, blunted, or restricted affect, which can be referred to as the "negative" symptoms of the disorder. *Congruency:* Does the mood match the situation, or topic – that is, is the person's mood congruent or mood incongruent? *Lability:* A "labile" person swings abruptly from low to high mood or vice-versa.
- THOUGHT CONTENT: This refers to evidence of delusions, obsessions/compulsions, phobias, and suicidal or homicidal intentions. Delusions may take many forms, including beliefs about persecution, special signs or omens, special powers or abilities, or thoughts that the individual is being controlled by external forces. Beliefs that do not apparently reach the threshold of delusion may be referred to as over-valued ideas.[1]

- THOUGHT FORM: This refers to the rate of thoughts, how they flow and are connected. "Normal" would tend to be tight, logical, and linear, coherent and goal directed, whereas abnormal would mean that associations between thoughts are not clear, organized, or coherent. Examples of thought form disorder include circumstantiality (taking a long time and many detours before getting to the point), tangentiality (moving away from, and never getting to, the point), echolalia (repetition of other people's words or phrases), loosening of associations (no logical connection between parts of speech), thought blocking, neologisms (creation of new words), flight of ideas, and "word salad."
- PERCEPTIONS: This refers to hallucinations, which may be auditory, visual, or olfactory, and to other disturbances, such as heightened perception and depersonalization (e.g., feeling as if one is in a dream).
- COGNITION: This refers to attention, concentration, memory, and ability to think abstractly (versus concretely). Clients are typically rated on their orientation to time (what year, month, day is it?), place, and person (usually referring to individuals in the immediate proximity, such as family members). There may be assessment of memory, both short-term (e.g., by having the client repeat three words given earlier in the interview) and long-term (by seeing if recollection of childhood events is consistent with other sources of information). Concentration may be assessed by asking the person to subtract serial sevens from one hundred. Cognitive deficits are often assessed with a tool called the "mini-mental status exam," more commonly given to older clients who are suspected to have dementia.
- INSIGHT/JUDGMENT: "Judgment" has been defined as the ability to anticipate the consequences of one's behaviour and to make decisions to safeguard one's well-being and that of others. "Insight" is a somewhat controversial term since it is based on the client's not agreeing with the professional, and it is defined as not having an awareness of one's illness or one's situation. In practice someone with "no insight" does not agree that she or he has a psychiatric disorder or that there is anything wrong with her/ him (and thus that she/he does not need medication, for example).

Rating Scales and Other Structured Instruments

A practice document suggests that, during assessments, "semistructured interviews and the use of standardized clinical rating scales are recommended, since they increase diagnostic reliability, ensure consistent coverage, quantify symptom severity, permit later comparisons, and are useful for program evaluation" (Mental Health Evaluation and Community Consultation Unit 2002, 6). In considering the use of these instruments, the following should be noted: first, scales are created for different purposes and are not necessarily designed for assessment or clinical applications. Some, such as the Brief Psychiatric Rating Scale and the Positive and Negative Syndrome Scale (PANSS), are more commonly used in research, in which reliability and comparability of results is the foremost concern. An example of a scale used for diagnostic purposes is the Structured Clinical Interview for Axis I *DSM*-IV Disorders (SCID) (see First et al. 2002). Second, some scales have been thoroughly evaluated for validity and reliability, while others have not. Third, some scales are in the public domain, while use of others may require permission of the copyright holder. And fourth, some scales require trained raters, some do not; and some are self-reports.

A large number of scales and structured instruments have been developed that can be applied in community mental health settings, and it is impossible to list them all here (the interested reader may refer to published compendia and evaluations [e.g., Baer and Blais 2010; Ehmann and Hanson 2004a; Health Canada 2001a; Ralph 2009]). Scales have been developed for each of the major categories of mental disorder as well as for clients with drug or alcohol addiction. These tools can be helpful as a screening device, used to "flag" issues that can then be explored in more depth.

Health authorities may use clinical outcome scales that are mandated by provincial funding bodies as a means to greater accountability. An example of one of these is the HoNOS (Health of the Nation Outcome Scales), developed in the UK as a means to track the health and social functioning of persons with serious mental disorders and now being used in Canada (Kisely et al. 2008a). The client is rated from zero (no problem) to four (severe problem) on twelve scale items, which include aggression, self-injury, substance misuse, psychosis, depression, and interpersonal difficulties (see http://www.gpcare.org/outcome%20measures/HONOS.html). The measure is cross-sectional, applying to the time period immediately prior to the assessment, and is given at least every six months. The instrument is copyrighted.

Rating scales are often used by practitioners working with older clients to test and track cognitive impairment and dementia over time (Lorentz, Scanlan, and Borson 2002). One test commonly used with clients when dementia is suspected is the Mini-Mental Status Exam (MMSE), scored out of thirty, which provides a quick assessment of orientation, attention, recall, and use of language. A longer version of this test is the Modified Mini-Mental Status Exam (3MS), which is scored out of one hundred. Evaluations of the MMSE have found it useful as a screening tool to rule out dementia in community and primary care populations but that other tests may offer greater sensitivity in specialist (psycho-geriatric) settings (Ismael, Rajji, and Shulman 2009; Mitchell and Malladi 2010; Molloy, Standish, and Lewis 2005). While tests of cognition have typically been used with possible cases of dementia, interest in recent years in remediating the cognitive deficits seen in younger adults with schizophrenia (e.g. Wykes et al. 2011) means that there may be wider application of neuro-cognitive tests in community settings.

Suicide Assessment

Persons suffering from serious mental disorders – notably schizophrenia, depression, and borderline personality disorder – are more likely to experience suicidal thinking and to attempt and complete suicide than members of the general population (Centre for Applied Research in Mental Health and Addiction 2007b; Edwards et al. 2008; Heisel 2006; Johnson 2011; Mamo 2007; Skodol et al. 2002). For example, a study of a large Canadian community mental health program found that, over a three-year period, the forty-three documented completed suicides on the part of clients of the program represented a rate twenty-five times higher than that seen in the general public (Davis 2000). Concerning suicide attempts, data from a 2010 survey of Canadian hospitals found about seven in ten hospitalizations for self-injury to have been associated with a diagnosis of mental illness (Canadian Institute for Health Information 2011a).

Because their clients are at higher risk, clinicians in community mental health settings need to be able to address the question of suicide and carry out risk assessments, and managers need to consider this a core competency area. Accreditation Canada (2008) standards dictate that mental health programs assess and monitor clients for risk of suicide and gives the following tests for compliance:

- The organization assesses each client for risk of suicide at regular intervals, or as needs change.
- The organization identifies clients at risk of suicide.
- The organization addresses the clients immediate safety needs.
- The organization identifies treatment and monitoring strategies to ensure client safety.
- The organization documents the treatment and monitoring strategies in the client's health record.

Despite this imperative, there is evidence that practitioner training in this area is inadequate (McNiel et al. 2008). For example, a survey of Canadian mental health practitioners found that while 83 percent used "no suicide agreements", 43 percent had received no formal training in their use (Page and King 2008).

There are a number of myths surrounding suicide, such as the idea that suicidal people do not give warning signs (Centre for Applied Research in Mental Health and Addiction 2007b). Another common misconception, held as well (unfortunately) by some mental health practitioners, is the belief that talking about suicide will "plant the idea in the person's head." In fact, broaching the subject can come as a *relief* to the client, and it shows the worker to be serious and engaged (American Psychiatric Association 2003). One also encounters worries about liability (i.e., the expectation that suicidal events can be predicted), so rather than risk a "false negative" – which makes the worker look bad – it is better to not raise the issue at all. Apart from being irresponsible, this attitude is also misguided. As noted by Bryan and Rudd (2006, 186), "predicting low base-rate phenomena such as suicide with reliability is not possible ... [T]he clinician's task is not to predict suicide, but to recognize when a patient has entered into a heightened state of risk (risk assessment) and to respond appropriately."

How does one assess suicide risk? Briefly, this involves a consideration of *risk factors* and *protective factors*, the latter including coping skills that may be developed with the clinician's help. Some risk factors – such as gender – are "actuarial" and thus cannot be changed. They are known to be predictive of suicide but only in a statistical sense, and while they do not tell you the likelihood of the person in front of you attempting suicide, they should at least be in the back of the clinician's mind. Other factors are more dynamic and fluctuate over time. For structured interview guidelines in suicide risk assessment, see Centre for Applied Research in Mental Health and Addiction (2007b).

The following categorization derives from several sources (American Psychiatric Association 2003; Bryan and Rudd 2006; Canadian Institute for Health Information 2011; Centre for Applied Research in Mental Health and . Addiction 2007b; Davis 2000; Public Health Agency of Canada 2006).

Risk factors
(1) Vulnerable populations: this includes males (re. suicide completion), persons with a mental illness, youth, First Nations people, the elderly, widowers, gay males, and those suffering from a painful, chronic, or terminal physical illness.
(2) Historical factors: previous attempts, history of suicide in the family or among friends, history of abuse or trauma, history of impulsivity, and the proximity of anniversaries of significant events, such as the birthday of a child who was taken away.
(3) Current risk factors:

- acute symptoms of mental illness, such as "command" hallucinations or delusions that support suicide;
- loss of a job, social standing, or relationship (or anticipation of same);
- living alone or in isolation;
- recent death by suicide of another significant person;
- rigid, "black-and-white" thinking, and/or perfectionism;
- recent discharge following a hospitalization for psychiatric reasons;[2]
- use of substances that are depressive or disinhibiting (such as alcohol);
- access to lethal means, including firearms and large quantities of medication.[3]

(4) Current thinking: hopelessness (assess severity and duration); thoughts of suicide that are frequent, persistent, and specific; a concrete plan; lethality of intent.

Protective factors

Generally, "social connectedness [and] a strong sense of competence and optimism in coping with life's problems" (Centre for Applied Research in Mental Health and Addiction 2007b, 29) are protective. Protective factors include:

- social support, including peer support (a sense of belonging);
- children present in the home and/or sense of family responsibility;
- pets;
- skills with respect to coping, problem-solving, and relationships or a history of competence to draw upon;
- optimistic outlook;
- sense of humour;
- religious affiliation;
- access to employee assistance programs;
- a positive therapeutic relationship and active participation in treatment.

Persons assessed as a high risk for suicide may require a structured and protective environment, such as a hospital. Others may be managed at home provided there are caregivers present and accessible crisis response. Intensity of treatment is typically proportional to degree of risk (i.e., higher risk needing more frequent contact). In all cases, workers should develop with clients and significant others a safety plan, which includes emergency contacts, as well as a list of activities that may calm or comfort, and reasons for living.

Sometimes workers will use "no harm" or "no suicide" agreements, a "contract" wherein the client states that he or she will not harm him- or herself, or at least contact someone should she/he feel unable to maintain safety. There is no compelling evidence to support the use of these agreements (Bryan and Rudd 2006). For example, a Canadian survey of mental health personnel found that 31 percent of respondents had had the experience of a client's attempting or completing suicide while an agreement was in place (Page and King 2008). These contracts may be more reassuring to the worker than the client, and in any case suicide specialists do not recommend their use (Centre for Applied Research in Mental Health and Addiction 2007b).

With respect to longer-term clinical involvement, the following are considered important for recovery (Michel et al. 2002):

- a steady therapeutic relationship with (at least initially) frequent contact
- a treatment approach that "works the ambivalence" of the client
- an approach that puts behaviour in historical and biographical context
- the development of coping and problem-solving skills
- the building of a supportive network outside of the mental health program

Violence Risk Assessment

Sometimes mental health professionals may be asked by the courts, or other bodies, to comment specifically on an individual's likelihood of committing future violent acts. This may arise in the case of persons found "not criminally responsible" because of mental disorder (a special Criminal Code verdict) or in pre-sentence reports, which may arise in the context of domestic violence or sexual assault. In these cases the assessors are usually psychiatrists or clinical psychologists with a forensic specialty. Interestingly, Canada has produced a number of internationally recognized experts in the field of violence risk assessment. On this subject interested readers may refer to authors such as Stephen Hart, Robert Hare (creator of the "Psychopathy Checklist"), Vernon Quinsey, and Chris Webster (the last three holding an "emeritus" status).

A risk assessment tool designed for mentally ill persons that has been used quite widely in Canada and elsewhere is the "HCR-20" (Douglas et al. 2001; Webster et al. 1997).[4] This instrument contains twenty items: ten historical ("H"), which include previous violence; five current or clinical ("C"), which include active symptoms; and five referring to risk management ("R"), which incorporate the environment and support system awaiting the individual post-discharge. For a bibliography on the HCR-20 see Douglas et al. (2010). Another tool used in clinical practice, and also developed in Canada, is the Violence Risk Appraisal Guide (Harris, Rice, and Camilleri 2004).

More routinely, risk-screen tools may be used by staff in community settings who work alone and make home visits. In these situations, employers must be mindful of liability and risk management, and they are accountable in this respect to unions, accreditation bodies, and workers' compensation boards. The screening here pertains not just to the person being visited but also to the environment, other residents, animals, lighting, infestation, and so on.

Functional and Needs Assessments

The more clinically oriented assessments described above may need to be supplemented with assessments of social functioning. For example, a practice guidelines document on interventions with clients experiencing a first psychotic break notes that a psychosocial assessment should obtain information on the following (Mental Health Evaluation and Community Consultation Unit 2002):

- the status of social relationships, including school, work, and recreation;
- activities of daily living, including money management, self-care, and domestic roles;
- strengths and intact functions to support self-efficacy;
- the rate of change of these functions;
- cognitive and intellectual status;
- stressors, coping abilities, and beliefs about illness;
- developmental, academic, occupational, and social histories.

Appraisals of activities of daily living are sometimes called "functional assessments," and these address a client's ability to perform tasks such as cooking, shopping, budgeting, and use of transit, all of which are skill areas that may need to be developed or "recharged" among more disabled clients. Such assessments may also inform decisions about residential placement or the need for more intensive services.

While social functioning may be addressed, at least in part, in the initial assessment, typically in multidisciplinary programs, psychosocial and functional assessments are carried out by an occupational therapist, who may refer to structured instruments or rating scales for this purpose. For example, the Canadian Occupational Performance Measure is described by Kirsh and Cockburn (2009, 171) as a tool that "supports goal setting and the assessment of change" and "is designed to foster partnership between clients and practitioners." There are both advantages and disadvantages with this functional assessment being handled by the occupational therapist (OT). The OT is a rehabilitation specialist, with a skill set and orientation well-suited to work with persons with psychiatric disabilities; there is a focus on function, as opposed to diagnosis, and OTs try to identify what a client *can* do as opposed to what she or he cannot do. However, involvement with an OT may require a referral from a case manager, a gate-keeping arrangement that means a client may miss out on important rehab services unless the case manager him- or herself systematically identifies rehab goals or the agency has a practice of new clients all having some initial contact with an OT. There is also sometimes the tendency to diminish the importance of the rehab role as "non-clinical," which Kopelowicz and Liberman (2003, 1491) point out involves fallacious reasoning in that "there are no conceptual or operational differences between 'treatment' and 'rehabilitation.'" Three authors from Yale University suggest that *all* members of a multidisciplinary team need to be involved in client-centred care planning; the alternative is "continuing to treat the illness as if it took place in a vacuum [which] perpetuates the narrowly-defined, practitioner-driven model of care that people with mental illnesses routinely identify as a major barrier in their recovery" (Tondora, Miller, and Davidson 2012, 412).

In addition to functional assessments, clinicians should consider an appraisal of *client-identified* needs and interests at the outset of the therapeutic engagement and periodically thereafter. This is important for several reasons:

- Interests and domains of life important to the client may otherwise go unaddressed.
- Unmet needs have been associated with a lower quality of life (Slade et al. 2005).
- Client-identified needs have been shown to differ from those identified by health care providers (e.g. Trauer, Tobias and Slade 2008).
- Addressing client-identified needs can promote a stronger therapeutic alliance. For example, studies by Calsyn et al. (2006) and Junghan et al. (2007) found that client ratings of the strength of the relationship was a function of whether or not they felt their needs were being met. In turn, a stronger therapeutic alliance is associated with improved health outcomes (Couture et al. 2006).

The Province of Ontario has led the implementation of standard needs-based tools, which historically in most Canadian jurisdictions have either not been used or have been used in an inconsistent fashion. In 2006, Ontario piloted the use of a common intake assessment tool and, for persons activated at a mental health program, a common needs assessment tool, the OCAN

(Ontario Common Assessment of Need) (Zosky et al. 2010). The rationale for this was: (1) to provide an assessment that was comprehensive, holistic, and informed by client self-appraisal; (2) to consequently identify gaps in service, at both the individual and system level, to better inform planning; and (3) to try to ensure a common data standard across jurisdictions so that clients and staff were starting from the same place regardless of where an individual contacted the system. Fundamentally, a needs assessment answers the question: "How do you determine what interests the person has that he or she might like to pursue?" (Tondora, Miller, and Davidson 2012, 413).

A Strengths Perspective

Many assessment approaches in psychiatry are deficit-oriented. The mental status exam considers signs of pathology, assessments for disability income look at obstacles to independent functioning, and so on. By contrast, and very much congruent with the recovery perspective, the need for *strengths-based* assessments has been increasingly emphasized. A strengths perspective is characterized by Maguire (2002, 29) as a move "toward recognizing the client's own positive resources as well as that of his or her social system," so that this individual is seen as "a very active partner in the helping process." A useful document in this regard is "100 Ways to Support Recovery," authored by British psychologist Mike Slade (2009). Slade suggests that the assessment process be used as a means for developing and validating personal meaning ("writing a new script"), amplifying strengths, fostering personal responsibility (e.g., by goal-setting), supporting a positive identity, and developing hope. Slade (2009, 13) identifies elements of a more strengths-based mental health assessment as follows:

- *Current strengths and resources:* What keeps you going? Consider spirituality, social roles, cultural/political identity, self-belief, life skills, toughness, resilience, humour, environmental mastery, support from others, ability to express emotion artistically.
- *Personal goals:* How would you like your life to be different? What are your dreams now? How have they changed?
- *Past coping history:* How have you got through the tough times in your life? What supports have you found useful? What do you wish had happened?
- *Inherited resources:* Is there any history of high achieving in your family? Any artists, authors, athletes, or academics?
- *Family environment:* When you were growing up, was there anyone you really admired? What important lessons did you learn during childhood?

- *Learning from the past:* What have these experiences taught you? Are there any positive ways in which you have changed or grown as a person? Consider gratitude, altruism, empathy, compassion, self-acceptance, self-efficacy, meaning.
- *Developmental history:* What was life like for you when you were growing up? What did you enjoy? What's your best memory? What skills or abilities did you discover you had?
- *Valued social roles:* What would someone who knew you really well and liked you say about you? What would you like them to say? How are you useful or of value to others?
- *Social supports:* Who do you lean on in times of trouble? Who leans on you?
- *Personal gifts:* Has anyone ever paid you a compliment? What things that you've done or ways that you've behaved make you feel really proud of yourself?

An even more extensive strengths assessment is offered in Rapp and Goscha's (2012) book *The Strengths Model*. A*spirations, competencies* and *confidence* are seen by these authors as key elements underpinning the strength and resilience of an individual.

Assessments through a Cultural Lens

Practitioners need to be sensitive about the age, literacy, and cultural background of the clients they are assessing. Some "standardized" assessment instruments may have been validated with a different population than that of a particular minority client. Alverson and colleagues (2007) note that, in an era of client-centred care, collaboration between client and practitioner becomes particularly important, and to this end, there is an onus on clinicians working with clients from various cultural backgrounds to be aware of the differences in how individuals experience their illness. For example, mental distress may be more likely to be expressed as a physical ailment – "somaticized" – among Chinese or East Asian clients than among Westerners.

Kleinman and Benson (2006) talk about conducting a "mini-ethnography" when working with clients from other cultures, which starts by considering ethnic identity and whether this matters for the client (i.e., whether it is an important part of her/his sense of self). A second step is to determine what is at stake for the individual or her/his family, for example concern about marriage prospects should the client be identified as mentally ill. Next is to try to determine the illness narrative, or explanatory model, which involves answering the following questions:

- What do you call this problem?
- What do you believe is the cause of this problem?
- What course do you expect it to take? How serious is it?
- What do you think this problem does inside your body?
- How does it affect your body and your mind?
- What do you most fear about this condition?
- What do you most fear about the treatment?

In a paper on cross-cultural assessment, Mushquash and Bova (2007) offer several suggestions to make the process more valid and relevant:

- For the clinician to make a preliminary assessment of his or her own assumptions and biases (practitioners in training may address this through "reflection papers").
- Where English ability is limited, to arrange for an interpreter. Ideally, this would be a trained person, and in any case, family members or friends would not be in the best position to provide this service.
- To use a multi-method approach to assessment, including interviews and collateral information from various sources.
- To be cautious in the use and interpretation of standardized measures.

For more on cultural context see Chapter 6.

Diagnosis and the *DSM*

Assessments undertaken by clinicians inform diagnosis. The psychiatric diagnostic system used in almost all Canadian settings is the *Diagnostic and Statistical Manual*, published by the American Psychiatric Association. The other major system in use is the International Statistical Classification of Diseases and Related Health Problems (ICD), published by the World Health Organization. While attempts have been made to harmonize these two systems, there are differences in the criteria and definitions used, and where diagnostic criteria are used in this book they will refer to the *DSM*. What follows in this section is a brief, critical overview of elements and assumptions of the *DSM* model.

Reliability and Validity

The classification system articulated in the *DSM* has been evolving for over fifty years, with ongoing disputes about the validity and reliability of the definitions listed in the various revisions of this publication (Genova 2003; Duncan, Miller, and Sparks 2004). An apparent problem with the early versions of the *DSM* was a lack of specificity regarding how the disorders were defined, which, in turn, led to poor inter-rater agreement when making diagnoses. As reviewed by Eaton (2001), studies on the *DSM*'s diagnostic reliability conducted between 1950 and 1980, using a value of the kappa statistic of 0.50 as the minimum acceptable standard,[5] found not one study that was able to attain values above 0.50 for all diagnostic categories. Schizophrenia was diagnosed more reliably, relatively speaking, with kappa values above 0.50 being achieved in five of seven studies, while rates of agreement on personality disorders were so low as to be considered unacceptable.

To address problems with reliability, the *DSM* system changed radically, with its third edition in 1980, to a descriptive approach, which provided clinicians with a "checklist" of operational criteria, which did improve diagnostic reliability (Eaton 2001). As well, later editions of the *DSM* have been deliberately atheoretical, avoiding reference to the aetiology of disorders, apparently to obviate disagreements that might arise between different factions in the psychiatric community. However, concerning the checklist approach, critics have suggested that the *DSM* still "falls short of using fully operational criteria" – that is, still lacks specificity – pointing out that "terms such as 'often' and 'easily' are used without guidance about the severity of the problems they represent" (Nietzel, Bernstein, and Milich 1998, 367).

Concerning validity, Duncan, Miller, and Sparks (2004) note that *DSM* categories do not offer any predictive power with respect to how a client will succeed in treatment, nor in fact to they specify any particular treatment. They note that, to be comparable to medical diagnoses, *DSM* categories would need to be supported by "biomarkers" or have defining criteria that are distinct from neighbouring syndromes, neither of which can really be claimed (see also Patten 2006). Similarly, the validity and reliability of disorder *subtypes*, such as the subcategories of schizophrenia listed previously in the *DSM* – paranoid schizophrenia being an example – have been questioned (Amador 2009). In a review of the subject, Helmes and Landmark (2003, 702) conclude that "subtypes may have little utility when the variability of symptoms over the longitudinal course of the [schizophrenic] illness is considered." In response to this, schizophrenia subtypes were eliminated in the fifth edition of the *DSM*, published in 2013.

Syndrome Inclusion and Threshold

How are disorders included in the *DSM*? Historically, psychiatric syndromes have been included largely on the basis of clinical judgment and "expert consensus" – a lower standard of evidence upon which to base decisions than empirical research. Because of the potential for bias inherent in this approach, starting with the *DSM-IV* in 1994, experts were organized into working groups, which were to incorporate empirical as well as clinical literature and which also conducted field trials using the proposed diagnostic criteria. Despite these efforts, some have expressed concern that there is still too much reliance on consensus and hence lobbying in creating diagnostic categories – that is, that the process is more political than scientific (Kleiner 2011). In an interview, University of Toronto professor Edward Shorter observes that the *DSM* is "a consensus document and consensus always involves a lot of horse-trading: 'I'll put in your favourite diagnosis if you put in mine'" (quoted in Kirkey 2010). On the consequences of this, Canadian psychologist Paula Caplan has suggested that the predominantly male caucus that revises the *DSM* has produced a document that manifests a gender bias, among other things (Caplan 1995). It has also been argued that this process may be contributing to diagnostic "expansionism," with more and more categories being included in each revision of the *DSM* without a sound scientific rationale (Spiegel 2005; Wente 2009).

By its very name, the *DSM* is meant to be a compendium of "disorders." In examining this assumption, critics have suggested that some of the categories included are actually just variants of normal perception or experience that do not meet the threshold of disorder.[6] For example, in the *Canadian Journal of Psychiatry*, Wakefield, Horwitz, and Schmitz (2005) argue that diagnosing social phobia is in effect "overpathologizing the anxious." In commenting on the approach used in the *DSM*, Fauman (2002, 11) suggests that differentiation between persons with pathological and mild symptoms is achieved by adhering to the general diagnostic principle that the disorder must be one that causes "clinically significant distress or impairment in social, occupational, or other important areas of functioning."

Category or Continua?

Some of the problems described above could, in theory, be dealt with by changing from a categorical system to a continuum or dimensional model. In such a model, intervention decisions would be based on the severity of symptoms and functional impairment rather than on the category under which the symptoms fall.

There are several arguments supporting a change to a dimensional model (Skodol and Bender 2009; Stip 2009). For one thing, despite advances made in genetic research, there are still no biological markers upon which to distinguish psychiatric categories. Further, neither symptoms nor treatments have been found to be specific for particular categories. For example, persons with bipolar disorder and schizophrenia, two apparently discrete categories, may experience similar symptoms (e.g., psychosis, grandiosity) and may be treated with the same medications (Vieta and Phillips 2007). The same could be said to apply to bipolar II vis-à-vis borderline personality disorder. Also, co-morbidity (possessing features of more than one syndrome) is common among the mentally ill and is probably the rule rather than the exception. Clients may present with a range of symptoms, which makes problematic the presumption that clinical entities are separate, or "primary," as implied in a diagnostic formulation (Ballou and Brown 2002; Harris and Fallot 2001). Finally, the case can be made that we are in effect using dimensional thinking anyway, to cope with the inadequacies of a categorical system. Examples are (1) the construct of schizoaffective disorder, which may represent an intermediate position on a continuum between schizophrenia and mood disorders (Cheniaux et al 2008); (2) the bifurcation of bipolar disorder into bipolar I and II; and (3) the use of "overvalued ideas" as a symptom to be placed on a continuum between obsessions and delusions (O'Connor 2009). A criticism of dimensional systems is that they run the risk of pathologizing a wider tract of normal experience and behaviour (Pierre, 2010). Kleiner (2011, 34) notes that this could "lead to some symptoms being classified as below the threshold needed for diagnosis ... but still severe enough to be a problem," resulting in diagnoses like "pre-psychotic syndrome."

It should be noted that Canadian health care settings are already using severity rating scales, an example being the HoNOS system referred to earlier in this chapter. Another example is the Minimum Data Set (MDS), a tool developed in the US and now used in Canada to determine eligibility for long-term care services (Kane, Ouslander, and Abrass 2004).

Using the DSM

Starting with its third edition in 1980 and continuing to its 2000 edition, the *DSM* used a multi-axial system for diagnostic formulations, which was intended to give a fuller picture of a client's psychological, physical, and social functioning, and to encourage "thoroughness in evaluation" (American Psychiatric Association 2000, 29). The diagnostic formulation also included reference to psychosocial or environmental problems, and a scale – the Global Assessment of Functioning (GAF) – that was intended to capture the degree of functional impairment experienced at the time of the assessment.[7] The GAF ranges from 1 to 100, with the highest number indicating "superior functioning in a wide range of activities." The multi-axial system changed with the *DSM-5* in 2013 (see below).

Assessors enter psychiatric diagnoses according to the criteria provided in the *DSM*. When no condition is present, this is coded as "none," and where more information is needed the practitioner may enter "deferred." Concerning personality disorders, the *DSM* offers the option of recording personality *traits* that do not meet the threshold for a full-blown disorder. The formulation created will often include differential diagnoses – that is, other conditions that need to be ruled in or out before a more specific diagnosis can be made.

Prior to the *DSM-5*, each diagnostic group also contained a "not otherwise specified" (NOS) option, categories that were to serve as "catch-all diagnoses that can be used when a patient does not fit a more specific diagnosis" (Fauman 2002, 12). "Psychosis NOS" was not infrequently seen in the case of persons briefly admitted to a hospital emergency where there is little background information available on the client and, presumably, no time to gather this collateral data. In the Study Guide to the *DSM-IV-TR* (12), Fauman (2002) concedes that the NOS option is problematic since persons so diagnosed will be a heterogeneous group and, therefore, the diagnosis will offer "little predictive value for response to treatment or illness prognosis." He goes on to say that "every effort should be made to gather the necessary clinical information to make a more specific diagnosis" and that the NOS option should be used "as little as possible." To force clinicians to be more specific, the NOS option was dropped in the *DSM-5*.

The *DSM-5*
Prior to the *DSM-5*, personality disorders were put into a different axis ("Axis II") than other mental disorders, such as bipolar disorder and schizophrenia ("Axis I"). This, according to the *DSM*, was so that: "consideration will be given to the possible presence of personality disorders ... that would otherwise be overlooked when attention is directed to the usually more *florid* Axis I disorders" and that it "should not be taken to imply that their pathogenesis or range of appropriate treatment is fundamentally different from Axis I conditions" (American Psychiatric Association 2000, 28, emphasis added). In other words, despite their being – to quote the *DSM* – less "florid," putting them into a different axis was not meant to give personality disorders an inferior status, so to speak. Unfortunately, this is exactly what happened in that personality disorders were often regarded by practitioners as less serious than the conditions coded on the other axis. The significance of this, as we saw in Chapter 3, is that decisions on service eligibility often hinge on the perceived "seriousness" of a person's condition. Suggesting that the multi-axial system was at least partly to blame, a professor of psychiatry at McGill noted that "ironically, whereas a separate axis for personality was created to encourage practitioners to take these forms of pathology into account, it has often led only to their isolation in an Axis II ghetto" (Paris

1998, 135). To resolve this, Canadian psychiatrist John Livesley (1998) concluded that, because of the potential for discrimination, personality disorders should be coded on the same axis as other mental disorders. This in fact is what was resolved with the publication of the *DSM-5* in 2013: the multi-axial system was removed and former Axis I and II disorders, along with medical conditions formerly listed under Axis III, are now combined, with separate notations for psychosocial factors (previously Axis IV) and disability (previously Axis V).

While elimination of the multi-axial system is arguably a positive development, concern has been expressed that the *DSM-5* continues to expand the jurisdiction of psychiatry by adding new diagnostic categories and lowering the threshold for others. Hoarding and premenstrual dysphoric disorder are now included as *DSM* diagnoses, and "disruptive mood dysregulation disorder" is now included as a diagnosis for persons under 18, the latter, according to the APA, "to address concerns about potential overdiagnosis and overtreatment of bipolar disorder in children" (American Psychiatric Association 2013, 4). The *DSM-5* also removes the two-month "bereavement exclusion" for a diagnosis of depression; now, short-term depression following the death of a loved one may be considered pathological.

Notes

1 While definitions of these terms are provided in psychiatric texts, it should be said that the distinction between "delusion," "obsession," and "overvalued idea" is not always easily made.

2 There are different hypotheses attempting to explain this association: (1) that clients are being discharged prematurely, while still in a psychologically fragile state; (2) conversely, that an illness – typically a psychosis – has been *successfully* treated, so the person now sees her/his very limited prospects more clearly; (3) that the person become reliant upon, or used to, the milieu of the hospital, so that post-discharge isolation is relatively more difficult. Concerning the association between hospital discharge and suicide, psychiatrist Sarah Mourra (2013) notes: "People who have just recovered from psychosis often experience depression afterwards. Added to this, a psychiatric hospitalization by its very definition involves a loss of control, which is not always, but often, uncomfortable and traumatic for someone trying to process the internal realization of not being able to trust their own appraisal of reality. These experiences often raise philosophical questions, identity questions, emotions, and fears that the inpatient unit is sadly unequipped to deal with. Unless there is a particularly invested trainee, nurse, or other staff member, patients are often alone with their thoughts, and before long discharged home."

3 The reference to "medication" implies a need to be cautious with the length of a prescription, but in truth there is nothing preventing an individual from gaining access to large quantities of over-the-counter drugs, which may be just as lethal in overdose.

4 As this was being written, the HCR-20 was under revision with a third edition said to be forthcoming.

5 The kappa statistic is used to measure agreement between different raters and runs below zero if agreement is less than would occur by chance, to zero at chance agreement, and to one at perfect agreement.

6 There is evidence that even psychotic symptoms, generally considered the clearest sign of a mental disorder, are more commonly seen in the general population than we may have assumed (O'Connor 2009; Stip and Letourneau 2009).

7 The precision and reliability of the GAF has been called into question (Söderberg, Tungström, and Armelius 2005; Vatnaland et al. 2007).

Other Resources

Canadian Association for Suicide Prevention: www.suicideprevention.ca.
The Suicide Prevention Resource Center: http://www.sprc.org.
The Centre for Suicide Prevention: http://suicideinfo.ca.

Medical Management

15

"Medical management" is used here to refer to a process, led by a psychiatrist or physician, that involves the treatment and stabilization of acute psychiatric symptoms, primarily with the use of medications. Non-pharmacological approaches to treatment – education, skills training, and psychotherapy – are described in Chapter 16. The separation of pharmacological and non-pharmacological treatments is an artifact of this book's construction: in reality, clients of mental health teams may simultaneously receive services from a prescribing physician and one or more other care providers, involving (for example) occupational therapy or cognitive behavioural therapy. That being said, the fact remains that, in some cases, mental health clients do not receive more than "medical management," despite their own wishes and despite evidence that other types of treatment and education are effective (Barkil-Oteo 2013). There are three main reasons for this. The first is ideological, reflecting the dominant position of biological approaches in North American psychiatry. The second has to do with training: not all practitioners have been exposed to, for example, cognitive-behavioural approaches. The third has to do with resource allocation: family physicians and practitioners on mental health teams generally have large caseloads, with clients being booked at short intervals, so brief assessments and medication renewals are favoured over longer counseling sessions. A related issue, which mainly applies to GPs, is that medical insurance policies may create a financial disincentive for persons providing longer counselling sessions.[1]

This chapter provides an overview of psychopharmacological treatment, pros and cons, as well as some brief comment on the use of lab tests and electroconvulsive therapy (ECT). Discussing the use and effects of medication is fraught with difficulty because of the speed with which new products are developed and because our understanding of the benefits and costs associated with their use is constantly changing. As a result, the reader is strongly advised to consider other sources of information, such as the *Compendium of Pharmaceuticals and Specialties,* published annually by the Canadian Pharmacists Association.

Lab Tests

Practitioners may be asked: "Is there a blood test or imaging technique you can administer to determine whether someone has a mental illness?" While researchers continue to look for "biomarkers" in psychiatry, at present the answer to this question is "no."[2] Tests and scans may be used to *rule out* other causes of unusual behaviour, which include toxicity (drug-induced effects), trauma (e.g., concussion or subdural bleeding), infection (e.g., meningitis or syphilis), brain tumours, epilepsy, endocrine dysfunction (e.g., hyper-thyroidism), and electrolyte imbalance. Tests of liver and kidney function may also be conducted to ensure that drugs, prescribed by the mental health practitioner, can be *metabolized* safely. If a person has a liver disease, this may mean prescribing in lower doses or discontinuing the medication. The safe use of certain psychiatric medications requires that blood tests be conducted periodically, two well-known examples being clozapine and lithium. Lithium, an anti-mania drug, must have its levels monitored for signs of toxicity (which is also assessed clinically). Clozapine, an antipsychotic, may in some cases cause suppression of white blood cells – meaning the body is more vulnerable to infection – so white cell count must be monitored. Despite this problem, clozapine may be used when other antipsychotic drugs have failed since it still has the greatest impact on symptoms such as delusions and hallucinations.

Psychotropic Medication

The medications used in psychiatry are referred to as "psychotropic," which is defined (not very helpfully) as "having an effect on the mind" (Andrews et al. 2000, 110). Since the 1950s, the number and type of medications used in psychiatry have increased dramatically, and currently in Canada they form the cornerstone of the treatment offered to persons with mental disorders. To quote the editor of the *Canadian Journal of Psychiatry,* "while many areas have made significant contributions [to psychiatric practice], the area of psychopharmacology has been in the forefront since the introduction of chlorpromazine for schizophrenia" (Rae-Grant 2002, 513). However, some would argue that our reliance on drug therapy has become an over-reliance, with one professor of psychiatry stating flatly that "psychiatry in practice is mostly psychopharmacology" (Ghaemi, 2010, p. 110). The counter-argument is that, until acute symptoms, such as psychosis and mania, are stabilized, which usually requires the use of medication, the individual will, in any case, be unable to avail him- or herself of other, complementary treatments.

Even specialists in psychosocial approaches to rehabilitation concede that "psychosocial services are of little value unless the client is adhering to maintenance antipsychotic, mood stabilizer, and antidepressant regimens" (Kopelowicz and Liberman 2003, 1492). The use of medication as the *sole* treatment is more difficult to defend, especially when one is talking about non-psychotic and non-manic disorders.

What is the mechanism by which psychotropic drugs achieve their effect? There is still uncertainty about the answer(s) to this question as well as some controversy, for example, with the serotonin-deficit theory.[3] But in very general terms, it is understood that psychotropic drugs work by affecting the activity of neurotransmitters, which are chemicals that transmit nerve impulses across the synapse (gap) between nerve cells by attaching to receptor sites on the neighbouring cell. A number of different neurotransmitters are believed to play a role in psychiatric disorders, including dopamine, serotonin, acetylcholine, norepinephrine, and gamma aminobutyric acid (GABA). Psychotropic drugs modify natural physiological events in several ways: (1) they may alter presynaptic activity to prompt neurotransmitter release; (2) they may alter postsynaptic activity by affecting the binding at the receptor site; (3) they may interfere with normal neurotransmitter reuptake processes; and (4) they may alter the manufacture of the receptor cells. These medications can be classified as agonists, which means that they increase neurotransmitter effects, or as antagonists, which means that they decrease these effects. How exactly neurotransmitter activity affects the manifestation of psychiatric disorders is not clearly understood, but it appears that dopamine plays a role in psychotic disorders, with antipsychotic drugs achieving their effect in part by blocking dopamine receptors (Owens 1999). In the case of mood disorders, it is hypothesized that low serotonin levels play a role in depression, with antidepressants achieving their effect in part by boosting synaptic levels of this neurotransmitter.

Drugs differ with respect to *half-life*, which refers to how quickly they are metabolized and clear the system. Injectable antipsychotic drugs, for example, stay in the system for a long time (they may be injected as infrequently as every four weeks), which has advantages with respect to administration but which is a concern if the drug is producing an adverse reaction. Other drugs have short half-lives: the anti-anxiety agent lorazepam (Ativan) has a shorter half-life than other drugs in its class, which means less daytime sedation and decreased risk of psychomotor impairment but, at the same time, more pronounced withdrawal symptoms and greater likelihood of rebound anxiety (Andrews et al. 2000).

Psychotropic drugs, like all medications, have side effects. While these may diminish with time, it is unfortunately the case that some side effects are persistent and unpleasant enough to deter clients from taking the medication (Gumpp 2009). When this happens, the practitioner must consider alternatives, such as reducing the dose, switching to a different agent, or adding another medication to deal with the side effects. The practitioner is often struggling with a cost-benefit situation while attempting, through trial and error, to arrive at a medication regimen that is the least complicated and that provides maximum therapeutic benefit with minimum side effects. One great difficulty concerns the fact that medication response is very idiosyncratic, meaning that a practitioner can never be certain that any two individuals with the same diagnosis will respond to a medication in the same way (Davis and Leucht 2008) (for a discussion of the difficulties of applying "global evidence" from drug trials – "average effects" – to individual cases, see Kravitz, Duan, and Braslow 2004). Psychotropic drug response may also differ as a function of age or of genetic differences both within and between ethnic groups (Campbell et al. 2008; Kirkey 2004). While newer medications in psychiatry are often marketed with the promise of a better side-effect profile, it is almost certainly the case that dealing with side effects will continue to be a preoccupation of clients, practitioners, and family members.

Some of the most commonly encountered side effects seen with the use of psychotropic medications include:

- Extrapyramidal symptoms (EPS), most often associated with the use of older antipsychotic drugs, such as haloperidol. EPS refers generally to movement disorders, which can include akathisia (a feeling of restlessness in the legs), dystonia (a muscular spasm that can affect the neck, jaws, back, or eyes – the latter referred to as an "oculogyric crisis"), Parkinsonism (stiffness, tremor, loss of facial expression, drooling, or stooped posture), and tardive dyskinesia (enduring involuntary movements, usually in the facial muscles, such as the lips and tongue). "Tardive" by definition refers to a late onset; thus, a tardive dystonia, for example, is one appearing after sixty days, whereas an acute dystonia is one that manifests right away.
- Anticholinergic effects, which can include dry mouth, blurred vision, and constipation. These are seen particularly with older antipsychotic and antidepressant medications.
- Gastrointestinal effects, including constipation, diarrhea, and nausea. These are seen with a wide range of drugs, including mood stabilizers and antidepressants, although effects are transient in many cases.
- Weight gain, seen particularly with the use of lithium (a mood stabilizer) and newer antipsychotic drugs, in particular olanzapine and clozapine. The weight gain and onset of type II diabetes associated with the newer antipsychotic medications, a cluster of symptoms called "metabolic syndrome,"

has in fact become a source of great concern (Abidi and Bhaskara 2003; Kisely, et al. 2009; Mitchell et al. 2013; Saari et al. 2004).

- Sedation, seen with a range of different medications (response can be idiosyncratic).
- Diminished sex drive and performance, seen with antidepressant drugs such as the selective serotonin reuptake inhibitors (SSRIs).
- Anxiety and insomnia, seen sometimes with the use of antidepressant medications.
- Rarer, but potentially serious, conditions such as (1) neuroleptic malignant syndrome, which is seen with the use of older antispychotics and which can lead to muscle rigidity, fever, and in some cases death; (2) agranulocytosis, which refers to the diminishing of white blood cells and, consequently, of the body's ability to fight infection, and which is a particular concern with the use of the newer antipsychotic clozapine.

Helping a client to talk about and manage side effects, a crucial role for practitioners, is addressed later in this chapter.

In the following description of different drug categories, the reader is reminded that medications have both a generic and a trade name, an example being the antidepressant fluoxetine, which is better known by the trade name Prozac. (Drug companies may manufacture generic forms of a drug originally produced by another company once the patent protection has expired.) In most cases the references here will be to the generic name.

Antipsychotics

Currently, antipsychotic medications (previously known as neuroleptics) are classified as either older generation ("typical") or newer generation ("atypical").[4] The first generation commenced with the discovery by French researchers in the early 1950s of the antipsychotic properties of chlorpromazine, a drug that is still in (limited) use today. Building from this discovery, other agents were developed, including thioridazine, fluphenazine, haloperidol, and loxapine, all of which are now available in generic form. These medications have been found to be effective treatments for the positive symptoms of psychosis – delusions, hallucinations, and thought disorder – although it is estimated that about one-third of clients will show only a partial response or no response (Kane et al. 2011). In the jargon of psychiatry, persons who do not respond are said to be *refractory* to a particular type of treatment.

Concerning the mechanism of these agents, it has been found that stimulating the activity of the neurotransmitter dopamine increases symptoms of psychosis and that antagonist medications such as chlorpromazine work against this by blocking dopamine at neural receptor sites. Unfortunately, as dopamine blockade increases so does the likelihood of extrapyramidal side effects (EPS), which take the form of movement disorders (see above) (Blin 1999). It is believed that EPS is due to the non-specific action of this class of drugs, which block dopamine in areas of the brain (the basal ganglia) that are related to movement disorders. Further, in about 5 percent of cases a year, clients may develop tardive dyskinesia, a movement disorder that may be irreversible even after the discontinuation of the medication (Tollefson et al. 1997). To address this problem, most mental health settings now require physicians to assess persons on antipsychotic medication regularly with tests for involuntary movement, an example being the Abnormal Involuntary Movement Scale (AIMS). Other problems associated with using first-generation antipsychotics include over-sedation, particularly with "low potency" drugs such as chlorpromazine and thioridazine, as well as hormonal effects (Andrews et al. 2000). Finally, while beneficial for positive symptoms, the first-generation antipsychotics have been found to have little or no impact on the negative symptoms of schizophrenia – such as apathy, blunted affect, and lack of spontaneous speech (Kane and Mayerhoff 1989).

Since the 1980s a number of "atypical" antipsychotics have been developed, including clozapine, risperidone, olanzapine, quetiapine, ziprasidone, amisulpride, aripiprazole, and paliperidone. "New generation" drugs inevitably become less new, so, for example, in 2011 paliperidone was touted as a promising new medication even though it is a derivative of the now "old" drug risperidone. (Clozapine is considered a newer drug when, in fact, it was developed in the 1960s: its more widespread use was delayed for some years because of concerns about side effects.) It has been found that these agents achieve a therapeutic effect at a lower level of dopamine blockade than is the case with the first-generation antipsychotics, a result being that the newer medications are less likely to produce extrapyramidal side effects and tardive dyskinesia (Correll, Leucht, and Kane 2004; Ehmann and Hanson 2004; Margolese et al. 2005). The new drugs came with the promise of being better than the old ones; that is, of being at least as effective in treating psychosis but also ameliorating a wider range of symptoms (negative, affective, and cognitive), producing better functional outcomes, and having a superior side effect profile (Blin 1999; Green, Marshall, and Wirshing 1997; Woodward et al. 2005). Unfortunately, most of these claims have not been supported: with the exception of clozapine, the newer-generation drugs are no more effective than the older ones with respect to the positive symptoms, and any reduction in EPS side effects is compensated for by the problems they create with respect to weight gain and glucose and lipid metabolism (Arbuckle et al. 2008; Hogan 2008; Sutton 2008; Whitaker 2010).[5] A major study looking at this issue is the Clinical Antipsychotic Trials of Intervention Effectiveness (CATIE), a multi-site project that was not sponsored by the drug companies and hence is considered less biased (Lieberman et al. 2005). The study recruited almost fifteen hundred subjects and compared treatment failure rates between an older antipsychotic and four newer-generation drugs. "Treatment failure" was defined as discontinuation of treatment, which could be due to lack of efficacy, intolerability, or the subject's decision to quit the trial. The assumption had been that the newer drugs would be better tolerated, but the finding was that three of the four "atypicals" in fact had *higher* treatment failure rates than the older drug, perphenazine. Olanzapine, a newer drug, had a better retention rate but was associated with higher rates of weight gain and metabolic syndrome. (A secondary finding was that close to *three-quarters* of all subjects had dropped out of the trial by eighteen months, which, if nothing else, shows the high rate of non-adherence and/or poor tolerability associated with antipsychotic medication; see also Leucht et al. [2003].)

Concerning other areas of potential benefit, subsequent research has not supported claims that the new-generation drugs improve cognition (Goldberg et al. 2007; Gonzalez-Blanch et al. 2008),[6] help with depression (Mauri et al. 2008), improve quality of life (Jones et al. 2006), or lead to better functional outcomes (Swartz et al. 2007). In summarizing the research, psychiatrists at the University of Toronto conclude that "second generation antipsychotics, except clozapine in the treatment-resistant population, offer little, if any, clinical benefits, and moreover harbour their own significant side effects" (Foussias and Remington 2010, 117). An editorial in the medical journal the *Lancet* added that "the time has come to abandon the terms first-generation and second-generation antipsychotics, as they do not merit this distinction" (Tyrer and Kendall 2009, 5).

There is some hope, and evidence, that three of the newest antipsychotics – aripiprazole, ziprasidone, and paliperidone (the latter available in long-acting injection form) – have fewer adverse effects with respect to metabolic syndrome (Addington et al. 2009).[7] As noted, clozapine is the one newer-generation drug that has been found to be superior with respect to the positive symptoms of schizophrenia. Clozapine is not a first-line treatment because one of its side effects is aganulocytosis, although severe adverse effects are rare (Abidi and Bhaskara 2003). Current guidelines are that a switch to clozapine be undertaken following poor treatment response to two other antipsychotics. Persons taking clozapine in Canada are required to have regular blood tests, starting weekly, then moving to monthly, which may be a challenge for clients who are very disorganized or disabled.[8]

As noted, an association has been established between atypical antipsychotic medication use and weight gain. A study in the UK found that the more negative self-identity that formed among young adults entering the psychiatric system was in part related to their change in appearance (i.e., becoming more obese due to the medication) (Lester et al. 2011). Canadian health authorities are now implementing policies concerning the metabolic monitoring of their clients, something not traditionally within the scope of psychiatric practice. Arguably, this is an ethical imperative, given that the treatment being given is contributing to the problem, with some taking the position that failing to do this constitutes negligence (Radke, Parks, and Ruter 2010). At this author's program, clients are routinely measured for blood pressure, weight, waist circumference, and body mass index and are given requisitions to have glucose and lipid levels tested.

Antipsychotic medication is available in oral form (pills and in some cases liquid) and in long-acting injectable ("depot") form. Injections are intramuscular, usually given in the buttock, and are administered at intervals of two to four weeks. The compounds reach a peak plasma level, depending on the product, in two to nine days and have single injection half-lives ranging from four to twenty-one days. The choice of injection over oral administration usually has to do with a client's history of poor adherence with the oral form and may be recommended for persons who are forgetful or disorganized. The newer-generation antipsychotics were initially only available in oral form, but several are now available as an injection.

Antidepressants

It is believed that the majority of antidepressant medications achieve their effect by enhancing the action of neurotransmitters such as serotonin and noradrenaline. As with antipsychotics, antidepressants can be classified as older and newer generation. One class of older antidepressants is the monoamine oxidase inhibitors (MAOIs), which include phenelzine and tranylcypromine and which work by inhibiting enzymes that break down serotonin and noradrenaline. Problems with this class of drugs include their toxicity in overdose, which is always a concern when prescribing for depressed persons, and the potential for a hypertensive crisis, which, in rare cases, can be fatal (Andrews et al. 2000). The risk of this reaction is partly managed by dietary restrictions. MAOIs can also be problematic with respect to drug interactions, so the use of other medications must be monitored closely by a physician, possibly including a "washout" period. MAOIs are now rarely prescribed, although a newer class of antidepressant, reversible MAOIs, has been developed, which does not have the dietary restrictions and which is safer in overdose. Another major class of older-generation antidepressants is the tricyclics, which include amitriptyline (Elavil), clomipramine, and doxepin (all available as generics) and that work by blocking the reuptake of neurotransmitters that include noradrenaline and serotonin. The most common side effects are anticholinergic (see above), and this class is highly toxic in overdose due to cardiac complications.

More recently, since the late 1980s, a number of new antidepressant agents have been developed that come with the promise of acting more specifically on neurotransmitters, having fewer side effects, and being safer in overdose.[9] These newer products are now first-line treatments for depression (BC Ministry of Health Services 2008). One class that remains widely prescribed at the time of writing is the SSRIs, which include fluoxetine (Prozac), fluvoxamine (Luvox), paroxetine (Paxil), and sertraline (Zoloft). The longer-term side effects of this group include lethargy and, in 30 to 70 percent of cases, sexual dysfunction (Nurnberg et al. 2003). Bupropion (Wellbutrin), a newer agent of the class noradrenaline dopamine modulator (NDM), has fewer sexual side effects (this product has been marketed in Canada as a smoking cessation medication under the trade name Zyban).

Antidepressants, unlike some other classes of medication, can take some time to achieve a therapeutic effect, often several weeks, which can result in frustration and early termination of treatment. With poor treatment response, clinicians may consider switching to a different antidepressant or augmenting with another drug (see BC Ministry of Health Services 2008). While primarily used for the treatment of depression, the SSRIs may also be prescribed for other conditions, such as obsessive-compulsive disorder, panic disorder, and other anxiety disorders.

There have been several controversies associated with antidepressant medication usage. First, there is the *extent* of their use: in BC, for example, per capita utilization more than doubled from 1996 to 2004 (Raymond, Morgan, and Caetano 2007), a finding that does not apparently reflect an increase in the incidence of depression or a change in help-seeking behaviour but, rather, "a change in practice patterns, which could be related to changes in the prescribing patterns of physicians or to greater public acceptance of these medications" (Patten and Beck 2004; see also Harman, Edlund, and Fortney 2009). Estimates of the number of people taking antidepressants have been as high as 15 percent of all middle-aged persons in North America (Smith 2011). Harvard University psychiatrist Joseph Glenmullen (2000) suggests that this is the result of the medications being prescribed for non-serious matters, in "as many as 75% of patients ... for mild, even trivial, conditions" (11), and because family doctors are more commonly prescribing antidepressants now than they were historically. A large-scale survey of Alberta residents concluded that the increasing use of antidepressants was due at least in part to "use of these medications for reasons other than depression" (Esposito et al. 2007, 780). Antidepressant use has increased among the elderly as well: Newman and Schopflocher (2008) report on a prescription rate increase of close to 60 percent among senior citizens in Alberta between 1997 and 2004.

A second area of concern is the possible association between the use of SSRIs and increased incidence of suicidal/parasuicidal behaviours (Fergusson et al. 2005). It has been hypothesized, variously, that these drugs may produce akathisia (a side effect that some find intolerable), disinhibition, increased energy, or induction of mania, any of which could in theory contribute to suicidal thinking (Brent 2009). In 2003, concerns about adverse effects of SSRIs and about the lack of an evidence base to support their use in children with depression led, in the UK, to restrictions being placed on the use of most SSRIs with juveniles. Since then, other studies and reviews have concluded that the associated increased risk is small (Brent 2009) and that, overall, with respect to prescribing these medications to juveniles, the benefits outweigh the costs (Bridge et al. 2007). Current practice, based on advisories

All in Your Mind? The Placebo Effect

Antidepressant medications do seem to work for many people, with results from clinical trials suggesting that 65 to 75 percent of clients show clinically significant improvement and that 50 to 60 percent achieve a full recovery (BC Ministry of Health Services 2008). The question of *how* these drugs achieve this result becomes more complicated when one considers the fact that most of their benefit is apparently due to a placebo effect (Johnson 2006). For example, a meta-analysis of data submitted to the United States Food and Drug Administration covering the years 1987 to 1999 found that approximately 80 percent of the response to SSRI medications was duplicated in placebo control groups (Kirsch et al. 2002; see also Vedantam 2002). In other words, hopefulness, or expectation, or some other apparently intangible aspect of the treatment process – unrelated to the drug itself – is accounting for much of the benefit. The greatest non-placebo effect of antidepressant medication is seen among the 13 percent of persons suffering from severe depression, with mildly to moderately depressed persons gaining little or no benefit above that from placebo (Begley 2010; Kirsch et al. 2008). As large as it is, we may still be underestimating the placebo effect: persons in the treatment arm of a medication trial (i.e., the ones getting the "real" drug) may perceive that medication's side effects and become even more hopeful because they know they are not on placebo, thus exaggerating the drug's apparent benefits (Begley 2010). Interestingly, there is evidence that the placebo effect operates at the level of populations, not just individuals: Goldacre (2008, 81) notes that the placebo response to antidepressant medication has actually increased over time, "perhaps as our expectations of these drugs have increased." We have also found out that the placebo effect is not just "all in the mind" in that it brings about measurable physiological changes (Motluck 2001).

This leaves the clinician with a dilemma. A benefit is still a benefit, regardless of whether it is due to a pharmacological agent or a placebo. However, treatment on this basis would appear to violate the ethical principle of "do no harm" (see Chapter 18) by exposing an individual to risks (e.g., side effects) when the benefit is apparently being achieved by something other than the treatment itself. One possible solution to this conundrum is to use a response known as "watchful waiting," whereby the physician continues to reassess the client at regular intervals but holds off on prescribing antidepressants. Watchful waiting, based on the finding that many depressive episodes resolve themselves without intervention, is a practice recommended by the National Health Service in the UK for cases of less severe depression. This practice arguably promotes client-centred care by "allowing for patient preference when there is no definitive treatment choice" (Meredith et al. 2007, 72). It is likely that watchful waiting would be less successful among clients who strongly buy into the medical model and the belief that there is "a pill for every ill." Other persons, however, may be reassured that their careprovider will stick with them and continue to provide support even without an "active intervention."

There are a number of interesting implications that flow from this. The placebo effect points out the importance of *hope* in the treatment process, which, as we saw in Chapter 5, is a critical factor in recovery. It also underlines the benefit of somebody "doing something," although at the same time it calls into question the significance of the particular intervention being applied. While acknowledging that good rapport and continuity are aspects of successful treatment, we have still tended to believe, very reasonably, that it is the intervention – the antidepressant drug, for example – that is critical for a successful outcome. What the placebo effect suggests is that, in less serious cases of depression, positive, ongoing support from a helper can be equally important.

from Health Canada, is that physicians weigh risks and benefits before pre-scribing to juveniles and, once started, that medication effects be closely monitored for the first several months of treatment.[10]

A third controversy has to do with the efficacy of antidepressant drugs, based on findings that benefit seems to be largely due to a placebo effect (see box).

Mood Stabilizers

Mood stabilizers are used for the acute treatment of mania and hypomania and for the ongoing management of bipolar disorder. These may be pre-scribed for other conditions in which there is a mood component, such as schizoaffective disorder. A trio of drugs has been used for some time as the main pharmacological treatments for bipolar disorder: lithium (in the form lithium carbonate) and two anti-seizure agents, carbamazepine (Tegretol) and valproic acid (Valporade). Lithium is a naturally occurring element that was found to have antimania properties by an Australian psychiatrist in 1949, although the physiological mechanism by which this is achieved re-mains unclear. Lithium, while clearly effective for mania, can become toxic at relatively low levels, which can, in some cases, lead to kidney damage, coma, and even death. As a result, blood levels need to be monitored regu-larly to ensure that the serum concentration is not below or above the therapeutic range. Apart from overdose, use of lithium may in the longer term produce a fine tremor and weight gain. Side effects associated with the other two medications include gastrointestinal problems and some less common but potentially serious effects, such as agranulocytosis in the case of carbamazepine (Andrews et al. 2000). The medication lamotrigine may be used as an adjunctive treatment for the depression experienced by persons with bipolar disorder (Gorman 2003).

Benzodiazepines

The benzodiazepines are the class of drugs most commonly used as anti-anxiety agents, although they may be prescribed for a number of other conditions, including insomnia and alcohol withdrawal; as a treatment for extrapyramidal side effects; and as an adjunctive treatment for schizophre-nia, bipolar disorder, and other mood and anxiety disorders. Benzodiazepines are among the most widely used medications in Canada (Hermann 2002), with studies finding that, despite the recommended short duration of use, prescriptions often run for long periods of time (Valenstein et al. 2004). There are a large number of products in this class, examples being diazepam (Valium), lorazepam (Ativan), oxazepam (Serax), and clonazepam (Rivotril), all now available as generics. Physiologically, these agents are thought to act by achieving more complete bonding of the neurotransmitter GABA to its receptor sites. The key difference between the various benzodiazepines has to do with their half-lives. Longer half-life drugs such as clonazepam require less frequent doses, have more stable plasma concentrations, and have milder withdrawal symptoms; however, they cause more daytime sedation, a greater accumulation of the drug in the body, and more psychomotor impairment (Andrews et al. 2000). Benzodiazepine use, in the long term, can lead to dependency and tolerance, which refers to the need to keep increasing the dose to achieve the same effect. Long-term use means that the body's natural benzodiazepine compounds diminish, so when the drug is withdrawn, particularly if this is done abruptly, a withdrawal syndrome can occur, symptoms of which include "rebound" insomnia, anxiety, restlessness, and irritability. Among the elderly – a group that is frequently prescribed benzo-diazepines – use of these drugs has also been blamed for falls and broken bones as well as incontinence (Hogan et al. 2003).

Stimulants

Stimulant medications are most often associated with the treatment of attention-deficit hyperactivity disorder (ADHD), although they may be pre-scribed for other conditions, such as depression and narcolepsy. Studies of the use of these drugs with schoolchildren have found that they improve concentration and academic performance (Sadock and Sadock 2007), with one review concluding that "the effectiveness of stimulants for the short-term treatment of ADHD is well documented and constitutes the largest body of evidential literature in child psychiatry pharmacology" (McClellan and Werry 2003, 1,392). The exact mechanism of action of these compounds is not clearly understood; one hypothesis is that stimulant drugs increase central nervous system activity in parts of the brain that are responsible for inhibition (Nathan, Gorman, and Salkind 1999; Volkow et al. 2008). Examples of drugs in this category are methylphenidate (Ritalin), dextroamphetamine (Dexadrine), and modafinil (Provigil). Side effects, which can be seen as exaggerations of the main effects, include agitiation, tremor, and tachycardia. Other effects include weight loss (which is a desired effect when the drug is in the form of a diet pill), mood changes, and in some cases, psychosis, with one Canadian study finding that, in 6 percent of cases, children with ADHD who were prescribed stimulants developed psychotic symptoms (Cherland and Fitzpatrick 1999). Because of the potential for abuse and addiction, use of these medications must be monitored closely (medication orders require a triplicate prescription). Despite concerns about the use of these compounds, a survey of Alberta psychiatrists found that almost half – 47 percent – of respondents were prescribing stimulants to adult patients, a result that the authors concluded was "higher than expected" (Beck et al. 1999).

Special Considerations

How drugs are absorbed, metabolized, and excreted is affected by the age, gender, ethnicity, and physical health of the client, and these factors need to be taken into account when psychotropic medications are being considered. For example, it has been found that persons of Asian ancestry metabolize psychotropic medications more slowly and need to be given lower doses (Janicak et al. 2006). Metabolism also changes with age, meaning that elderly people are generally more sensitive to psychotropic agents, necessitating lower doses. Since older adults are also more likely to be on other types of medication, drug interactions may be a problem. A basic principle in prescribing for the elderly is "start low, go slow, and avoid multiple medications" (Andrews et al. 2000, 152).

Smoking can also affect how drugs are metabolized and can lower the blood levels of some antipsychotic medications by up to 50 percent (Mental Health Evaluation and Community Consultation Unit 2002).

Another area of concern is the client who is, or may be, pregnant. The approach in this situation is summarized by Andrews and colleagues (2000, 15): "In general, unnecessary use of medication is to be discouraged during pregnancy and, wherever possible, all medication is to be avoided during the first 12 weeks of pregnancy. However, in some cases medication is considered necessary and will be prescribed if the benefits ... outweigh all possible risks. For example, the risks associated with untreated psychosis or affective illness are generally higher than the risks of taking drugs."[11] While not all drugs may be harmful, drugs that are associated with fetal malformation include lithium, carbamazepine, valproic acid, and clonazepam. There is no indication that antipsychotic medications such as olanzapine and clozapine cause birth defects (Gentile 2004), although the evidence base for the newest drugs in this class is lacking. While antidepressant use has not been associated with foetal malformation, there is evidence that it increases the risk of spontaneous abortion (Einarson et al. 2009; Nakhai-Pour, Broy, and Berard 2010).

Off-Label Prescribing

"Off-label" prescribing refers to medications being ordered for conditions or populations not specified within the product's monograph or licence and, by extension, where the evidence base for doing so is unclear. By all accounts this practice is not uncommon and may be driven by the challenge of persons "whose symptoms have proven resistant to a range of treatment approaches"

(Baldwin and Kosky 2007, 415). For instance, the atypical antipsychotics, currently indicated for schizophrenia and bipolar disorder, have also been trialed for use with anxiety disorders (Depping et al. 2010). In another example, Quetiapine (Seroquel), the most sedating of the atypicals, may be used to aid with sleep when there is concern that other drugs will be dependency-producing, even though there is no evidence to support this usage (see http:// www.ti.ubc.ca/letter79). A 2012 report using data from the US Food and Drug Administration determined that off-label prescribing of "atypical" antipsychotics had doubled between 1995 and 2008 so that, by 2008, more than half of all prescriptions were off label, being used in cases of anxiety, insomnia, ADHD, dementia, and behavioural problems in children (Boodman 2012). It has been argued that off-label prescribing is also influenced by the marketing of drug companies, who have an incentive to claim more "turf" for their product. An example is the drug Neurontin (gabapentin), used to treat neuropathic pain, which was additionally promoted by the manufacturer Warner-Lambert as a treatment for, among other things, bipolar disorder. In 2004, Warner-Lambert was fined \$430 million by the US government after admitting there was no evidence base for these claims (Roslin 2008). Off label may also refer to prescribing at a dose higher than that given in the product licence; in doing this, physicians need to weigh clinical benefit against diminishing therapeutic returns and increased side effects.

A controversial area of off-label medication use concerns the number of prescriptions being written for children and adolescents (Boodman 2012; McClellan and Werry 2003; Parens and Johnston 2008). American data showed a dramatic increase in psychotropic drug use from the 1990s to the 2000s among children and adolescents, a population for which few such medications are approved (Olfson et al. 2006a; Thomas et al. 2006). Concerning the more widespread use of schizophrenia drugs among children, who are presumably too young in most cases to manifest the condition, one US study found a more than doubling of young persons being prescribed atypical antipsychotics from 2001 to 2005, with 41 percent of new users having "no diagnosis for which treatment was supported by a published study" (Pathak et al. 2010, 123). Canadian data similarly showed a significant increase in antidepressant prescriptions for persons under eighteen from the 1990s to the 2000s (Branham 2004; Mitchell et al. 2008). As with the study by Pathak and colleagues, researchers in Manitoba (Alessi-Severini et al. 2008, 2012) found a substantial increase in antipsychotic prescriptions given to young persons, from 1.9 per 1,000 in 1999 to 7.4 per 1,000 in 2008, despite there being no clear diagnostic indication (other than "aggressive behaviour") in a number of cases. Data from the US suggest that some of the increase in antipsychotic prescriptions is a result of the controversial practice of diagnosing bipolar disorder in children, in some cases, re-diagnosing young persons previously considered to have ADHD (Boodman 2012).

Prescribing for young persons carries with it a particular set of practical and ethical concerns (such as diagnostic uncertainty), given that psychiatric syndromes may only manifest clearly in adulthood. Another concern is that the safety and efficacy of psychotropic drugs with this age group has not been adequately tested because children have not traditionally been included in research trials (Garland 2004; McClellan and Werry 2003). Should they be? There is the argument that, without such an evidence base, children may be deprived of potential benefits from these medications or, conversely, exposed to unknown side effects and unnecessary risks (Matsui et al. 2003). The counter-arguments include questions about the capacity of a child to give informed consent for participation in trials as well as concern that differences in metabolism and pharmacokinetics between younger and older persons constitute an unreasonable exposure to harm (Baldwin and Kosky 2007). It would appear, in any case, that the inclusion argument has won, given that children and adolescents are now being recruited for psychotropic drug trials (e.g. Pierson 2009).[12]

The Issue of Medication Non-Adherence[13]

It has been well established that a significant number of clients will alter or discontinue a regimen of psychotropic medication, often after only a very short period of time (Olfson, Marcus and Ascher-Svanum 2007). As noted above, three-quarters of participants in the large-scale CATIE trials discontinued antipsychotic medication by eighteen months. Similarly, a study from Quebec, using data from the provincial health insurance plan, found that about 60 percent of clients discontinued using antipsychotic medication in the first year of treatment (Cooper et al. 2005). Non-adherence, particularly to antipsychotic medication, is often viewed by practitioners as a sign of "poor insight," and, indeed, there is evidence from clinical and research settings that a lack of awareness or denial of mental illness is a major reason for discontinuation (Arango and Amador 2011; Kessler et al. 2001; Olfson et al. 2006b). For some, the issue is not so much unawareness as actually enjoying the effects of the disorder, such as the client who told this author that medication "prevents me from having a religious experience." Notably, persons in a manic state may often enjoy the "high" that they are feeling.

It has been argued that "unawareness" is part of the underlying pathology of the disorder itself ("anosognosia") and, hence, is beyond the individual's control (see box). The Treatment Advocacy Center, a medically oriented organization that promotes involuntary treatment options, goes a step further down the path of biological fatalism to suggest that, for persons so affected, there is no point investing a lot of resources to make service systems attractive and culturally relevant: "Such individuals will not voluntarily utilize psychiatric services, no matter how attractive those services are, because they do not believe that they have an illness" (Treatment Advocacy Center

Anosognosia

Anosognosia is a term that comes from neurology and refers to unawareness of an obvious deficit, an unawareness that presumably is a result of damage to the brain, such as someone not being able to recognize a paralyzed limb as their own following a stroke (Steingard 2012). More recently this concept has been applied to mental illness, with psychologist Xavier Amador (Amador 2009; Arango and Amador 2011) writing about the "lack of insight" (unawareness) sometimes seen in persons with schizophrenia as also being a form of anosognosia, distinguishing unawareness from *denial*. The Treatment Advocacy Center (TAC) (2005), a conservative US lobbying group, has taken up this hypothesis, suggesting that 50 percent of persons with schizophrenia have anosognosia and using this claim to support more widespread use of involuntary treatment since, presumably, affected persons cannot help themselves. The empirical basis for this has been the subject of heated debate, with psychiatrist Sandra Steingard (2012) arguing that the studies being used to support the claim offer equivocal results and that importing the term "anosognosia" into psychiatry "confers a certain sophistication of understanding and knowledge that is not supported by the data." Writing for TAC, Torrey (2012) offers a rebuttal, concluding – unequivocally – that "anosognosia is caused by damage to the brain caused by the schizophrenia disease process" and that "mental health professionals who deny that schizophrenia is a brain disease ... are simply demonstrating their ignorance." The difficulty with this message – that unawareness of illness is in many cases "hard wired" and intractable – is that it may have the effect of supporting the stigmatizing "us-versus-them" distinction that is applied to mentally ill persons since any of us may engage in denial, but only an unfortunate few (apparently) have a form of unawareness that is biologically based. At this writing, the jury is still out on the legitimacy of anosognosia in the context of schizophrenia, and it is a concept still relatively unknown in mental health settings.[14]

2009b, 2). When lack of awareness of a confirmed mental illness results in non-adherence and dangerous behaviour, clinicians may consider other methods of drug administration, such as injection.

Interestingly, "resisting medicine" is not unique to persons being prescribed psychotropic drugs: researchers have found high drop-out rates, close to 50 percent, according to one estimate (Pound et al. 2005), among *all* persons being treated for long-term illnesses. This is a significant finding since it suggests there is something in the "human condition," common to all of us, that makes medicine-taking a challenge. In a literature review on this subject, starting from the perspective that research in this area has lacked qualitative approaches and neglected the client perspective, Pound and colleagues (2005) found the following:

- Taking medication is an evaluative process, involving the weighing of costs and benefits, which includes a consideration of adverse effects and the complexity of the regimen. As part of this evaluation, people may stop taking medication to "see what happens." It may be difficult for some to face the idea of taking a drug(s) indefinitely, particularly if there is perceived uncertainty of diagnosis. Self-dosing and experimenting with medication may also speak to the need for a sense of control in one's life, control that is diminished by a lengthy drug regimen (see also Gumpp 2009).
- Non-adherence may have to do with personal identity. If taking a medication is associated with having a mental illness, some may be unwilling to accept this identity. This is more than simply unawareness or "anosognosia," and may have to do with the substantial stigma associated with a psychiatric label.
- Medicine-taking can have a coercive aspect to it, related to the need to "fit in." The authors note that people on antipsychotic medication "perceive the existence of an unwritten social contract; take the medicine in order to be tolerated by the community [and] felt that medicine was used to control them and make them acceptable to society" (Pound et al. 2005, 146).

In working with persons who benefit from psychotropic medication, practitioners need to actively identify the client's concerns. While clinicians may feel sure that they know what the issues are, studies comparing clients' and physicians' responses to a "reasons-for-stopping-medication" survey have found, in many instances, a low level of agreement between the two groups (Pope and Scott 2003). One obvious area of concern is side effects, which can include movement disorders, weight gain, and diminished sex drive – matters no one should take lightly (Goldacre 2008; Gumpp 2009). As reviewed by Andrews and colleagues (2000), practitioners should closely monitor these effects and, where necessary, consider changing the medication, reducing the dose, prescribing divided doses, making sure medications are taken with appropriate food, or adding a medication to treat the side effects. Strategies can also be employed for particular side effects, concerning diet, exercise, and alcohol and caffeine intake. As noted above, another area of concern may be the complexity of the medication regimen, which may require taking a number of different pills at various times of the day and night. (Hospitals may initiate regimens to which adherence is difficult in community settings.) Administration orders should be streamlined as much as possible (ideally to once-a-day), and clients may be assisted by having medications put in blister packs or dosette containers. Valenstein and colleagues (2011) describe an effective "pharmacy-based intervention" involving dosettes, education, and early notification of both client and clinician. A third area of concern is the client who works or goes to school and finds that the drugs impair concentration. There is no easy solution here since improved concentration must be weighed against the additional stress of returning to employment, stress that may be compensated for, at least in part, with medication. In sum, practitioners need to be aware of activities and abilities that are important to the client and that are affected by medication use since not addressing these will only increase ambivalence (Deegan 2007).

In some cases clients will make the unilateral decision to stop taking medication. Often, because of fear of judgment, they will not disclose this to the attending doctor, who may find out later by accident. Concerns about stopping medication must be put in the context of the known likelihood and degree of risk should the client become ill and the speed with which this may happen (on this matter see the useful decision-making guide developed by Toronto psychiatrists Christopher Tam and Samuel Law [2007]). When aware that their client has stopped medication "against medical advice" practitioners should strive to keep communication channels open and maintain contact rather than shutting down the therapeutic relationship, which has been known to happen.[15] The advantage here, apart from the ability to monitor the health and safety of the client when off medication, is that the client will, it is hoped, see the worker as someone who will stick with him or her in good times and in bad. As Tam and Law (2007, 459) suggest, this "may help in the development or repair of a therapeutic alliance over the long term." By way of example, Canadian author Victoria Maxwell (2012), in describing her own experiences with mental illness, offers appreciation for the enduring, non-judgmental support offered by her parents even when she was refusing treatment: "When the time came and I finally realized I needed help, the unwavering acceptance they had shown allowed me to reach out to them for that help."

This again points to the importance of the therapeutic relationship, referring to active listening, being respectful, and trying to involve the client in treatment decisions. Not surprisingly, a poor therapeutic alliance has been found to be associated with greater medication non-adherence (Day et al. 2005). A qualitative study by Vancouver author Ruth Gumpp (2009) found that trust in the prescribing doctor was critically important for mental health clients, in particular when treatment seemed like trial-and-error, and that it made listening to and trying out the doctor's suggestions more likely. The study also found that trust:

- took time to develop;
- was *enhanced* by the physician's taking enough time and addressing all the issues raised;
- was enhanced by the belief that the doctor was acting in the client's best interests;
- was enhanced by the belief that the doctor *also trusted the client;* and
- was *diminished* by not "getting better," by experiencing too many side effects, or by the perception that the doctor was not telling tell the truth.

Ideally, decision making about medications should be a shared process between client and practitioner, a practice consistent with the ultimate goal of self-management of medical conditions (Bilsker, Goldner, and Jones 2007). However, shared decision making with reference to *psychiatric* medication use, especially with persons diagnosed with psychotic conditions, has been an idea generally greeted with skepticism. Seale and colleagues (2006, 2,862) note that paternalistic modes of decision making may be justified "when insight is impaired" but that, given the pessimistic attitudes about schizophrenia held by practitioners, there may be "an inappropriate readiness to reach a judgment of incompetence." Tools and guidelines to support shared decision making have been developed, and, on this topic, the reader is directed to the work of Patricia Deegan (e.g., Deegan 2007; Deegan et al. 2008).

Other Physical Treatments

ECT
Electroconvulsive therapy (ECT) involves inducing a minor brain seizure by the application of a brief electric current to sites on the scalp. The procedure has been in use since the mid-1930s, when it was administered to individuals with schizophrenia, this based on the observation that schizophrenic symptoms decreased after a seizure and on the (unfounded) belief that schizophrenia and epilepsy could not coexist in the same person.

A major problem with early versions of ECT was the discomfort that it produced and the fact that some seizures were severe enough to result in broken bones. With improvements in anaesthesia and muscle relaxants, these severe consequences have largely been eliminated, and, despite a negative public image, the technique is now considered safe and effective (Andrews et al. 2000; Fink 2011; Mathew et al. 2007). The most common side effects of ECT are short-term headaches and muscle pain; a more significant side effect is memory impairment, although this is transient in most cases.

Nowadays, ECT is primarily used for persons suffering from depression, particularly when other treatments (medication and psychotherapy) have failed or when there is an increased risk of self-neglect or suicide, and it seems to be especially effective with forms of depression in which somatic or psychotic symptoms are present. The exact mechanism by which this is achieved is still not fully understood (see Fink 2011). Treatments are usually administered three times a week for one to five weeks. This is sometimes done on an outpatient basis, but usually the patient is hospitalized. ECT is more commonly given to older adults (Rapoport, Mamdani, and Herrmann 2006).

RTMS
A relatively new treatment for depression, which has some parallels with ECT, is repetitive transcranial magnetic stimulation (RTMS). This technique, developed in the mid-1980s, has moved from experimental status, to being offered in private clinics, to now being offered through public health systems, including those in Toronto and Vancouver. The procedure involves a hand-held electrical coil, which is positioned on the scalp and creates a magnetic pulse that passes through the brain. An advantage of RTMS is that it is non-invasive, does not require a general anaesthetic, and does not produce seizures, possibly offering some advantages to frail patients (Haynes 2002). In the September 2008 edition of the *Canadian Journal of Psychiatry*, several articles were devoted to evaluating the efficacy of RTMS, with the general conclusion that this technology was promising but that "further studies are needed before RTMS can be considered as a first-line monotherapy treatment" (Lam et al. 2008). In the author's health region, RTMS is offered on an outpatient basis for persons with mild to moderate depression who are not candidates for ECT and who have experienced a poor response to medications.

Limbic Surgery
A procedure called limbic surgery is used – in rare circumstances – as a treatment of last resort for persons with severe forms of obsessive-compulsive disorder and depression. This procedure involves positioning the patient's

head in a metal frame, bilaterally drilling small holes in the skull, then using a heated instrument to produce a small lesion (about the size of a pea) in the brain tissue. Eligibility criteria are very strict: persons accepted for surgery must have been suffering from severe incapacitation for at least five years (which often means chronic suicidality) and must have tried and failed every other available treatment (Haynes 2002).

Notes

1 Regarding the US situation, see Harris's (2011) report, "Talk Doesn't Pay, So Psychiatry Turns Instead to Drug Therapy."
2 Biological psychiatrist Jeffrey Lieberman (2011), speaking about the *DSM-5* incorporating biomarkers and laboratory tests to augment existing diagnostic criteria, concludes: "Sadly, this has proved to be beyond the reach of the current level of evidence," although adding that "this time is not far off." For example, researchers working with the private American company RBM have claimed that a test of fifty-one protein-based biomarkers can help confirm a diagnosis of schizophrenia (Schwarz et al. 2010). In another example, researchers with Kings College in the UK used pattern-recognition techniques with MRI scans and concluded that this approach could help distinguish patients with bipolar disorder from healthy individuals (Rocha-Rego et al. 2013).
3 The claim that low mood is caused by insufficient serotonin levels has been disputed, for example, by Lacasse and Leo (2005), who state that "there is not a single peer-reviewed article that can be accurately cited to directly support claims of serotonin deficiency in any mental disorder." In a review, Whitaker (2010) notes that the low serotonin (depression) and high dopamine (psychosis) hypotheses predict different metabolite levels from "normals," but this has not been borne out. See also Begley (2010) and Johnson (2006).
4 There is disagreement as to whether the newer generation drugs are truly atypical with reference to their mechanism of action, and some have argued that it is presumptuous to consider them as "novel" in this respect (e.g., Owens 1999).
5 It may be that *subjectively* the side effect of weight gain (manifested in some cases as cravings) is tolerated better than EPS.
6 Grohol (2007) notes that the positive effects on cognition touted by previous studies were found to be artifacts of the study design.
7 Paliperidone is a metabolite of the older antipsychotic risperidone (see Chapter 8).
8 Protocols for how often tests are required, or whether they are required at all, vary from country to country.
9 While the newer drugs may be safer in overdose, their side effects – such as sexual dysfunction – may nonetheless be significant (see Goldacre 2008; and Begley 2010). For a description of other, under-recognized adverse effects, see Glenmullen (2000).
10 This last point is based on the idea that increased suicidal events tend to occur early on in treatment (Jick, Kaye, and Jick 2004), a claim that has been disputed. See Mittal, Brown, and Shorter (2009).
11 For example, there is some evidence that maternal depression during pregnancy is a risk factor for premature birth and lower birth weights (Picard 2009a).
12 In 2009, the US FDA approved the use of the antidepressant Lexapro with twelve- to seventeen-year-olds, although this was based on just four trials, with two of the four showing the product to be ineffective (Pierson 2009).
13 "Adherence" is used here in preference to "compliance," again recognizing the limitations of the language used in psychiatry. "Concordance" has also been used in this respect.

14 I raised the concept of anosognosia in a paper at a 2011 conference on mental health ethics (Davis 2011) and found that virtually no one in the audience – made up mostly of service providers – was familiar with the term.

15 This is a complicated matter in truth, and it may be related to fears of liability should the doctor be seen to be endorsing non-treatment and then have something go wrong. Agencies may have policies around closing files expeditiously when no treatment is being given, although note that this in effect defines "treatment" purely in pharmacological terms.

Education, Skills Training, and Cognitive-Behavioural Approaches

16

Philosophies about psychiatric treatment have shifted considerably over the past half-century, from Freudian theory and the practice of psychoanalysis in the 1950s and 1960s, to the rise of biological psychiatry and pharmacotherapy in the 1970s and 1980s, to the more recent influence and incorporation of cognitive-behavioural approaches as a first-line intervention – even for persons suffering from psychotic disorders. At the same time, and of equal if not greater significance, the *belief system* underlying our treatment approaches has been challenged, particularly the idea of the client as a dependent, passive recipient of professional wisdom and of the practitioner as a detached, expert/authority figure. In considering the growing emphasis on approaches to treatment and rehabilitation other than, or complementary to, pharmacotherapy, one can point to several contributing factors:

- *The limitations of medication.* While pharmacotherapy is often an important component of treatment, the fact remains that – for a number of reasons – not all persons with mental disorders benefit from taking medications. For example, it is estimated that one-third of persons with positive symptoms of schizophrenia will experience a poor response to antipsychotic medication (Stone et al. 2010). Regarding antidepressant drugs, as was described earlier in this book, systematic reviews of clinical trials have found a large proportion of treatment response to be duplicated in placebo control groups, making the specific benefit of the pharmaceutical agent difficult to determine. Given that conditions such as depression are often *multidetermined*, by social and lifestyle factors as well as by biology, this result may not be all that surprising. As one depression treatment manual concludes: "Medication is seldom a *complete* treatment" (Paterson et al. 1997, 8, emphasis in the original). Even if effective in one domain, medications may not be effective in others: studies of antipsychotic drug benefits have found little to suggest that these medications improve quality of life

(Jones et al. 2006) or functional outcomes (Swartz et al. 2007). Finally, an argument can be made to use alternative, psychological treatments in cases of early psychosis – when a diagnosis of schizophrenia is not yet established – because of the downsides of starting the client on medication (such as side effects).

- *Empirical support.* It can now be said that a number of non-pharmacological treatments and programs are evidence-based – that is, have been shown to be beneficial using randomized controlled trials (Dixon et al. 2010). This was not always the case in that earlier evaluations of psychotherapy and psychoanalysis (most famously, a review by British psychologist Hans Eysenck in 1952) either showed outcomes no better than those achieved with placebo or, more often than not, were impossible to conduct because of difficulties in operationalizing the concepts under consideration.[1] Currently, the evidence supporting the use of cognitive-behavioural approaches in the treatment of depression and anxiety disorders appears to be quite strong (Reger and Gahm 2009; Somers 2007).
- *Concerns of clients and advocacy groups.* A report from the Mental Health Advocate for British Columbia concluded that the government needed to "develop the workforce" – that is, improve the skill sets of mental health practitioners so that the system could move beyond a "custodial" approach to mental health care (Hall 2000, 31). In particular, the lack of staff training and service availability in the area of anxiety disorders – which are often responsive to behavioural treatments – came in for criticism. The mental health advocate noted that "the limited treatment strategies available through the regional system and fee for service medicine are not evidence-based and create dependencies" (14). Similarly, the President of AnxietyBC notes that "evidence-based interventions [for anxiety disorders] are received by only a minority of individuals who seek treatment ... unfortunately, many practitioners do not have the appropriate training to deliver evidence-based treatments" (quoted in AnxietyBC 2010). As another example, in an editorial entitled "Changing the Paradigm," a psychiatric service user criticizes the system's preoccupation with pharmacotherapy and speaks about the need for "medical coverage for non-drug medical support" such as "counseling, 'talk therapy' ... and coping skills education" (Thor-Larsen 2002, 4). Another service user observes, similarly, that few public mental health programs "offer any kind of in-depth counseling, a piece in the puzzle of recovery that is indispensible" (Carten 2006, 52).

This chapter gives an overview of the counselling and educational approaches most commonly used in public mental health programs in Canada. Admittedly, this is very ambitious, and interested readers are encouraged to pursue individual topics in more detail, with the references here serving as a preliminary guide. Psychodynamic treatments, such as psychoanalysis, are not covered here for several reasons: (1) these interventions are used predominantly by private practitioners; (2) they are used with individuals less disabled than those typically seen at public mental health centres;[2] and (3) there is uncertainty about the evidence base and benefits of a treatment such as psychoanalysis (Paris 2005a; Shorter 1997). It is assumed, and should be a given, that practitioners have some training in basic interviewing skills.

For the sake of clarity, this chapter is organized into separate sections on the various approaches. This may give the false impression that interventions are discrete entities, when in fact there are common elements. For example, separating "education and skills training" from "cognitive-behavioural approaches" is a false dichotomy in that many cognitive-behavioural approaches explicitly *involve* skills training and education. Finally, discussion on the implications for service delivery – staff training, mandates, how interventions should be offered and by whom – is included at the end of the chapter.

Education and Skills Training

While the importance of educating clients about their mental disorder may seem obvious, the idea that this is a necessary component of a treatment and recovery plan has been historically underappreciated. This was the result of several factors: (1) a model of "professional as authority/expert" that apparently did not include empowerment of clients; (2) during the mid-1900s, influential psychodynamic theories that placed the root of clients' psychiatric problems in the *unconscious* mind, meaning that self-help was by definition not possible; (3) clinical pessimism about the prognosis of disorders such as schizophrenia; and (4) evolution of a service delivery structure in which there was an over-reliance on pharmacotherapy to the neglect of other interventions. As an illustration, Canadian author Pavlina Vagnerova (2003a, 19) describes her frustration concerning information about her condition that was not forthcoming from treating professionals:

> Another turning point was when I was finally provided information about schizophrenia: the first diagnosis my doctors gave me. I asked them repeatedly for it, but for some reason they were reluctant to give it to me until almost the end, when they deemed I was "ready." Once I held this information in my hands and was able to read academic text – just like I used to for my classes at university – I realized that all the delusions of grandeur, paranoias and hallucinations I experienced had also been shared by many others before me. I also realized that I was not as special as I thought I was,

in the grand scheme of things, and that I would be able to lead the normal life I wished.

Self-described psychiatric survivor Pat Capponi (2003, xvi) summarizes the client perspective as follows: "The challenge for psychiatric survivors, then, is the same for anyone with a chronic illness: learn anything you can about what it is you're supposed to have; don't let it consume you; pay attention to triggers, learn what eases the pain; and understand how frustration and behavior can sometimes undermine you."

Practitioners can assist clients, and their friends and family, by imparting to them our best current understanding of treatment and rehabilitation issues. To this end, often the most useful service is telling people what something is *not*, since misconceptions about mental disorders continue to be widespread. Examples of these include the theory that depression is a sign of character weakness (see Chapter 6), that schizophrenia is a form of multiple personality, or that young persons in the early stages of a psychotic illness are simply being wilful and disobedient. There are a number of good sources for mental health information, such as the websites of organizations like Health Canada, the Canadian Mental Health Association, and the Schizophrenia Society of Canada, as well as books written for clients, families, and non-specialists, including some written by persons themselves recovering from psychiatric disability. Some periodicals, such as the *Psychiatric Rehabilitation Journal*, will routinely publish clients' accounts of their own struggles with mental disorder and other existential concerns.

While a newer development in psychiatry, Mueser and colleagues (2002) observe that educational approaches with clients suffering from chronic illnesses – such as diabetes, cancer, and heart disease – have been used for some time in medical practice. In extending this to the area of mental health, these authors note that the goal is "helping people collaborate with professionals in managing their mental illness while pursuing their personal recovery goals" (1,272). Canadian psychologist Dan Bilsker (2003, 4) describes this *self-management* model as

> an active engagement of the health care consumer in dealing with his or her disorder, meaning that the person with the disorder is an active participant in care, rather than someone who simply follows recommendations and complies with the treatment plan developed by a health professional ... [Clients are given] a central role in determining their care, one that fosters a sense of responsibility for their own health. Using a collaborative approach, providers and patients work together to define problems, set priorities, establish goals, create treatment plans and solve problems along the way.[3]

Responding to the argument that persons with mental disorders are too uninsightful or cognitively impaired to "self-manage," Bilsker concludes that, notwithstanding transitory periods of incapacity, "individuals with mental disorders have a considerable and *largely untapped* capacity to engage in self-management practices" (5, emphasis added).

Education may be delivered in a number of formats, including by the practitioner (either one-on-one or in the presence of friends and family) and through groups led or co-led by a practitioner, staff from a partner agency (such as the Schizophrenia Society), family members, or clients and peer-support workers. Presentations that include the insider perspective of a client are particularly powerful. Groups may be either less structured and more supportive or more structured and specialized, with sequences of "modules" covering particular topics. Of increasing concern in recent years has been the need to disseminate mental health information to the ethnic and immigrant community, preferably by persons familiar with the language and cultural values of this group.

Concerning who delivers the service, Mueser and colleagues (2002, 1,273) make a distinction between professionally led and peer-led education programs, noting that the former are "conducted in the context of a therapeutic relationship in which the teacher ... is responsible for the overall treatment," unlike the client's relationship with a peer. These authors describe the peer approach as an important alternative to the professional relationship, which may be perceived as hierarchical (see also Chapter 17). As noted above, the aim in self-management is a collaborative approach to recovery, something very much consonant with the current emphasis on shared decision making in psychiatric care (Drake and Deegan 2009). Concerning the evidence base, a systematic review of forty-four evaluative trials of schizophrenia psychoeducation programs found a participant benefit with respect to reduction in relapses and hospital length of stay, and improvement in medication adherence, although the authors noted that the studies were variable in quality (Xia, Merinder, and Belgamwar 2011).

Education inevitably overlaps with skills training, which is defined here as techniques, either cognitive or behavioural, that assist an individual in coping with or managing the effects of a disorder. "Effects" refers both to particular symptoms and to social situations that may be made difficult or more stressful because of deficits created by the disorder or because of responses by others to the disorder. A more detailed rationale for social skills training is given as follows:

> Almost by definition and by diagnostic criteria, an individual with a
> mental disability is likely to demonstrate deficits in social skills and social

adjustment. Sometimes this arises ... because the mental illness intervened early in adolescence or adulthood, before critical interpersonal and independent living skills could be acquired. Other deficits occur because of ... intrusion of positive and negative symptoms of psychosis or depression, current lack of environmental stimulation and learning opportunities, and cognitive impairments. With social functioning being a prime diagnostic indicator of long-term outcome of mental disorders, it becomes incumbent upon practitioners to teach social skills to the severely mentally ill. (Liberman 1998, 5)

In speaking about schizophrenia, Kopelowicz, Liberman, and Zarate (2006, S13) note that "social skills and social competence can be viewed as protective factors in the vulnerability-stress ... model of schizophrenia. Strengthening [these skills] can ... attenuate and compensate for the ... effects of cognitive deficits, neurobiological vulnerability, stressful events and social maladjustment."

In many instances, persons with mental disorders will come up with their own coping strategies in an attempt to confront, reframe, or deflect intrusive symptoms. While some will resort to using drugs and alcohol, credit must be given to the clients who have arrived at constructive strategies and lifestyle choices without the intervention of mental health professionals. Indeed, it can be argued that what we call "skills training" is simply a somewhat more systematic application of principles that clients have already been using in many cases.

Below are overviews of four potential problem areas commonly encountered in mental health practice and corresponding strategies that clients may employ to deal with them: (1) relapse prevention, (2) dealing with anxiety, (3) being assertive, and (4) structured problem solving.[4]

Relapse Prevention

"Relapse prevention" refers to a client's recognition of the *early warning signs* of a particular disorder, attention to *high-risk situations* that may exacerbate the disorder, and putting into action *early intervention strategies* that may head off potential problems. Signs that a client may be "slipping" are specific and unique to that person. Since the practitioner typically has more limited contact with the individual, he or she needs to rely on the client's self-report or, failing that, on the report of someone with intimate knowledge of the client, such as a spouse or parent. Self-detection of early signs is not always easy: in some cases the onset is so gradual that the client will not feel that anything is wrong or different. In other cases, the "window of opportunity" is extremely small: a client with bipolar disorder told this author that she tripped over into mania so quickly that there was no chance to respond other than to "go along for the ride." One client, diagnosed with bipolar disorder, describes the early warning signs as follows:

> I began to see patterns to my illness. There were certain reliable early signs of relapse that I could identify. I learned that an early symptom of my pending mania would be increased excitement and decreased need for sleep. The immediate effect of this would be fatigue. The fatigue manifested itself in several ways: a cold sore, a facial tic, hand tremor and neck stiffness. As the mania progressed, I developed racing thoughts, pressured speech and severe insomnia. Gradually I would turn the night into day – staying up all night, and sleeping only during the day. My apartment and my car would be a mess, and I would stay up nights writing poetry. Friends would comment that I didn't look myself, and that would embarrass or irritate me. (Winram 2002)

Once identified, the warning signs need to be articulated in some fashion, which may be done with a template that lists the signs and the planned responses (see below).

High-risk situations are those that are known to be associated with a worsening of the disorder or some other negative outcome. The logic here is often applied to persons with addictions, who learn to recognize that certain individuals or locations may prompt a return to substance use. For persons with mental disorders, a number of situations may be significant, such as reminders of loss (e.g., anniversary dates, visits to a previous residence) or stressful events (e.g., family reunions). Where possible clients should keep a journal and note when, where, and under what circumstances symptoms appear to get worse (Maguire 2002).

Early intervention strategies are those that the client can put into place before, or without, having to seek assistance from the mental health system – which may not be immediately available. Again, these strategies will be specific to the individual and can be written down for future reference. The client with bipolar disorder, cited above, speaks about his "emergency kit":

At the onset of hypomania, my "emergency kit" consists of:

- Taking a few days off work.
- Taking a sleeping pill (extra sleep early in the mania is the key).
- Increasing my mood-stabilizing medication and my antipsychotic medication.

- Phoning my psychiatrist to arrange for an emergency visit (but taking my increased medication immediately without waiting for the appointment).
- Reduce stress (it's not the time for me to contemplate romances or finances).
- Regular sleep, regular exercise, regular meals, reduced caffeine, no cigarettes or alcohol.
- Increased walking and listening to classical music to relax.
- I avoid the news or upsetting television.
- I stop driving my car (because of sedation from the medication or impulsively from the mania) (Winram 2002).

An example of a personal relapse prevention/crisis plan, adapted from a model created by Eric Macnaughton of the Canadian Mental Health Association (British Columbia Partners for Mental Health and Addictions Information 2003a), is as follows:

Signs that suggest I am doing well:

Events or situations that triggered relapses in the past:

Early warning signs that I experienced in the past:

Effective ways that I can cope if I experience early warning signs:

What early warning signs indicate that I need help from others:

Who I would like to assist me (names):

What I would like them to do:

If in crisis:

    Ways that I can manage stress, regain balance, or calm myself:
    People that I can call and their phone numbers:
    Resources that I can use (agencies, support groups):
    Things that I or other people can do that I find helpful:
    Medications that have helped in the past:
    Medications that have not helped or that have caused an adverse reaction:
    Medications that I am currently on:

Relaxation Training

Relaxation exercises are used to cope with symptoms such as panic attacks and are also used within the context of cognitive-behavioural treatments such as graded exposure (see below), in which the individual is deliberately exposed to anxiety-producing stimuli. One common technique for dealing with acute anxiety is to breath into a paper bag, which helps steady the level of carbon dioxide in the blood. A preferred method is a slow breathing exercise, which is used at the first signs of panic and at other times during the day for practice. The exercise takes about five minutes and involves the following steps (Andrews et al. 2000): (1) hold your breath and count to five; (2) at five, breathe out and say the word *relax*; (3) breathe in for three seconds, and out for three, saying *relax* with each outward breath; (4) at the end of each minute (ten breaths) hold your breath for five seconds; (5) continue until the anxiety subsides. This exercise may be used on its own or as the lead-in to progressive muscle relaxation, which takes about another fifteen minutes. This involves alternately tensing (for about ten seconds) then relaxing (for about ten seconds) in sequence: the hands, lower arms, upper arms, shoulders, neck, forehead and scalp, eyes, jaw, tongue, chest, stomach, back, buttocks, thighs, calves, and feet.

Assertiveness Skills

Clients may lack the ability to communicate opinions, needs, and feelings in an effective manner. In particular, communication styles may be overly passive or overly aggressive. In the former case, one runs the risk of being taken advantage of, and in the latter, there is the danger of antagonizing and alienating others. While communication may be a problem area for any of us, mental health clients may be more likely to have deficits for a number of reasons: (1) the onset of the disorder may have interrupted the normal course of developing relationship skills; (2) clients may come from chaotic family backgrounds in which role models were either absent, negligent, or abusive; (3) clients may be estranged from family, socially isolated, and have no way to practice conversation skills; (4) clients disproportionately reside in inner-city, skid-row, and institutional settings, where "getting by" requires placing a premium on toughness; and (5) alternately, passive styles may be fostered in psychiatric hospital, residential, and treatment settings, in which the professionals "call the shots."

When teaching assertiveness, the costs of staying with the present style of interaction need to be weighed against the benefits, with at some point – it is hoped – the scales being tipped in favour of more effective communication. (This can be done with the use of a two-by-two "decisional balance grid.") For example, the client may acknowledge that being passive is a way of avoiding conflict but, with encouragement, may see that this has a cost in terms of self-respect, respect from others, and independence. Common myths about assertiveness can be described to clients (Andrews et al. 2000): (1) the myth of humility – "be humble at all costs" – which may lead to putting oneself down all the time and creating a poor self-image; (2) the myth of the good friend, which is the idea that companions should somehow know intuitively what you want, when, more often than not, open discussion is needed; (3) the myth of anxiety, referring to avoiding anxiety-producing situations – such as being assertive – at all costs, when in reality some degree of anxiety is normal; (4) the myth of obligation, which holds that you must always grant a favour to an associate when asked; and (5) the myth of sex roles – "it's not feminine (or masculine) to do that" – an example being the woman as "nagging wife" who stands up for herself. Andrews and colleagues (2000) list what they call "protective skills," to be used as a last resort in extreme situations when nothing seems to be working. These include:

- *"Broken record"*: repeating an answer over and over – without explanation – to someone who is not prepared to let you say "no" gracefully, such as a pushy salesman.
- *"Selective ignoring"*: not responding when someone continues to badger you about something despite a clear message that you no longer wish to discuss the topic.
- *"Disarming anger"*: stating that you will not respond until the person calms down.
- *"Separating issues"*: for example, "It's not that I don't care for you, it's just that I don't wish to lend you money."
- *"Dealing with guilt"*: Don't let people guilt-trip you, and, in particular, don't use the phrase "I'm sorry" unless there are good reasons to apologize.

In assertiveness training, clients may be given scenarios in which they role play or describe what they would do before practising these in real-world situations, later getting feedback from the practitioner or group.

Structured Problem Solving

Structured problem solving is a process by which clients learn to identify for themselves problem areas and optimal solutions. While the concepts may seem straightforward, it must be emphasized that for some clients the ability to focus and prioritize will be impaired by symptoms that can include thought disorder, anxiety, depression, rumination, perseveration, and diminished concentration. The steps involved are as follows (Andrews et al. 2000):

- *Identifying problems or goals.* One rule here is that problems/goals should be considered one at a time; additional problems may be addressed on another occasion. Another guideline is that goals should be specific, realistic, and achievable and that the client – not the practitioner – should "own" the goal. If someone sets a goal at a high level and does not achieve it (e.g., because he or she is depressed), this failure represents another setback that may further reduce morale and motivation. For this reason, where possible, working towards an ultimate goal in small steps – "mini-goals" – is recommended (Paterson 1997).

- *Generating ideas through brainstorming.* The individual comes up with as many alternative solutions as possible without worrying at this point about how useful they may be.
- *Evaluating solutions.* What are the pros and cons of each? How feasible are they?
- *Choosing the best solution.* Often it is better to choose something that can be implemented sooner rather than later: even if the results are mixed, the individual may still learn something useful from the experience.
- *Planning.* What specifically needs to be done to put this into action?
- *Review.* What went right (or wrong)? What alternatives might now be tried?

Here the practitioner should be encouraging, and outcomes should be framed as partial successes rather than as failures.

BRIDGES and WRAP

There are several education models that incorporate components such as assertiveness, relapse prevention, and crisis planning. An example of a program offered in Canada through the Schizophrenia Society, created and led by service users rather than professionals, is BRIDGES (Building Recovery of Individual Dreams and Goals through Education and Support). BRIDGES has the following format (BC Schizophrenia Society 2010):

CLASS 1: The Foundation of BRIDGES (Emotional Stages of Recovery, Principles of Support)

CLASS 2: Mood Disorders: Depression, Bipolar Disorder (Coping Skills: Excerpts from WRAP~Wellness Recovery Action Plan)

CLASS 3: Thought Disorders: Schizophrenia (Relapse Prevention)

CLASS 4: Anxiety Disorders and Mini Module Chosen by Class (Use and Misuse of Diagnosis)

Module Subjects to Choose from:
- Personality Disorders
- Eating Disorders
- Attention Deficit Disorder
- Concurrent Disorder
- Dissociative Identity Disorder

CLASS 5: Helpful Support (Circle of Support, Mental Health Services, *Crisis Planning, Suicide Prevention*)

CLASS 6: Medications and the Brain (Talking to Your Doctor about Medications)

CLASS 7: Problem Management Method

CLASS 8: Communication (Active Listening, Non-Verbal Communication, Reflective Response and Assertive Communication)

CLASS 9: Module Chosen by Class (Healthy Spirituality, Self-injury)

CLASS 10: Advocacy and Graduation (Patients' Rights, Do's and Don't's of Advocacy)

Another influential curriculum, being disseminated in a number of North American settings, is WRAP (Wellness Recovery Action Plan), conceived by Mary Ellen Copeland, an American educator and someone who herself was treated and hospitalized for bipolar disorder (see website at http://mentalhealthrecovery.com/). Like BRIDGES, WRAP is designed to be taught by service users, with the intent of creating an individualized plan/document with which to better manage stressors and crises. WRAP modules include creating a "wellness toolbox" and a daily maintenance plan, identifying "triggers" and early warning signs, and crisis planning.

What is the evidence base for mental health education programs? An evaluation of BRIDGES was conducted by Cook and colleagues (2012) in a study where 428 subjects were randomly assigned to BRIDGES or to a service-as-usual waiting list. Following the course completion, it was found that, compared to controls, BRIDGES participants had significantly greater improvement in measurements of self-perceived recovery and hopefulness. The effectiveness of WRAP was examined in a study by Cook and colleagues (2011), in which 519 persons were randomly assigned to either the intervention or a control group. The outcome measures were symptom profiles, hopefulness, and quality of life, "outcome areas that are widely acknowledged to be indicators of recovery" (8), assessed using established self-report instruments at the end of the program and six months later. It was found that the benefits to WRAP participants compared to control subjects reached statistical significance across all three measures and persisted for at least six months.[5] More generally, a review of studies of education programs targeting persons with schizophrenia found them to be effective: Xia, Merinder, and Belgamwar (2011) undertook a systematic review of published studies up to 2010, with forty-four meeting the standard of randomized controlled trials, incorporating 5,142 (mostly hospitalized) participants. The authors concluded that there were benefits from education with respect to reducing relapse and re-admission, reducing the length of hospital stay, and adherence to medication regimens. Studies that have looked at the acquisition, retention, and transfer of social skills have produced more mixed results (see Canadian Psychiatric Association 2005). In a review, Kopelowicz, Liberman, and Zarate (2006, S15) note that published studies found "substantial improvements in participants' knowledge and behaviors as the result of training" but that the findings concerning transferability of skills were more discouraging. This may change, at least in the vocational domain, with newer models that emphasize learning skills specific to a particular work environment (see Becker and Drake [2003], and also Chapter 17).

Cognitive Remediation
We now know that for people suffering from an illness like schizophrenia, cognitive deficits cause problems with respect to functioning at school, work, and in relationships and may be more significant even than positive symptoms in this respect (Carter 2006; Eack and Keshavan 2008; Medalia, Revheim, and Herlands 2009). Previously, cognitive symptoms were believed to be secondary to other features, such as psychosis; we now understand them to be a primary symptom that may persist even when the psychosis is under control. Responding to this can involve *adaptations*, which may include memory aids, visual cues, and recording devices; *compensatory strategies*, which include mnemonic aids to help with memory; and *remediation* techniques. Cognitive remediation methods vary, but usually include drills and exercises using computerized software, paper and pencil tasks, and group activities (Aldhous 2009; Medalia, Revheim and Herlands 2009). In addition to adults with psychotic disorders, there is evidence that cognitive remediation benefits older adults with cognitive impairment associated with aging (Belleville et al. 2006).

An example of a cognitive remediation program is given by Fisher and colleagues (2009). In this study, fifty-five clinically stable clients diagnosed with schizophrenia were randomly assigned to either fifty hours of computerized auditory training or to a control condition using computer games. The training consisted of daily, progressively more difficult exercises, designed to improve the speed and accuracy of auditory information processing. Relative to the control group, subjects who received active training showed significant gains in global cognition, verbal working memory, and verbal learning and memory. A different approach is described by Wykes and colleagues (2007), consisting of forty face-to-face sessions, each involving a number of paper and pencil tasks that provided practice in a variety of cognitive skills set out in a manual. In their evaluation these authors found that, compared to a control group receiving "treatment as usual," participants showed durable improvements in working memory, which, in turn, predicted improvement in social functioning. Cognitive remediation approaches have expanded from information processing to "reality monitoring" – the ability to distinguish internal from external cues – with a group of American researchers finding that a computer-based cognitive training curriculum was able to improve reality monitoring compared to those in a computer games control condition (Subramaniam et al. 2012). A meta-analysis (Wykes et al. 2011) concluded that cognitive remediation is beneficial for persons with schizophrenia, particularly when participants are clinically stable, and even more so when the therapy is provided in a coordinated fashion with other psychiatric rehabilitation interventions. Currently, cognitive remediation is considered a "promising practice," having a body of supportive evidence but not yet achieving the full status of "evidence-based" (Dixon et al. 2010).

Group Delivery

Skills-training and cognitive behavioural treatments may be carried out with individuals but in many cases are conducted in a group format. The rationale for group delivery is quoted here at some length:

> For many reasons ... group therapy is the principal modality for doing social skills training. Training patients in a group is more cost effective, enhanced by the cohesion established among the participants, augmented by having peers serve as models and reinforcers for each other, providing an opportunity for self-help and peer support, and a context for participants to learn from each other's real-life experiences and efforts at problem solving. Training is often defined in a non-stigmatizing fashion as education, with the patients being able to tell their friends and families that they are attending a class in human relations or community life. (Kopelowicz, Liberman, and Zarate 2006, S15)

Lecomte and Lecomte (2002, 54) highlight the potential advantage of *normalization* that is offered in groups: "In therapy, learning that one's problems are not unique is a powerful source of relief ... Cognitive-behavioral therapy, especially in a group format, validates the client's experience through the sharing of similar symptoms, distress and coping strategies." Randomized trials have found that group treatments, for example to manage bipolar disorder, can be as effective as individual counselling (Parikh et al. 2012).

The Trans-Theoretical Model and Motivational Interviewing

Motivational interviewing (MI) is introduced here because it is an influential treatment model, originally used in the addictions field, that is seen as having broad applicability across a number of counselling and psychiatric rehabilitation settings (Miller and Rollnick 2009; Westra, Aviram, and Doell 2011). Having at least some understanding of the principles of MI is now seen as a core competency for clinicians working in mental health settings. That said, it is not a method that is easily described or learned, and interested readers are referred to other sources for a fuller explication (e.g., Miller and Rollnick 2009; Rosengren 2009; Naar-King and Suarez 2011).

Motivational interviewing starts with the premise that most clients approach the relationship with the practitioner with *ambivalence* – indeed, while in some cases they may have sought help voluntarily, in others they may have been cajoled or coerced. This ambivalence is seen as a natural state of affairs in that people rarely want to give up control over their lives, but it is not necessarily an indication that the client is unwilling to change. In the case of someone misusing drugs or alcohol, the substances may not initially be perceived as a problem but as the *solution* to a person's problems. For example, a survey of untreated heavy drinkers published in the journal *Addiction Research and Theory* found that, despite what others might think, perceived benefits of drinking outweighed the drawbacks for the subjects themselves (a fact that the authors noted "challenges ... health promotion efforts") (Orford et al. 2002, 347). Not accounting for this ambivalence may be an obstacle to engaging or keeping a person in treatment.

Motivational interviewing is associated with what is called the *trans-theoretical model of change* (TTM), originally developed by Prochaska and DiClemente (1984). Miller and Rollnick (2009, 130) make the distinction that the trans-theoretical model is a conceptual model of how and why changes occur, whereas MI is a "specific clinical method to enhance personal motivation for change." The TTM makes explicit the observation that people entering treatment systems may not be ready for change and that interventions should be adjusted to the person's level of readiness. In this model people are seen as being at one of five stages:

- *Precontemplation:* not thinking of making a change.
- *Contemplation:* thinking of making a change but undecided.
- *Preparation:* prepared to take action – for example, "within the next thirty days."
- *Action:* engaged in doing things to change their behaviour.
- *Maintenance:* have made changes, and are working to stay on track.

The client may move through these changes or may in fact relapse and fall back to an earlier stage. In each stage the practitioner's tasks are somewhat different, with motivational interviewing used more commonly in the first two stages to move the person towards action.

- With precontemplation, the worker's task is to raise doubt and to increase the client's perception of the risks and problems associated with current behaviours.
- With contemplation, the worker is endeavouring to "tip the balance," evoke reasons to change and the risks of not changing, and support client self-efficacy.
- With preparation, the worker gives the client options and helps him or her to determine the best course of action to take in seeking change (see "structured problem solving" above).
- With action, the worker helps the individual to take these first steps.
- With maintenance, the worker helps the client to identify and use strategies to prevent relapse (see discussion on "relapse prevention" above).
- With relapse, the worker helps the client to renew the process and to address possible demoralization.

Motivational interviewing, according to the two clinical psychologists credited with developing it, is a "collaborative, person-centered form of guiding to elicit and strengthen motivation for change" (Miller and Rollnick 2009, 137). Expanding on this, these authors speak about "the assumption and honoring of personal autonomy," and the goal of "eliciting the person's own inherent arguments for change, not imposing someone else's" (131). When engaged in motivational interviewing, the practitioner should be guided by the following principles:

- *Express empathy:* the worker should be accepting rather than judgmental, use reflective listening, and recognize that ambivalence is normal.
- *Develop discrepancy:* the worker contrasts client goals and values with current behaviours, develops the discrepancy between where the client is and where he or she wants to be, makes the person aware of consequences, and allows the client to present arguments for change.
- *Avoid argumentation:* arguments and confrontation breed defensiveness and denial; resistance may be a signal to change strategies.
- *Roll with resistance:* opposing resistance may only reinforce it; instead, validate the client's perspective and use the individual as a resource for finding solutions.

- *Support self-efficacy:* the client is ultimately responsible for choosing and carrying out change strategies.

There is still some question as to mechanism – that is, how exactly MI produces changes in behaviour (Westra, Aviram, and Doell 2011). MI sessions are based around the therapist promoting "change talk" and moving the client away from what is called "sustain talk," which refers to arguments for keeping things the way they are. To do this, a number of strategies are used for evoking change talk ("how would you go about this?") and responding to it (affirmation, asking for elaboration), and these can be observed and coded in MI training sessions. As reviewed by Miller and Rose (2009, 533), based on empirical evaluation, it does appear that (1) the MI method influences change talk, and, in turn, (2) "the natural language utterances of clients do predict behaviour change." These authors suggest that change talk has some parallels with the symbolic importance of an engagement between two romantic partners, as a public commitment that is accompanied by shifts in self-perception.

A second major component of MI, also found to be empirically related to positive outcomes, concerns the client-counsellor relationship, in particular the skills of collaboration and empathic understanding (Miller and Rose 2009).[6] Conversely, there are clinician behaviours that may evoke resistance to change: argumentation, paternalism, being the "expert," shaming, labelling, and being in a hurry (getting ahead of the client's readiness) (Miller and Rollnick 2009).

Cognitive-Behavioural Therapies
Cognitive-behavioural therapy (CBT) in its various forms is increasingly being used to address a wide range of mental health problems and has become the predominant non-pharmacological approach to treating and managing psychiatric disorders in public mental health programs in North America and other Western countries. Originally used in the treatment of depression and anxiety disorders, its application has expanded to include schizophrenia and bipolar disorder, which is "noteworthy ... because it challenges what has, until recently, been a dominance of biological approaches to these disorders" (Lynch, Laws, and McKenna 2010, 9). According to Somers (2007, 1) CBT "holds a unique status in the field of mental health [in that it] is effective for many psychological problems, is relatively brief, and is well-received by individuals." CBT treatments are now available online, with a meta-analysis of published trials finding this modality to be as effective as in-person treatment (Reger and Gahm 2009).[7]

What is CBT? "[It] is less like a single intervention and more like a family of treatments and practices" (Somers 2007, 3). Some approaches may be more "behavioural," some more "cognitive," and others a combination of these two. Common features are that it is time-limited, follows a structured style of intervention, focuses on the present, and is practical or problem-focused (versus, for example, psychoanalytic approaches that look for underlying psychic "root causes") (Somers 2007). CBT in some cases may be delivered in a self-help or guided self-help format. Called "low-intensity CBT," this approach is more suited to persons experiencing mild to moderate levels of distress (Livingston et al. 2009). CBT has been adapted for use with other cultures and languages, and a report on its application with Chinese-Canadian clients found, interestingly, that elements particular to the approach – being time-limited, practical, and having an educational focus – were especially well received by this population (Kam and Ng 2009). Concerning the "structured style of intervention," fidelity to treatment protocols is encouraged in CBT: a commentator notes that persons who talk about having "failed" at CBT may in fact have been exposed to something "CBT-like" that fell short of a systematic application of the complete model (Lott 2001). What follows is an overview of CBT treatments and their evidence base, as applied to different syndrome areas.

Behavioural Techniques

Behavioural techniques are based on principles of conditioning and social learning first articulated by psychology pioneers such as John Watson, B.F. Skinner, and Albert Bandura. These techniques have traditionally been used with persons with anxiety disorders, behavioural problems, and sexual disorders such as pedophilia. Behavioural methods are also used in the treatment of autism (Cooper, Heron, and Heward 2007). A key underlying principle here is that the consequences of a client's behaviour will be either reinforcing or not. Based on this, a clinician can design contingencies to diminish unwanted responses, such as severe anxiety in anticipation of being in a public place.

Using the treatment of phobias as an example, the approach used will usually involve either *graded exposure* – exposure to a graduated hierarchy of situations that the client finds anxiety-provoking – or prolonged exposure ("flooding") until there is a recognition that no harm will come to the person. An example of the latter would be a person extremely fearful of germs being asked to continue touching a "contaminated" object until the anxiety dissipated (see Abramowitz 2006); an example of the former would be gradually – over a period of weeks – increasing the distance travelled from home for someone suffering from agoraphobia. To help manage the anxiety, clients are taught techniques such as slow breathing or muscle relaxation, used at the beginning of the session to try to ensure that the individual is calm and during the session if anxiety rises. Through conditioning – since the relaxation response is incompatible with anxiety – anxiety symptoms will, it is hoped, be extinguished. For more detailed descriptions of these types of interventions see, for example, Andrews and colleagues (2000) and Canadian Psychiatric Association (2006). While behavioural treatments of anxiety disorders have traditionally been done *in vivo*, more recently, virtual reality technologies have been used to create three-dimensional representations of anxiety-producing stimuli, with the results of these "virtual" exposure therapies apparently being generalizable to the real world (MacDonald 2002). This technique may be particularly beneficial in treating children.

Other behavioural techniques, referred to as "contingency management," involve systems of rewards and punishments designed to elicit positive, and to extinguish, negative behaviours, an example being the concept of the "token economy," which was formerly used in psychiatric hospitals. Such methods may be applied in institutional settings with very disabled persons, such as children suffering from severe forms of autism. This approach has also been used in addiction treatment programs, in which participants with negative drug screens are rewarded by being given vouchers with monetary value (Roll et al. 2006).

Because behavioural treatments have been shown to be effective in diminishing distressing thoughts and behaviours, adherents have been able to argue that tracing a symptom back to its psychic origins, as per psychodynamic theory, is unnecessary. As one text concludes: "Behavior therapies will have a secure and valued position in the history of psychology because they helped lay to rest the hallowed notion of *symptom substitution* ... as a result, the avenue was opened for the development of specific techniques for dealing with specific patient complaints" (Phares and Trull 1997, 399, emphasis in original).

CBT and Depression

Cognitive treatments consider the ways that distorted thinking – irrational, unrealistic, or self-defeating beliefs and interpretations – can affect an individual's mental and emotional state. In other words, how a person feels and acts depends more on what she or he *thinks* is going on than on what, more objectively, is happening. Pioneered by clinicians such as Aaron Beck and Albert Ellis, and originally designed for persons with mood and anxiety disorders (particularly depression), cognitive approaches have become increasingly influential and have been extended and modified for use with clients with personality and psychotic disorders.

As summarized by Nietzel, Bernstein, and Milich (1998), the strategies employed in Beck's model for the treatment of depression include: (1) helping the client recognize the connections between cognitions, affect, and behaviour; (2) monitoring occurrences of cognitive distortions; (3) examining the evidence for and against these distortions; (4) substituting more realistic interpretations; and (5) giving clients homework assignments focused on practising new thinking strategies and more effective problem solving. Examples of this approach are as follows (Paterson and Bilsker 2002):

- Clients are asked to write about events that have been upsetting as well as about their *interpretations* of the events and their *responses*. A client might write about how a friend cancelled a lunch date, which was interpreted as "He doesn't like me; no one likes me; I'll always be alone" and which was responded to with "Stayed at home alone, felt sad." The practitioner works with the client to come up with alternative, more realistic interpretations.
- Clients are asked to write down "put-downs" – statements or thoughts such as "I'm so stupid" – each time they occur and to make note of how they affect their mood. They are asked to substitute a more realistic phrase, such as "I may not like this, but I'll get through it."
- Similarly, clients are asked to write down *automatic thoughts* – negative thoughts that seem to arise spontaneously – as well as problem beliefs, such as "everything I do must be absolutely perfect; otherwise, I am a failure." They may then be asked to identify the thought or belief that has had the biggest impact on them, describe the impact, then come up with ways to challenge the belief.
- Clients are asked to "catch themselves" using various forms of biased thinking, such as over-generalizing ("It's always going to be like this"), disqualifying the positive ("Anyone can do what I just did"), mind-reading ("She thinks I'm stupid"), fortune-telling ("I'm sure to fail this course"), and catastrophizing (being stood up for a date means I'll spend my entire life alone). Clients are asked to come up with more reality-based ways of thinking and may be provided with axioms, such as "I need to pay attention to the whole picture."

Depending on the individual client, overcoming negative thinking can involve:

- Awareness of the distorted thoughts – so that they are no longer "automatic" and can instead be critically evaluated.
- Thought-challenging: for example, keeping a journal in which the client writes about situations, automatic thoughts associated with the situation,

and more realistic appraisals of the situation – which can then be read aloud or kept for future reference.

- Thought-stopping, which involves a routine in which the client orders him- or herself to stop ruminating by standing up, clapping his or her hands, and shouting "Stop!" Eventually, the sequence of three actions is reduced to one and then replaced by a mental image of a stop sign.
- Worrying time. The client writes down issues that are worrying but defers dealing with them until a set, limited time when he or she will not be distracted.
- Worry inflation. The logic here is for the client to exaggerate his or her fears until they become ridiculous and implausible so that the original problem shrinks in size.

While the psychological treatment of depression involves cognitive techniques, therapists specializing in this approach will often incorporate other components of recovery, including education about depression and stress, lifestyle choices (diet, sleep, physical activity, use of substances, recreation), assertiveness training, and building a supportive social network.

Evaluations of CBT suggest that it is highly effective for unipolar depression and, moreover, that these effects persist in the longer-term, defined by number of relapses (Boudreau, Moulton, and Cunningham 2010; Butler et al. 2006; Kuyken, Dalgleish, and Holden 2007; Lynch, Laws, and McKenna 2010).[8] In looking at predictors of a better response, a review by Somers (2007) concludes that "individuals with less severe illness, shorter length of illness, later age of onset and fewer previous episodes tend to respond well to CBT." Given this conclusion, and the finding that the greatest non-placebo benefit with medication is found in cases of more severe depression, CBT as an alternative to pharmacotherapy may be a viable option when symptoms are in the mild to moderate range.

CBT and Personality Disorder

As noted earlier, practitioners frequently approach clients who have been diagnosed with borderline personality disorder with great apprehension and ambivalence. The belief that these persons are untreatable may become a self-fulfilling prophecy because of the clinician's strong response to the client's apparent manipulative and provocative actions. In her approach to working with persons diagnosed with BPD, psychologist Marsha Linehan (1993a, 1993b) takes this into account, noting that, before anything can be accomplished, the clinician needs to accept some basic assumptions: (1) that the patient wants to change and, despite appearances, is trying to do his or her best; (2) that the behaviour is understandable given the person's background and life circumstances; (3) that, while the client may not be entirely to blame for the way things are, it is his or her responsibility to make them different; (4) that clients cannot fail in therapy – rather, if things are not improving it is the treatment that is failing; and (5) that the clinician must avoid thinking or talking about the client in pejorative terms since this will work against the therapeutic alliance and feed into problems that have led to the development of BPD in the first place. Linehan strongly cautions against using terms like "manipulative," which implies a degree of skill in managing other people or from which one can infer intentionality, both of which are likely incorrect conclusions.

Linehan's influential model for working with clients diagnosed with BPD, described as a "modified CBT approach" (Hadjipavlou and Ogrodniczuk 2010), is outlined here, although interested readers are advised to consult the original manuals (Linehan 1993a, 1993b) and later publications (e.g., Miller, Rathus and Linehan 2007). The approach is called dialectical behaviour therapy (DBT), the term "dialectical" referring to the tension (or balance) between *acceptance,* on the one hand (i.e., validation of the client) and *change,* on the other (i.e., achieving the goals of skill acquisition and learning more adaptive ways of dealing with problems). It is noted that *invalidating environments* are those in which the client experiences rejection and in some cases punishment or in which problems and solutions are oversimplified – responses not infrequently encountered in health care settings. A consequence of these sorts of system responses is that the client may be retraumatized (Harris and Fallot 2001) or that, because undesired behaviours are inconsistent and erratic, they may unintentionally be reinforced. Interestingly, an Australian study found that DBT could have a consciousness-raising effect on otherwise skeptical staff: researchers found that, following a workshop on this model, staff expressed a "significant shift in the meanings associated with borderline personality disorder, with a pervasive therapeutic pessimism being displaced by more optimistic understandings and outlooks" (Hazelton, Rossiter. and Milner 2006, 120).

The two main modes of treatment in DBT are individual therapy with a clinician, and skills training, which is conducted in a group format. The client is required to attend both. In the skills training component, four groups of skills are described: (1) "core mindfulness skills," which are "techniques to enable one to become more clearly aware of the contents of experience and to develop the ability to stay with that experience in the present moment" (Kiehn and Swale 1995, 7); (2) "interpersonal effectiveness skills," which have some parallels with assertiveness skills and which aim to have the client maintain self-esteem in interactions with other people; (3) "emotion modulation skills," which are ways of changing distressing emotional states and which involve examining the *misinterpretation* of events (such as over-generalizing and catastrophizing, similar to the logic seen in CBT with depressed persons); and (4) "distress tolerance skills," techniques for putting up with emotional states if they cannot be changed for the time being, this involving skills such as "distracting," "self-soothing," "improving the moment," and "thinking of pros and cons."

Individual treatment is approached in stages: stage one focuses on stabilizing suicidal and "therapy interfering" behaviours (which is necessary before advancing to later stages and could involve distress tolerance and other skills); stage two deals with problems related to post-traumatic stress; and stage three focuses on self-esteem and individual treatment goals. Clients are given homework, which includes recording targeted behaviours in journals. Core strategies in treatment are (1) validation of the client's behaviours as understandable in relation to his or her life situation and (2) problem solving, meaning the establishment of necessary skills. Treatment involves creating a crisis plan, using cognitive and graded exposure techniques (see above), and, in some cases, using medication. In the course of treatment, behaviour is examined through a "chain analysis," which looks at the sequence of events leading to unwanted behaviours while generating hypotheses about factors that may be controlling the behaviour. Subsequently, alternative ways of dealing with situations are considered before being put into place and compared. The clinician tries to promote self-efficacy rather than doing everything for the client (such as intervening with other care providers). Kiehn and Swale (1995, 9-10) conclude: "Particular note should be made of the pervading application of contingency management throughout the therapy, using the relationship with the therapist as the main reinforcer. In the session-by-session course of therapy care is taken to systematically reinforce targeted adaptive behaviors and to avoid reinforcing targeted maladaptive behaviors." From this one can note how DBT has elements in common with, and pulls together, other approaches described in this chapter: education, skills teaching, crisis planning, graded exposure, contingency management, and motivational interviewing. One may also note that DBT is an elaborate treatment model, which, in turn, has implications for staff training and support.

Linehan's original evaluation of DBT involved a study that compared two groups of twenty-two clients, one group receiving DBT and the other "treatment as usual" (TAU) (which could constitute a variety of outpatient situations). The outcome measures were frequency of parasuicidal behaviours, number of hospital days, and attrition rate from therapy (a frequent problem for persons with BPD). Results showed that the group receiving DBT did better on all three indicators, having fewer suicidal behaviours, lower therapy attrition rates (16.7 percent versus 50 percent), and fewer days spent in hospital (eight days per year compared to over thirty-eight for the TAU group) (Linehan et al. 1991). Later evaluations of DBT by other authors have found it to be effective, particularly with respect to self-harming behaviours (Lynch et al. 2007). A 2006 study co-authored by Linehan compared outcomes for persons receiving DBT with persons treated by psychiatrists, considered to be experts in borderline personality, but not using DBT (Linehan et al. 2006). While participants in both groups showed improvement, the DBT group had superior outcomes with respect to suicide attempts, hospital visits and admissions, and treatment dropout. The largest trial to date evaluating DBT (n = 180), conducted in Toronto, involves a comparison with "general psychiatric management" (GPM), the latter consisting of weekly counselling, case management, and medication (McMain et al. 2009). Both groups showed improvements in most clinical outcomes, including self-harming behaviour, but neither modality was shown to be superior, contrary to the original expectations of the researchers. In discussing this, the authors note that the result could not be explained by "inferior delivery" of DBT, based on fidelity ratings taken during the trial, but could be attributed to GPM being more efficacious than the psychological controls used in previous studies, such as "treatment as usual." The authors conclude that the study helped "dispel the myth that borderline personality disorder is untreatable and supports the thesis that this population can benefit from specific specialized interventions" (McMain et al. 2009, 1,372). The study also points out that, while DBT is currently the best-known treatment model for borderline personality disorder, other psychotherapies may also be effective (see Hadjipavlou and Ogrodniczuk 2010) and that optimal therapeutic "fit" may have to do with characteristics and preferences of both worker and client. For example, there is some evidence that clients with BPD who are expressing greater anger and hostility may be less able to tolerate the DBT model (Rusch et al. 2008).

CBT and Psychosis
In recent years, cognitive-behavioural techniques have been utilized in the treatment of persons with psychotic disorders such as schizophrenia and bipolar disorder (Buccheri et al. 2004; Lam et al. 2003; Lynch, Laws, and McKenna 2010; Rollinson et al. 2007; Zaretsky et al. 2008). This represents a major change in thinking, given that these disorders were previously considered contraindications for CBT, having been relegated to the category of "biological" or "brain" conditions that were only appropriately managed with medications (Kingdon 1998; Lam et al. 2003). As a review article in

the *Canadian Journal of Psychiatry* summarizes, for some time the prevailing view had been "that psychotic symptoms resulted from a core neurophysiological dysfunction or dysfunctions that [were] not amendable to a talking therapy" (Norman and Townsend 1999, 245), a view supported by findings that psychodynamic therapies were of apparently little utility in the treatment of psychotic disorders (Fenton 2000; Gunderson et al. 1984). Clinical staff in mental health programs (such as this author) were often instructed not to challenge or even discuss the content of a client's delusions or hallucinations (except to conduct risk assessments) since, so the reasoning went, the "beliefs [would only] be reinforced by such exploration" (Kingdon 1998, 177) or "talking about voices could only make them worse" (Row 2003, 27).

Notwithstanding this legacy, there has been increasing interest in the use of cognitive treatments for clients with psychotic disorders. The impetus for this comes from several directions (Norman and Townsend 1999):

- The finding that a number of clients, on their own, have for some time been developing coping strategies for dealing with psychotic symptoms (Vagnerova 2003a).[9] While "anecdotal," personal accounts offer the prospect that, at least in some cases, confronting delusional beliefs may be beneficial,[10] as one service user attests: "One last lesson I took from all this was that it does not hurt to argue with a schizophrenic. I wanted to tell my story, and when people did object to parts of it, it did *force me to think*. And eventually, as I got better, their arguments made more sense. Recovery to me means that, even if the delusions are not completely gone, I am able to function as if they are. I am even able to joke about something that obsessed me for almost 20 years" (Cohen 2008, 407, emphasis added). Similarly, Ellen Saks, a woman with schizophrenia who went on to become a professor of law, found from her own research that people, like her, who had succeeded despite the diagnosis, had all developed cognitive, deflecting, and distracting techniques "to keep their schizophrenia at bay" (Saks 2013).
- Evidence of the success of these techniques in other clinical domains, such as the treatment of depression.
- Evidence of the importance of psychosocial factors in rehabilitation and the development of the stress-vulnerability model; while CBT approaches cannot solve the question of vulnerability, they can be useful in reducing the stress that may lead to breakthrough of symptoms (Kopelowicz, Liberman, and Zarate 2006).
- The finding, as noted earlier, that a significant number of persons do not achieve a full benefit from antipsychotic medications.

- Recognition that psychological and pharmacological approaches can be viewed as complementary rather than incompatible.

What goes into CBT as it is applied to psychotic conditions? Models of delivering treatment have been found to vary, with some focusing more on coping strategies and others more on what is called *schema* work (Lecomte and Lecomte 2002; Morrison and Barratt 2010; Rollinson et al. 2007; Wykes et al. 2008). Since approaches need to be tailored to the degree of disability and ability and "to the needs and circumstances of individual patients" (Norman and Townsend 1999, 246), it may be the case that a single, uniform approach is neither possible nor desirable at this point. Somers (2007, 78), in his review, suggests that most approaches incorporate "the main principles of CBT." He notes the potential for difficulties in engagement and relationship-building when, for example, the main symptom is paranoia, and the importance of treating delusional beliefs with respect and empathy. Somers also suggests that both the practitioner and the client should "have a shared understanding of the illness and its causes and consequences" (79), a significant element since a number of people affected by psychosis – and a majority in the acute phase – may not be able to meet this pre-condition.

Concerning the components of treatment, therapy with persons diagnosed with psychotic disorders incorporates stress reduction, belief modification, distraction/disruption techniques, and behavioural methods. Concerning stress reduction, Norman and Townsend (1999) identify several skills to be taught as part of the CBT approach, such as: (1) "reframing psychosis," which is explanation and reinforcement of the stress-vulnerability model so that clients will see "the possible role of their social and physical environment as triggers" (246); (2) "identifying triggers for psychosis" (discussed under "relapse prevention" earlier in this chapter); (3) "reducing physiological arousal" by means of muscle relaxation and breathing techniques; and (4) "improving general coping skills," such as assertiveness, conflict resolution, and knowing when and how to withdraw from stressful situations. The more cognitive components of treatment include belief modification, whereby client and clinician examine the client's evidence for apparently false beliefs or perceptions, consider alternative explanations, and "empirically [test] their relative validity" (247); and, "disrupting symptoms," whereby clients are encouraged to move their attention away from symptoms by means of other activities such as "listening to music, watching television, humming, and engaging in social interaction" (247). Belief modification may incorporate behavioural methods: Somers (2007, 79) notes: "Similar to the exposure techniques used with other types of disorders, attempts are made to test disordered thoughts and beliefs, enabling the individual to gradually face feared situations and to begin to regard psychotic symptoms as less threatening." Using CBT for persons with psychotic disorders will not necessarily eliminate positive symptoms; rather, the rationale is that environmental stressors *leading* to increased symptomatology are alleviated through enhanced coping strategies and that the emotional *consequences* of psychotic symptoms are reduced. Manuals for CBT with psychosis include those by Kingdon and Turkington (2005), and Morrison and colleagues (2004).

Evaluations of CBT have looked mainly at effects on positive symptoms and relapse rates; there is a presumption that reduction in psychosis then positively affects other symptom domains and, indeed, functioning, in general. More recently, efforts have been made to apply cognitive approaches to negative symptoms as well (Grant et al. 2011). In brief, the evidence base for CBT with psychosis is not as strong as it is with other syndromes, depression in particular. Reviews of randomized trials have found the impact on positive symptoms to be modest, and when methodologically weaker studies – for example those with inadequate "blinding" – are excluded, the effect size of the intervention is smaller still (Lynch, Laws, and McKenna 2010; Somers 2007; Wykes et al. 2008). Wykes and colleagues (2008) note that there is still work to be done in determining which specific components of CBT are effective with psychosis and that there may be a convenience bias at play, with staff favouring some treatment elements simply because they are easier to implement. Concerning which clients benefit the most, a review by Somers (2007) suggests that persons with a shorter duration of illness, less severe symptoms, fewer negative symptoms, and some degree of insight (ability to consider the possibility that they might be mistaken about their delusional beliefs) have a better response with CBT. Conversely, persons with apparently fixed delusional beliefs and those who have not been able to experience a good working relationship with professionals would be poorer candidates. CBT for psychosis may be a useful tool, but it is one that should be part of a comprehensive rehabilitation approach that also addresses social health determinants, such as adequate food and shelter.[11]

Treatments for Trauma-Related Conditions

An increased demand for resources to respond to trauma-related conditions has come from greater recognition of the extent and impact of child abuse, domestic violence, the residential school experience of Aboriginal persons, and combat-related mental health problems among the military. By 2012, the federal government had opened ten "operational stress injury" clinics in Canada to assist current and discharged military personnel (see also Chapter 1).

The aetiology of a post-trauma condition is complex, and not all persons will develop PTSD following even a highly disturbing event, which speaks to individual differences in vulnerability and resilience (Briere 2002; Kluft, Bloom, and Kinzie 2000). Concerning the aftermath of trauma and possible need for treatment, Regehr and Glancy (2010, 113) note, first, that symptoms do tend to diminish on their own over time and, second, that denial/avoidance – behaviours sometimes seen by clinicians as problematic – may in fact "be highly adaptive because they can assist people to contain arousal and intrusion symptoms." These authors suggest that a possible response sequence to trauma involves, first, crisis intervention to help with focusing and decision making, then, if symptoms persist, the application of cognitive-behavioural strategies and, later, the consideration of approaches such as DBT (see above). Techniques include anxiety management (training in relaxation and breathing, positive self-talk, assertiveness, and thought-stopping), cognitive therapy (challenging beliefs such as self-blame), and exposure therapy (confronting situations that remind the person of the trauma) (Van der Kolk 2002). Concerning exposure therapy, Regehr and Glancy (2010) note that treatment inclusion criteria for this modality are more selective, that there should be an established strong therapeutic alliance, and that CBT techniques without exposure are otherwise an option. Systematic reviews of cognitive-behavioural treatments for trauma-related conditions suggest that they are a promising practice (Cary and McMillen 2012; Powers et al. 2010).

Service Provision

There have been a number of promising developments in psychological treatments for the mentally ill, and a rebirth – in a form different from earlier conceptions – of the idea and practice of "talk therapy." Education and self-management programs and resources, such as BRIDGES and WRAP, have rolled out and are starting to establish an evidence base. That said, access to psychological treatment, in particular to CBT, remains quite limited in Canada and elsewhere (Layard et al. 2007; Livingston et al. 2009; Mental Health Commission of Canada 2012; Rhodes et al. 2010; Wilk et al. 2006). The Mental Health Commission of Canada (2012, 62) notes that "there are some publicly funded psychotherapies and clinical counseling in Canada in hospitals and mental health centres, but the waiting lists are very long and the criteria to access these services can be very restrictive."

As reviewed by Newton and Yardley (2007, 1,497), barriers to service provision include "a lack of suitably qualified practitioners to provide training, insufficient training programs, a lack of support from managers to implement training programs, financial constraints, limited time availability for training, and ... a change-averse culture." Adopting new interventions means accommodating the greater complexity of some approaches (particularly when compared to treatment based mainly on medication administration), which more generally speaks to the issue of *knowledge exchange*: convincing clinicians that new approaches are feasible and can be applied in ordinary practice settings (Liberman 1998).

Concerning the financing of psychological services, the Canada Health Act stipulates that "medically necessary" expenses be covered, this referring mainly to hospital and physician services. While some additional benefits may be provided by the provinces, in most cases psychological treatment is not covered by medical service plans, except in the case of psychologists employed by health authorities at hospitals and public clinics. And there are very few of these: for example, this author worked in a large urban health authority in which *none* of the adult community mental health teams employed PhD-level psychologists. Psychotherapy may be covered on a limited basis by employee assistance programs and some victim assistance programs, but in most cases seeing a clinical psychologist is a private-pay arrangement.

What about the training of other disciplines in CBT? It is hard to disagree with the conclusions of two McGill University authors that "students of all mental health disciplines should receive training in CBT" (Myhr and Payne 2006, 668), and, further, that this should include rehabilitation specialists (Kopelowicz and Liberman 2003). In theory, psychiatrists could be an important resource since their services to clients are covered (for the most part) by provincial government medical plans. However, historically CBT has not been a major part of psychiatric training; while this is changing, Myhr and Payne (2006, 668) note that "few Canadian programs offer exposure adequate for proficiency." For example, in a survey of Vancouver-area psychiatrists conducted in 2010, only 30 percent of respondents, when asked if they could provide CBT, answered "yes" (Goldner, Jones, and Fang 2011). To this end, Gunter and Whittal (2010, 197) suggest "using clinical practice guidelines to meet quality assurance criteria for training program accreditation." For now, exposure to CBT training comes after graduation for many mental health practitioners. This has been helped, in the example of Toronto, by the creation, within the Centre for Addiction and Mental Health, of the Intermediate Cognitive Therapy Institute, which is aimed at enhancing practice skills of health care practitioners who have had some "didactic" exposure to the principles of CBT. Students within this program may also complete a diploma in CBT practice.

Presently, for the most part, it has fallen on health authority employers and managers to "add on" CBT training for their staff in the form of workshops and symposia, and more advanced training for a smaller, presumably more interested and committed group of individuals. This method obviously has its limitations since proficiency in psychotherapy requires, first of all, that it be put into practice, which often does not happen, and, further, that there be ongoing support, feedback, and mentoring with like-minded colleagues, which is difficult to arrange. Skills introduced in workshops that are not practised, unsurprisingly, will soon be lost. Further, workshops usually just cover basic principles and not the nuances of the actual therapy: this author was told by a workshop leader certified in motivational interviewing that a two-day training could "barely scratch the surface" of the subject, for example.

What about advanced training for a few? An interesting discussion of this topic, as it applies to the implementation of DBT, is provided in an article by Herschell and colleagues (2009). Thirteen senior administrators from the State of Pennsylvania took part in discussions and interviews concerning the challenges faced in bringing this best practice model to their programs. A number were concerned about the complexity of the training and of the DBT model itself (see also Perseius et al. 2007) and about how much it would take clinicians away "from direct service provision." There was also the question of which staff should be chosen for the training and what criteria should be used – for example, seniority, credentials, diversity, and whether the person volunteered. There was ambivalence about picking young, enthusiastic persons since the managers' experience was: "Young people are interested in attending the training to advance their careers but will then move on after they've received it which doesn't help the agency" (Herschell et al 2009, 991). While readers may see this as a rather mundane point, it does speak to the real problem of trying to maintain continuity of care and program skill sets in the face of high staff turnover, something that will be familiar to Canadian managers of mental health teams (see also Frankel and Gelman 2004). Theoretically, this problem could be helped by worker specialization; that is, instead of expecting clinicians to be competent in a range of therapeutic modalities, personnel could be hired (for example) *either* as case managers *or* as group therapists, not both.

While CBT approaches are more labour-intensive than a medical management model (which, in its starkest form, consists of a GP prescribing antidepressant medication after a ten-minute interview), a cost-benefit argument can be made in favour of these interventions. In justifying the hiring by the National Health Service of more CBT therapists to treat depression and anxiety, a group of British authors (Layard et al. 2007) argued that any additional costs would be recovered in two to five years at the outside, based on the claim of high treatment success rates (50 percent), low therapy costs relative to benefits gained in client employment and tax revenue, and savings in incapacity benefits. What about DBT, more specifically? Some studies suggest additional costs in outpatient treatment are more than offset by savings in hospital bed days and emergency department visits (Mental Health Center of Greater Manchester 1998), but a systematic review of available DBT trials concludes that there is not yet strong evidence of cost-effectiveness (Brazier et al. 2006) (which should not be confused with *clinical* effectiveness). Another way of addressing cost and access to CBT is through the (increasing) development of internet-based programs, which may be used with or without guidance from a professional and which are aimed at persons experiencing mild to moderate levels of distress (Livingston et al. 2009).[12] The cost-effectiveness of CBT may in fact improve with time and experience as methods are better tailored to meet the needs of target populations, efficiencies are developed, and the most important components of treatment packages identified (Norman and Townsend 1999). Finally, there is some preliminary evidence that the benefits achieved with more intensive and expensive one-on-one CBT interventions may also be achieved with group psycho-education sessions, which, if confirmed, would have significant implications for service delivery in public sector settings (Parikh et al. 2012).

Notes

1 Concerning evaluation, the Canadian Psychoanalytic Society states: "Psychoanalysis has pioneered ... techniques for eliciting, gathering and interpreting, *but not measuring* information about the way different human personalities are organized and function" (emphasis added). See http://www.psychoanalysismontreal.com/psychoanalysis-FAQ.html.

2 The website of the Toronto Psychoanalytic Society and Institute notes: "To undergo psychoanalysis, a person must have achieved some important satisfaction in life, and have a sufficiently stable lifestyle to meet the requirements of the treatment. This person may have already achieved important satisfactions – with friends, in marriage, in work, or through special interests and hobbies." See http://www.torontopsychoanalysis.com/what_is_psychoanalysis.php. Psychoanalysis has been seen as contraindicated in the case of persons suffering from serious conditions such as a psychotic disorder (Fenton 2000; Norman and Townsend 1999).

3 Unfortunately, terminology in this area is unnecessarily confusing. Educational approaches in psychiatry have been referred to as "psychoeducation," a rather loaded term that is not used in this book. Further, Mueser et al. (2002) make a distinction between "illness management" and "self-management," defining the latter as peer led services and the former as professional-led; however, these definitions are not shared by others (e.g., Bilsker 2003).

4 See also Hourston's (2010) article on "five tools for resilience."

5 The study had a number of methodological limitations, and effect sizes were not in fact large. Interestingly, scores for control subjects also improved across all three outcomes, possibly

due to an "anticipation effect," as they had been promised an opportunity to receive WRAP at the end of the study. This last finding would mean that the relative benefits of WRAP may in fact have been underestimated.

6   This is not a surprising or novel finding: previous research has found that an empathic therapeutic relationship is more predictive of a positive outcome than the particular treatment model being used (Duncan, Miller, and Sparks 2004; Lambert and Barley 2001).

7   For an example, see "Beating the Blues" at http://www.beatingtheblues.co.uk. This program was adopted by the employee assistance program at the Vancouver Coastal Health Authority to help those staff coping with depression and anxiety.

8   This conclusion is qualified in the review by Lynch, Laws, and McKenna (2010), which determined that, when analysis was limited to "well-controlled" studies – ones that used psychological controls (such as supportive therapy or relaxation) as opposed to no treatment – a benefit was still found but the effect size diminished.

9   In some settings in Canada "Hearing Voices" groups are being set up as a peer-led initiative to help persons cope with bothersome hallucinations. In a conversation with Ron Coleman, one of the founders of this network, I was told that the techniques used in CBT can indeed be seen as similar to those taught in his groups.

10 Nobel Prize-winning mathematician John Nash, who resisted medical treatments for his schizophrenic illness, in a *60 Minutes* interview, attributed his eventual recovery to becoming "disillusioned with the delusions" – that is, being able to understand them as abstract entities that could be examined for veracity.

11 It is a truism that clients need to have established some stability and supports in other areas of their life in order for psychological approaches such as CBT to be effective: a three-year study of clients in Pittsburgh who had received support and training in interpersonal skills and stress reduction found lower relapse rates and better social functioning among those in the treatment group, *except* for those among the fifty-four individuals in the study who lived alone or with non-family members. The conclusion was that, for these persons, securing shelter, food, and clothing was so demanding that meeting other treatment requirements proved to be overwhelming (Hogarty et al. 1997).

12 An example is the "Bounce Back" program offered through the CMHA: http://www.cmha.bc.ca/bounceback.

Other Resources

The "MoodGYM" is an online course that helps individuals gain knowledge and skills to manage depression: http://moodgym.anu.edu.au/welcome.

Occupation

17

Psychiatric rehabilitation specialists use the term "occupation" in a broad sense, going beyond paid employment to refer to a range of activities that give meaning to an individual's life. Occupation can be defined as an "active process of living: from the beginning to the end of life ... all the active processes of looking after ourselves and others, enjoying life, and being socially and economically productive over the lifespan and in various contexts" (Crepeau et al. 2009, 16). The significance of occupation was identified in a quality-of-life study by researchers in London, Ontario, who found that clients in their survey "emphasized the importance of 'making the choice to be part of things' and being socially active on a regular basis [which] could mean competitive employment or volunteer work ... [or] activity of any kind as a way of keeping themselves healthy, building self-confidence and feeling useful" (Corring and Cook 2007, 242). One Canadian service user observes, poignantly, that with "no occupation to take pride in ... [we] find little love in a world that shuns the idle" (Carten 2006, 111).

Within occupation are a number of life-domains, including work, self-care, and education, which are discussed in more detail below. It will be noted that a historical pessimism about job prospects for the seriously mentally ill is starting to shift, in light of new approaches to vocational rehabilitation.

Personal Life

Mental disorders such as schizophrenia, because of the timing of their onset in the lifecycle, the degree of impairment produced, and their duration, can result in life skill deficits. In some cases these skills are never learned; in some cases they are learned but fall into disuse, an outcome contributed to by care providers who discourage independent thought and action.

Rehabilitation in the area of "personal life" refers to "services that help an individual gain or regain practical skills in the areas of personal care, home management, relationships and use of community resources" (British Columbia Ministry of Health 2002f, 3). Components of personal life include the following:

- Personal care: grooming and hygiene, physical health, relaxation, coping strategies and skills, fitness, nutrition, stress management, sleep, illness education (similar to relapse prevention), personal safety, drug and alcohol use, financial management, sexuality, smoking, and weight control.
- Home management: home safety, meal preparation, telephone skills, laundry, and household maintenance.
- Relationships: interpersonal skills, communication skills, self-advocacy, friendships, building social networks, assertiveness, anger management, sexuality (dating skills, healthy relationships), intimacy, and family relationships and support.
- Community resources: hearing about resources, transportation, local community resources – including health, social, and financial services – and accessibility issues.

Some deficits in the area of personal life may have more to do with resources than with personal failings. For example, a client's poor hygiene may be due to the fact that laundry facilities are inaccessible or unaffordable. This, in turn, speaks to the need to visit clients on their own "turf" in order to get an appreciation of local resources and the obstacles they face.

From the bulleted list above "relationships" is arguably an area of considerable need among clients, and one that has not been adequately met by program response. Surveys on the topic of sexuality, for example, have found service users both willing to articulate their hopes and beliefs in this area and open to support from practitioners, even if the latter group has historically been uncomfortable with addressing this domain (McCann 2010).

While practitioners will form general impressions of a client's skill deficits, there may be the need for a more systematic assessment – for example, at the time of hospital discharge or a change of residence. The assessment method may involve a self-report, an interview, observation, a task, or a combination of these. An evaluation instrument may also be used (Naccarato, DeLorenzo, and Park 2008). For example, a "money management assessment" involves the following: (1) client self-report (clients are asked about how they manage their finances); (2) knowledge of currency (clients are asked to identify the name and worth of units of currency); (3) purchasing task, requiring calculation (staff persons give clients change from purchase, asking if amount given is correct); (4) knowledge of source of income (government pension, income assistance, inheritance, etc.); (5) description of assets and debts; (6) use of the banking system (name and location of bank, type of account, can client write a cheque, use a bank machine, etc.); (7) bill payment (can client identify what bill is for, amount, due date, and where payment is made); (8) budgeting (for essential and leisure items); (9) taxes (who prepares tax return and where can the client get assistance); and (10) comparison shopping (task involves comparing two items with different prices and sizes).

Practitioners need to be reflective and tactful when appraising the life skills of clients. The issues being addressed are very sensitive; none of us, after all, wants to appear incompetent. Further, clients should not be held to unreasonably high standards, standards that the average person does not always live up to. Practitioners have to balance, on the one hand, the need to encourage and model healthy behaviours with, on the other hand, the right of clients to be free from excessive interference and from the imposition of personal morality or excessive paternalism.

Skill deficits may be addressed in a number of settings. Functional assessments may be performed by occupational therapists in hospitals or at community mental health clinics. Skills training may be offered by clinical and rehab staff at mental health clinics in either individual or group format. Skills training may also be offered through a number of community organizations, self-help groups, and clubhouses (see box). In situations in which a client has a case manager or primary worker who is not a rehabilitation specialist, that worker should be alert to "personal life" problems, be aware of rehabilitation resources, and make linkages where appropriate. To this end, the assessment process for new clients should be as holistic as possible, incorporating interests and needs across various life domains.

Employment

Work is "central to self-identity, self-esteem and well-being" (Scheid and Anderson 1995 164), and clients themselves have for some time spoken about the importance of employment:

> Told, upon the advent of my being diagnosed with bipolar affective disorder, that I may never work again, I rebelled. Whatever else I imagined myself to be before my diagnosis was contingent upon my ability to work and be a productive citizen. This fact was ingrained within the value system I inherited. It was part of myself that no doctor could diagnose away, or make disappear. This sense of who "I" was in relation to myself and the world would prove stronger than any psychotropic drug I had ever ingested or any mental illness I supposedly had. (Molnar 2004, 7)

The Clubhouse

Clubhouses were originally self-help initiatives, and the genesis of what became the clubhouse model can be traced to the 1940s in New York, where a group of clients who had been patients at the same state hospital, and who had found little support in the outside world, formed a mutual-aid organization called WANA (We Are Not Alone). This eventually became Fountain House (http://www.fountainhouse.org), which has served as the model for a number of other organizations in the United States and Canada, usually run as non-profit societies. According to the International Center for Clubhouse Development (ICCD - http://www.iccd.org/) clubhouses are "a place where people with serious mental illness – who are known as 'members' – participate in their own recovery process by working and socializing together in a safe and welcoming environment" and are a "community-based approach that complements available psychiatric treatment." In addition to providing social support, clubhouses have provided employment training through work units that can – for example – involve food preparation and meal service to members and also the prospect of paid placements through a model called transitional employment (described in more detail below).

The clubhouse is an example of a "separate" program, with respect to both physical space and mandate, catering only to mental health clients. This has its advantages, in that the program may serve as a sanctuary and low-stress environment for persons feeling overwhelmed, and disadvantages, in that others may want a normalized environment in which they are not so easily identified as "different" (Drake et al. 2003). Traditionally clubhouses have not made long-term competitive employment a priority, which some service users have seen as an outmoded approach (Scardillo 2012) but that also speaks to the importance of having a *range* of vocational programs available for clients. Other challenges faced by clubhouses in the present era include maintaining an approach complementary to – and not dominated by – the professional/medical model and ensuring that staff co-option is resisted and that client members are seen as equal partners. To this end, the ICCD has developed a set of standards to be used for accreditation (http://www.iccd.org/quality.html#rel), including, for example, the requirement that "all clubhouse space [be] accessible ... [and that there be] no staff-only or member-only spaces." At this writing there are twenty clubhouses in Canada accredited by the ICCD, including Crossroads in Sydney, Nova Scotia (http://www.crossroadscapebreton.ca/).

A best-practices document concludes that, for mental health clients, "improvements in symptoms, lower hospitalization rates, greater social interaction, decreased anxiety, enhanced self-esteem and self-confidence, and reduced stress are all potential benefits from engagement in a work setting" (British Columbia Ministry of Health 2002f, 17).[1] In addition to benefits to the clients themselves, employing persons with mental disorders can provide benefits to the organizations that employ them, particularly when these are mental health programs. As reviewed by Bainbridge (1998, 23), these include the dispelling of negative myths about clients, the fact that "acknowledgement of the value of consumer roles in service provision makes explicit statements about the overall worth of consumers," and the positive influence that clients can have on service philosophy and practice.

While acknowledging these potential benefits, it must be said that employment data from North America and British Commonwealth countries have not been promising, showing an unemployment rate for persons with a serious, persistent mental disorder ranging from 70 to 95 percent (British Columbia Partners for Mental Health and Addictions Information 2003b; Burns et al. 2007; Crowley-Cyr 2008; Eklund, Hansson, and Ahlqvist 2004; Killeen and O'Day 2004; Mental Health Commission of Canada 2012; Salkever et al. 2007).[2] This situation may be improving with the advent of new employment initiatives, discussed in more detail below. Apart from specialized vocational programs, there is evidence that adequate clinical support in and of itself will improve employment outcomes: a study of 3,370 ACT clients in Ontario found that, while fewer than 10 percent of clients were employed at admission, this figure increased to 23 percent after four years with the program ("employment" in this study could include unpaid as well as sheltered work) (Lurie, Kirsh, and Hodge 2007). This is noteworthy in that ACT programs target the most disabled individuals.

Unemployment among persons with a serious mental disorder is affected by:

- The disabling impact of the illness, with more disabling conditions predicting greater employment interruption (Russinova, Bloch, and Lyass 2007; Salkever et al. 2007). There is definite evidence of a mental health *benefit* to mentally ill persons from being employed (e.g., Bush et al. 2009; Hutchinson et al. 2006; Kirsh et al. 2009; Mee, Sumsion and Craik 2004), but, at the same time, there needs to be careful consideration of the additional stress inherent in a competitive workplace and whether (for example) accommodations or part-time work should be considered. Illness impact also means that, in most cases, clients will have lower educational attainment (Cook 2006).

- Potential loss of benefits. Provincial disability plans may contain disincentives for persons considering re-entry into the workforce, such as loss of medical, dental, and transportation benefits, and claw-backs of earned income (Gram 2008; Mental Health Commission of Canada 2012). Disincentives are even greater in countries with no universal medicare, such as the US, where loss of disability benefits may mean losing health insurance altogether (Bond, Xie, and Drake 2007; Cook 2006).
- Discrimination. A report from the Ontario Human Rights Commission (2010, 13) notes: "Mental illness is a 'hidden' disability. In workplaces, housing or services, where the need to accommodate people with physical disabilities is understood, there is often reluctance or even refusal to accommodate people with mental health disabilities." Despite the fact that the Charter of Rights and human rights codes in Canada prohibit discrimination in hiring decisions with disabled persons,[3] there is evidence that complaints on this basis are increasing (Dranoff 2005). Unfortunately, ostensible statutory protections may be insufficient and sometimes circumvented: reviewing the application of the Americans with Disabilities Act in the US, Petrila (2009) notes that courts in that country have adopted an "increasingly constricted" interpretation of the statute, necessitating the passage of new, more strongly worded legislation.
- Lack of effective services. Many persons with psychiatric disabilities do not have access to what are considered best practice approaches to vocational rehabilitation, if in fact they have access to any vocational services at all (Cook 2006; Marshall et al. 2008). For example, an Ontario study looking at employment outcomes determined that the poor results in one ACT program – which did have a vocational worker – were due to the lack of guidelines or mandate about the employment *model* to be used (Lurie, Kirsh, and Hodge 2007).
- Staff attitudes. Given the impairments associated with a disorder such as schizophrenia, clinicians may assume that high rates of unemployment are natural and inevitable. The counter-argument is that people will tend to live up to expectations and that our expectations of clients have been consistently and unreasonably very low (Becker and Drake 2003; Carten 2006; Killeen and O'Day 2004; Kruger 2000). Lieberman and colleagues (2008, 490) note that, in the institutional era, "patients with schizophrenia experienced profound atrophy of social, vocational and basic living skills as a result of prolonged isolation and exposure to neglectful, stultifying conditions." Concerning client potential, a 2007 in-house survey of 482 clients of Vancouver's Midtown Mental Health Team found 37 percent of clients to be currently engaged in either paid (full-time and part-time) or volunteer work, 23 and 14 percent, respectively – figures more promising

than those reported in other studies.[4] Interestingly, this "baseline" snapshot came *prior* to the implementation of a supported employment program and was used, in part, for consciousness-raising among staff skeptical about the employability of their clients.

Employment Programs

Our thinking about vocational rehabilitation in mental health settings has changed considerably in a relatively short period of time (Drake et al. 2003). A review by Menear and colleagues (2011) traces developments in Canada, from sheltered workshops in the 1960s and 1970s, to skills training programs and social enterprises in the 1980s, to supported employment programs in the 1990s, the latter necessitated by the poor outcomes from earlier approaches with respect to actual job placement. Becker and Drake (2003, 4) are blunt in their appraisal of these earlier models:

> Approaches to vocational rehabilitation generally have reflected our paternalistic treatment models. According to the diathesis-stress model, competitive employment is often seen as a high expectation stress to be avoided, at least until the individual has been stable for many years. Many mental health professionals still believe that competitive employment represents a dangerous experiment ... Most vocational rehabilitation programs have been anything but liberating ... Sheltered workshops and day rehabilitation programs emphasized structure, protection by close oversight, slow stepwise approaches to prepare people for the community, and low expectations. The sheltered workshop approach was recognized as "deadening" many years ago ... [The] explicit goal was to provide stabilization, and the implicit goal was to help people become "good patients" instead of good citizens.

These authors argue that older, sheltered models of vocational rehabilitation were unable to match the skills taught with those needed in future placements, did not match work tasks with actual client interests, and resulted in people losing interest and motivation during the training.

So what do we know about "what works"? The accumulated evidence suggests the following program elements relating to better employment outcomes (Becker and Drake 2003; Kirsh, Cockburn, and Gewurtz 2005):

- An explicit focus on work as part of the agency's mission.
- Inclusion of an employment specialist on the mental health team, rather than (a) relying on an allied vocational agency or (b) simply making this a part of existing team staff's range of responsibilities. (This can be a hard

sell when colleagues argue that limited funding should be spent on clinical rather than on vocational resources.)

- Respecting client preference concerning the type of job, which is associated with greater satisfaction and longer tenure.
- Ongoing support. The evidence suggests that "place-train" models have better outcomes than the older "train-place" models, whereby the client loses contact with a job coach or counsellor after placement.
- Rapid placement, so that on-the-job training can be individualized to a specific worksite.
- Pay for work.

The model that currently adheres most closely to these principles is *supported employment* (SE), which focuses on competitive work, consumer choice, rapid job search and placement, and integration within mental health treatment teams (Menear et al. 2011). Within SE are IPS (individual placement and support) staff, vocational specialists who follow the client after placement in a time-unlimited fashion and coordinate services within the team so that the client does not get contradictory messages from staff from different disciplines. Becker and Drake (2003) suggest that an IPS unit consist of a supervisor and two or more employment specialists with twenty to twenty-five clients each. In this model program eligibility is primarily determined by client preference and interest; that is, anyone expressing a desire to work should have access to SE "regardless of job readiness factors" (Dartmouth IPS Supported Employment Center 2011, 2).

SE has accumulated a large evidence base, and a number of studies and reviews of studies across North America, Europe, and Asia have found it to be a successful model with respect to job acquisition and tenure, with results superior to other vocational models regardless of factors such as unemployment rates or individual clinical and demographic characteristics (Bond, Drake, and Becker 2008; Burns et al. 2007; Burns and Catty 2008; Campbell, Bond, and Drake 2011; Salyers et al. 2004; Wong et al. 2008). Supported employment is now considered an evidence-based practice (Dixon et al. 2010).

Some clients may have an interest in exploring vocation short of competitive employment, and to this end pre-employment programs may be considered (British Columbia Ministry of Health 2002f). These include:

- Sheltered workshops.
- Vocational assessment and career counselling.
- Pre-employment and work readiness training. In this area, clients are given skills training, work experience, and job search services; goals are to increase

confidence and "work tolerance" and to help individuals "grow into" a job (British Columbia Ministry of Health 2002f, 22-3).

- Volunteer work. Compensations here are not financial (apart from honoraria) but rather may be in the form of verbal and written recognition or enhancement of an individual's sense of purpose and self-esteem. Volunteer work may be an end in itself or an opportunity to develop skills and gain work experience in a safer environment. Mental health programs may partner with existing volunteer services or develop their own service. Volunteer experience increasingly includes agency committee work by clients.

- Transitional employment. This is defined as a "time-limited series of placements in community jobs for the purpose of gaining work experience and building self-confidence" (British Columbia Ministry of Health 2002f, 26). Placements usually involve on-the-job training, and participants are paid at the going rate. This has traditionally involved a partnership between a mental health clubhouse program and an employer, with positions being held for mental health clients who, if unable to work for a period, would be replaced by another client from the clubhouse (thus alleviating the problem of staff turnover for the employer) (Johnson 1997).

A caveat: not everyone is work-ready, and while better models of supported employment have been an important and necessary development, it must be acknowledged that persons recovering from a serious mental disorder in some cases need a lower-expectation setting. For example, authors of a study conducted with mental health clubhouse members in Calgary concluded: "While it is often assumed that work-orientated rehabilitation programs are suitable for anyone recovering from a mental illness, member feedback suggests that some people are more appropriately served in a [lower expectation] drop-in centre environment (Schiff, Coleman and Miner 2008, 72). These authors found clubhouse members appreciative of a place that offered support but not high demands for persons feeling pressured, overwhelmed, and "too sick."

Peer Initiatives

Increasingly, in a number of mental health settings in Canada, services are being provided by peer workers. In trying to define "peer support," O'Hagan and colleagues (2010, 14) write: "At the most basic level, it may described as support provided by peers, for peers; or any organized support provided by and for people with mental health problems." As noted, the support provided is organized, as opposed to what might be called "befriending." The recognition of peer support as an essential component of mental health services was identified as a priority by the Mental Health Commission of Canada (2012).

Peers have a credibility borne from personal experience that the practitioner may not share; thus, they are in a unique position with respect to a helping engagement. As Bainbridge (1998, iii) notes: "Consumers have an in-depth knowledge of the system and can share insights with non-consumer providers and clients from the position of having been there. The consumer provider's credibility is magnified in the eyes of clients when they can relate a specific issue to their own personal experience." In addition to instrumental support, peers who have "endured, and overcome adversity can offer ... encouragement, hope, and perhaps mentorship to others facing similar situations" (Davidson et al. 2006b, 443; see also Davidson 2012).

The evolution of peer support has come from two different directions: (1) self-help, an example being Alcoholics Anonymous, and (2) more recently the creation of peer services *within* the formal mental health system. While similar, there may also be some significant differences with respect to roles in these different settings. Peer support formed outside of the formal system is often in response to the inadequacies of that system and thus comes from an advocacy orientation, in some cases, more critical and civil-rights oriented. Conversely, peers working "inside" the formal system – sometimes called "prosumers" – are contracted to provide services within a model aligned more closely with professional practice, for example emphasizing the importance of boundaries between persons delivering and receiving service. Some working in the field of peer support take issue with the latter approach, arguing that peers should de-emphasize differences and "responsibly challenge the assumptions about mental illness ... and a strong sense of identity as 'mental patient' ... by practicing relationships in a different way" (Mead, Hilton, and Curtis 2001, 136).

There are a wide range of peer support initiatives, and a report to the Mental Health Commission of Canada reviews their philosophical and organizational differences (O'Hagan et al. 2010). For the purposes of their report, these authors identify "four main structures in which peer support take place":

- Informal grassroots self-help groups run by volunteers, with a Statistics Canada (2003) survey determining that 5 percent of persons identified with a mental illness or addiction sought support from a self-help group, either in person, online, or via the phone.
- Independent peer-run organizations, staffed and governed by clients, which may provide advocacy and/or support. In Canada, it is noted that Quebec

has been a leader in developing innovative models of peer support advocacy organizations; in Ontario, a multi-site study found that peer-run organizations in that province were "an important complement or alternative to formal services provided by professionals" (Goering et al. 2006, 367).

- Peer-support programs in mainstream agencies.
- Peer support workers employed or contracted by mainstream services.

Peer support workers have become an important component of the services provided at a number of formal mental health programs in Canada, despite the initial trepidations of professional staff. In the Vancouver Coastal Health Authority, the first cohort of these workers started placements in 1997, with eighty-three contracts operating by 2011.[5] A contract is normally for twenty hours a month, at remuneration somewhat higher than minimum wage, to work one-on-one with other clients on mutually identified goals (Richard, Jongbloed and MacFarlane 2009). In its strategy document, the Mental Health Commission of Canada (2012, 41) recommends the creation of "opportunities for people living with mental health problems and illnesses to take up positions at all levels within the mental health workforce."

Evaluations of peer initiatives have found benefits for the workers, the clients they see, and the sponsoring organizations (Bradstreet and Pratt 2010). For example, a US study comparing persons randomly assigned to "usual care" or "usual care plus peer support" found a significant reduction in hospitalizations and hospital days among clients receiving peer support (Sledge et al. 2011). In a study that compared peer-based and traditional case management services, peer workers, by revealing their own experiences, were found to be more effective at engaging alienated, hard-to-reach clients early in treatment (Sells et al. 2008). A literature review by Repper and Carter (2011) found that PSWs appeared to be more successful than professional staff in promoting hope, belief in recovery, self-esteem, self-management, and increased social networks. For professional staff, being exposed to peer workers at the worksite can have a consciousness-raising, humanizing effect, and the organization can also be seen as "walking the walk" when it comes to promoting employment of persons with mental health problems.

Challenges remain, particularly with respect to interpersonal relationships in peer support settings. In some cases professional staff may view peer appointments as tokenism and minimize or trivialize their roles and responsibilities. Non-client staff may also question the skills and "professionalism" of client co-workers (e.g., the ability to maintain confidentiality). Some of these concerns were identified in a Canadian study that involved in-depth interviews with five peer support workers in Vancouver (Richard, Jongbloed, and MacFarlane 2009). In their accounts, the peer workers spoke about feeling excluded by professional staff (e.g., not being invited to some social events and, even when invited, being left by themselves), not feeling valued for their client work, and being treated not as a colleague but rather as a mentally ill person. Significant individual differences were noted, with "some professionals ... still not comfortable ... [while] others [were] very progressive, very relaxed about it" (106). Frustration was also expressed about limited career prospects available in the contract model being used and limited access to educational opportunities.

Peer support workers may also encounter some tensions with respect to their relationships with clients. These can include the prejudice among service recipients that only a "qualified professional" can assist them or the view that client service providers are no longer true "peers" once they become employees. In the worst-case scenario, the client-employee becomes marginalized from both reference groups – professionals and peers. This role complexity is summarized in the following passage, entitled "Working within the System," written by a client who became a member of the board of directors of the Coast Foundation, a non-profit mental health agency:

> At first I was suspicious of the professionals I worked with [on the board]. But I came to realize that, ultimately, they weren't different from me. They actually cared. I learned that, just because you think some people have more power than you, that doesn't make them the enemy. When I was on [the agency's] board, *I* became suspect. I was perceived by my friends who were consumers as having sold out to management. Staff people who had been my friends [now] saw me as a threat. And some board members were afraid of consumers. There was a handful of other consumers on the board, and a couple of them just couldn't get past their anger. (Gagnon 2011, 8)

As noted earlier, a tension particular to this role concerns the appropriate use of boundaries (which are emphasized in professional-client relationships) versus self-disclosure, given that the peer worker's own experiences are considered to be a potentially important tool in her/his engagement with clients. As noted by Repper and Carter (2011, 398), PSWs "are not only allowed, but also in fact are expected to disclose personal information and to share intimate stories from their own lives." On the one hand, there is the view that "without ... flexible and individually negotiated boundaries we perpetuate the power structure of a more formal professional relationship" (Mead, Hilton, and Curtis 2001, 139); on the other hand, one can point to a study on coping methods in which peer support workers spoke about the need to set clear boundaries at times so as not to feel overwhelmed in their roles (Silver 2004). It may be that programs hiring peer workers need to more clearly define ethical issues, including use of self-disclosure, that relate to this difficult role (O'Hagan et al. 2010).

Mental Illness in the Workplace

The discussion so far has concerned clients of the mental health system, persons identified as having a mental disorder, and ways to support their employment. There is another, less visible population: persons already employed in regular work settings who have or may develop a mental disorder, and who may be uncertain about where to turn for help or nervous about disclosing their mental health issues to their employer (Proudfoot 2007).

It should not be surprising that mental disorder in the workplace is relatively common, given what we know about prevalence rates in the general population, and a CMHA publication refers to this as "the largest untreated epidemic facing the Canadian workforce" (Steinke and Dastmalchian 2009, 6). The extent of the problem is reflected in the considerable number of sick days taken because of illnesses such as depression (Conference Board of Canada 2008), and the substantial proportion of short-term and long-term disability claims attributable to mental health and addiction issues, which have become the fastest growing category of claims (Government of Canada 2007; Shain 2008). Clearly, there is a business case to be made for supporting psychiatric disability in the workplace.

A good illustration of the challenges faced by employees with mental health concerns comes from a Canadian study of the experiences of health care staff returning to work after a leave related to mental illness or addiction (Glasgow 2007). An interesting aspect of this was that these individuals were working *in the mental health system*, where one might reasonably expect a more sympathetic, coherent response. However, participants disclosed that they in fact experienced considerable shame and stigma within their own service. Glasgow (2007) also found that stigma varied, with anxiety and depression triggering less of a response while psychosis and addiction produced the greatest negative reaction. Participants also spoke about:

- confusion with respect to the many departments and individuals involved in the return-to-work process and how it all seemed under-resourced;
- polices and procedures being oriented to physical rather than psychiatric disabilities;
- a lack of accommodations;
- the importance of trust and having someone who believed in you;

- the importance of leadership and of having the supervisor be someone who could potentially be a role model in supporting and welcoming the employee.

Glasgow concludes by underlining the importance of early intervention, before mental health worsened, and to this end highlighted the need for management training (see also Galt 2006).

On the question of training, some employers and educational institutions are building mental health awareness into their curricula. In a report on this subject, Galt (2006) cites examples such as the Toronto Dominion Bank offering employees on maternity leave information on postpartum depression, and McGill University requiring all MBA students to attend a seminar entitled "Mental Health and Productivity: Sustainable Performance in a Brain-Based Economy." Another example is the conferences convened by the CMHA for business, government, and union leaders on the subject of workplace mental health (Rossi 2006). In 2011, the Mental Health Commission announced it would start a process to produce a set of best practice standards for workplace mental health, making Canada the first country to do so (Minsky 2011).

A substantial section of the 2006 Kirby Report is devoted to mental illness in the Canadian workplace. The authors talk about primary and secondary prevention measures, with primary measures designed to "eliminate, or at least reduce, factors in the workplace that have a negative impact on the mental health of the workforce" (Standing Senate Committee on Social Affairs, Science and Technology 2006, 180). It is noted that certain management practices can "precipitate or aggravate mental health problems" (182), and these include unreasonable work demands, providing no credit for accomplishments, allowing no use of discretion, and tolerating an atmosphere of uncertainty and ambiguity. Secondary intervention involves "strategies designed principally to reduce the effects of stressful work situations by improving the ability of individuals to adapt to and to manage stress" (180). These would include disability management and employee assistance programs, and workplace accommodations. Accommodations can involve specific arrangements such as scheduling, workspace layout, and location, but this also refers to the larger organizational culture. Concerning workplace culture, acceptance and inclusion need to be the guiding philosophies of practice for programs to be considered inclusive (Bainbridge 1998). To this end, Curtis and Smith (1996) speak to the need for clarity and consistency in ethical and practice standards, which are communicated clearly and often through words *and* action. One key area of accommodation concerns flexible scheduling, which can refer to allowing more time for orientation and for the completion of specific tasks, modifying hours of work, and allowing time off to accommodate medical and counselling appointments. Bainbridge (1998, 31) notes that scheduling in many instances is the most crucial accommodation but one that is "difficult to arrange," which speaks to the reality of co-workers expressing resentment about someone "unfairly" being favoured and, in turn, the invisibility of psychiatric, as opposed to physical, disabilities.

For persons in pre-vocational and supported employment settings staff may need to consider providing coverage for absences due to hospitalization, a feature of the transitional employment model (see above). Other considerations include the provision of an advocate for advice and support, a job coach, or an employee willing to act as a mentor (this, in fact, is a standard feature of supported employment models).

Education

As noted, the impact of mental illness means that persons affected will often have lesser educational attainment than their peers. American surveys have determined that fewer than 40 percent of persons categorized as having "severe emotional disturbance" graduate from high school (Cook 2006) and that 86 percent of students with mental illnesses withdraw from college before completing a degree, compared to 37 percent for the general population (Salzer, Wick, and Rogers 2008). Surveys have also found a substantial proportion of those living with a mental illness expressing the desire to return to school and complete postsecondary education (Corrigan et al. 2008).

However, for persons struggling with a mental disorder, the prospect of entering or returning to school can be daunting. Potential barriers also include the attitudes of mental health practitioners, teachers, and administrators as well as the effects of the disorder itself:

People with psychiatric disabilities often exhibit cognitive, perceptual, affective and interpersonal deficits intrinsic to or resulting from the mental illness. In addition, there can be feelings of anxiety, hopelessness and guilt combined with perceptual problems, difficulty in processing and/or retaining information, effects of learning disabilities and limited attention span. Individuals with serious mental illnesses cannot predict when they might become ill or how long they might be away from a classroom setting because of relapse. When medications are prescribed, it frequently takes time to determine the dosage that is most effective at allowing full participation in an educational setting. (British Columbia Ministry of Health 2002f, 14)

Canadian data on campus mental health come from a survey of four thousand students at Simon Fraser University near Vancouver (the response rate in this study was about 38 percent) (Whiting 2008). In this survey, 17.5 percent of respondents reported experiencing depression, and 12.2 percent reported an anxiety disorder, both figures somewhat higher than prevalence rates for the general population (BC Ministry of Health Services 2008), possibly suggesting an exacerbation of symptoms in a stressful environment. Of those reporting depression, one in five were taking psychotropic medication. Eighteen percent of respondents (270 persons) reported that a mental health condition affected their academic performance, and among this group, 55 percent reported feeling "hopeless," 40 percent stated it was "difficult to function," and 11 percent reported seriously considering attempting suicide.

While symptoms of mental illness can of course exist before entering university, there are a number of aspects of campus life that may trigger an underlying psychiatric vulnerability (Whiting 2008):

- the transition from living with family to managing on one's own;
- managing a change of locale (e.g., a new city or in some cases a new country);
- financial pressures;
- juggling work and studies;
- the pressure to compete and succeed, for example, gaining entry to professional schools.

What sort of support can students with mental health problems expect? In some cases preparatory programs may be offered by mental health professionals (e.g., Gutman 2008). For those going on to postsecondary education there will, in most cases, be programs for persons with disabilities at those institutions, although students with mental health concerns may not be aware of these services and, in some instances, may be too embarrassed to use them. Concerning the effectiveness of these programs, a large-scale US survey of college students reporting mental health problems found the situation had improved somewhat over earlier periods, with respect to knowledge of and access to disability services and accommodations, but that a number of challenges and barriers remained (Salzer, Wick, and Rogers 2008). In the study, among the group who had requested academic supports for a mental disorder, over half reported feeling embarrassed about disclosing their status to, or being stigmatized by, a faculty member; 42 percent found faculty to be uncooperative or unreceptive; 41 percent were fearful of being stigmatized by other students; and 27 percent had difficulty in obtaining documentation to receive the support. One of the most significant findings of the study was that, even when disability offices were available, students would end up trying to negotiate support directly from the course instructor rather than enrolling in the specialized program. This speaks to the importance of educating all stakeholders about gaining access to appropriate services and accommodations, which, in the words of Enid Weiner (2008, 24) at York University in Toronto, "are [a] right, not a privilege."

Academic accommodations can take various forms and are described by a York University administrator as "changes made to the academic environment that level the playing field so that students with disabilities can perform in a way that best reflects their potential" (Weiner 2008, 24). Accommodations may refer specifically to ways of completing assignments but should also consider preventative measures and stress reduction (e.g., stress reduction may be addressed by taking a reduced course load). Examples of accommodations include (Vagnerova 2003b; Weiner 2008):

- classroom accommodations, such as preferential seating, permitting beverages (to help with medication side effects such as sedation and dry mouth), and assistance with note taking (such as having another student or a friend take notes or allowing use of a tape recorder);
- studying accommodations, such as texts on tape, tutoring, mentoring, and the creation of peer-support groups;
- assignment accommodations, such as delays granted due to hospitalization (or other mental health concerns), more time for completion, and assistance in completing assignments during hospitalization;
- alternate forms of evaluation, for example, creation of a video, in place of an oral presentation;
- examination accommodations, such as altering the format, allowing the use of a computer, if handwriting is made difficult because of side effects, allowing more time to write the exam, allocation of a separate room, and giving a (different) take home exam;
- administrative accommodations, such as flexibility in determining full-time status for the purposes of financial aid and health insurance as well as offering an incomplete grade, rather than a failure, if the student suffers a relapse.

Finally, readers may utilize resources such as the Canadian Mental Health Association's online *Guide to College and University for Students with Psychiatric Disabilities*, which includes discussion on topics such as disclosure, advocacy, funding, accommodations, support networks, and illness management (http://www.cmha.ca/youreducation).

Notes

1 In assessing employment benefits, researchers must address confounding factors such as the direction of effect (i.e., are benefits due to the impact of employment or is it that persons functioning at a higher level are more able to work?).

2 The figures are somewhat lower in studies using a broader definition of mental illness (e.g., the Canadian Community Health Survey [cycle 2.1], which screened for mood and anxiety but not psychotic disorders) (Alberta Mental Health Board 2007).

3 Under Canadian law, a disability may be grounds for non-hiring if it can be argued that the condition prevents the person from safely and competently carrying out the job. Employers may have a legal duty to provide accommodations for disabled persons when the disability does *not* affect job performance, *if* the accommodations can be made without causing the employer "undue hardship" (Dranoff 2005).

4 This survey was not published but is available from this author.

5 A worker could hold more than one contract, so the actual number of workers in this example was fewer than eighty-three.

Other Resources

Workplace Mental Health Promotion is a website created by CMHA Ontario that provides tools to help create mentally healthy workplaces: http://wmhp.cmhaontario.ca/.

The Legal and Ethical Context of Mental Health Practice

18

As we have seen, mental health practitioners in the course of their work may interfere with the liberty of individuals, such as when they arrange for the involuntary detention and treatment of someone in a hospital psychiatric ward or when they are supervising a community treatment order. At this point, we turn to the legal and ethical basis for curtailing freedom, asking: "How and when is it justified?"

A few have suggested that it is never justified. This extreme version of civil libertarianism is reflected in the writings of the late American author and critic of psychiatry Thomas Szasz (see box), who argued that, since no biological "markers" can be found to distinguish persons diagnosed with schizophrenia, their situations cannot be compared to other persons disabled by "real" medical conditions – in short, "mental illness" is an invention of psychiatry. A more legitimate concern with the overreach of psychiatry had to do with the argument that, in the earlier part of the twentieth century, statutory committal criteria were too broad, meaning a greater likelihood of the involuntary hospitalization of persons whose behaviour involved no real harm to themselves or others.

Because of the temptation to become involved with persons for "their own good," and the associated threats to individual dignity and autonomy, ethicists have tended to conclude that, while we may at times have to interfere with the liberty of individuals, "interference always stands in need of justification" and that "the onus of justification always lies on those who want to interfere" (Browne et al. 2002, 285). This view is associated with English philosopher John Stuart Mill, who in his famous essay *On Liberty*, published in 1859, argues that state intervention, no matter how well intentioned, leads inevitably to the *infantilization* of the subjected person. Mill recognized that the state had a right to intervene to prevent an individual from harming *others* (police powers), but he applied a higher standard when the issue was (apparent) *self*-harm. While not speaking specifically to what we now call mental illness, Mill also recognized that not all adult citizens could be held to the same standard of responsibility and that some were "encumbered" due to lack of information, duress, or particular emotional states (Browne et al. 2002).

If one assumes, then, that a mental disorder constitutes a form of encumbrance that may compromise a person's ability to care for him- or herself, justifying an intervention, there is still the question: At what point do we intervene? One problem with focusing on the *prevention* of harm is that it necessitates the prediction of future behaviour, an exercise fraught with difficulty. Indeed, some – often family members – complain that this requirement may mean waiting until it is "too late" (Hall 2000). An alternative position is that mental health practitioners have an obligation to look after individuals who are apparently unable to look after themselves *before* they come to harm. This viewpoint, supported by family advocacy organizations (such as the National Alliance on Mental Illness in the US), is in legal terms referred to as the *parens patriae* powers of the state – "government as parent."

Thomas Szasz and the Myth of Mental Illness

When considering psychiatry and civil rights, it is impossible not to refer to the views of American author Thomas Szasz, who, although himself a psychiatrist, was a steadfast critic of psychiatric practices. In a number of publications (e.g., *The Myth of Mental Illness* [1974]; *Schizophrenia: The Sacred Symbol of Psychiatry* [1976]; *Psychiatric Slavery* [1977]) and on his website (http://www.szasz.com), he argued that "mental illness" has no basis in physical reality and that labelling individuals "schizophrenic" is simply a means by which society controls persons exhibiting undesirable behaviours. This position appears to fly in the face of increasing evidence that disorders such as schizophrenia do have a biological basis, and it has also been criticized as a heartless stance in that the logical outcome is the abandonment of individuals who cannot look after themselves. In Szasz's writings there is an emphasis on personal accountability and a dismissal of the idea of mental illness as an excuse for unacceptable behaviour. Notably, his website is called the "Cybercenter for Liberty and Responsibility." Szasz, who died in 2012, was influential for some time and is still cited as an authority by critics of psychiatry and some psychiatric consumers (e.g., Shimrat 1997), although an opponent suggests that his theories finally "have been relegated to the shelf of quirks of medical history" (Torrey 1988, 165).

Intervention decisions can thus be seen as falling somewhere on a continuum, from a narrow standard for intervention (e.g., imminent physical danger to self or others) to a broad standard, which may refer to the welfare of the individual, need for treatment, "best interests," or the potential for future deterioration. Decisions are based, in part, on the individual practitioner's own comfort level, or risk tolerance, and also on the criteria in provincial mental health statutes, which may refer to "protection," "harm," or "safety" as the basis for the involuntary admission of persons with a mental illness (described in more detail below). Readers should also be aware that the intervention standard that any jurisdiction adopts must be viewed in historical, social, and political context. In the 1970s, reflecting issues being raised by the civil rights movement, legislation was amended in some provinces to narrow committal criteria and to consider treatment refusal. By the 2000s, the pendulum had swung back somewhat, with broader committal criteria and community treatment orders being introduced (Gray, Shone, and Liddle 2008). There is some concern that these more recent legislative developments are the product of an increased preoccupation with "protection of the public" and that media accounts of violent behaviour on the part of psychiatric patients have swayed popular and political opinion (Davis 2002).

There are three main areas of law in Canada that apply to mental health practice:

- provincial mental health acts, which deal with involuntary hospital admission;
- provincial guardianship laws, which contain provisions for adults and older adults who may suffer from abuse or neglect or who may be unable to make decisions (especially health care and financial decisions) in their best interests;
- The federal Criminal Code, which has a set of provisions for accused persons believed to have a mental disorder.

These are reviewed separately below, following a necessary introduction to the Charter of Rights and Freedoms.

The Charter of Rights and Freedoms

Before looking at Canadian mental health statutes, it is necessary to consider the impact of the Charter of Rights and Freedoms. Enacted in 1982, this is Canada's supreme law, one that, with some exceptions,[1] takes precedence over other existing federal and provincial statutes, including mental health laws. New laws must conform with the Charter, and existing laws must be applied in accordance with the Charter or risk being challenged on that basis (Gray, Shone, and Liddle 2008). If a law appears to infringe one or more of the Charter rights and a challenge is made, the government must be able to show that any infringement was in accordance with the principles of fundamental justice, procedural fairness, and a balancing of the interests of the individual and society or that the law can be "saved" by section 1 of the Charter, which states that the rights therein are "subject only to such reasonable limits prescribed by law as can be demonstrably justified in a free and democratic society." In practice, section 1 refers to a legal test developed in a court case called *Oakes*,[2] which requires the following: the infringing law must pursue an objective that is "pressing and substantial"; there must be a rational connection between how the law works and its objective; the law must infringe upon Charter rights as little as is reasonably possible; and there must be proportionality between the effects of an infringing law and the objective of the law. If a challenge is successful, the provision in question is ruled invalid by the Court, necessitating the passage of new or amended legislation. In anticipation of the potential impact of the Charter, in 1987 an inter-provincial committee drafted the Uniform Mental Health Act to comply with Charter guarantees, with the hope that this would lead to greater standardization of the various provincial and territorial mental health acts (Davis 1995a).

Several sections of the Charter may have application in considering the reasonableness of the involuntary detention and treatment of mentally disordered persons. These include:

- s. 7: Right to life, liberty, and security of the person;
- s. 9: Right not to be arbitrarily detained or imprisoned;
- s. 10: Right to be given the reasons for any detention and to have the validity of that detention challenged in court;
- s. 12: Right not to be subjected to any cruel and unusual treatment or punishment;
- s. 15: Right to equal protection of the law without discrimination, including discrimination based on mental disability.

Some specific Charter challenges are discussed below, but for a more comprehensive picture, the reader is directed to Gray, Shone, and Liddle's excellent 2008 text, *Canadian Mental Health Law and Policy*. (In this book the authors, who favour access to treatment, discuss not only "negative" freedoms – i.e., protection from interference – but also how the Charter could be used to *gain* access to services that otherwise might be denied.)

Provincial Mental Health Acts and Involuntary Hospitalization

With health care a provincial jurisdiction in Canada, each province and territory has an act (or acts) that governs the involuntary detention ("committal" or "certification") and treatment of persons presumed to have a mental disorder. This section reviews (1) the criteria for involuntary admission, (2) the procedures used in committals, (3) the issue of treatment refusal, (4) mandatory outpatient treatment, and (5) legal protections for the patient. The reader is cautioned that the laws referred to here were current as this book went to press but that the relevant statutes would need to be consulted concurrently regarding possible revisions.

Criteria for Involuntary Admission

As noted above, in the 1970s, with increasing recognition of the civil rights of psychiatric patients, detention criteria shifted away from "need for treatment" – felt to be an overly broad and paternalistic standard – and began to refer to physical danger as the basis for certification. This started in Ontario, with Alberta and the Northwest Territories following not long after (Gray, Shone, and Liddle 2008). While these three retain the standard of physical or bodily harm in their statutes, and while other jurisdictions modified their admission criteria (e.g., BC dropped the "welfare" test), it is noteworthy that currently only three of thirteen jurisdictions (the Northwest Territories, Nunavut, and Quebec) refer to physical harm exclusively. For example, Prince Edward Island includes *mental* harm as a basis for committal, while a number of provinces now include *deterioration* (mental or physical) in their laws. In summarizing more recent events – and the swinging of the pendulum – concerning involuntary admission criteria, Gray, Shone, and Liddle (2008) note that four provinces *broadened* their committal criteria between 2000 and 2007.

Gray, Shone, and Liddle (2008) offer a number of critiques of physical dangerousness as the sole basis for involuntary hospitalization: (1) neither the Charter nor the courts in their decisions has required exclusive bodily harm as the certification standard; (2) such a standard does not address, for example, the case of a manic person who is causing untold financial harm in a spending spree but who cannot be hospitalized unless he/she becomes violent; (3) this standard may contribute to criminalization of the mentally ill when the option of diverting a non-violent mentally ill person charged with a crime is closed off; (4) hospitalization is now much briefer, and conditions better, than the days of *One Flew Over the Cuckoo's Nest*, meaning the "ideological origins of the criterion no longer apply" (137); (5) clinicians end up "bending the rules" anyway, by continuing to commit to hospital persons who (apparently) would benefit from treatment but who may not meet the dangerousness criterion. This is based on findings from a number of US studies, which show that, in jurisdictions that narrowed committal standards, patients continued to be sent to hospital at the same rate as they had been prior to the change in the law (Appelbaum 1994). These studies found not only clinicians but also judges concluding that the dangerousness criterion was unworkable.

Canadian mental health acts make reference to "safety," "protection," or "harm" (to self or others) as the basis for intervening with mentally disordered persons. In some cases these terms are qualified – for example *imminent* harm in New Brunswick and *serious* harm in Ontario – but in others they are not, leaving it to other parties (academics and, in some cases, the courts) to interpret them. For example, the standard of "safety" used in Prince Edward Island has been interpreted more broadly by legal analysts to include non-physical harms (Robertson 1994). There is also the question of whether admission criteria *should* be qualified in law: concerning the possible ambiguity of the dangerousness standard used in Alberta, a government task force concluded that it would be best not to qualify the meaning of the term; that, rather, there should be "latitude for the exercise of professional discretion and clinical acumen" (Government of Alberta 1983, 56). Such a conclusion would likely be reassuring for many clinicians, and less so for civil rights advocates.

In British Columbia, the standard of "protection" was challenged using the Charter of Rights in the 1993 BC Supreme Court case *McCorkell v. Director of Riverview Hospital Review Panel*,[3] where the plaintiff argued that the standard was "vague and overbroad" and that, consequently, committed persons were being denied their liberty (s. 7) and subjected to arbitrary detention (s. 9), contrary to Charter guarantees. In dismissing this action, Justice Donald wrote that, "given the purpose of the Act – the treatment of the mentally disordered who need protection and care – the language must permit the exercise of some discretion." He further stated that "protection" could refer to "social, family, vocational or financial harm" (beyond simply physical danger), thereby giving a very broad interpretation of the committal standard. The BC Mental Health Act was undergoing a revision at the time, and this court decision was seen as a victory for those concerned about restricting access to treatment for the mentally ill (Davis 1995a).

Finally, in looking at certification standards, some comment must be made on how decision making is affected by resource availability. As noted earlier in the book, in many larger urban centres in Canada, there is great pressure on psychiatric beds in general hospitals. Consequently, it has become more difficult to get patients admitted, with hospital staff feeling the pressure to move current patients out as new cases arrive at the front door. Doctors in the community are of course aware of this and know that, even though a particular patient might be certifiable by the letter of the law, he or she may not be detained or may be discharged quickly if there are others arriving at the hospital who are apparently more in need. In other words, while a particular certification standard may appear broad in theory (notably that given in the *McCorkell* court decision in BC), a narrower standard will be applied in *practice* if hospital beds are in short supply.

Procedures Used in Committals

There are four mechanisms by which a person can be hospitalized involuntarily in Canada. The first and most frequent method involves obtaining a certificate signed by a health care professional. In all jurisdictions, except Nova Scotia, only one certificate is required.[4] The initial certificate gives authority to have the person taken to an inpatient unit for further examination. The person certifying is usually a physician, not necessarily a psychiatrist. Exceptions to this have been made in some jurisdictions, presumably because of more limited access to physicians. So, in Nunavut and the Northwest Territories, a psychologist may certify if a delay would be "unreasonable"; in the Yukon, a nurse may, under his or her authority, detain a person for observation for twenty-four hours (although she/he must consult with a physician by some means); and, in Newfoundland and Labrador, a nurse practitioner may complete the initial certificate. The single certificate authorizes detention of the person for twenty-four to seventy-two hours, depending on the jurisdiction. Beyond this time, a second certificate must be signed at hospital for the person to be detained longer. Statutory or common law provide for involuntary treatment of the patient during this initial period if the circumstances can be considered an emergency.

The second method of involuntary hospitalization involves apprehension by a police officer, which exists in all Canadian jurisdictions.[5] This often occurs during evenings or on weekends when medical offices may be closed, and, by statute, there is a presumption that gaining access to a physician in these cases would be impossible or impractical. Concerning the criteria used by police for apprehension, in some jurisdictions they are the same as for a physician, in others they are narrower, with the latter usually referring to physical harm or endangerment.

The third method, available in all Canadian jurisdictions, involves obtaining a judge's warrant. This method, used presumably because no other mechanisms are available, involves a citizen approaching (depending on the jurisdiction) a judge, magistrate, or justice of the peace and making a statement that a person is apparently mentally ill, is refusing help, and apparently meets the certification criteria. A warrant may then be issued to the police.

The fourth method, existing only in Nunavut and the Northwest Territories, involves a "citizen's arrest," whereby a person who has "reasonable and probable grounds" to believe the police criteria are met may take the individual in question involuntarily to a physician or hospital. The law presumes that this would be a last resort (i.e., no police officer available).

The Issue of Refusal of Psychiatric Treatment

"Certification" for the most part refers to involuntary *detention* and does not necessarily refer to treatment, which, currently in Canada, is a separate issue in most jurisdictions. This was not always the case. As reviewed by Gray, Shone, and Liddle (2008), prior to the 1960s, the question of psychiatric treatment refusal by involuntary patients did not arise since the discretion to impose treatment was granted as part of the authority to commit persons to hospital. Following the 1960s, however, more legal protections were built into mental health acts, a reflection of greater societal recognition of patients' rights. The impetus for this came from several directions. For one thing, it was suggested that psychiatric treatments could have deleterious effects – electroconvulsive therapy, in particular, received much bad publicity. Further, there is the fact that *non*-psychiatric patients have the right to refuse medical treatments and procedures, notwithstanding their potential benefits and necessity – although this is complicated by the question of whether the patient is of "sound mind" (more on this in a later section). It has also been argued that the issue of competency in one area of decision making should not automatically extend to another; for example, just because an individual has a mental illness, one cannot assume that he or she is incapable of making financial decisions. While few would disagree with the logic of this example, it becomes more challenging in the case of mental health laws (such as exist in Ontario) that permit treatment refusal when the certified patient has already been found incapable with respect to decisions about the need for hospitalization since these two areas of decision making seem closely tied together.

Concerning the right to refuse treatment, a landmark decision on this issue came out of the 1991 Ontario Court of Appeal case *Fleming v. Reid*.[6] Under the Mental Health Act at that time,[7] a review board would receive the expressed wishes of the patient, made when apparently competent, but was not obliged to follow the wishes (in the case of treatment refusal) and instead could apply a "best interests" standard. The Court ruled in this case that the relevant provisions in the act were in violation of the Charter and thus invalid.

The judgment read: "Although the right to be free from nonconsensual psychiatric treatment is not an absolute one, the state has not demonstrated any compelling reason for entirely eliminating this right, without any hearing or review." This means that previously expressed wishes against treatment, made when competent, cannot be simply overridden or ignored. While court decisions in one province are not binding in another, this ruling suggests that statutes, such as British Columbia's Mental Health Act, that do not provide a mechanism for considering the competency of patients concerning their treatment wishes are likely in violation of Charter guarantees, such as the rights to life, liberty, and security (s. 7) and to freedom from discrimination on the basis of mental disability (s. 15).

Currently, Canadian provinces handle the question of involuntary treatment quite differently (Gray, Shone, and Liddle 2008). Generally, if a certified person is deemed incompetent to make treatment decisions, she or he can be treated involuntarily. However, in BC, the issue of competent treatment refusal is not even addressed in the Mental Health Act: the certification itself provides authority for treatment (making BC's the most "paternalistic" statute). In three other provinces – Saskatchewan, Nova Scotia, and Newfoundland and Labrador – dealing with competent treatment refusal does not arise because, by law, competent persons cannot be admitted involuntarily. In other words, competency is addressed before admission rather than after. Four jurisdictions – Alberta, Yukon, New Brunswick, and Quebec – permit treatment refusal by a competent patient but provide mechanisms for overriding the refusal, through a review board, tribunal (New Brunswick), or judge (Quebec). The standard applied by these decision makers is based on a "best interests" test, which addresses whether or not the patient is likely to improve with or without the proposed treatment and whether the treatment benefits outweigh the risks. Finally, five jurisdictions – Manitoba, Ontario, PEI, Nunavut, and the Northwest Territories – do not allow competent treatment refusal to be overridden, meaning that indefinite detention is possible if it is felt that releasing the patient would be unsafe.

Using Ontario as an example (Regehr and Glancy 2010), a person certified to hospital may refuse treatment, but then her/his competence to do so would be assessed. If found competent, no treatment is ordered. If found *not* competent, the next question is whether she or he has a substitute decision maker (SDM). If she/he does, the SDM is consulted and has two options: (1) if the SDM knows of a patient's previously expressed wish, made while competent, she/he must act in accordance with it; (2) if she/he does not know of an applicable wish, she/he must act in the patient's best interests. If the patient does not have an SDM, treatment refusal is considered by the Consent and Capacity Review Board, which makes a determination. Finally, under the Health Care Consent Act, there are some avenues for appealing no-treatment decisions.

As the above example shows, authorizing involuntary treatment in some jurisdictions is a cumbersome matter, with lengthy delays being possible. The idea that patients committed to a psychiatric facility should have a right to refuse treatment, in particular by way of advance directives, is controversial and has been criticized by family members and clinicians (Tibbetts 2003; O'Reilly 2008), with some referring to it as the "right to remain psychotic" (McCaldon, Conacher, and Clark 1991). One argument is that the comparison with treatment refusal by *non*-psychiatric patients is spurious since, in the case of psychiatric patients, the organ that is used to make decisions – the brain – is the very one impaired by illness. Concerning advance directives, it is possible that circumstances may change, thus a University of Toronto professor of psychiatry talks about "the danger of advance directives being applied in a circumstance that a person could not foresee" (Hoffman 1997, 84). Finally, perhaps the most compelling argument is that not offering treatment to a hospitalized patient may mean that the individual will have to be detained longer than would otherwise be the case and that further mental and physical deterioration, and greater risk to staff and other patients, will be the result (Kelly et al. 2002). Gray, Shone, and Liddle (2008) discuss this at some length, referring to the potential for increased patient suffering, increased use of restraints and seclusion, longer stays, poorer prognosis, and additional financial burdens. These authors refer to the high-profile court case *Starson v. Swayze* (2003), wherein the Supreme Court of Canada upheld the right of amateur physicist Scott Starson to refuse medication, which Justice Major wrote in the majority decision had a "dulling effect on his thinking." Starson subsequently became increasingly psychotic, thinking the hospital was poisoning him, and starved himself until he was near death.

Mandatory Outpatient Treatment

As we have seen, "certification" refers to involuntary hospitalization, an *in*patient status. However, in recent years, there has been greater utilization of – and debate about – statutes that provide for *outpatient* certification, which authorize mandatory treatment from a community clinic, with "treatment" almost always including medication. Should conditions – such as attendance at the clinic – be "breached," the individual may be sent to hospital. Provisions of this sort have been implemented in a number of British Commonwealth countries, several Canadian jurisdictions, and most US states (Gray, Shone, and Liddle 2008).[8]

In Canada, there are three ways in which mandatory outpatient treatment may be imposed under civil law (Gray, Shone, and Liddle 2008). First, a number of mental health acts include a *leave* provision, whereby the patient leaves the hospital but is not formally discharged and is still under certification. For example, in BC, patients on "extended leave" have their care transferred, through forms contained in the Mental Health Act, to a community physician, who then takes over treatment and supervises the conditions of the leave (along with colleagues at the treatment program). Extended leave must be initiated in hospital, but the community physician does have the authority to discharge the person from leave. Second, a more recent development is the *community treatment order*, first brought in by Saskatchewan in 1994, which, unlike leave provisions, may be initiated in the community. Other provinces have followed suit, with Ontario (2000), Nova Scotia (2005), Newfoundland and Labrador (2006), and Alberta (2007) also introducing provisions for community treatment orders. There are a number of differences in procedures between these jurisdictions, but all require some evidence of prior "treatment failure" (as does extended leave), which usually refers to repeated hospitalization. Third, other legal mechanisms that empower a guardian or substitute decision maker to authorize health care decisions include mandatory outpatient treatment. Such mechanisms also include committeeship (referring to someone appointed by a court), adult protection laws (used in cases of self-neglect), and representation agreements, through which the client may appoint someone to make treatment decisions.

Why do we have mandatory outpatient treatment? The main justification is to prevent what has been called the "revolving door syndrome," whereby a person discharged from a psychiatric unit repeatedly fails to follow through with treatment in the community and becomes re-hospitalized. Using BC as an example, that province's *Guide to the Mental Health Act* (British Columbia Ministry of Health 2005, 29) states:

Extended leave may be considered suitable for an involuntary patient who:

- requires reinforcement of/support for compliance once out of hospital, and
- has had repeated relapses as a result of repeated non-compliance with medication and other care arrangements, and/or
- exhibits non-compliance which is intentional and/or due to lack of insight into the nature and severity of his/her illness.

Notably, the same document also states that extended leave should be considered "only when the patient will be provided appropriate services in the community" (30), which could be a problem in small, remote locations, and also that extended leave should not be used to reduce "length of stay in hospital when the patient is still in need of inpatient care" (29). This second point is significant in that it addresses one of the criticisms of mandated outpatient treatment; namely, that it is used to compensate for inadequate resources, in particular insufficient hospital beds, which leads to the premature discharge of persons who are still unwell. As a policy analyst puts it: "Coercion will not lead to more effective treatment if the treatment system itself is inadequate" (Diamond 1996, 60; see also Stainsby 2000).

The use of outpatient certification remains an issue that produces strong divisions of opinion. The Vancouver mother of a mentally ill woman states that, if a psychotic person cannot understand the need for treatment, then there are "no other logical options" than enforced treatment through community treatment orders (CTOs) (Inman 2011c). Supporters argue that studies evaluating CTOs clearly show positive outcomes, in particular, better engagement with treatment and support services, reductions in hospital admissions and lengths of stay, and reduced arrest rates (e.g., Hunt et al. 2007; Jaffe 2012; Link et al. 2011; New York State Office of Mental Health 2005; Treatment Advocacy Center 2009a). Others have questioned this conclusion, arguing that the studies used to support the reduced hospitalization claims are methodologically weak, with a shortage of randomized controlled trials (although randomized trials would be ethically problematic in this instance) (Kisely and Campbell 2006; Swartz 2010).[9] Proponents of CTOs also point out that they are, by definition, less restrictive than hospitalization since the person remains in the community. While this seems to make sense, a counterargument is that, being on a probation order, in effect, *indefinitely* (most forms of outpatient certification can be renewed and have no end date) might seem somewhat intrusive. Another criticism of CTOs is that they hurt the therapeutic relationship since the community practitioner's policing function is emphasized (Davis 2002), with a British review finding anywhere from one-third to two-thirds of psychiatrists surveyed opposed in principle to CTOs (Lawton-Smith 2008). With CTOs, there is also the implication, which some say reinforces the stereotype, that the mentally ill are so dangerous that they need tight controls. It is noteworthy, for instance, that the Ontario community treatment legislation was named "Brian's Law," after a sportscaster who was killed by an apparently mentally ill assailant. Similar pieces of legislation in New York and California were referred to, respectively, as "Kendra's Law" and "Laura's Law," following homicides in those jurisdictions.[10]

What do clients themselves say about being on CTOs? Concerning *inpatient* detention, studies have found a significant proportion of clients recognizing that their committal was justifiable in hindsight (O'Reilly et al. 2006). Should we expect this with CTOs? Perhaps not, if we assume that CTOs are used primarily with individuals who have, to quote again from the *BC Guide to the Mental Health Act*, "a lack of insight into the nature and severity of [their] illness." In an evaluation of the New York ("Kendra's") law, researchers interviewed seventy-six persons receiving court-ordered treatment in New York City (New York State Office of Mental Health 2005).[11] They found that just over half reported feeling "angry" or "embarrassed" by the experience but that 62 percent reported that, "all things considered," court-ordered treatment had been a good thing for them. A clear majority reported that the program had helped them stay well (81 percent), gain control over their lives (75 percent), and made them more likely to keep appointments and take medication (90 percent). Finally, 87 percent said they were confident in their case manager's ability to help them. What about Canada? The 2000 Ontario community treatment law underwent a mandatory evaluation, with a report published by a consulting firm in 2005 (Dreezer and Dreezer Inc. 2005). A number of stakeholders were interviewed, and family members in particular expressed satisfaction with the law. However, the forty-seven CTO clients interviewed were apparently more critical of the program (although response percentages were not given). While clients interviewed did report positive results, such as staying out of hospital and maintaining housing, they also spoke about loss of autonomy, not being consulted, not being treated with respect, and a loss of dignity. Some also voiced the opinion that CTOs are best applied "selectively," with a "small group of needy clients" (Dreezer and Dreezer Inc. 2005, 84). A survey of stakeholders was also conducted in Saskatchewan, with similar results (i.e., enthusiasm on the part of family members and ambivalence on the part of clients who had been/were on CTOs) (O'Reilly et al. 2006). The authors noted: "many patients in our study were initially resentful of being placed on a CTO but reported that this reaction lessened with time"; however, they conceded that positive responses may have been due to sampling bias, with those agreeing to participate (only two in five of those approached) possibly "having reached some level of insight" (522). Despite limitations in these studies, these client observations are important food for thought: working within coercive contexts is likely to be an enduring reality for community practitioners, with, as noted, more jurisdictions in North America implementing mandatory treatment orders.[12]

Legal Protections

Provincial and territorial mental health acts provide some safeguards and protections whereby involuntary treatment or detention is reviewed and may be challenged (Gray, Shone, and Liddle 2008). As noted above, with the exception of BC, provinces and territories must address the question of the patient's competency to make treatment decisions before imposing treatment. Involuntary patients may also request a second opinion about their treatment in Manitoba, BC, and the Northwest Territories (although this opinion is not binding on the treating physician). In Saskatchewan, two medical opinions are required before ECT can be administered. In BC, persons on extended leave (mandatory outpatient treatment) undergo an automatic review of their involuntary status once a year even if they do not request it.

For patients seeking to be discharged, the most common method by which they may challenge certification is through an application to a *review board*, which is available in all Canadian jurisdictions except the Northwest Territories and Quebec, where a court performs this function. The review board is supposed to function as an independent tribunal, which does not cost the patient anything and which is normally less formal than a court hearing. The composition of and procedures used by these boards vary somewhat from jurisdiction to jurisdiction, and for more on this the reader is referred again to Gray, Shone, and Liddle (2008). Review boards make decisions about the continuation of an involuntary status, either inpatient our outpatient, and they have the authority to overturn a certification and discharge the patient. In jurisdictions in which treatment refusal may occur, the role of the review board can include addressing the question of the patient's competency. Generally, the criteria used by the board are the same as those used in certification, so the question being asked is: "Do these criteria still apply?" Data from BC show that, in 2004, patients successfully appealed their detention in 23 percent of cases when the appeal was heard; however, two-thirds of review applications never got to that stage, being suspended, rejected, or cancelled (British Columbia Ministry of Health Services 2005).

A second, less common method of challenging certification involves going through the courts. Patients may be deterred from this approach because of the time and potential costs involved, although some advocacy organizations take on cases without charge. One means of challenging a detention is by way of *habeas corpus,* a right in common law that allows the detained person (or representative) to request that a court determine the validity of the detention. This right in common (non-statutory) law is also upheld in section 10 of the Charter of Rights, which states: "Everyone has the right on arrest or detention ... to have the validity of the detention determined by way of *habeas corpus* and to be released if the detention is not lawful." In practice, a challenge of this type in psychiatry would mean seeing if the certification forms were completed correctly (e.g., signed, correctly dated, and referring to the appropriate legal criteria). Review board decisions may also be appealed to the courts. In theory, habeas corpus can also be used if involuntary patients are not informed of their rights; again, referring to section 10, detained persons have the right "to be informed promptly of the reasons therefore ... [and] to retain and instruct counsel without delay and to be informed of that right."

Competency and Adult Guardianship

The legislation and procedures pertaining to competency and adult guardianship are complex. Generally, these are laws, court orders, and, in some cases, voluntary arrangements that address the situation of adults who may be suffering from abuse, neglect, or self-neglect, and who are apparently unable to look after themselves. Referring to neglect, this could be due to the symptoms of a mental illness (which is where we start to move towards the domain of provincial mental health acts), or a dementia, a physical disability, intoxication, duress (coercion or manipulation by a third party), or inaccurate/incomplete information. Areas of need could include health care, personal care, or finances. Gray, Shone, and Liddle (2008) note that legislation in this area was pioneered in Canada in the Maritimes, starting with Newfoundland and Labrador's Neglected Adults Welfare Act, 1990.

Laws concerning the protection of vulnerable adults, similar to child protection laws, place an onus on designated persons to respond (i.e., authorities *must* investigate reports of abuse or neglect).[13] While there is an emphasis in adult protection on "least intrusive" options being considered first, the investigation process can ultimately result in the issuance of court orders authorizing, for example, treatment of a serious medical condition.

Living with Risk

In working with vulnerable adults, practitioners must struggle with the question of how much risk is tolerable. While there is an obligation to investigate cases of neglect, there is also an ethical imperative to intrude as little as possible and to protect individual dignity. Tolerance is determined to a considerable extent by the assessed *capacity* or *capability* of the client to live with risk (more on this below). The following points may also be considered:

- All of us live with some degree of risk in our lives; on any given day we may meet with misfortune, in a traffic accident for example. Hence, in considering risk, it is better to speak about risk *reduction* than risk elimination.
- Risk can be seen as a function of both the degree of harm that may result and the probability that it will happen. For example, concerns about an elderly relative falling in her apartment may be related to the frequency

with which this occurs, but even when the event is infrequent, concern may be raised if the individual has osteoporosis and is more likely to sustain a serious injury.

- Risk is seen as applying to specific situations – for example, risk of starting a fire, risk of being evicted, or risk of malnutrition.
- In assessing risk, Silberfeld and Fish (1994) suggest that care providers consider several factors, such as: Is the risk new or old? Are there actual concrete instances of harm (or is this supposition)? Is the risk imminent or remote? Can the assessment be considered "objective?" Is the risk chosen or accidental? And is the risk to self or others? A stronger case can be made for intervening if the individual is putting others at risk. On the other hand, Browne and colleagues (2002) note that "worry to relatives" is insufficient to support an intervention without additional information.

Competency

In trying to assist vulnerable adults, practitioners in most cases must address the question of *competency*, which Silberfeld and Fish (1994) define as having sufficient ability to perform a specific task, as opposed to actions that are beyond an individual's control. Disability may in some situations be pervasive, affecting a number of domains of decision making. A person severely affected by Alzheimer's disease might be an example of this. On the other hand, individuals may be competent in one sphere, such as financial planning, but not in another, such as the safe operation of a motor vehicle. Laws in this area generally *presume* adults to be competent with respect to decision making and, as per the definition above, incompetence – if found – should be specific to a particular domain. O'Connor (2010) notes that, since the mid-1990s, there has been a move away from a global concept of competence to one that considers capacity as multiple functional abilities along a continuum, which can vary over time and also according to context.

Competency assessments typically have a medical/psychiatric component and a functional component, the latter involving task-specific tests, preferably performed in a real world setting (e.g., at the person's residence or a financial institution). Competency assessment instruments are used in some jurisdictions (e.g. Kershaw and Webber 2008). In an overview of standardized tests, O'Connor (2010) notes that a tool used to assess decisions about treatment, the MacCAT-T,[14] is becoming a "gold standard," that tools related to financial decisions are being developed, but that the Mini Mental Status Exam has not been useful or specific enough for capacity decisions.

Depending on the gravity and complexity of the decisions, competency assessments may be multidisciplinary conferences that include an ethicist.

Clinical decisions concerning competence should not be taken lightly, given that they may necessitate restrictions of an individual's liberty – restrictions that can be wide-ranging. Further, being *wrongly* deemed incompetent can cause considerable psychological and practical harms for the individual so assessed.

What about competence and mental illness? While these are two separate issues, persons working in the mental health field may sometimes encounter the belief that "mental illness" *equals* "incompetence." This may arise when a concerned friend or family member argues with a practitioner that, because the person in question has schizophrenia (for example), she or he is "by definition" not able to make decisions about her/his health care or finances. This is a problematic and patronizing assumption and is not supported in law. That said, working with concerned family members, when the loved one has a mental illness and a neglected medical condition, is clearly an ethical challenge.

Consent to Health Care

Suppose a mental health practitioner becomes aware that a client is neglecting a medical condition but refusing to have it treated – what then? Generally, in Canadian law, a medical procedure may not be performed on any individual without her or his consent.[15] For the consent to be valid:

- It must be voluntary, that is "free of coercion ... [which] may include financial incentives, unnecessary fear, or influence created by the therapeutic alliance between the patient and the health care provider" (Regehr and Kanani 2006, 66).
- It must be informed, with the care provider explaining the main risks and benefits.
- The person must have the capacity or capability to consent.

How is capability determined? As Regehr and Kanani (2006, 61) summarize, "people must be able to understand the information that is provided to them and how that information applies to their specific situation." More specifically, the client needs to understand the condition for which the health care is proposed, the procedures involved, the risks and benefits, any alternative approaches, and the outcomes that could be (reasonably) anticipated should they have or not have the treatment. In practice, making an assessment of this nature is difficult. It is possible that an interview with a client may reveal that the treatment refusal is delusionally based, supporting a finding of incapability. However, if a client expressed anxiety about a surgical procedure an assessor would have to be able to argue that the anxiety was "abnormal" or pathological, beyond the anxiety that most people would experience in anticipation of surgery. A further complication is that a person's capability may fluctuate and change over time. And there are practical issues beyond simply applying the law, such as how to get the non-consenting client to the treatment location and how to manage any after-care, which may involve dressing changes, medication, and so on. Assessors have to determine whether the complications and aftermath of the treatment might outweigh the benefits, even if the person lacks the capacity to consent. If it is a question of life or limb, this determination may be easier; if not, the equation changes.

There are some exceptions to the consent rule, one being emergency situations. For example, the BC Health Care Consent and Care Facility Admission Act (s. 12) states that treatment may be given without consent "in order to preserve the adult's life, to prevent serious physical or mental harm or to alleviate severe pain." There is a presumption here that gaining access to a guardian would result in an unreasonable delay.

Health care consent legislation also provides for substitute decision making in the case of incapable adults. Using the BC statute as an example again, the hierarchy of decision makers from which the health care provider must choose, sequentially, is: the adult's spouse, the adult's child, the adult's parent, the adult's brother or sister, anyone else related by birth or adoption to the adult, or the public guardian and trustee. In some cases substitute decision makers are appointed in advance. This can be what is called a *committee*, which is a person appointed by a court to make medical decisions for an incapable adult, or a *representative*, which is a person voluntarily chosen by the client to make treatment decisions.[16]

Finally, case law and legislation in Canada dictate that advance directives cannot be ignored by health care providers (as we saw earlier with *Fleming v. Reid*). For example, in the 1990 Ontario Court of Appeal case *Malette v. Shulman*,[17] hospital staff were found liable by the Court for giving a blood transfusion to a Jehovah's Witness patient against her stated (written) wishes. For a statutory example, the BC consent law (s. 12.1) states: "A health care provider must not provide health care ... if the health care provider has reasonable grounds to believe that the person, while capable and after attaining 19 years of age, expressed an instruction or wish applicable to the circumstances to refuse consent to the health care."

Newcomers to this area of law must be excused for finding this confusing, particularly since different statutes and provisions appear to be addressing similar issues. For example, hospital admission is authorized by provincial mental health acts but could also be mandated by adult protection laws, committees, or representation agreements. In fact, it can be argued that, with these more recent legal developments, it is no longer necessary to have separate mental health legislation (Szmuckler and Holloway 1998). That said, as reviewed by Gray, Shone, and Liddle (2008), there are a number of disadvantages to using these other mechanisms to support non-consensual treatment: (1) guardianship orders can be complex, time consuming, and expensive; (2) their complexity, and an aversion to using the courts, make "business as usual" – the use of mental health acts – a more attractive, expedient option for practitioners; (3) guardianship arrangements offer fewer protections of individual autonomy; (4) guardianship orders may be unenforceable (even if a process eventually results in a court order, an attending physician may consider a particular non-consensual procedure to be infeasible and refuse on practical and/or ethical grounds). Concerning representation agreements – which conceivably are a means by which family members could be more involved in the care of their relative – a barrier to their utilization is the fact that clients, not uncommonly, are estranged from or hostile towards family members, or simply resent what they see as interference.

Mental Disorder and the Criminal Code
So far we have been talking about the legal basis for involuntary interventions coming from the area of *civil* law. Readers should be aware that the Criminal Code, a federal statute, also contains provisions concerning the detention, assessment, and (under limited conditions) treatment, before the criminal courts, of persons who are apparently suffering from a mental disorder. The need for such provisions becomes more apparent when one considers the evidence that substantial numbers of the seriously mentally ill in Canada are, unfortunately, being caught up in the criminal justice process, as was discussed earlier.

To begin with, the Criminal Code gives a judge the authority to order a psychiatric assessment of an accused person, which is intended to address that person's *fitness to stand trial* and/or whether she or he may be *not criminally responsible* on account of mental disorder (NCRMD).[18] This assessment may be conducted in custody, usually at a psychiatric facility. The Code stipulates that in-custody fitness assessments should not be more than five days' duration, although there are provisions for extending this period. "Fitness to stand trial" refers to the accused person's mental state while at court and whether he or she can competently participate in an adversarial criminal proceeding. The test, according to the Criminal Code, is to determine whether the accused can understand the nature or object of the proceedings, understand the possible consequences of the proceedings, or communicate with defence counsel. Canadian courts may try to avoid applying too high a standard of fitness in such cases because of the delays and possible deprivations of liberty that may ensue, given that a finding of unfitness may result in the accused's being held in custody until fitness is restored. Of particular concern are those individuals suffering from apparently intractable conditions such as fetal alcohol syndrome since there is the prospect that, once declared unfit, they will never be found competent to stand trial (Department of Justice Canada 2003). The Criminal Code also authorizes, following a finding of unfitness, involuntary psychiatric treatment of the accused to restore fitness, an unusual exception to the rule that medical treatment is a provincial jurisdiction, to be governed by provincial or territorial statutes. Historically, the pretrial psychiatric assessment, while ostensibly addressing fitness, has been used in Canada as a mechanism whereby mentally ill persons charged with less serious offences have been "diverted" – that is, transferred to psychiatric facilities with charges being dropped. This is a practice that has had both its proponents and its critics (e.g., Menzies 1989), and one that is on the decline in any case because of the downsizing of psychiatric hospitals and because of changes to the Criminal Code in 1992 that restrict the duration and scope of pretrial assessments (Davis 1994).

The Court (or the accused) may also request an assessment of criminal responsibility. The test here is that the accused, at the time of the act or omission, must have been suffering from a mental disorder "which made him or her incapable of appreciating the nature and quality of the act or omission, or of knowing that it was wrong" (Criminal Code, s. 16.1). For judicial interpretations of this test, the reader is referred to more specialized texts (e.g., Verdun-Jones 2010). Historically, defence lawyers in Canada have been reluctant to use (what was then called) the "insanity defence," particularly for lesser offences, because it could result in a lengthy detention in a psychiatric hospital, a longer period in many cases than typical jail sentences for similar offences (Davis 1994). The Criminal Code at that time mandated the automatic and indeterminate detention of an insanity acquittee and did not provide specific criteria by which the person's status, including consideration of discharge, would be reviewed. These provisions were found to be in violation of the Charter of Rights and were ruled invalid in the landmark 1991 Supreme Court of Canada decision in *Regina v. Swain.*[19] This decision necessitated the passage of new legislation in 1992. Following *Swain,* for people found NCRMD, the Criminal Code specified that a review board was to make a disposition that was the "least onerous and least restrictive to the accused" and that, if the accused was not deemed to be a "significant threat" (Criminal Code, s. 672.54) to the safety of the public, he or she was to be given an absolute discharge.[20] Persons not given an absolute discharge could be detained in hospital or granted a conditional discharge whereby they would report periodically to an outpatient clinic. A statistical report from the Department of Justice Canada (2006) determined that there had been a substantial increase in the number of persons using the NCRMD defence and being found NCRMD in the period from 1994 to 2004, probably not surprising given that the consequences of this special verdict were now less onerous.[21]

The situation changed again in 2013 when the federal government introduced Bill C-54, amending the "not criminally responsible" sections of the Criminal Code. Bill C-54 represented, apparently, a swinging of the pendulum away from the rights of the accused and back toward "safety of the public." The act saw the wording in the Code revised so that public safety became the *paramount* consideration in disposition orders, whereas previously this had to be balanced with the reintegration, mental condition, and other needs of the accused. There would be a new category of "high-risk" individuals – based on the person's index offense – who would only be eligible to apply for conditional discharge every three years. The new legislation also broadened the definition of "significant threat," which did not necessarily have to be related to violence. The proposed changes in the law were consistent with the federal Conservative government's stance on "law and order" and were likely influenced by high-profile NCRMD cases featured in the media (see Chapter 4). While Bill C-54 was protested as contributing to the stigmatizing association of mental illness and violence, for example by the Canadian Alliance on Mental Illness and Mental Health, the tendency of Canadians to view "mental disorder defences" skeptically remains. For example, a study by Justice Canada published in 2010 found that nearly 40 percent of respondents thought that mentally ill persons should still be subject to the same criminal sanctions as anyone else despite their being incapable of knowing that what they were doing was wrong (Butler 2010).[22]

Apart from the questions of fitness and criminal responsibility, an individual's mental state may be an issue at the point of sentencing, thus requiring, for example, that the person attend psychiatric treatment as a condition of probation. In the 1990 BC Court of Appeal case *Regina v. Rogers*,[23] it was ruled that medication compliance cannot be enforced through a probation order, so in this respect a criminal court order is probably not as effective as a community treatment order. Monitoring a mentally ill person via probation is a cumbersome process in any case since a breach of the probation condition may only have the effect of the person's being sent back to court. As well, mental health practitioners are often very reluctant to deal with persons under a court order unless they are mandated to do so (i.e., work at a specialized forensic unit). Indeed, clients with histories that combine "madness" and "badness" are often doubly stigmatized, both by the public and sometimes by treating professionals.

Ethical Decision Making

As we have seen, practitioner decision making is mandated, limited, and circumscribed by a number of federal and provincial laws. However, on a day-to-day basis, these laws cannot speak specifically to all the situations a mental health practitioner may face, and they provide only a very rough guide to action. In short, practitioners still have to utilize judgment and discretion and, in doing so, will feel the tensions between competing ethical perspectives. Arguably, these tensions are more challenging than ever in the present environment.

Why? On the one hand, we are in an era of recovery, which in the mental health context means that client autonomy and risk-taking are emphasized and are to be facilitated whenever possible. For example, an article on practitioner competencies in the *Psychiatric Rehabilitation Journal* lists the following as desired attitudes or approaches for persons working with the seriously mentally ill (Coursey et al. 2000):

- Encourage independent thinking.
- Support consumers' freedom to make their own mistakes.
- Support choices and risk-taking as leading to growth.
- Avoid controlling behaviours.

This is echoed in writings by consumers of psychiatric services, such as Patricia Deegan (2000), who, in her article "Recovering Our Sense of Value after Being Labeled Mentally Ill," speaks eloquently about the *dignity of risk*.

On the other hand, there are professional duties, practice approaches, and organizational factors that appear to work against the goal of promoting client autonomy (see Chapter 7). Clinicians have a duty of care to their clients, which must be taken very seriously (even if there may be some debate about what this term means). In part this may be driven by fear of liability should something go wrong: a US survey of mental health administrators found that the top concern about the potential impact of the recovery movement was that it would increase service-providers' exposure to risk and liability (Davidson et al. 2006a). Family members may also react negatively if they sense their loved one is being exposed to unnecessary risk of if they have the perception that the practitioner is not doing enough to look after the individual. On this point, the former Mental Health Advocate for BC wrote in her annual report:

> Advocates for people with mental illness did not always have the same perspective as family advocates ... The central and most controversial point was the role of coercion in the treatment system. Relatives of ill people,

typically with schizophrenia, tended to see their family member as having little insight into his or her illness and requiring compulsory treatment. Consumer advocates, on the other hand ... saw coercion as a strategy that reduces self-esteem and dignity and ultimately drives people out of the treatment system. (Hall 2000, 20)

And there is the organizational context to consider since most corporations are "risk-averse." "Risk managers" are employed to help steer a cautious course through ethically perilous waters, and there are audits and critical incident meetings to look forward to should something go wrong. Finally, practitioners must try to reconcile recovery principles with the development and greater use of more coercive practices, in particular assertive/intensive case management models, broader committal criteria, and mandated out-patient treatment (described earlier in this chapter). Referring to what they see as the inherently controlling and paternalistic aspects of "assertive" treatment models, Spindel and Nugent (1999, 2) suggest that this "flies in the face of the progress which has been achieved ... in recent years."

So, how can practitioners attempt to reconcile these competing perspectives? While there is no easy answer to this question, the following points can be made. First, in considering a basis for risk-taking among clients, practitioners should recall other practice approaches referred to in this book in which self-efficacy is emphasized and recognized as an important part of the recovery process. These include cognitive-behavioural techniques, motivational interviewing, and more generally, the move towards self-management of health care conditions.

Second, while practitioners may need to be paternalistic and directive at times of crisis, we should recognize this as a *phase* of the intervention and not a permanent state of affairs. Therapy models (not to mention Maslow's Hierarchy of Needs) recognize that safety and containment (both physical and emotional) must be addressed first, but once these have been established, the aim should be to move further down the path of growth and recovery.

Third, while it might be said that the recovery perspective is new, the values underlying it are not. Four key principles are generally seen as underpinning ethical practice in health care (e.g., McCormick 1998):

- Autonomy, which involves respecting people's preferences and avoiding controlling influences, much in line with the desired practitioner attitudes and approaches listed above. The concept of autonomy incorporates *informed consent* (providing the necessary information to make an informed choice); *veracity* (telling the truth); *privacy* (respecting the client's preferences around information-sharing); and *fidelity* (keeping your promises).

- Beneficence, which refers to doing good and preventing or removing harm.
- Non-maleficence – "do no harm." In mental health, there are a number of ways that a practice approach may be harmful, despite the best intentions of the practitioner.[24] Recall the survey of persons on community treatment orders (above), with respondents speaking about loss of dignity. Consider also that assertive outreach programs that do a lot "for" the client may risk making the client more, rather than less, dependent. As one ethicist puts it, "if adults are prevented from making their own decisions, they revert to being children" (Browne et al. 2002).
- Justice: be fair; treat like cases alike.

But, the reader may ask, how can these ethical standards be achieved when some forms of involvement are *explicitly* involuntary (community treatment orders) or assertive (ACT)? As one policy analyst notes, when first conceived in the 1970s, "consumer empowerment was not a serious consideration [with ACT programs]" since ACT "was designed to 'do' for the client what the client could not do for himself or herself" and that, while times have changed, "a clear articulation of the underlying ethical principles of these 'new teams' [still] does not yet exist" (Diamond 1996, 53). Because of this, it can be argued that greater attention needs to be paid to guidelines for dealing with ethical issues arising out of approaches that appear to be inherently coercive (Davis 2002).

In wrestling with this, it is important to try to define what we mean by "coercion" – a loaded term with which most practitioners are uncomfortable.[25] Szmuckler (1999) writes about practitioner influence existing on a continuum:

- Persuasion: an "appeal to reason" (332).
- Leverage: exploiting the relationship between worker and client, more likely if the client has become emotionally dependent.
- Coercion: a proposal that would make the client worse off, a threshold referred to as the "moral base line" (333). Coercion would involve removing something to which the client is entitled, whereas a "perk" not being given would in this analysis not cross the line since the client is no worse off: the former imposes a penalty, the latter a reward.

In practice, these distinctions are not so easily made. For one thing, the client may still feel manipulated and sense a loss of control, and, further, establishing a baseline above and below which the client may be said to be "better" or "worse" off is in reality a difficult task.

Some general guidelines for coercive practices are offered by Monahan and colleagues (1996) as follows: (1) use positive approaches, such as persuasion, as the strategies of choice; (2) use negative approaches, such as threats, only as a last resort; (3) be explicit about what you are doing and why, allow clients to tell their side of the story, and seriously consider this information. Some useful tools for collaboratively managing risk in community mental health practice have been developed: see, for example, Burns-Lynch, Salzer, and Baron (2010).

Finally, practitioners should try to draw from, and help develop, organizational resources. Implementing recovery-oriented services will work best in an organizational structure and culture that encourage open group discussion and feedback regarding complex and difficult treatment scenarios. Curtis and Hodge (1995, 54-55) note that "managers have a responsibility to help line staff make thoughtful decisions, and to develop an environment where staff can safely and comfortably raise such questions [about ethical decisions] ... In some organizations, it is difficult for many staff to raise questions about ethics or relationship boundaries, or even to admit they have concerns, since doing so may imply a failing in judgment." There may be formal supports available, such as ethicists, guardianship consultants, and clinical supervisors. Individuals may also need to consider creating informal supports, such as like-minded colleagues and mentors getting together at "brown bag" lunch meetings.

Notes

1 For instance, the "notwithstanding clause," although rarely used, permits federal or provincial governments to declare that a law shall remain in force despite the Charter.
2 *R. v. Oakes*, [1986] 1 S.C.R. 103.
3 *McCorkell v. Riverview Hospital*, [1993] 8 W.W.R. 169, 81 B.C.L.R. (2d) 273 (S.C.).
4 Requiring two persons to certify instead of one provides (arguably) greater protection of a client's civil rights, but from the clinician's viewpoint this was said to be too cumbersome when the situation required a prompt response. When the BC Mental Health Act was amended in 1999, changing the number of physicians required to certify from two (unaffiliated) to one, this was interpreted as a progressive move by some and as a retrograde move by patients' rights advocates.
5 In Quebec, the police officer's involvement is more restricted and must be initiated in consultation with other parties (Gray, Shone, and Liddle 2008).
6 82 D.L.R. (4th) 298 (Ont C.A.).
7 In 1996, the provisions for authorizing treatment were removed from the Ontario Mental Health Act and put into the Health Care Consent Act.
8 The Treatment Advocacy Center in the US keeps an updated list of states with mandatory outpatient laws, which totalled forty-four as of 2011. See http://www.treatmentadvocacycenter.org/solution/assisted-outpatient-treatment-laws.
9 In 2012, the Department of Justice in the US certified assisted outpatient treatment as an "effective crime prevention program" (Jaffe 2012).

10 On this matter, Balko (2011) suggests that "laws named after crime victims ... are usually a bad idea" since "they play more to emotion than reason."

11 Without knowing more details of the study method, one can note that there is a potential problem in interviewing persons who are *still under* a court order, as was apparently the case here, since these subjects may feel more pressure to give positive feedback.

12 In Vancouver, the number of cases of persons required to report to a mental health team as a condition of extended leave increased from about one hundred in 2002 to almost four hundred in 2010.

13 Nova Scotia's Adult Protection Act goes one step further, placing a *duty to report* on any citizen with information concerning abuse or neglect.

14 The MacArthur Competence Assessment Tool for Treatment.

15 For the purposes of the discussion here, "medical procedure" does not include psychiatric treatment.

16 See the BC Representation Agreement Act at http://www.bclaws.ca/EPLibraries/bclaws_new/document/ID/freeside/00_96405_01.

17 72 O.R. (2d) 417 (C.A.).

18 Previously referred to as "not guilty by reason of insanity."

19 (1991), 63 C.C.C. (3d) 481 (C.C.C.).

20 This section of the Code, and in particular the interpretation of the term "significant threat," has been debated in a number of court cases in recent years, some at the level of the Supreme Court of Canada. See Broderick (2006). Generally, the courts have held that dispositions must be "least restrictive" and that there is an onus on boards of review to discharge persons unless they are certain about the threat potential.

21 One might assume increased NCRMD applications would be driven by the defence lawyers, but in conversations this author (Davis 1994) had with crown counsel in the early days of the new law it was suggested that this would increase options for the prosecution as well.

22 As this book went to press the new legislation had not yet been enacted.

23 61 C.C.C. (3d) 481 (B.C.C.A.). In this case the Court ruled that enforcing medication compliance through probation was "an unreasonable restraint upon the liberty and security of the accused person" (re. s. 7 of the Charter) and thus unlawful.

24 In *the consequentialist* school of ethics (which includes John Stuart Mill) actions are judged only by their outcomes, not by the actor's intentions.

25 The author's in-house survey of 108 clinical staff at Vancouver Coastal Health found a majority stating that coercion was "never" used, despite the fact that, among other things, the agency had close to four hundred clients on outpatient certification orders.

Afterword:
Lessons Learned and Future Challenges

At this point a brief overview of some of the major "take away" messages is offered. These comments draw, in part, from the author's own experience, and it is hoped that the reader will be forgiving if they stray somewhat into the realm of editorial.

In taking stock of where we are in community mental health in Canada, there is reason for optimism and still some cause for concern. More stakeholders have been given a voice, but some would argue that theirs is still a token input. Co-option by practitioners needs to be resisted. Promising evidence-based housing, vocational, treatment, and support models have been developed, but in many cases the actual availability of these is limited. The recovery vision is making inroads, but not all stakeholders understand it or support some of its more contentious elements. To reiterate a comment from the introduction, these are indeed interesting times and, potentially, a time of opportunity.

Mental Health and Mental Illness

Conceptually, it is useful to see mental health and mental illness as being on two separate continua. In this conception a person may have a significant genetic vulnerability to mental illness yet still have relatively good mental health, with medical treatment, stress management, meaningful activity, and supportive relationships. Conversely, a person may not be manifesting signs of mental illness yet still have poor mental health, a condition sociologist Corey Keyes refers to as "languishing." The challenge here is that this second group, the "languishers," has not historically been seen as the priority population, and, indeed, some stakeholders have expressed the concern that shifting resources towards mental health promotion will mean taking resources away from the most seriously disabled. While acknowledging this concern, health promotion still makes sense if it can be seen as increasing resilience among persons with mental illness so that their likelihood of relapse is diminished.

Program Eligibility

Eligibility for mental health services needs to be based on functional impairment, coping skills, and subjective distress, not just diagnosis. Even with schizophrenia, it can be argued that persons continuing to experience symptoms – despite medical treatment – may not need long-term specialized psychiatric care if these symptoms are manageable and not upsetting. Instruments measuring quality of life and functional impairment exist (or can be adapted) for this purpose but are presently under-utilized.

Prevention

Can we prevent mental illnesses from happening? While currently we lack the knowledge to do this at the level of individuals, there is evidence that promotion initiatives that improve health and reduce illness among expecting mothers and their children, especially in marginalized groups, will decrease morbidity at the level of populations. Such initiatives should be supported.

Stigma

Stigma is one of the greatest challenges faced by persons diagnosed with a mental illness, and we have seen that prejudicial attitudes among the public have been very difficult to shift. It has been noted that explanatory models that connote *differentness*, biogenetic explanations in particular, may not be helpful in this respect.

Future practitioners need to be mindful about the creation of stigma within the health care system, our own "back yard" so to speak. To this end, persons entering the field need to reflect on their own attitudes about mental illness and addictions, and whether they can be empathetic towards someone whose actions may be seen as willful, as is the case with the borderline personality diagnosis. How individuals who are distressed or suicidal are handled at our emergency wards is both a cause for concern and an opportunity for learning. Those working in the field need to remember the importance of hope and to recognize and celebrate client success stories. *Contact* is an important mechanism for diminishing stigma, and within the system the visible example of peer workers effectively providing services will, it is hoped, be enlightening for practitioners.

Recovery

The recovery vision is gaining a tentative foothold but, as of this writing, has not been implemented in Canadian settings in a comprehensive sense and is still not well understood. Outstanding issues include:

- the question of evaluating recovery at the aggregate/system level, or applying fidelity scales, when recovery is seen as *subjectively* defined and hence difficult to operationalize;
- whether recovery can take place in involuntary settings, as with a person certified to a psychiatric unit;
- the problem with an approach that promotes risk-taking when the practitioner operates in a culture that is risk-averse;
- the concern that a practitioner promoting self-determination may appear to be negligent;
- whether the vision, and the idea that recovery may occur without professional involvement, is realistic or ethical when the client's thinking is seriously affected by mental illness;
- the question of "anosognosia" (see Chapter 15).

In considering these concerns the following points are made:

- Recovery should be approached with reference to a needs hierarchy, with safety and survival needs always being the first consideration. Safety plans need to be written in all cases and shared between the client, practitioner and other supporters.
- Practitioners cannot assume a common understanding of recovery: being client-centred and transparent are crucial.
- Assessments should be as holistic as possible.

Elements of the recovery vision can be brought in that do not require a radical restructuring of service delivery. At the program level, policies and practices that support client choice and continuity of care should be developed and implemented. Restrictive eligibility rules, and preconditions to program involvement, should be reconsidered. And peer placement and advancement should be developed. In addition to peer support positions, efforts should be made to place clients on committees with voting authority, on hiring panels, and on program evaluation teams.

Cultural Sensitivity

Practitioners need to exhibit curiosity and practise humility when working with persons whose culture and/or explanatory models are different. The role of family, the significance of stigma, the expression of distress, the historical context, and the meaning of illness are all issues that may need to be explored.

Families

Relationships among clients, families, and practitioners are complicated and at times strained. Families may experience guilt and feel that they are being judged by clinicians, and, indeed, there is the historical context of family-blaming arising out of aetiological theories such as the "double-bind" and the "schizophrenogenic mother." We need to acknowledge the challenges family members face and the fact that, in a number of instances, they bear the major brunt of care-provision without any additional resources being provided. We need to understand that, for them, safety is paramount and that this may not coincide with the practitioner's promoting client independence. And there is the fact that our codes of ethics and confidentiality policies may have the effect of excluding families from the treatment process. This may happen as a result of practitioner indifference but can also have to do with that person maintaining a trusting therapeutic relationship when the client has not given permission to involve others. Minimally, however, family members should be able to bring forward their concerns and to have these received respectfully.

The Continuum of Services

We need to be thoughtful about the entry into, journey through, and exit from the mental health system. Mental health services should, as much as possible, be normalized with respect to their location and appearance. Hospital care is a necessary last resort, but there is no reason for other services to be based in or attached to hospitals. Intensive outreach programs, whether through an ACT or home-based psychosis treatment model, have been shown to be effective and less traumatizing than certification to hospital involving police and ambulance. At the other "end," there is the question of transitions out of the formal mental health system. Planned exits from the system are necessitated by the need to accommodate new referrals and are seen by some as an essential part of the journey towards recovery. Not all clients, however, are comfortable with losing the services of a team that may provide social, recreational, and vocational resources in addition to treatment and case management. Indeed, the drop-off seen at this transition point – from specialized program to family doctor – may be severe and abrupt. As we have discussed, getting support from a GP alone may be sufficient in some cases, but not in others. Shared care models that support GPs working alone have been developed but are not widely available. Another consideration is to provide a more *graduated* exit from the formal system by de-linking rehabilitation services from treatment, so that a client may attend groups at the mental health program even if his or her medical care is provided through a GP. There is a potentially significant role for peers here, either through "alumni groups" or one-on-one support, to provide an intermediate, less-intense transition away from specialized care.

Housing
Safe, affordable housing that offers a measure of privacy gives clients a stake in society and is arguably the single greatest social determinant of health. As the Mental Health Commission of Canada (2012, 72) concludes: "More adequate, affordable housing needs to be made available, and individualized housing options should be promoted."

Staff Skill Sets
The evidence base continues to accumulate in mental health, and in a number of areas best or better practices have been established. Yet in many instances these interventions are not available for clients. Students entering the field are not always getting adequate exposure to, for example, cognitive behavioural methods, and it may be that university curricula are not sufficiently informed by clinical practice guidelines and accreditation standards, which may be the case when faculty are not currently engaged in clinical work. After graduates enter the workforce, employers may struggle to effectively train staff and disseminate research evidence. To this end, an effective knowledge exchange approach is needed, with dedicated educators who have credibility as clinicians and who understand real-world contingencies. "One-off" training sessions, with no follow-up and support, are usually not effective. This, then, gets to the heart of the question of whether mental health clinicians can sustain their skills as generalists or whether systems need to consider greater staff specialization. For example, clients who have endured severe trauma or who have significant problems with distress tolerance may benefit from seeing counsellors trained in techniques such as dialectical behaviour therapy. To support this, health authorities may consider hiring trauma specialists rather than attempting to retrain persons from other orientations (although all staff should at least be trauma-*aware*). Those with a similar interest and training could then form a clinical interest group for debriefing and mentoring, or be co-located, to best maintain their skills.

Working with Clients
In reviewing the evaluation data, Hubble, Duncan, and Miller (1999) conclude that the therapeutic model itself is only one of four major elements that account for the improvement seen in counselling interventions. The other three they found to be significant are:

- Client factors – that is, the resources and strengths a client brings with her/him to the therapeutic relationship. There are implications here with respect to practitioners *identifying* and *building* on these strengths.
- The relationship with the practitioner. Unsurprisingly, clinicians who were seen as caring, empathetic, warm, and accepting were found to be more effective. This is probably even more the case with seriously mentally ill persons, who have had difficulty maintaining relationships and establishing trust.
- Placebo/hope/expectancy. We have encountered this factor earlier in the book, in the case of the large placebo effect seen with antidepressant medication, and in the example of the recovery vision's emphasis on hopefulness in relationships with clients. Practitioners need to be hopeful, or "hold hope," particularly early in the engagement or trajectory of illness, which is a critical time wherein the service user may engage further or turn away.

What about working with persons with serious psychotic illnesses, who may "lack insight?" How can we engage with these individuals? In addressing this challenge, Davidson (2012) notes that this can be seen as working with someone who does not share the same explanatory model, and, rather than trying to "convert" the individual, we need to meet that person "where they are at." He suggests we do this:

> First, by *not* insisting on acceptance or acknowledgment of having a mental illness as a precondition to providing concrete and practical assistance with *their concerns*. Second, by finding out what those everyday concerns and needs are ... and offering concrete and practical assistance to address those concerns and meet those needs ... Third, by taking a *strength-based* (as opposed to an illness-based) approach to addressing the identified concerns and needs. And fourth, both for the person in need and the practitioner's sake, it is important to understand the engagement process will likely take time before producing tangible results. (emphasis in original)

Davidson's comments about a therapeutic relationship taking time are reflected in a study conducted by Canadian author Ruth Gumpp (2009), who carried out in-depth interviews with persons in psychiatric treatment, exploring with them "what worked." A common theme that emerged was how trust in the clinician took time to develop and that this continuity was crucial and in fact compensated for other deficiencies in the relationship. When continuity broke down – through staff turnover or the client's being transferred to another program – the thought of starting from square one, of having to tell the story all over again, was daunting. Trust was enhanced, according to the participants, by the clinician's giving enough time for the story to be told, by their believing that the other person was acting in their best interests, and by their getting the sense that the clinician trusted them as well.

References

Abbey, S., et al. 2011. Stigma and discrimination. *Canadian Journal of Psychiatry* 56: insert 1-9.

Abbott, A. 2011. City living marks the brain. *Nature News*. http://www.nature.com/news/2011/110622/full/474429a.html.

Abdel-Baki, A., et al. 2011. Schizophrenia, an illness with bad outcome: Myth or reality? *Canadian Journal of Psychiatry* 56: 92-101.

Abidi, S., and S. Bhaskara. 2003. From chlorpromazine to clozapine: Antipsychotic adverse effects and the clinician's dilemma. *Canadian Journal of Psychiatry* 44: 749-55.

Aboriginal Nurses Association of Canada. 2009. Cultural competence and cultural safety in nursing education. http://www2.cna-aiic.ca/cna/documents/pdf/publications/First_Nations_Framework_e.pdf.

Abramowitz, J. 2006. The psychological treatment of obsessive-compulsive disorder. *Canadian Journal of Psychiatry* 57: 407-16.

Accreditation Canada. 2008. Risk assessment. http://www.accreditation.ca/uploadedFiles/suicide%20prevention.pdf?n=3772.

–. 2011. Community-based mental health services and supports standards. Ottawa: Accreditation Canada.

Addington, D., et al. 2009. A comparison of ziprasidone and risperidone in the long-term treatment of schizophrenia: A 44 week, double-blind, continuation study. *Canadian Journal of Psychiatry* 54: 46-54.

Afifi, T., B. Cox, and J. Sareen. 2005. Perceived need and help-seeking for mental health problems among Canadian provinces and territories. *Canadian Journal of Community Mental Health* 24: 51-61.

Alberta Mental Health Board. 2006. Aboriginal mental health: A framework for Alberta. http://www.albertahealthservices.ca/MentalHealthWellness/hi-mhw-aboriginal-framework.pdf.

–. 2007. Mental health economic statistics. http://www.ihe.ca/documents/AMHB_Statistics_pktbk07_eng.pdf

Aldhous, P. 2009. Mind gym helps people live with schizophrenia. *New Scientist*, 18 June, 35.

Alegria, M., et al. 2008. Disparity in depression treatment among racial and ethnic minority populations in the US. *Psychiatric Services* 59: 1264-72.

Alessi-Severini, S., et al. 2008. Utilization and costs of antipsychotic agents: A Canadian population-based study, 1996-2006. *Psychiatric Services* 59: 547-53.

–. 2012. Ten years of antipsychotic prescribing to children: A Canadian population-based study. *Canadian Journal of Psychiatry* 57: 52-58.

Alexander, B. 2008. *The Globalisation of Addiction: A Study in Poverty of the Spirit*. New York: Oxford University Press.

–. 2009. Direct-to-consumer drug ads losing their punch. NBC News. http://www.nbcnews. com/id/28584952/ns/health-health_care/t/direct-to-consumer-drug-ads-losing-their -punch/#.UTttqDedhu8.

Aleccia, J. 2011. Smoking-pill suicides overlooked in missing reports. NBC News. http://www. nbcnews.com/id/43187290.

Allen, T. 2000. *Someone to Talk To: Care and Control of the Homeless*. Halifax: Fernwood.

Amador, X. 2009. About poor insight and diagnosis. *SZ Magazine*, Summer, 36-37.

American Association of Community Psychiatrists. 2010. LOCUS: Level of care utilization system for psychiatric and addiction services. http://www.communitypsychiatry.org/ publications/clinical_and_administrative_tools_guidelines/LOCUS%20Instrument% 202010.pdf.

American Psychiatric Association. 2000. *Diagnostic and Statistical Manual*. 4th ed. Washington, DC: APA.

–. 2003. Practice guidelines for the assessment and treatment of patients with suicidal behaviors. *American Journal of Psychiatry* 160 (November supplement).

–. 2013. Highlights of changes from DSM-IV-TR to DSM-5. http://www.psych.uic.edu/ docassist/changes-from-dsm-iv-tr–to-dsm-5l.pdf.

American Psychological Association. 2006. Stress weakens the immune system. http://www. apa.org/research/action/immune.aspx.

Andreasen, N., et al. 2005. Remission in schizophrenia: Proposed criteria and rationale for consensus. *American Journal of Psychiatry* 162: 441-49.

Andres-Lemay, V., E. Jamieson, and H. MacMillan. 2005. Child abuse, psychiatric disorder and running away in a community sample of women. *Canadian Journal of Psychiatry* 50: 684-88.

Andrews, G., E. Goldner, S. Parikh, and D. Bilsker, eds. 2000. *Management of Mental Disorders, Canadian edition*. Vancouver: Mental Health Evaluation and Community Consultation Unit, University of British Columbia.

Angell, B., A. Cooke, and K. Kovac. 2005. First-person accounts of stigma. In *On the Stigma of Mental Illness*, ed. P. Corrigan, 69-98. Washington, DC: American Psychological Association.

Angell, M. 2004. The truth about the drug companies. *New York Review of Books*. http://www. nybooks.com/articles/17244?email.

Angermeyer, M., M. Beck, and H. Matschinger, H. 2003. Determinants of the public's preference for social distance from people with schizophrenia. *Canadian Journal of Psychiatry*, 48: 663-68.

Anthony, W. 1993. Recovering from mental illness: The guiding vision of the mental health service system in the 1990s. *Psychosocial Rehabilitation Journal* 16: 11-21.

Anthony, W., E. Rogers, and M. Farkas. 2003. Research on evidence-based practices: Future directions in an era of recovery. *Community Mental Health Journal* 39: 101-14.

Anxiety Disorders Association of Ontario. 2010. Terminology. http://www.anxietydisorders ontario.ca/.

AnxietyBC. 2010. AnxietyBC's president's address. http://www.anxietybc.com/anxietybcs -presidents-address.

Appelbaum, P. 1994. *Almost a Revolution*. New York: Oxford University Press.

Arango, C., and X. Amador. 2011. Lessons learned about poor insight. *Schizophrenia Bulletin* 37: 27-28.

Arboleda-Florez, J. 1998. Mental illness and violence: An epidemiological appraisal of the evidence. *Canadian Journal of Psychiatry* 43: 989-96.

–. 2003. Considerations on the stigma of mental illness. *Canadian Journal of Psychiatry* 48: 645-50.

Arbuckle, M., et al. 2008. Brief reports: Psychiatric opinion and antipsychotic selection in the management of schizophrenia. *Psychiatric Services* 59: 561-65.

Asarnow, J. 1988. Children at risk for schizophrenia: Converging lines of evidence. *Schizophrenia Bulletin* 14: 613-31.

Aubrey, T., and J. Myner. 1996. Community integration and quality of life: A comparison of persons with psychiatric disabilities in housing programs and community residents who are neighbours. *Canadian Journal of Community Mental Health*, 15: 5-19.

Aviv, R. 2010. Which way madness lies: Can psychosis be prevented? *Harper's Magazine*, December, 35-43.

Bachrach, L. 1994. Deinstitutionalization: What does it really mean? In *Schizophrenia: Exploring the Spectrum of Psychosis*, ed. R. Ancill, S. Holliday, and J. Higenbottam, 21-34. Chichester, UK: John Wiley and Sons.

–. 1996. What do patients say about program planning? Perspectives from the patient-authored literature. In *Schizophrenia: Breaking down the Barriers*, ed. S. Holliday, R. Ancill, and G. MacEwan, 17-37. New York: John Wiley and Sons.

Baer, L., and M. Blais, eds. 2010. *Handbook of Clinical Rating Scales and Assessment in Psychiatry and Mental Health*. New York: Humana Press.

Bainbridge, L. 1998. *Consumer Involvement in the Workplace: A Literature Review*. Report prepared for the Greater Vancouver Mental Health Services Society.

Baldwin, D., and N. Kosky. 2007. Off-label prescribing in psychiatric practice. *Advances in Psychiatric Treatment* 13: 414-22.

Balko, R. 2011. Why "Caylee's Law" is a bad idea. *Huffington Post*. http://www.huffingtonpost.com/2011/07/11/caylees-law-casey-anthony-_n_893953.html.

Ballou, M., and L. Brown, eds. 2002. *Rethinking Mental Health and Disorder: Feminist Perspectives*. UK: Guilford Press.

Barkhimer, R. 2003. Breaking the silence of stigma. *Schizophrenia Digest*, Spring, 22-28.

Barkil-Oteo, A. 2013. The paradox of choice: When more medications mean less treatment. *Psychiatric Times*. http://www.psychiatrictimes.com/apa2013/paradox-choice-when-more-medications-mean-less-treatment.

Barranco-Mendoza, A., and D. Persaud. 2012. In *Health in Rural Canada*, ed. J. Kulig and A. Williams, 178-96. Vancouver: UBC Press.

Barrett, J. 2010. Suffering in silence. *Vancouver Courier*, 2 December, 13.

Barry, K., J. Zeber, F. Blow, and M. Valenstein. 2003. Effect of strengths model vs. assertive community treatment model on participant outcomes and utilization: Two year follow-up. *Psychiatric Rehabilitation Journal* 26: 268-77.

Beardsley, W., P Chien, and C. Bell. 2011. Prevention of mental disorders, substance abuse, and problem behaviors: A developmental perspective. *Psychiatric Services* 62: 247-54.

Beck, C., P. Silverstone, K. Glor, and J. Dunn. 1999. Psychostimulant prescriptions higher than expected: A self-report survey. *Canadian Journal of Psychiatry* 44: 680-84.

Beck, P. 2000. The confidentiality of psychiatric records and the patient's right to privacy. Canadian Psychiatric Association. https://ww1.cpa-apc.org/Publications/Position_Papers/Records.asp.

Becker, D., and R. Drake. 2003. *A Working Life for People with Severe Mental Illness*. New York: Oxford University Press.

Begley, S. 2010. The depressing news about antidepressants. *Newsweek*. http://www.newsweek.com/2010/01/28/the-depressing-news-about-antidepressants.html.

Bekelman, J., Y. Li, and G. Gross. 2003. Scope and impact of financial conflicts of interest in biomedical research. *Journal of the American Medical Association* 289: 454-65.

Bellett, G. 2010. Vancouver property crime plummets: Police. Global TV Calgary. http://www.globaltvcalgary.com/vancouver+property+crime+plummets+police/75466/story.html.

Belleville, S., et al. 2006. Improvement of episodic memory in persons with mild cognitive impairment and healthy older adults: Evidence from a cognitive intervention program. *Dementia and Geriatric Cognitive Disorders* 22: 486-99.

Ben Noun, L. 1996. Characteristics of patients refusing professional psychiatric treatment in a primary care clinic. *Israel Journal of Psychiatry* 33: 167-74.

Berenson, A. 2006. Disparity emerges in Lily data on schizophrenia drug. *New York Times,* 21 December.

–. 2008. Lilly settles Alaska suit over Zyprexa. *New York Times.* http://www.nytimes.com/2008/ 03/26/business/26cnd-zyprexa.html?adxnnl=1&adxnnlx=1318637064-p31HoG5TTlb6a YlH7morDg.

Beresford, P. 2006. A service-user perspective on evidence. In *Choosing Methods in Mental Health Research,* ed. M. Slade and S. Priebe, 223-30. London: Routledge.

Bertram, L. 2008. Genetic research in schizophrenia: New tools and future perspectives. *Schizophrenia Bulletin* 34: 806-12.

Bilsker, D. 2003. Self-management in the mental health field. *Visions: BC's Mental Health Journal* 18: 4-5.

Bilsker, D., E. Goldner, and W. Jones. 2007. Health service patterns indicate potential benefit of supported self-management for depression in primary care. *Canadian Journal of Psychiatry* 52: 86-94.

Birchwood, M., P. Todd, and C. Jackson. 1998. Early intervention in psychosis: The critical period hypothesis. *British Journal of Psychiatry* 172 (suppl. 33): 53-59.

Birchwood, M., and K. Brunet. 2004. Delay in secondary mental health services constitutes a major component of DUP in the UK. Paper presented at the 4th International Conference on Early Psychosis, Vancouver, BC, 29 September.

Bird, V., et al. 2010. Early intervention services, cognitive-behavioural therapy and family intervention in early psychosis: Systematic review. *British Journal of Psychiatry* 197: 350-56.

Bisetty, K. 2004. One-third of police killings are "suicide by cop": Study. *Vancouver Sun,* 4 October.

Blake, C. 2003. Ethical considerations in working with culturally diverse populations: The essential role of professional interpreters. *Canadian Psychiatric Association Bulletin* 35, 21-23.

Blanchflower, D., and A. Oswald. 2008. Is well-being U-shaped over the life cycle? *Social Science and Medicine* 66: 1733-49.

Blin, O. 1999. A comparative review of new antispychotics. *Canadian Journal of Psychiatry* 44: 235-44.

Blitz, C., N. Wolff, and J. Shi. 2008. Physical victimization in prison: The role of mental illness. *International Journal of Law and Psychiatry* 31: 385-93.

Block, R., et al. 2008. The impact of integrating mental and general health services on mental health's share of total health care spending in Alberta. *Psychiatric Services* 59: 860-63.

Blumner, K., and S. Marcus. 2009. Changing perceptions of depression: Ten-year trends from the general social survey. *Psychiatric Services* 60: 306-12.

Bogart, T., and P. Solomon. 1999. Procedures to share treatment information among mental health providers, consumers and families. *Psychiatric Services* 50: 1321-25.

Bond, G., H. Xie, and R. Drake. 2007. Can SSDI and SSI beneficiaries with mental illness benefit from evidence-based supported employment? *Psychiatric Services* 58: 1412-20.

Bond, G., R. Drake, and D. Becker. 2008. An update on randomized controlled trials of evidence-based supportive employment. *Psychiatric Rehabilitation Journal* 31: 280-90.

Bonsack, C., et al. 2005. Difficult to engage patients: A specific target for time-limited assertive outreach in a Swiss setting. *Canadian Journal of Psychiatry* 50: 845-50.

Boodman, S. 2012. Docs. Antipsychotics often prescribed for "problems in living." NBCNews. com. http://vitals.msnbc.msn.com/_news/2012/03/18/10724080-docs-antipsychotics often-prescribed-for-problems-of-living.

Borch-Jacobsen, M. 2011. I'm bipolar, you're bipolar. *Adbusters.* http://www.adbusters.org/ magazine/94/im-bipolar-youre-bipolar.html.

Borg, M., and K. Rasmussen. 2004. Recovery-oriented professionals: Helping relationships in mental health services. *Journal of Mental Health* 13: 493-505.

Boudreau, R., K. Moulton, and J. Cunningham. 2010. *Self-Directed Cognitive Behavioural Therapy for Adults with Diagnosis of Depression: Systematic Review of Clinical Effectiveness, Cost-Effectiveness, and Guidelines.* Ottawa: Canadian Agency for Drugs and Technologies in Health.

Bourgeois, M., et al. 2004. Awareness of disorder and suicide risk in the treatment of schizophrenia: Results of the international suicide prevention trial. *American Journal of Psychiatry* 161: 1494-96.

Bowman, M. 1999. Individual differences in posttraumatic distress: Problems with the DSM-IV model. *Canadian Journal of Psychiatry* 44: 21-33.

Boydell, K., and B. Everett, B. 1992. What makes a house a home? An evaluation of a supported housing project for individuals with long-term psychiatric background. *Canadian Journal of Community Mental Health* 10: 109-23.

Boydell, K., B. Gladstone, and E. Crawford. 2002. The knowledge resource base: Beginning the dialogue. *Canadian Journal of Community Mental Health* 21: 19-33.

Boydell, K., B. Gladstone, and T. Volpe. 2006. Understanding help seeking delay in the prodrome in first episode psychosis. *Psychiatric Rehabilitation Journal* 30: 54-60.

Boyle, T. 2010. Class action settlement in drug for schizophrenia. *Toronto Star.* http://www.thestar.com/article/830750–class-action-settlement-in-drug-for-schizophrenia.

Bradford, D., et al. 2008. Access to medical care among persons with psychotic and major affective disorders. *Psychiatric Services* 59: 847-52.

Bradstreet, S., and R. Pratt. 2010. Developing peer support worker roles: Reflecting on experiences in Scotland. *Mental Health and Social Inclusion* 14: 36-41.

Branham, D. 2003. Drugs for kids need scrutiny. *Vancouver Sun,* 12 December.

–. 2004. 6200 BC children on unapproved medication. *Vancouver Sun,* 4 February.

Brannen, C., et al. 2012. Rural mental health services in Canada: A model for research and practice. In *Health in Rural Canada,* ed. J. Kulig and A. Williams, 240-57. Vancouver: UBC Press.

Brass, G. 2009. Respecting the medicines: Narrating an Aboriginal identity. In *Healing Traditions: The Mental Health of Aboriginal Peoples in Canada,* ed. L. Kirmayer and G. Valaskakis, 355-80. Vancouver: UBC Press

Brazier, J., et al. 2006. Psychological therapies including DBT for borderline personality disorder: A systematic review and preliminary economic evaluation. *Health Technology Assessment* 10: 1-136.

Brean, J. 2010. Mental block: Opposers of mad pride protest anti-psychiatrist. Social Policy in Ontario. http://spon.ca/mental-block-opposers-of-mad-pride-protest-anti-psychiatrist/ 2010/12/19/.

–. 2011. Mental Health Commission struggles to find balance in developing strategy. *National Post.* http://news.nationalpost.com/2011/10/08/mental-health-commission-struggles-to -find-balance-in-developing-strategy/.

Brenner, R., et al. 2010. Primary prevention in schizophrenia: Adult populations. *Annals of Clinical Psychiatry* 22: 239-48.

Brent, D. 2009. Selective serotonin reuptake inhibitors and suicidality: a guide for the perplexed. *Canadian Journal of Psychiatry* 54: 72-74.

Bridge, J., et al. 2007. Clinical response and risk for reported suicidal ideation and suicide attempts in pediatric antidepressant treatment: A meta-analysis of randomized controlled trials. *Journal of the American Medical Association* 297: 1683-95.

Briere, J. 2002. Treating adult survivors of severe childhood abuse and neglect: Further developments of an integrative model. In *The APSAC Handbook on Child Maltreatment,* 2nd ed., ed. J. Myers, L. Berliner, J. Briere, C. Hendrix, T. Reid, and C. Jenny. Newbury Park, CA: Sage.

Brink, J., D. Doherty, and A. Boer. 2001. Mental disorder in federal offenders: A Canadian prevalence study. *International Journal of Law and Psychiatry* 24: 339-56.

Brink, J., et al. 2011. *A Study of How People with Mental Illness Perceive and Interact with the Police*. Calgary: Mental Health Commission of Canada.

British Columbia Medical Association. 2008. Improving access to acute care services. http://www.sem-bc.com/joomla/component/option,com_docman/task,doc_view/gid,62/Itemid,77/.

British Columbia Ministry of Health. 2002a. *Best Practices: Psychosocial Rehabilitation and Recovery*. Victoria: BC Ministry of Health.

–. 2002b. *Best Practices: Housing*. Victoria, BC: BC Ministry of Health.

–. 2002c. *Best Practices: Inpatient/Outpatient Services*. Victoria: BC Ministry of Health.

–. 2002d. *Best Practices: Family Involvement and Support*. Victoria: BC Ministry of Health.

–. 2002e. *Best Practices: Assertive Community Treatment*. Victoria: BC Ministry of Health.

–. 2002f. *Best Practices: Consumer Involvement and Initiatives*. Victoria: BC Ministry of Health.

–. 2005. *Guide to the Mental Health Act*. http://www.health.gov.bc.ca/library/publications/year/2005/MentalHealthGuide.pdf.

British Columbia Ministry of Health Services. 2005. *Mental Health Act Review Panels Statistical Report*: 2004. Victoria: BC Ministry of Health.

–. 2008. *Family Physician Guide for Depression, Anxiety Disorders, Early Psychosis and Substance Use Disorders*. Victoria: BC Ministry of Health Services.

–. 2010. *Healthy Minds, Healthy People: A Ten Year Plan to Address Mental Health and Substance Use in British Columbia*. http://www.health.gov.bc.ca/library/publications/year/2010/healthy_minds_healthy_people.pdf.

British Columbia Partners for Mental Health and Addictions Information. 2003a. *Mental Disorders Toolkit: Information and Resources for Effective Self-Management of Mental Disorders*. http://www.relatedminds.com/wp-content/uploads/2011/06/mdtoolkit.pdf.

–. 2003b. Unemployment and mental health and addictions. http://www.heretohelp.bc.ca/sites/default/files/Unemployment2010web.pdf.

–. 2003c. Concurrent disorders: Addictions and mental disorders. http://www.cmha-bc.org/content/resources/primer/32-stigma.pdf.

British Columbia Psychogeriatric Association. 2012. *Meeting Seniors' Mental Health Care Needs in British Columbia*. http://www.viha.ca/NR/rdonlyres/05F21EFF-D217-4395-8BC1-65A6B421ACDE/0/meetingseniorsmentalhealthcareneeds.pdf.

British Columbia Schizophrenia Society. 2010. BRIDGES education and support program. http://www.bcss.org/programs/2007/05/bridges-education-and-support-program/.

Broderick, L. 2006. The disposition of not criminally responsible accused persons in British Columbia: The impact of the *Winko* case on the decision-making process of the British Columbia Review Board. MA thesis, Simon Fraser University.

Brook, P. 2003. Crazy: The inside story. *Vancouver Sun*, 5 April.

Brown, A., and J. McGrath. 2011. The prevention of schizophrenia. *Schizophrenia Bulletin* 37: 257-61.

Brown, A., and P. Patterson. 2011. Maternal infection and schizophrenia: Implications for prevention. *Schizophrenia Bulletin* 37: 284-90.

Brown, M., P. Ridgway, W. Anthony, and E. Rogers. 1991. Comparison of outcomes for clients seeking and assigned to supported housing services. *Hospital and Community Psychiatry* 42: 1150-53.

Browne, A., M. Blake, M. Donnelly, and D. Herbert. 2002. On liberty for the old. *Canadian Journal on Aging* 21: 283-93.

Browne, G., and M. Courtney. 2004. Measuring the impact of housing on people with schizophrenia. *Nursing and Health Sciences* 6: 37-44.

Brunette, M., et al. 2003. Benzodiazepine use and abuse among patients with severe mental illness and co-occurring substance use disorders. *Psychiatric Services* 54: 1395-401.

Bryan, H. 2004. Policing the policing of psychiatric patients. *Georgia Straight*, 10-17 June, 41.

Bryan, C., and D. Rudd. 2006. Advances in the assessment of suicide risk. *Journal of Clinical Psychology* 62: 185-200.

Bryant, T. 2003. The current state of housing in Canada as a social determinant of health. *Policy Options,* March, 52-56.

Buccheri, R., et al. 2004. Long-term effects of training behavioral strategies for managing persistent auditory hallucinations. *Journal of Psychosocial Nursing:* 42: 19-27.

Buchanan, L. 2011. Letter to the CEO of the Mental Health Commission of Canada, 24 October. http://www.cfact.ca/cfactletterOct.pdf.

Bula, F. 2004. There's no place like homelessness. *Vancouver Sun,* 24 January.

Bula, F., and C. Skelton. 2004. The best strategy: Caring for the mentally ill. *Vancouver Sun,* 31 January.

Burgess, P., et al. 2010. *Review of Recovery Measures.* Australian Mental Health Outcomes and Classification Network. http://amhocn.org/static/files/assets/80e8befc/Review_of_ Recovery_Measures.pdf.

Burns, T., and J. Catty. 2008. IPS in Europe: The EQOLISE trial. *Psychiatric Rehabilitation Journal* 31: 313-17.

Burns, T., et al. 2007. The effectiveness of supported employment for people with severe mental illness: A randomized controlled trial. *Lancet* 370: 1146-52.

Burns-Lynch, B., M. Salzer, and R. Baron. 2010. *Managing Risk in Community Integration: Promoting the Dignity of Risk and Supporting Personal Choice.* Philadelphia, PA: Temple University Collaborative on Community Inclusion of Individuals with Psychiatric Disabilities.

Bush, P., et al. 2009. The long-term impact of employment on mental health service use and costs for persons with severe mental illness. *Psychiatric Services* 60: 1024-31.

Butler, A., et al. 2006. The empirical status of cognitive-behavioral therapy: A review of meta-analyses. *Clinical Psychology Review* 26: 17-31.

Butler, D. 2010. Mental health matters when it comes to crime, survey finds. *Montreal Gazette.* http://www.montrealgazette.com/news/Mental+health+matters+when+comes+crime+ survey+finds/3262140/story.html.

Butters, M., et al. 2004. The nature and determinants of neuropsychological functioning in late-life depression. *Archives of General Psychiatry* 61: 587-95.

Calsaferri, K., and Jongbloed, L. 1999. Three perspectives on the rehabilitation needs of consumers. *Canadian Journal of Community Mental Health* 18: 199-210.

Calsyn, R., et al. 2006. Predictors of the working alliance in assertive community treatment. *Community Mental Health Journal* 42: 161-75.

Campbell, W. 2003. Addiction: A disease of volition caused by a cognitive impairment. *Canadian Journal of Psychiatry* 48: 669-74.

Campbell, D., et al. 2008. Ethnic stratification of the association of RGS4 variants with antipsychotic treatment response in schizophrenia. *Biological Psychiatry* 63: 32-41.

Campbell, K., G. Bond, and R. Drake. 2011. Who benefits from supported employment: A meta-analytic study. *Schizophrenia Bulletin* 37: 370-80.

Campbell-Orde, T., et al. 2005. *Measuring the Promise: A Compendium of Recovery Measures.* Vol. 2. National Empowerment Center Inc. http://www.power2u.org/downloads/pn -55.pdf.

Canada Mortgage and Housing Corporation. 1999. *Best Practices Addressing Homelessness.* Ottawa: Canada Mortgage and Housing Corporation.

–. 2011. Canada's rental vacancy rate decreases. http://www.cmhc-schl.gc.ca/en/corp/nero/ nere/2011/2011-06-09-0815.cfm.

Canadian Alliance on Mental Illness and Mental Health. 2007. *Mental Health Literacy in Canada: Phase One Report.* http://www.camimh.ca/files/literacy/MHL_REPORT_Phase_ One.pdf.

Canadian Centre on Substance Abuse. 2010. Substance abuse in Canada: concurrent disorders. http://www.ccsa.ca/Eng/KnowledgeCentre/OurPublications/Pages/Concurrent_Disorders. aspx.

Canadian Counselling Association. 2007. *Code of Ethics.* Ottawa: Canadian Counselling Association.

Canadian Housing and Renewal Association. 2002. *On Her Own: Young Women and Homelessness in Canada.* Ottawa: Status of Women Canada.

Canadian Institute for Health Information. 2007. *Improving the Health of Canadians: Mental Health and Homelessness.* Ottawa: Canadian Institute for Health Information.

–. 2008a. *Improving the Mental Health of Canadians: Mental Health, Delinquency and Criminal Activity.* Ottawa: Canadian Institute for Health Information.

–. 2008b. *Hospital Mental Health Services.* http://secure.cihi.ca/cihiweb/products/Hmhdb_annual_report_2008_e.pdf.

–. 2010. *Health Services - Hospital Mental Health Services.* http://www.cihi.ca/cihiweb/dispPage.jsp?cw_page=statistics_results_topic_mentalhealth_e&cw_topic=Health%20Services&cw_subtopic=Hospital%20Mental%20Health%20Services.

–. 2011a. Health indicators. http://secure.cihi.ca/cihiweb/products/health_indicators_2011_en.pdf.

–. 2011b. Drug expenditure in Canada, 1985 to 2010. http://secure.cihi.ca/cihiweb/products/drug_expenditure_2010_en.pdf.

Canadian Medical Association. 2004. *CMA Code of Ethics.* http://policybase.cma.ca/PolicyPDF/PD04-06.pdf.

–. 2008. *Eighth Annual National Report Card on Health Care.* http://www.cma.ca/multimedia/CMA/Content_Images/Inside_cma/Annual_Meeting/2008/GC_Bulletin/National_Report_Card_EN.pdf.

Canadian Medical Association Journal. 2004. Editorial: The "file drawer" phenomenon: Suppressing clinical evidence. *Canadian Medical Association Journal* 170: 437.

Canadian Mental Health Association. 2001. Submission to the Commission on the Future of Health Care in Canada. http://www.ontario.cmha.ca/submissions.asp?cID=2590.

–. N.d. Meaning of mental health. http://www.cmha.ca/bins/content_page.asp?cid=2-267-1319&lang=1.

Canadian Mental Health Association, BC Division. 1998. The BC Early Intervention Study. http://www.cmha.bc.ca/files/ei_fin.pdf.

–. 1999. *Where Does Stigma Live?* (brochure). Vancouver: Canadian Mental Health Association.

–. 2003. Study in blue and grey: Police interventions with people with mental illness – A review of challenges and responses. http://www.crpnbc.ca/policereport.pdf.

Canadian Mental Health Association, Ontario. 2009. Rural and northern community issues in mental health. http://www.ontario.cmha.ca/backgrounders.asp?cID=289773.

Canadian Mental Health Association, Thunder Bay Branch. 2001. Mental Health Diversion Program. http://www.cmha-tb.on.ca/mhdiversion.htm.

Canadian Patient Safety Institute. 2006. *Canadian Root Cause Analysis Framework.* http://www.patientsafetyinstitute.ca/English/toolsResources/rca/Documents/March%202006%20RCA%20Workbook.pdf.

Canadian Psychiatric Association. 2005. Canadian clinical practice guidelines for the treatment of schizophrenia. *Canadian Journal of Psychiatry* 50 (suppl. 1): 7S-56S.

–. 2006. Clinical practice guidelines: Management of anxiety disorders. 51 (suppl. 2): 7S-91S.

Canadian Psychological Association. 2009. Summary position on health human resource and access to health services. http://www.cpa.ca/cpasite/userfiles/Documents/Practice_Page/CPA_position_HHR_Access.pdf.

Canadian Study of Health and Aging Working Group. 1994. Canadian study of health and aging: Study methods and prevalence of dementia. *Canadian Medical Association Journal* 150: 899-913.

Canadian Task Force on Preventive Health Care. 2013. Recommendations on screening for depression in adults. *Canadian Medical Association Journal* 185: 775-82.

Canadian Therapeutic Recreation Association. 2003. About CTRA. http://www.canadian-tr.org/About.

Cantor-Graae, E. 2007. The contribution of social factors to the development of schizophrenia: A review of recent findings. *Canadian Journal of Psychiatry* 52: 277-86.

Caplan, P. 1995. *They Say You're Crazy: How the World's Most Powerful Psychiatrists Decide Who's Normal*. Reading, MA: Addison-Wesley.

Capponi, P. 1992. *Upstairs in the Crazy House*. Toronto: Penguin.

–. 2003. *Beyond the Crazy House: Changing the Future of Madness*. Toronto: Penguin.

Caras, S. 1998. Personal accounts: The downside of the family-organized mental illness advocacy movement. *Psychiatric Services* 49: 763-64.

Carey, B. 2011. Expert on mental illness reveals her own fight. *New York Times*. http://www.nytimes.com/2011/06/23/health/23lives.html?pagewanted=all.

Carlson, R. 2011. Communication deviance, expressed emotion, and family cohesion in schizophrenia. University of Miami Libraries, Scholarly Repository. http://scholarly repository.miami.edu/oa_dissertations/615.

Carrigg, D. 2002. Double trouble. *Vancouver Courier*, 30 January, 4-5.

–. 2003. Backpack hostel conversions blamed for homelessness. *Vancouver Courier*, 20 July, 8-9.

–. 2004. Health authority streamlining help for addicts. *Vancouver Courier*, 21 January, 23.

Carten, R. 2006. *The AIMS Test, Mad Pride, and Other Essays*. Victoria: Keewatin Books.

Carter, C. 2006. Understanding the glass ceiling for functional outcome in schizophrenia. *American Journal of Psychiatry* 163: 356-58.

Cary, C., and C. McMillen. 2012. The data behind the dissemination: A systematic review of trauma-focused cognitive behavioral therapy for use with children and youth. *Children and Youth Services Review* 34: 748-57.

Cassels, A. 2008. Victoria double-cross on pharma watchdog. *Georgia Straight*. http://www.straight.com/article-147390/victoria-doublecross-pharma-watchdog.

Castel, S., et al. 2007. Screening for mental health problems among patients with substance use disorders: Preliminary findings on the validation of a self-assessment instrument. *Canadian Journal of Psychiatry* 52: 22-26.

Centre for Addiction and Mental Health. 2001. Police and nurses team together. http://www.camh.net/journal/journalv4no2/in_brief.html.

Centre for Addiction and Mental Health. 2004. *Putting Family-Centered Care Philosophy into Practice*. http://camh.net/Care_Treatment/Community_and_social_supports/Social_Support/FCCI/FCC_Better_Practices_PDF.pdf.

Centre for Applied Research in Mental Health and Addiction. 2007a. *Housing and Supports for Adults with Severe Addictions and/or Mental Illness in BC*. http://www.health.gov.bc.ca/library/publications/year/2007/Housing_Support_for_MHA_Adults.pdf.

–. 2007b. *Working with the Client Who Is Suicidal*. http://www.health.gov.bc.ca/library/publications/year/2007/MHA_WorkingWithSuicidalClient.pdf.

–. 2007c. *Integration of Mental Health and Addiction Services in BC: A Provincial Scan*. Burnaby, BC, Simon Fraser University Faculty of Health Sciences.

Chacon, F., et al. 2011. Efficacy of lifestyle interventions in physical health management of patients with severe mental illness. *Annals of General Psychiatry*. http://www.annals-general-psychiatry.com/content/10/1/22.

Chaimowitz, G. 2012. The criminalization of people with mental illness. *Canadian Journal of Psychiatry* 57: Insert, 1-6.

Chaimowitz, G., and Glancy, G. 2002. The duty to protect. https://ww1.cpaapc.org/Publications/Position_Papers/duty.asp.

Chaimowitz, G., R. Milev, and J. Blackburn. 2010. The fiduciary duty of psychiatrists. *Canadian Journal of Psychiatry* 55: Insert 1, 1-6.

Chamberlin, J. 2010. Confessions of a non-compliant patient. National Empowerment Center Inc. http://www.power2u.org/articles/recovery/confessions.html.

Chandler, M., and C. Lalonde. 2009. Cultural continuity as a moderator of suicide risk among Canada's First Nations. In *Healing Traditions: The Mental Health of Aboriginal Peoples in Canada*, ed. L. Kirmayer and G. Valaskakis, 221-48. Vancouver: UBC Press.

Chansonneuve, D. 2005. Reclaiming connections: Understanding residential school trauma among Aboriginal people. Aboriginal Healing Foundation. http://www.ahf.ca/downloads/healing-trauma-web-eng.pdf.

Charbonneau, M., et al. 2010. The psychiatrist's role in addressing stigma and discrimination. *Canadian Journal of Psychiatry* 55: Insert, 1-2.

Charlton, J. 1998. *Nothing about Us without Us: Disability, Oppression and Empowerment.* Berkeley: University of California Press.

Chavis, S. 2010. Depression stigma higher in medical students. PsychCentral. http://psychcentral.com/news/2010/09/21/depression-stigma-higher-in-medical-students/18468.html.

Chen, A., et al. 2010. Mental health service use by Chinese immigrants with severe and persistent mental illness. *Canadian Journal of Psychiatry* 55: 35-42.

Cheniaux, E., et al. 2008. Does schizoaffective disorder really exist? *Journal of Affective Disorders* 106: 209-17.

Cherland, E., and R. Fitzpatrick. 1999. Psychotic side effects of psychostimulants: A five-year review. *Canadian Journal of Psychiatry* 44: 811-13.

Choe, J., L. Teplin, and K. Abram. 2008. Perpetration of violence, violent victimization, and severe mental illness: Balancing public health concerns. *Psychiatric Services* 59: 153-64.

Chue, P., P. Tibbo, E. Wright, and J. Van Ens. 2004. Client and community services satisfaction with an ACT subprogram for inner-city clients in Edmonton, Alberta. *Canadian Journal of Psychiatry* 49: 621-24.

Clark, C., and T. Krupa. 2002. Reflections on empowerment in community mental health: Giving shape to an elusive idea. *Psychiatric Rehabilitation Journal* 25: 341-49.

Clarke Institute of Psychiatry. 1997. Best practices in mental health reform: Discussion paper. Report prepared for the Federal/Provincial/Territorial Advisory Network on Mental Health.

Codony, M., et al. 2009. Perceived need for mental health care and service use among adults in Western Europe: Results of the ESEMeD project. *Psychiatric Services* 60: 1051-58.

Cohen, M. 2008. Emerging from schizophrenia. *Schizophrenia Bulletin* 34: 406-7.

Cohen, S. 1985. *Visions of Social Control.* Cambridge, UK: Polity Press.

Coldwell, C., and W. Bender. 2007. The effectiveness of assertive community treatment for homeless populations with severe mental illness: A meta-analysis. *American Journal of Psychiatry* 164: 393-99.

Coley, N., et al. 2008. Dementia prevention: Methodological explanations for inconsistent results. *Epidemiologic Reviews* 30: 35-66.

College of Family Physicians of Canada. 2007. *National Physician Survey 2007.* http://www.cfpc.ca/English/cfpc/research/janus%20project/nps2007/default.asp?s=1.

Commission on the Future of Health Care in Canada. 2002. *Building on Values: The Future of Health Care in Canada.* Saskatoon: Commission on the Future of Health Care in Canada.

Committee on Addictions of the Group for the Advancement of Psychiatry. 2002. Responsibility and choice in addiction. *Psychiatric Services* 53: 707-13.

Condon, S. 2006. Doctors' work conditions turn critical. *Vancouver Courier,* 23 February.

Conference Board of Canada. 2008. Western workplace health 2008: Mental health, productivity, and performance. http://secure.conferenceboard.ca/conf/jun08/health/default.asp.

Cook, J. 2006. Employment barriers for persons with psychiatric disabilities: Update of a report for the President's Commission. *Psychiatric Services* 57: 1391-405.

Cook, J., et al. 2009. Apples don't fall far from the tree: Influences on psychotherapists' adoption and sustained use of new therapies. *Psychiatric Services* 60: 671-76.

–. 2011. Results of a randomized controlled trial of mental illness self-management using Wellness Recovery Action Planning. *Schizophrenia Bulletin.* http://schizophreniabulletin.oxfordjournals.org/content/early/2011/03/14/schbul.sbr012.full.pdf?keytype=ref&ijkey=LFsLUgMpqsVNV1q.

–. 2012. Randomized controlled trial of peer-led recovery education using Building Recovery of Individual Dreams and Goals through Education and Support (BRIDGES). *Schizophrenia Research* 136: 36-42.

Cook, T., and D. Campbell. 1979. *Quasi-Experimentation: Design and Analysis Issues for Field Settings*. Boston: Houghton Mifflin.

Cooper, D., et al. 2005. Ambulatory use of olanzapine and risperidone: A population-based study on persistence and the use of concomitant therapy in the treatment of schizophrenia. *Canadian Journal of Psychiatry* 50: 901-6.

Cooper, J., T. Heron, and W. Heward. 2007. *Applied Behavior Analysis*. 2nd ed. Columbus, OH: Pearson/Merrill Prentice Hall.

Correctional Investigator of Canada. 2009. *Annual Report of the Correctional Investigator.* Ottawa: Correctional Investigator of Canada.

Correll, C., S. Leucht, and J. Kane. 2004. Lower risk for tardive dyskinesia associated with second-generation antipsychotics. *American Journal of Psychiatry* 161: 414-25.

Corrigan, P. 2003. Towards an integrated, structural model of psychiatric rehabilitation. *Psychiatric Rehabilitation Journal* 26: 346-58.

–. 2004. Target–specific stigma change: A strategy for impacting mental illness stigma. *Psychiatric Rehabilitation Journal* 28: 113-21.

–. 2005. Dealing with stigma through personal disclosure. In *On the Stigma of Mental Illness*, ed. P. Corrigan, 257-80. Washington, DC: American Psychological Association.

Corrigan, P., and B. Gelb. 2006. Three programs that use mass approaches to challenge the stigma of mental illness. *Psychiatric Services* 57: 393-98.

Corrigan, P., and A. Watson. 2005. Findings from the National Comorbidity Survey on the frequency of violent behaviour in individuals with psychiatric disorders. *Psychiatry Research* 136: 153-62.

Corrigan, P., et al. 2003. Perceptions of discrimination among persons with serious mental illness. *Psychiatric Services* 54: 1105-10.

–. 2008. The educational goals of people with psychiatric disabilities. *Psychiatric Rehabilitation Journal* 31: 67-70.

Corring, D., and L. Cook. 2007. Use of qualitative methods to explore the quality-of-life construct from a consumer perspective. *Psychiatric Services* 58: 240-44.

Coursey, R., et al. 2000. Competencies for direct service staff members who work with adults with severe mental illnesses: Specific knowledge, attitudes, skills and bibliography. *Psychiatric Rehabilitation Journal* 23: 370-89.

Couture, S., et al. 2006. Do baseline client characteristics predict the therapeutic alliance in the treatment of schizophrenia? *Journal of Nervous and Mental Disease* 194: 10-14.

Covell, N., et al. 2007. What's in a name? Terms preferred by service recipients. *Administration and Policy in Mental Health* 34: 443-47.

Craig, T., et al. 2008. Integrated care for co-occurring disorders: Psychiatric symptoms, social functioning and service costs at 18 months. *Psychiatric Services* 59: 276-82.

Craven, M., and R. Bland. 2006. Shared care. *Canadian Journal of Psychiatry* 51 (suppl. 1): 9S-11S.

Crepeau, E., et al. 2009. *Willard and Spackman's Occupational Therapy*, 11th ed. Philadelphia: Wolters Kluwer Health/Lippincott Williams and Wilkins.

Crocker, A., K. Hartford, and L. Heslop. 2009. Gender difference in police encounters among persons with and without serious mental illness. *Psychiatric Services* 60: 86-93.

Crowley-Cyr, L. 2008. Homelessness, mental illness and extreme suffering in Australia. PhD diss., University of Sydney (Australia).

CTV News. 2008. Military recruiting hundreds to combat PTSD. http://www.ctv.ca/CTVNews/CTVNewsAt11/20080306/PTSD_military_080306/.

Cuijpers, P., et al. 2008. Preventing the onset of depressive disorders: A meta-analytic review of psychological interventions. *American Journal of Psychiatry* 165: 1272-80.

Culhane, D., S. Metraux, and T. Hadley. 2002. Public service reductions associated with placement of homeless persons with severe mental illness in supportive housing. Projects for Assistance in Transition from Homelessness. http://pathprogram.samhsa.gov/resource/public-service-reductions-associated-with-placement-of-homeless-persons-with-severe-mental-illness-in-supportive-housing-23456.aspx.

Curtis, L., and M. Hodge. 1995. Ethics and boundaries in community support services: New challenges. *New Directions for Mental Health Services* 66: 43-59.

Curtis, L. and V. Smith. 1996. Old rules and new dilemmas: Relationship boundaries in community support services. Paper presented at the Annual Conference of the International Association of Psychosocial Rehabilitation Services. Detroit, June.

Cyranoski, D. 2011. More clues in the genetics of schizophrenia. http://www.nature.com/news/more-clues-in-the-genetics-of-schizophrenia-1.9270.

Dallaire, R., and B. Beardsley. 2003. *Shake Hands with the Devil: The Failure of Humanity in Rwanda*. Toronto: Random House Canada.

Daly, G. 1996. *Homeless: Policies, Strategies and Lives on the Street*. London, UK: Routledge.

Dartmouth IPS Supported Employment Center. 2011. 2011 SE Fidelity Review Manual. http://www.dartmouth.edu/~ips/page19/page49/page49.html.

Daumit, G., et al. 2006. Adverse events during medical and surgical hospitalizations for persons with schizophrenia. *Archives of General Psychiatry* 63: 267-72.

Davidson, K. 2008. *Cognitive Therapy for Personality Disorders*. 2nd ed. New York: Routledge.

Davidson, L. 2012. The issue of insight. International Initiative for Mental Health Leadership. http://www.iimhl.com/iimhlupdates/20120315a.pdf.

Davidson, L., and D. Roe. 2007. Recovery from versus recovery in serious mental illness: One strategy for lessening confusion plaguing recovery. *Journal of Mental Health* 16: 459-570.

Davidson, L., et al. 2006a. Top ten concerns about recovery encountered in mental health system transformation. *Psychiatric Services* 57: 640-45.

–. 2006b. Peer support among adults with serious mental illness: A report from the field. *Schizophrenia Bulletin* 32: 443-50.

–. 2009. Oil and water or oil and vinegar? Evidence-based medicine meets recovery. *Community Mental Health Journal*, 45: 323-32.

Davies, L. 2000. Housing is a human right: Responding to homelessness in Canada. *Visions: BC's Mental Health Journal* 10: 37-38.

Davis, J., and S. Leucht. 2008. Has research informed us on the practical drug treatment of schizophrenia? *Schizophrenia Bulletin* 34: 403-5.

Davis, S. 1987a. Four conceptualizations of schizophrenia as models for treatment. *Health and Social Work* 12: 91-100.

–. 1987b. The homeless mentally ill: A report from Vancouver. *Social Worker* 55: 10-13.

–. 1994. Exploring the impact of Bill C-30 on the handling of mentally disordered offenders. PhD diss., Simon Fraser University.

–. 1995a. Treating the mentally ill in British Columbia: Recent developments in policy and legislation. *British Columbia Medical Journal* 37: 400-2.

–. 1995b. Fitness to stand trial: A study of a change in the law concerning pre-trial psychiatric remands. *Health Law in Canada* 16: 33-38.

–. 1996. The trouble with closing the asylums. *Globe and Mail*, 18 March.

–. 2000. An analysis of suicide attempts and completions by consumers of Vancouver community mental health teams. Paper presented at the 11th Annual Conference of the Canadian Association for Suicide Prevention, Vancouver, BC, 12 October.

–. 2002. Autonomy vs. coercion: Reconciling competing perspectives in community mental health. *Community Mental Health Journal* 38: 239-50.

–. 2008. The "recovery" vision and risk-aversion in psychiatric service delivery: Thoughts on the reconciliation of competing perspectives. Paper presented at SFU Institute for the Humanities Conference on Madness, Citizenship and Social Justice, Vancouver, 12-15 June.

–. 2011. Family members and mental health practitioners: Disagreements and understanding the perspective of the other. Paper presented at the Fifth Journal of Ethics in Mental Health Conference on Ethics in Mental Health, Kelowna, BC, 13 May.

Dawson, D. 1988. Treatment of the borderline patient: Relationship management. *Canadian Journal of Psychiatry* 33: 370-74.

Day, J., et al. 2005. Attitudes toward antipsychotic medication. *Archives of General Psychiatry* 62: 717-24.

Deegan, P. 1988. Recovery: The lived experience of rehabilitation. *Psychosocial Rehabilitation Journal* 11: 11-19.

–. 1996. Recovery as a journey of the heart. *Psychiatric Rehabilitation Journal* 19: 91-97.

–. 2000. Recovering our sense of value after being labeled mentally ill. In *Readings for Diversity and Social Justice*, ed. M. Adams, 359-63. New York: Routledge.

–. 2007. The lived experience of using psychiatric medication in the recovery process and a shared decision-making program to support it. *Psychiatric Rehabilitation Journal* 31: 62-69.

Deegan, P., et al. 2008. Best practices: A program to support shared decision making in an outpatient psychiatric Medication Clinic. *Psychiatric Services* 59: 603-5.

Degenhardt, L., and W. Hall. 2006. Is cannabis use a contributory cause of psychosis? *Canadian Journal of Psychiatry* 51: 556-65.

Deiser, R. 2002. A personal narrative of a cross-cultural experience in a therapeutic recreation: Unmasking the masked. *Therapeutic Recreation* Journal 36: 84-96.

DeMello, J., and S. Deshpande. 2011. Career satisfaction of psychiatrists. *Psychiatric Services* 62: 1013-18.

Department of Justice Canada. 2006. *The Review Board Systems in Canada: An Overview of Results from the Mentally Disordered Accused Data Collection Study.* Ottawa: Department of Justice.

DePoy, E., and S. Gilson. 2008. *Evaluation Practice.* New York: Routledge.

Depping, A., et al. 2010. Second-generation antipsychotic drugs for anxiety disorders. Cochrane Collaboration. http://www2.cochrane.org/reviews/en/ab008120.html.

DesMeules, M., et al. 2012. Rural health status and determinants in Canada. In *Health in Rural Canada*, ed. J. Kulig and A. Williams, 24-43. Vancouver: UBC Press.

Dewa, C., et al. 2002. How much are atypical antipsychotic agents being used, and do they reach the populations that need them? *Clinical Therapeutics* 24: 1466-76.

–. 2003. Left behind by reform: The case for improving primary care and mental health system services for people with moderate mental illness. *Applied Health Economics and Health Policy* 2: 43-54.

–. 2004. Nature and prevalence of mental illness in the workplace. *HealthcarePapers* 5: 12-25.

Dewa, D., D. McDaid, and S. Ettner. 2007. An international perspective on worker mental health problems: Who bears the burden and how are costs addressed? *Canadian Journal of Psychiatry* 52: 346-56.

Diamond, R. 1996. Coercion and tenacious treatment in the community: Applications to the real world. In *Coercion and Aggressive Community Treatment*, ed. D. Dennis and J. Monahan, 51-72. New York: Plenum Press.

Dickinson, H. 2002. Mental health policy in Canada: What's the problem? In *Health, Illness and Health Care in Canada*, 3rd ed., ed. B. Bolaria and H. Dickinson, 372-88. Scarborough, ON: Nelson.

Didenko, E., and N. Pankratz. 2007. Substance use: Pathway to homelessness, or a way of adapting to street life? *Visions Journal* 4: 9-10.

Dieterich, M., et al. 2010. Intensive case management for severe mental illness. *Cochrane Database of Systematic Reviews.* Art. No. CD007906. http://www.ncbi.nlm.nih.gov/pubmed/20927766.

Dincin, J. 2001. The biological basis of mental illness. *New Directions for Mental Health Services* 91: 47-56.

Dinos, S., et al. 2004. Stigma: The feelings and experiences of 46 people with mental illness. *British Journal of Psychiatry* 184: 176-81.

Dixon, L., et al. 1994. Clinical and treatment correlates of access to Section 8 certificates for homeless mentally ill persons. *Hospital and Community Psychiatry* 45: 1196-00.

–. 1998. Severe mental illness in an outreach intervention. *Community Mental Health Journal* 34: 251-59.

–. 2001. Evidence-based practices for services to families of people with psychiatric disabilities. *Psychiatric Services* 52: 903-8.

–. 2007. Psychiatrists and primary caring: What are our boundaries of responsibility? *Psychiatric Services* 58: 600-2.

–. 2010. The 2009 schizophrenia PORT psychosocial treatment recommendation and summary statements. *Schizophrenia Bulletin* 36: 48-70.

–. 2011. Outcomes of a randomized study of a peer-taught family-to-family education program for mental illness. *Psychiatric Services* 62: 591-97.

Dobbs, D. 2009. Soldiers' stress: What doctors get wrong about PTSD. *Veterans Today: Military and Foreign Affairs Journal.* http://www.veteranstoday.com/2009/03/19/soldiers-stress-what -doctors-get-wrong-about-ptsd/.

Dodge, C. 2011. Caregiving and schizophrenia: The well sibling's perspective. MA thesis, University of Victoria.

Donnelly, M., J. McElhaney, and M. Carr. 2011. *Improving BC's Care for Persons with Dementia in Emergency Departments and Acute Care Hospitals.* Vancouver Island Health Authority. http://www.viha.ca/NR/rdonlyres/B50B77AC-A338-42B1-831E-BCE1DD87BF14/0/ improvingcaredementiahospital.pdf.

Donohue, J., M. Cebasco, and M. Rosenthal. 2007. A decade of direct-to-consumer advertising of prescription drugs. *New England Journal of Medicine* 357: 673-81.

Dore, G., and S. Romans. 2001. Impact of bipolar affective disorder on family and partners. *Journal of Affective Disorders* 67: 147-58.

Doroshow, D. 2007. Performing a cure for schizophrenia: Insulin coma therapy on the wards. *Journal of the History of Medicine and the Allied Sciences* 62: 214-43.

Dorrance, N. 2003. Police attitudes toward mentally ill belie stereotype. *Queens Gazette,* 27 January.

Doskoch, B. 2007. Tasers file: History, technology and controversy. CTV News. http://www. ctv.ca/CTVNews/Specials/20071018/tasers_background_071018/.

Douglas, K., et al. 2001. *HCR-20: Violence Risk Management Companion Guide.* Vancouver: Mental Health, Law, and Policy Institute, Burnaby, BC, Simon Fraser University.

–. 2010. *HCR-20 Violence Risk Assessment Scheme: Overview and Annotated Bibliography.* http:// kdouglas.files.wordpress.com/2007/10/hcr-20-annotated-biblio-sept-2010.pdf.

Drake, R., and P. Deegan. 2009. Shared decision-making is an ethical imperative. *Psychiatric Services.* http://ps.psychiatryonline.org/article.aspx?articleID=100639.

Drake, R., P. Deegan, and C. Rapp. 2010. The promise of shared decision making in mental health. *Psychiatric Rehabilitation Journal* 34: 7-13.

Drake, R., et al. 2003. The history of community mental health treatment and rehabilitation for persons with severe mental illness. *Community Mental Health Journal* 39: 427-40.

Dranoff, L. 2005. *Every Canadian's Guide to the Law.* Toronto: HarperCollins.

Drapalski, A., et al. 2012. Assessing recovery of people with serious mental illness: development of a new scale. *Psychiatric Services* 63: 38-53.

Dreezer and Dreezer Inc. 2005. Report on the legislated review of community treatment orders, required under s. 33.9 of the Mental Health Act. Ontario, Ministry of Health and Long-Term Care. http://www.health.gov.on.ca/english/public/pub/ministry_reports/ dreezer/dreezer.pdf.

Druss, B. 2007. Do we know need when we see it? *Psychiatric Services* 58: 295.

–. 2008. An orphan comes of age. *Psychiatric Services* 59: 833.

Druss, B., et al. 2001. Quality of medical care and excess mortality in older patients with mental disorders. *Archives of General Psychiatry* 58: 565-72.

Duncan, B., S. Miller, and J. Sparks. 2004. *The Heroic Client*. San Francisco: Jossey-Bass.

Duncan, D. 2004. Is "bad parenting" the chicken or the egg? *Visions: BC's Mental Health Journal* 2, 3: 12-13.

Dunn, J. 2000. Why housing? A framework for housing and mental health. *Visions: BC's Mental Health Journal* 10: 4.

–. 2003. *A Needs, Gaps and Opportunities Assessment for Research: Housing as a Socioeconomic Determinant of Health*. Report prepared for the Canadian Institutes of Health Research.

Dupuis, K. 2008. Mental illness and the medical student: The disturbing reality of medical student perspectives. *Journal of Ethics in Mental Health* 3: 1-2.

Durbin, J., et al. 2006. Does systems integration affect continuity of mental health care? *Administration and Policy in Mental Health* 33: 705-17.

Eack, S., and M. Keshavan. 2008. Foresight in schizophrenia: A potentially unique and relevant factor to functional disability. *Psychiatric Services* 59: 256-60.

Eaton, W. 2001. *The Sociology of Mental Disorders*, 3rd ed. Westport, CO: Praeger.

Eberle, M. 2001a. *Homelessness: Causes and Effects*. Vol. 1: *The Relationship between Homelessness and the Health, Social Services and Criminal Justice System – A Review of the Literature*. Victoria: Ministry of Social Development and Economic Security.

–. 2001b. *Homelessness: Causes and Effects*. Vol. 3: *The Costs of Homelessness in British Columbia*. Victoria: Ministry of Social Development and Economic Security.

–. 2001c. *Homelessness: Causes and Effects*. Vol. 4: *A Profile and Policy Review of Homelessness in the Provinces of Ontario, Quebec and Alberta*. Victoria: Ministry of Social Development and Economic Security.

Echenberg, H., and H. Jensen. 2008. Defining and enumerating homelessness in Canada. Ottawa: Parliamentary Information and Research Service, Social Affairs Division.

Edge, S., and R. Wilton. 2009. Reengineering residential care facilities: A case study of Hamilton, Ontario. *Canadian Journal of Community Mental Health* 28: 137-49.

Edwards, N., et al. 2008. Suicide in Newfoundland and Labrador: A linkage study using medical examiner and vital statistics data. *Canadian Journal of Psychiatry* 53: 252-59.

Egaland, G., et al. 2010. Food insecurity among Inuit preschoolers: Nunavut Inuit Child Health Survey, 2007-2008. *Canadian Medical Association Journal* 182: 243-48.

Ehmann, T., and L. Hanson, L. 2004. Pharmacotherapy. In *Best Practice in Early Psychosis Intervention*, ed. T. Ehmann, G. MacEwan, and W. Honer, 37-60. London, UK: Taylor and Francis.

Ehmann, T., J. Yager, and L. Hanson. 2004. "Early psychosis: A review of the treatment literature." Research report prepared for the BC Ministry of Children and Family Development.

Ehlers, A., et al. 2003. A randomized controlled trial of cognitive therapy, a self-help booklet, and repeated assessments as early interventions for post-traumatic stress disorder. *Archives of General Psychiatry* 60: 1024-32.

Einarson, A., et al. 2009. Incidence of major malformations in infants following antidepressant exposure in pregnancy: Results of a large prospective cohort study. *Canadian Journal of Psychiatry* 54: 242-46.

Einhaus, S. 2009. Personal accounts: My mother's schizophrenia – what I didn't know helped me. *Psychiatric Services* 60: 145-46.

Eklund, M., L. Hansson, and C. Ahlqvist. 2004. The importance of work as compared to other forms of daily occupations for wellbeing and functioning among persons with long-term mental illness. *Community Mental Health Journal* 40: 465-77.

El-Guebaly, N. 1997. Psychiatry 2000: Is it time for a sequel to "more for the mind?" http://ww1.cpa-apc.org:8080/publications/archives/bulletin/1997/feb/clinical.htm.

Emery, G. 2008. Drug trials with negative results unlikely to see print, team finds. *Vancouver Sun*, 18 January.

Engel, G. 1977. The need for a new medical model: A challenge for biomedicine. *Science* 196: 129-36.

Ernst, E. 1999. An evidence-based approach to acupuncture. BMJ Group. http://aim.bmj.com/content/17/1/59.full.pdf.

Esposito, E., et al. 2007. Frequency and adequacy of depression treatment in a Canadian population sample. *Canadian Journal of Psychiatry* 52: 780-89.

Essock, S., L. Frisman, and N. Kontos. 1998. Cost-effectiveness of assertive community treatment teams. *American Journal of Orthopsychiatry* 68: 179-90.

Essock, S., and L. Rogers. 2011. What's in a name? Let's keep on asking. *Schizophrenia Bulletin* 37: 469-70.

Estroff, S., C. Zimmer, W. Lachiotte, and J. Benoit. 1994. The influence of social networks and social support on violence in persons with serious mental illness. *Hospital and Community Psychiatry* 45: 669-79.

Everett, B. 1994. Something is happening: The contemporary consumer and psychiatric survivor movement in historical context. *Journal of Mind and Behavior* 15: 55-70.

Everett, B., et al. 2003. Recovery rediscovered: Implications for mental health policy in Canada. Canadian Mental Health Association. http://www.ontario.cmha.ca/admin_ver2/maps/recovery%5Frediscovered%2Epdf.

Eynan, R., et al. 2002. The association between homelessness and suicidal ideation and behaviors: Results of a cross-sectional study. *Suicide and Life-Threatening Behavior* 32: 418-27.

Fauman, M. 2002. *Study Guide to the DSM-IV-TR*. Washington, DC: American Psychiatric Publishing.

Fayerman, P. 2007. Pharmaceutical firms oppose cheap drug policy. *Vancouver Sun*, 9 August.

–. 2013. BCMA wants crackdown on online drug advertising. *Vancouver Sun*, 27 February.

Fenton, W. 2000. Evolving perspectives on individual psychotherapy for schizophrenia. *Schizophrenia Bulletin* 26: 47-72.

Fergusson, D., et al. 2005. Association between suicide attempts and SSRIs: Systematic review of randomized controlled trials. BMJ Group. http://bmj.bmjjournals.com/cgi/content/abstract/330/7488/396.

Ferris, L., et al. 2008. Defining the physician's duty to warn: Consensus statement of Ontario's Medical Expert Panel on Duty to Inform. *Canadian Medical Association Journal* 158: 1473-79.

Fikretoglu, D., et al. 2009. Predictors of likelihood and intensity of past-year mental health service use in an active Canadian military sample. *Psychiatric Services* 60: 358-66.

Fink, M. 2011. Electroconvulsive therapy resurrected: Its successes and promises after 75 years. *Canadian Journal of Psychiatry* 56: 3-4.

First, M., et al. 2002. *Structured Clinical Interview for DSM-IV-TR Axis I Disorders, Research Version, Patient Edition*. New York: Biometrics Research, New York State Psychiatric Institute.

Fischer, E., M. Shumway, and R. Owen. 2002. Priorities of consumers, providers and family members in the treatment of schizophrenia. *Psychiatric Services* 53: 724-29.

Fish, S. 1994. *There's No Such Thing as Free Speech, and It's a Good Thing, Too*. New York: Oxford University Press.

Fisher, D. 1999. Healing and recovery are real. National Empowerment Center Inc. http://www.power2u.org/articles/recovery/healing.html.

Fisher, M., et al. 2009. Using neuroplasticity-based auditory training to improve verbal memory in schizophrenia. *American Journal of Psychiatry* 166: 805-11.

Fisher, W., et al. 2011. Risk of arrest among public mental health services recipients and the general public. *Psychiatric Services* 62: 67-72.

Fitzpatrick, M. 2007. Ottawa establishes Canadian Mental Health Commission. *National Post*. http://www.canada.com/nationalpost/news/story.html?id=24b6fa78-4730-4338-aa89-7e9f0282b015&k=70506.

Fitzpatrick, M. 2008. Young Aboriginal women most likely to be overweight: Report. *Regina Leader Post*. http://www.canada.com/reginaleaderpost/news/story.html?id=f60c6a61-da7a-4871-8d62-83b2abad05ff&k=83264.

Flores, G., et al. 2002. The health of Latino children: Urgent priorities, unanswered questions and a research agenda. *Journal of the American Medical Association* 288: 82-90.

Fogel, J., and D. Ford. 2005. Stigma beliefs of Asian-Americans with depression in an internet sample. *Canadian Journal of Psychiatry* 50: 470-78.

Forchuk, C., G. Nelson, and G. Hall. 2006. It's important to be proud of the place you live in: Housing problems and preferences of psychiatric survivors. *Perspectives in Psychiatric Care* 42: 42-52.

Forchuk, C., et al. 2006. From psychiatric ward to the streets and shelters. *Journal of Psychiatric and Mental Health Nursing* 13: 301-8.

–. 2008. Developing and testing an intervention to prevent homelessness among individuals discharged from psychiatric wards to shelters and "NFA." *Journal of Psychiatric and Mental Health Nursing* 15: 569-75.

Foulkes, E. 2000. Advocating for persons who are mentally ill. *Administration and Policy in Mental Health and Mental Health Services Research.* 27: 353-67.

Fournier, S., and E. Crey. 1997. *Stolen from Our Embrace: The Abduction of First Nations Children and the Restoration of Aboriginal Communities*. Vancouver, BC: Douglas and McIntyre.

Foussias, G., and G. Remington. 2010. Antipsychotics and schizophrenia: From efficacy and effectiveness to clinical decision-making. *Canadian Journal of Psychiatry* 55: 117-25.

Frankel, A., and S. Gelman. 2004. *Case Management: An Introduction to Concepts and Skills,* 2nd ed. Chicago: Lyceum Books.

Freidson, E. 1994. *Professionalism Reborn: Theory, Prophecy and Policy.* Cambridge, UK: Polity Press.

Frese, F. 1997. The mental health service consumer's perspective on mandatory treatment. *New Directions for Mental Health Services* 75: 17-26.

Frueh, B., et al. 2006. Clinicians' perspectives on CBT treatment for PTSD among persons with severe mental illness. *Psychiatric Services* 57: 1027-31.

Fuller, C. 1998. *Caring for Profit: How Corporations Are Taking over Canada's Health Care System.* Ottawa: Canadian Centre for Policy Alternatives.

Fullerton, C., et al. 2011. Ten-year trends in quality of care and spending for depression. *Archives of General Psychiatry* 68: 1218-26.

Gabbard, G., and C. Nadelson. 1995. Professional boundaries in the physician-patient relationship. *Journal of the American Medical Association* 273: 1445-49.

Gaebel, W., and A. Baumann. 2003. Interventions to reduce the stigma associated with severe mental illness: Experiences from the Open the Door Program in Germany. *Canadian Journal of Psychiatry* 48: 657-62.

Gagnon, L. 2011. Working within the system. *Networker* (West Coast Mental Health Network publication). http://www.wcmhn.org/bulletin_files/Networker-FALL%202011%20wcmhn.pdf.

Gagnon, M., and J. Lexchin. 2008. The cost of pushing pills: A new estimate of pharmaceutical promotion expenditures in the United States. *PLoS Medicine* 5: 0029-0033. http://www.plosmedicine.org/article/fetchObject.action?uri=info%3Adoi%2F10.1371%2Fjournal.pmed.0050001&representation=PDF.

Galt, V. 2006. Out of the shadows: Mental health at work. Workopolis.com. http://www.mentalhealthroundtable.ca/mar_2006/Outoftheshadows.pdf.

Ganesan, S. 2000. Mental health and disorder in recent immigrants. *Visions: BC's Mental Health Journal* 9: 24.

Garland, E. 2004. Facing the evidence: Antidepressant treatment in children and adolescents. *Canadian Medical Association Journal* 170: 489-91.

Geller, J., and M. Harris, M. 1994. *Women of the Asylum.* New York: Anchor Books.

Genova, P. 2003. Dump the DSM. *Psychiatric Times* April, 72.

Gentile S. 2004. Clinical utilization of atypical antipsychotics in pregnancy and lactation. *Annals of Pharmacotherapy* 38: 1265-71.

Gerber, G., and P. Prince. 1999. Measuring client satisfaction with assertive community treatment. *Psychiatric Services* 50: 546-50.

Gerber, G., et al. 2003. Substance abuse among persons with serious mental illness in Eastern Ontario. *Canadian Journal of Community Mental Health* 22: 113-28.

Gerson, R., et al. 2009. Families' experiences with seeking treatment for recent-onset psychosis. *Psychiatric Services* 60: 812-16.

Ghaemi, S. 2010. *The Rise and Fall of the Biopsychosocial Model.* Baltimore: Johns Hopkins University Press.

Ghosh, S., and J. Greenberg. 2009. Aging fathers of adult children with schizophrenia: The toll of caregiving on their mental and physical health. *Psychiatric Services* 60: 982-84.

Gibson-Leek, M. 2003. Client vs. client. *Psychiatric Services* 54: 1101-2.

Gilbert, M., and D. Bilsker. 2012. *Psychological Health and Safety: An Action Guide for Employers.* Mental Health Commission of Canada. http://www.mentalhealthcommission.ca/Site CollectionDocuments/Workforce/Workforce_Employers_Guide_ENG.pdf.

Gilbody, S., P. Wilson, and I. Watt. 2004. Direct-to-consumer advertising of psychotropics. *British Journal of Psychiatry* 185: 1-2.

Gingell, C. 1991. The criminalization of the mentally ill: An examination of the hypothesis. PhD diss., Simon Fraser University.

Giron, M., et al. 2010. Efficacy and effectiveness of individual family intervention on social and clinical functioning and family burden in severe schizophrenia: A 2-year randomized controlled study. *Psychological Medicine* 40: 73-84.

Glannon, W. 2008. The blessings and burdens of biological psychiatry. *Journal of Ethics in Mental Health* 3: 1-4.

Glasby, J., and P. Beresford. 2006. Who knows best? Evidence-based practice and the service user contribution. *Critical Social Policy* 26: 268-83.

Glenmullen, J. 2000. *Prozac Backlash.* New York: Simon and Schuster.

Glasgow, J. 2007. Return to work from mental health and/or addiction related leave for Vancouver community mental health workers. MA thesis, Royal Roads University.

Glover, G., G. Arts, and K.S. Babu. 2006. Crisis resolution/home treatment teams and psychiatric admission rates in England. *British Journal of Psychiatry.* 180: 441-45.

Glyn, S., et al. 2006. The potential impact of the recovery movement on family interventions for schizophrenia: Opportunities and obstacles. *Schizophrenia Bulletin* 32: 451-63.

Goering, P., D. Wasylenki, and J. Durbin. 2000. Canada's mental health system. *International Journal of Law and Psychiatry* 23: 345-59.

Goering, P., et al. 1994. *Essential Service Ratios in a Reformed Mental Health System: Case Management.* Report submitted to the Ontario Ministry of Health.

–. 2006. Who uses consumer-run self-help organizations? *American Journal of Orthopsychiatry* 76: 367-73.

Goffman, E. 1961. *Asylums: Essays on the Social Situation of Mental Patients and Other Inmates.* New York: Anchor Books.

Goldacre, B. 2008. *Bad Science.* London, UK: Fourth Estate.

Goldberg, T., et al. 2007. Cognitive improvement after treatment with second-generation antipsychotic medications in first-episode schizophrenia: Is it a practice effect? *Archives of General Psychiatry* 64: 1115-22.

Goldbloom, D. 2003. Editorial: Language and metaphor. *Canadian Psychiatric Association Bulletin,* June: 3-5.

Golden, A., et al. 1999. *Report of the Mayor's Homelessness Action Task Force: Taking Responsibility for the Homeless: An Action Plan for Toronto.* City of Toronto: Mayor's Homelessness Action Task Force. http://www.toronto.ca/pdf/homeless_action.pdf.

Goldenberg, I., and H. Goldenberg. 1980. *Family Therapy: An Overview.* Monterey, CA: Brooks/ Cole Publishing Company.

Goldner, E., W. Jones, and M. Fang. 2011. Access to and waiting time for psychiatrist services in a Canadian urban Area: A study in real time. *Canadian Journal of Psychiatry* 56: 474-80.

Goldner, E., et al. 2000. Evidence-based psychiatric practice: Implications for education and continuing professional development. *Canadian Journal of Psychiatry* 46 (Insert 1): 1-6.

Gomoroy, T. 2001. A critique of the effectiveness of assertive community treatment. *Psychiatric Services* 52: 1394.

Gonzalez, H., et al. 2010. The epidemiology of major depression and ethnicity in the United States. *Journal of Psychiatric Research* 44: 1043-51.

Gonzalez-Blanch, C., et al. 2008. Lack of association between clinical and cognitive change in first-episode psychosis: The first 6 weeks of treatment. *Canadian Journal of Psychiatry* 53: 839-47.

Gordon, A. 1997. Psychiatric bed levels. *Canadian Psychiatric Association Bulletin* 29: 1-4.

Gorman, C. 2003. Finding a balance: Bipolar disorders. *Canadian Journal of Diagnosis* 20: 93-97.

Government of Alberta. 1983. *Report of the Task Force to Review the Mental Health Act.* Edmonton: Government of Alberta.

Government of Canada. 2007. Mental health, mental illness and addiction: Overview of policies and programs in Canada. http://www.parl.gc.ca/38/1/parlbus/commbus/senate/com-e/soci-e/rep-e/report1/repintnov04vol1part2-e.htm.

–. 2008. Issues and options for revisions to the *Tri-Council Policy Statement: Ethical Conduct for Research Involving Humans* (TCPS), Section 6: Research involving aboriginal peoples. http://www.pre.ethics.gc.ca/policy-politique/initiatives/docs/AREI_-_February_2008_-_EN.pdf.

Government of Manitoba. 2011. *Rising to the Challenge: A Strategic Plan for the Mental Health and Well-Being of Manitobans.* http://www.gov.mb.ca/health/mh/docs/challenge.pdf.

Gram, K. 2008. Willing to work. *Vancouver Sun.* http://www2.canada.com/vancouversun/news/westcoastnews/story.html?id=798dff2b-e622-4fc2-a187-cc6d3990b08c&p=3.

Grant, P., et al. 2011. Randomized trial to evaluate the efficacy of cognitive therapy for low-functioning patients with schizophrenia. University of British Columbia Library. http://archpsyc.ama-assn.org.ezproxy.library.ubc.ca/cgi/reprint/archgenpsychiatry.2011.129.

Gray, J., M. Shone, and P. Liddle. 2008. *Canadian Mental Health Law and Policy.* Markham, ON: LexisNexis.

Greater Vancouver Shelter Strategy. 2007. *Homeless Voices, Part 1: What We Heard from Metropolitan Vancouver Residents Who Have Experienced Homelessness.* http://www.gvss.ca/PDF/Including%20Homeless%20Voices%20report%20Oct%2011,%202007.pdf.

Green, M., B. Marshall, and E. Wirshing. 1997. Does risperidone improve verbal working memory in treatment resistant schizophrenia? *American Journal of Psychiatry* 154: 799-804.

Green, R., et al. 2003. Depression as a risk factor for Alzheimer disease: the MIRAGE Study. *Archives of Neurology* 60: 753-59.

Green, M., B. Marshall, and E. Wirshing. 1997. Does risperidone improve verbal working memory in treatment resistant schizophrenia? *American Journal of Psychiatry* 154: 799-804.

Greenberg, L. 2007. Grits hiding cost of autism treatment fight, MPP charges. *Ottawa Citizen.* http://www2.canada.com/ottawacitizen/news/story.html?id=3f1673b1-a160-4a90-95db-27b07b4767a1.

Greenfield, B., et al. 2006. Profile of a metropolitan North American immigrant suicidal adolescent population. *Canadian Journal of Psychiatry* 51: 155-59.

Griffiths, K., et al. 2004. Promoting consumer participation in mental health research: a national workshop. E-HUB, Australian National University. http://www.ehub.anu.edu.au/pdf/consumerworkshopreport.pdf.

Grohol, J. 2007. Are people with schizophrenia better off? PsychCentral. http://psychcentral.com/blog/archives/2007/10/09/are-people-with-schizophrenia-better-off/.

Grol, R. 2008. Knowledge transfer in mental health care: How do we bring evidence into day-to-day practice? *Canadian Journal of Psychiatry* 53: 275-76.

Grunier, A., et al. 2010. Frequency and pattern of emergency department visits by long term care residents. *Journal of the American Geriatrics Society* 58: 510-17.

Gucciardi, E., et al. 2004. Eating disorders. *BMC Women's Health* 4(suppl. L): S21

Gumpp, R. 2009. *Hope and Fear: Consumers, Psychiatric Medications and the Therapeutic Relationship.* CONKER Mental Illness, Vancouver. http://recoveryinmentalhealth.files.wordpress.com/2010/12/hope-and-fear-conker-report-september-20094.pdf.

Gunderson, J., et al. 1984. Effects of psychotherapy in schizophrenia, II: Comparative outcomes of two forms of treatment. *Schizophrenia Bulletin* 10: 564-98.

Gunter, R., and M. Whittal. 2010. Dissemination of CBT treatments for anxiety disorders: Overcoming barriers and improving patient access. *Clinical Psychology Review* 30: 194-202.

Gutman, S. 2008. Frontline reports: Supported education for adults with psychiatric disabilities. *Psychiatric Services* 59: 326-27.

Hadekel, P. 2011. Canada needs better patent protection for pharmaceuticals: CEO. *Montreal Gazette.* http://www.montrealgazette.com/business/Canada+needs+better+patent+protection+pharmaceuticals/4922806/story.html#ixzz1ZHqdA1aj.

Hadjipavlou, G., and J. Ogrodniczuk. 2010. Promising psychotherapies for personality disorders. *Canadian Journal of Psychiatry* 55: 202-10.

Haggarty, J., et al. 2000. Psychiatric disorders in an Arctic community. *Canadian Journal of Psychiatry* 45: 357-62.

Hall, N. 2000. *Pump up the Volume: A Report from the Mental Health Advocate of British Columbia.* Vancouver: Office of the Mental Health Advocate of British Columbia.

–. 2001. *Growing the Problem: The Second Annual Report of the Mental Health Advocate of British Columbia.* Vancouver: Office of the Mental Health Advocate of British Columbia.

Hall, N. 2008. Police are "brainwashed" by taser maker. *Vancouver Sun.* http://www.canada.com/vancouversun/news/story.html?id=28218a80-11db-47a3-baf9-90b7dc2618aa.

Hall, N., and C. Weaver. 2008. Keeping people with mental disorders out of trouble with the law. Canadian Police/Mental Health Liason. http://www.pmhl.ca/webpages/reports/Diversion%20Project%20-%20Keeping%20People%20Out%20of%20Trouble%20with%20the%20Law%20-%20Nov5.pdf.

Halley, D., R. Roine, and A. Ohinmaa. 2008. The effectiveness of telemental health applications: A review. *Canadian Journal of Psychiatry* 53: 769-78.

Hamid, S. 2000a. Culture-specific syndromes: It's all relative. *Visions: BC's Mental Health Journal* 9: 6.

–. 2000b. Overcoming NIMBY in Nelson: A lesson in perseverance and resourcefulness. *Visions: BC's Mental Health Journal* 10: 27-28.

Hanrahan, N., and D. Hartley. 2008. Employment of advanced-practice psychiatric nurses to stem rural mental health workforce shortages. *Psychiatric Services* 59: 109-11.

Harckham, R. 2003. Defining and servicing mental health in a remote northern community. MA thesis, University of British Columbia.

Hardiman, E., M. Theriot, and F. Hodges. 2005. Evidence-based practice in mental health: Implications and challenges for consumer-run programs. *Best Practices in Mental Health* 1: 105-21.

Harding, C., and J. Zahniser. 1994. Empirical correction of seven myths about schizophrenia with implications for treatment. *Acta Psychiatrica Scandinavica* 90 (suppl. 384): 140-46.

Harding, C., J. Zubin, and J. Strauss. 1992. Chronicity in schizophrenia revisited. *British Journal of Schizophrenia* 161 (suppl. 18): 27-31.

Harding, C., et al. 1987. The Vermont longitudinal study of persons with severe mental illness. *American Journal of Psychiatry* 144: 727-35.

Harman, J., M. Edlund, and J. Fortney. 2009. Trends in antidepressant utilization from 2001 to 2004. *Psychiatric Services* 60: 611-16.

Harnett, C. 2008. Shorter hospital stay a danger to schizophrenics, study reveals. *Victoria times Colonist*, 20 April.

Harris, G. 2011. Talk doesn't pay, so psychiatry turns instead to drug therapy. *New York Times*. http://www.nytimes.com/2011/03/06/health/policy/06doctors.html?_r=1&emc=eta1.

Harris G., M. Rice, and J. Camilleri. 2004. Applying a forensic actuarial assessment (the Violence Risk Appraisal Guide) to non-forensic patients. *Journal of Interpersonal Violence* 19: 1063-74.

Harris, M., and R. Fallot. 2001. Envisioning a trauma-informed service system: A vital paradigm shift. *New Directions for Mental Health Services* 89: 3-21.

Harrow, M., and T. Jobe. 2007. Factors involved in outcome and recovery in schizophrenia patients not on antipsychotic medications: A 15-year multifollow-up study. *Journal of Nervous and Mental Disease* 195: 406-14.

Hart, S. 2006. Mental illness and criminal justice: Where tolerance breaks down. *Visions Journal* 2: 4-5.

Hart, S., and J. Hemphill. 1989. Prevalence of and service utilization by mentally disordered offenders at the Vancouver Pre-Trail Services Centre: A survey. Unpublished report prepared for the British Columbia Ministry of the Solicitor General, Corrections Branch.

Hartman, A. 1994. *Reflections and Controversies: Essays on Social Work*. Washington, DC: NASW Press.

Hartocollis, A. 2008. Clinic treats mental illness by enlisting the family. *New York Times*. http://www.nytimes.com/2008/06/04/nyregion/04clinic.html?ref=bethisraelmedical center#.

Harvey, P., M. Lepage, and A. Malla. 2007. Benefits of enriched intervention compared with standard care for patients with recent-onset psychosis: A meta-analytic approach. *Canadian Journal of Psychiatry* 52: 464-72.

Haynes, D. 2002. Change your mind. *Trek: The Magazine of the University of British Columbia*. Spring, 19-24.

Hazelton, M., R. Rossiter, and J. Milner. 2006. Managing the "unmanageable": Training staff in the use of dialectical behaviour therapy for borderline personality disorder. *Contemporary Nurse* 21: 120-30.

Health Canada. 1997. *Review of Best Practices in Mental Health Reform*. Ottawa: Health Canada.

–. 2001a. *Best Practices: Concurrent Mental Health and Substance Use Disorders*. Ottawa: Health Canada.

–. 2001b. *National Program Inventory: Concurrent Mental Health and Substance Use Disorders*. Ottawa: Health Canada.

–. 2002a. *A Report on Mental Illnesses in Canada*. Ottawa: Health Canada.

–. 2002b. *Sharing the Learning: The Health Transition Fund*. Ottawa: Health Canada.

–. 2002c. Housing as a determinant of health. http://www.phac-aspc.gc.ca/ph-sp/oi-ar/09_housing-eng.php.

Health Council of Canada. 2012. Progress report 2012: Health care renewal in Canada. http://healthcouncilcanada.ca/tree/ProgressReport2012_FINAL_EN.pdf.

Healy, D. 2002. *The Creation of Psychopharmacology*. Cambridge, MA: Harvard University Press.

Hebert, P. 2008. The need for an institute of continuing health education. *Canadian Medical Association Journal* 178: 805-6.

Heisel, M. 2006. Suicide and its prevention among older adults. *Canadian Journal of Psychiatry* 51: 143-54.

Helmes, E., and J. Landmark. 2003. Subtypes of schizophrenia: A cluster analytic approach. *Canadian Journal of Psychiatry* 48: 702-8.

Hensley, M. 2006. Why I am not a "mental health consumer." *Psychiatric Rehabilitation Journal* 30: 67-69.

Hermann, Q. 2002. Addictive and over-prescribed. *Vancouver Sun,* 1 February.

Herschel, A., et al. 2009. Understanding community mental health administrators' perspectives on dialectical behavior therapy implementation. *Psychiatric Services* 60: 989-92.

Hewa, S. 2002. Physicians, medical profession, and medical practice. In *Health, Illness, and Health Care in Canada,* 3rd ed., ed. B. Singh Bolaria and Harley Dickinson, 55-81. Toronto: Harcourt, Brace, Jovanovich.

Hiday, V., and B. Ray. 2010. Arrests two years after exiting a well-established mental health court. *Psychiatric Services* 61: 463-68.

Hildebrandt, A. 2008. Canada's military suicide rate doubled in a year. CBC News. http://www.cbc.ca/canada/story/2008/04/18/suicide-rates.html.

Hillegers, M., et al. 2004. Impact of stressful life events, familial loading, and their interaction on the onset of mood disorders. *British Journal of Psychiatry* 185: 97-101.

Hilty, D., et al. 2003. The effectiveness of telepsychiatry: A review. *Canadian Psychiatric Association Bulletin* 35: 10-17.

Hoch, J., et al. 2009. Mental illness and police interactions in a mid-sized Canadian city: What the data do and do not say. *Canadian Journal of Community Mental Health* 28: 49-63.

Hodges, J., et al. 2003. Use of self-help services and consumer satisfaction with professional mental health services. *Psychiatric Services* 54: 1161-63.

Hodgins, S., and G. Cote. 1991. The mental health of penitentiary inmates in isolation. *Canadian Journal of Criminology* 33: 175-82.

Hoffman, B. 1997. *The Law of Consent to Treatment in Ontario,* 2nd ed. Toronto: Butterworths.

Hoffman, J., and M. Wilkes. 1999. Direct to consumer advertising of prescription drugs: An idea whose time should not come. *British Medical Journal* 318: 1301-2.

Hogan, D., et al. 2003. Prevalence and potential consequences of benzodiazepine use in senior citizens: Results from the Canadian study of health and aging. *Canadian Journal of Clinical Pharmacology* 10: 72-77.

Hogan, M. 2008. Transforming mental health care: Realities, priorities and prospects. *Psychiatric Clinics of North America* 31: 1-9.

Hogarty, G., et al. 1997. Three-year trials of personal therapy among schizophrenic patients living with or independent of family, II: Effects on adjustment of patients. *American Journal of Psychiatry* 154: 1514-24.

Holden, C. 2003. Getting the short end of the allele. *Science* 301: 291-93.

Hopper, K. 2008. Qualitative and quantitative research: Two cultures. *Psychiatric Services* 59: 711.

Hourston, S. 2010. Surviving change: Five tools for resilience. BC Coalition of People with Disabilities. http://bccpd.bc.ca/docs/transsummer10-web.pdf.

Howard, L., et al. 2008. Admission to women's crisis houses or to psychiatric wards: Women's pathways to admission. *Psychiatric Services* 59: 1443-49.

Howell, M. 2005. Counting the homeless. *Vancouver Courier,* 9 January, 4-5.

–. 2007. Recruits' mental health training adequate, says VPD. *Vancouver Courier,* 14 November, 13.

–. 2008. Harcourt pans "deinstitutionalization" of the 1980s. *Vancouver Courier,* 8 February, 16.

Hsu, G., et al. 2008. Stigma of depression is more severe in Chinese-Americans than Caucasian-Americans. *Psychiatry: Interpersonal and Biological Processes* 71: 210-18.

Hsu, J., et al. 2011. Incidence of diabetes in patients with schizophrenia: A population-based study. *Canadian Journal of Psychiatry* 56: 19-26.

Hubble, M., B. Duncan, and S. Miller. 1999. *The Heart and Soul of Change: What Works in Therapy.* Washington, DC: American Psychological Association.

Hucker, S. 1998. Editorial: Forensic psychiatry. *Canadian Journal of Psychiatry* 43: 456-57.

Human Resources and Skills Development Canada. 2008. Understanding homelessness. http://www.hrsdc.gc.ca/eng/homelessness/understanding_homelessness/index.shtml.

Human Rights Watch. 2003. United States: Mentally ill mistreated in prison. http://www.hrw.org/press/2003/10/us102203.htm.

Hume, M. 2007. Suicide rate crippling communities, doctor warns. *Globe and Mail,* 23 November.

Humphrey, S., and W. Townsend. 2005. The impact of culture on person/family centered planning. National Latino Behavioral Association. http://nlbha.org/PDFs/CulturePlanning.pdf.

Hunkeler, E., et al. 2000. Efficacy of nurse telehealth care and peer support in augmenting treatment of depression in primary care. *Archives of Family Medicine* 9: 700-8.

Hunt, A., et al. 2007. Community treatment orders in Toronto: The emerging data. *Canadian Journal of Psychiatry* 52: 647-56.

Hutchinson, D., et al. 2006. The personal and vocational impact of training and employing people with psychiatric disabilities as providers. *Psychiatric Rehabilitation Journal* 29: 205-13.

Hwang, S., et al. 2008. The effect of traumatic brain injury on the health of homeless people. *Canadian Medical Association Journal* 179: 779-84.

Hyman, I. 2004. Setting the stage: Reviewing current knowledge on the health of Canadian immigrants. *Canadian Journal of Public Health* 95: 4-8.

Inman, S. 2010. *After Her Brain Broke: Helping My Daughter Regain Her Sanity.* Dundas, ON: Bridgeross Communications.

–. 2011a. How can you support the parents of people with schizophrenia? University of British Columbia, Continuing Professional Development. http://www.ubccpd.ca/shared/assets/0900_Supporting_the_parents_Inman4082.pdf.

–. 2011b. Suppressing schizophrenia. *Tyee.* http://thetyee.ca/Opinion/2011/08/29/Review-Mental-Health-Strategy/.

–. 2011c. The right to be sane. *National Post.* http://fullcomment.nationalpost.com/2011/07/29/susan-inman-the-right-to-be-sane/.

Institute for Safe Medication Practices Canada. 2012. Analysis of harmful medication incidents involving psychotropic medications. *ISMP Canada Safety Bulletin* 12: 1-5.

Irwin, J. 2004. Who's to blame for homelessness? *Westender,* 24-30 June, 7.

Ismael, Z., T. Rajji, and K. Shulman. 2009. Brief cognitive screening instruments: An update. *International Journal of Geriatric Psychiatry* 25: 111-20.

Jacobs, P., et al. 2008. Expenditures on mental health and addictions for Canadian provinces in 2003 and 2004. *Canadian Journal of Psychiatry* 53: 306-13.

Jaffe, D. 2010. Mental health kills the mentally ill. Huffington Post. http://www.huffingtonpost.com/dj-jaffe/mental-health-kills-the-m_b_426672.html.

–. 2011. Book review: *Anatomy of an Epidemic* by Robert Whitaker. Huffington Post. http://www.huffingtonpost.com/dj-jaffe/book-review-anatomy-of-an_b_1071163.html.

–. 2012. Department of justice finds new program reduces violence by mentally ill. http://wroww.huffingtonpost.com/dj-jaffe/department-of-justice-fin_b_1380308.html.

Jamieson, M., et al. 2006. Developing empathy as a foundation of client-centred practice: Evaluation of a university curriculum initiative. *Canadian Journal of Occupational Therapy* 73: 76-85.

Janicak, P., et al. 2006. *Principles and Practice of Pharmacology.* 4th ed. Philadelphia: Lippincott, Williams and Wilkins.

Jarvis, G. 2007. The social causes of psychosis in North American psychiatry: A review of a disappearing literature. *Canadian Journal of Psychiatry* 52: 287-94.

Jenkins, J. 2010. More homeless off streets, counselors say. *Toronto Sun.* http://www.torontosun.com/news/torontoandgta/2010/05/11/13911721.html.

Jeste, D., O. Wolkowitz, and B. Palmer. 2011. Divergent trajectories of physical, cognitive and psychosocial aging in schizophrenia. *Schizophrenia Bulletin* 37: 451-55.

Jick, H., J. Kaye, and S. Jick. 2004. Antidepressants and the risk of suicidal behaviors. *Journal of the American Medical Association* 292: 338-43.

Joa, I., et al. 2008. The key to reducing duration of untreated psychosis: Information campaigns. *Schizophrenia Bulletin* 34: 466-72.

Jobe, T., and M. Harrow. 2005. Long-term outcome of patients with schizophrenia: A review. *Canadian Journal of Psychiatry* 50: 892-900.

John Howard Society of Alberta. 2002. Sex offender treatment programs. http://www.johnhoward.ab.ca/pub/respaper/treatm02.pdf.

Johnson, C. 1997. Recovery through employment. *Visions: BC's Mental Health Journal* 2: 8.

Johnson, G. 2006. Some say hope is the best antidepressant. *Georgia Straight*, 27 July, 34.

–. 2010. Thinking beyond prostates and penises. *Georgia Straight*, 13 May, 42.

–. 2011. Borderline disorder triggers turmoil and rage. *Georgia Straight*, 17 February, 38-39.

Jones, C. 2005. Supporting the families of the mentally ill. *Canadian Public Policy* 31, supplement: S41-S45.

Jones, D., et al. 2004. Prevalence, severity, and co-occurrence of chronic physical health problems of persons with serious mental illness. *Psychiatric Services* 55: 1250-57.

Jones, P., et al. 2006. Randomized controlled trial of the effect on quality of life of second vs. first-generation drugs in schizophrenia. *Archives of General Psychiatry* 63: 1079-87.

Judge, A., et al. 2008. Recognizing and responding to early psychosis: A qualitative analysis of individual narratives. *Psychiatric Services* 59: 96-99.

Jung, J. 2012. Cheaper drugs on the horizon. *Vancouver Sun*, 31 October.

Junghan, U., et al. 2007. Staff and patient perspectives on unmet need and therapeutic alliance in community mental health services. *British Journal of Psychiatry* 191: 543-47.

Kam, M., and K. Ng. 2009. CBT: Does it work well with the Chinese population in Vancouver? *Visions Journal* 6: 23-24.

Kane, J., and D. Mayerhoff. 1989. Do negative symptoms respond to pharmacological treatment? *British Journal of Psychiatry*, 155 (suppl. 7): 115-18.

Kane, R., J. Ouslander, and I. Abrass. 2004. *Essentials of Clinical Geriatrics.* New York: McGraw Hill.

Kane, J., et al. 2011. A double-blind, randomized study comparing the efficacy and safety of sertindole and risperidone in patients with treatment-resistant schizophrenia. *Journal of Clinical Psychiatry* 72: 194-204

Kaplan, A. 2004. Youth Violence Prevention Conference Explores Risk Factors, Interventions. *Psychiatric Times.* http://www.psychiatrictimes.com/display/article/10168/58786.

Kates, N., et al. 2010. The evolution of collaborative mental health care in Canada: A shared vision for the future. *Canadian Journal of Psychiatry* 56: 1-9.

Kelland, K. 2011. Nearly 40 percent of Europeans suffer mental illness. Reuters. http://www.reuters.com/article/2011/09/04/us-europe-mental-illness-idUSTRE7832JJ20110904.

Kelly, M., et al. 2002. Treatment delays for involuntary psychiatric patients associated with reviews of treatment capacity. *Canadian Journal of Psychiatry* 47: 181-85.

Kendall, P. 2010. *Investing in Prevention: Improving Health and Creating Sustainability.* Office of the Provincial Health Officer. http://www.health.gov.bc.ca/library/publications/year/2010/Investing_in_prevention_improving_health_and_creating_sustainability.pdf.

Kendlar, K. 2004. Editorial. Schizophrenia genetics and dysbindin: A corner turned? *American Journal of Psychiatry* 161: 1533-36.

Kennedy, M. 2004. Mental health system in a shambles, Senate says. *Vancouver Sun*, 20 November.

Keough, M., K. Timpano, and N. Schmidt. 2009. Ataques de nervios: Culturally bound and distinct from panic attacks? *Depression and Anxiety* 26: 16-21.

Kershaw M., and L. Webber. 2008. Assessment of financial competence. *Psychiatry, Psychology and the Law* 15: 40-55.

Kessler, R., et al. 2001. The prevalence and correlates of untreated serious mental illness. *Health Services Research* 36: 987-1007.

–. 2007. Prevalence, comorbidity, and service utilization for mood disorders in the US at the beginning of the 21st Century. *Annual Review of Clinical Psychology* 3: 137-58.

Keyes, C. 2002. The mental health continuum: From languishing to flourishing in life. *Journal of Health and Social Research* 43: 207-22.

–. 2005. Mental illness and/or mental health? Investigating axioms of the complete state model of health. *Journal of Consulting and Clinical Psychology* 73: 539-48.

–. 2007. Promoting and protecting mental health as flourishing: A complementary strategy for improving national mental health. *American Psychologist* 62: 95-108.

–. 2009. Keynote plenary address. Invited presentation at International Conference on Moving Mental Health and Wellness Promotion into the Mainstream, Toronto, 4-6 March.

Khashan, A., et al. 2008. Higher risk of offspring schizophrenia following antenatal maternal exposure to severe adverse life events. *Archives of General Psychiatry* 65: 146-152

Kiehn, B., and M. Swale. 1995. An overview of dialectical behavior therapy in the treatment of borderline personality disorder. MentalHelp.net. www.mentalhelp.net/poc/view_doc. php?type=doc&id=1020.

Kieseppa, T., et al. 2004. High concordance of bipolar I disorder in a nationwide sample of twins. *American Journal of Psychiatry* 161: 1814-21.

Kiesler, D. 1999. *Beyond the Disease Model of Mental Disorders.* Westport, CT: Praeger.

Killeen, M., and B. O'Day. 2004. Challenging expectations: How individuals with psychiatric disabilities find and keep work. *Psychiatric Rehabilitation Journal* 28: 157-63.

King, S., A. St. Hilaire, and D. Heidkamp. 2010. Prenatal factors in schizophrenia. *Current Directions in Psychological Science* 19: 209-13.

Kingdon, D. 1998. Cognitive-behavioural therapy of psychosis: Complexities in engagement and therapy, in *Treating Complex Cases: The Cognitive Behavioural Therapy Approach,* ed. N. Tarrier, A., Wells, and G. Haddock, 176-94. Chichester, UK: John Wiley and Sons.

Kingdon, D., and D. Turkington. 2005. *Cognitive-Behavioral Therapy of Schizophrenia.* New York: Guilford Press.

Kirk, S., and H. Hutchins. 1992. *The Selling of the DSM: The Rhetoric of Science in Psychiatry.* New York: Aldine de Gruyter.

Kirkbride, J., and P. Jones. 2011. The prevention of schizophrenia: What can we learn from eco-epidemiology? *Schizophrenia Bulletin* 37: 262-71.

Kirkey, S. 2004. "Socks sign" signals problem. *Vancouver Sun,* 11 June.

–. 2010. Non-conformity, creativity, quirkiness? There's a pill for that. *Vancouver Sun,* 30 April.

–. 2011. New ADHD rules could see kids as young as four on drugs. *Vancouver Sun.* http:// www.vancouversun.com/health/ADHD+rules+could+kids+young+four+drugs/5557398/ story.html.

–. 2013. Deaths reported in children prescribed newer generation antipsychotics. *Postmedia news.* http://www.ottawacitizen.com/health/family-child/Deaths+reported+children+ prescribed+newer+generation/8373683/story.html.

Kirmayer, L., L. Boothroyd, and S. Hodgins. 1998. Attempted suicide among Inuit youth: Psychosocial correlates and implications for prevention. *Canadian Journal of Psychiatry* 43: 816-22.

Kirmayer, L., G. Brass, and C. Tait. 2000. *The Mental Health of Aboriginal Peoples: Transformation of Identity and Community.* Report No. 10, Culture and Mental health research Unit, Division of Social and Transcultural Psychiatry, McGill University.

Kirmayer, L., G. Brass, and G. Valaskakis. 2009. Conclusion: Healing/intervention/tradition. In *Healing Traditions: The Mental Health of Aboriginal Peoples in Canada,* ed. L. Kirmayer and G. Valaskakis, 440-72. Vancouver: UBC Press.

Kirmayer, L., C. Fletcher, and R. Watt. 2009. Locating the ecocentric self: Inuit concepts of mental health and illness. In *Healing Traditions: The Mental Health of Aboriginal Peoples in Canada*, ed. L. Kirmayer and G. Valaskakis, 289-314. Vancouver: UBC Press.

Kirmayer, L., C. Tait, and C. Simpson. 2009. The mental health of Aboriginal peoples in Canada: Transformations of identity and community. In *Healing Traditions: The Mental Health of Aboriginal Peoples in Canada*, ed. L. Kirmayer and G. Valaskakis, 3-35. Vancouver: UBC Press.

Kirmayer, L., and G. Valaskakis, eds. 2009. *Healing Traditions: The Mental Health of Aboriginal Peoples in Canada*. Vancouver: UBC Press.

Kirmayer, L., et al. 2003. Cultural consultation: A model of mental health service for multicultural societies. *Canadian Journal of Psychiatry* 48: 145-52.

–. 2007. Use of health care services for psychological distress by immigrants in an urban multicultural milieu. *Canadian Journal of Psychiatry* 52: 295-304.

–. 2011. Common mental health problems in immigrants and refugees: General approach in primary care. *Canadian Medical Association Journal*. http://www.cmaj.ca/cgi/content/abstract/cmaj.090292v1.

Kirsh, B., and L. Cockburn. 2009. The Canadian Occupational Performance Measure: A tool for recovery based practice. *Psychiatric Rehabilitation Journal* 32: 171-76.

Kirsh, B., R. Gewurtz, and R. Bakewell. 2011. Critical characteristics of supported housing: Resident and service provider perspectives. *Canadian Journal of Community Mental Health* 30: 15-30.

Kirsh, B., et al. 2009. From margins to mainstream: What do we know about work integration for persons with brain injury, mental illness and intellectual disability? *Work* 32: 391-405.

Kirsch, I. 2002. The emperor's new drugs: An analysis of antidepressant medication data submitted to the FDA. *Prevention and Treatment* 5, 23: 1-11.

Kirsch, I., et al. 2008. Initial severity and antidepressant benefits: A meta-analysis of data submitted to the Food and Drug Administration. *PLoS Medicine* (a peer-reviewed open-access journal). http://www.plosmedicine.org/article/info:doi/10.1371/journal.pmed.0050045.

Kisely, S. 2010. Excess mortality from chronic physical disease in psychiatric patients – the forgotten problem. *Canadian Journal of Psychiatry*, 55: 749-51.

Kisely, S., and L. Campbell. 2006. Community treatment orders for psychiatric patients: The emperor with no clothes. *Canadian Journal of Psychiatry*, 51: 683-85.

Kisely, S., et al. 2005. Mortality in individuals who have had psychiatric treatment. *British Journal of Psychiatry* 187: 552-58.

–. 2008a. Routine measurement of mental health service outcomes: Health of the Nation Outcome scales. *Psychiatric Bulletin* 32: 1-3.

–. 2008b. Excess cancer mortality in psychiatric patients. *Canadian Journal of Psychiatry* 53: 753-61.

–. 2009. An epidemiologic study of psychotropic medication and obesity-related chronic illnesses in older psychiatric patients. *Canadian Journal of Psychiatry* 54: 269-74.

Kleiner, K. 2011. Mind games. *U of T Magazine*, Autumn, 33-36.

Kleinman, A., and P. Benson. 2006. Anthropology in the clinic: The problem of cultural competency and how to fix it. *PLoS Medicine* (a peer-reviewed open-access journal). http://www.ncbi.nlm.nih.gov/pmc/articles/PMC1621088/.

Kluft, R., S. Bloom, and J. Kinzie. 2000. Treating traumatized patients and victims of violence. In "Psychiatric Aspects of Violence: Issues in Prevention and Treatment," ed. C. Bell. *New Directions for Mental Health Service* 86: 79-102.

Knapp, M., D. McDaid, and M. Parsonage. 2011. *Mental Health Promotion and Mental Illness Prevention: The Economic Case*. London, UK: Department of Health.

Knapp, M., et al. 1998. Home-based versus hospital-based care for serious mental illness: Controlled cost-effectiveness study over four years. *British Journal of Psychiatry* 172: 506-12.

Kondro, W., and B. Sibbald. 2004. Drug company experts advised staff to withhold data about SSRI use in children. *Canadian Medical Association Journal* 170: 783.

Kopelowicz, A., and R. Liberman. 2003. Implementing treatment with rehabilitation for persons with major mental illnesses. *Psychiatric Services* 54: 1491-98.

Kopelowicz, A., R. Liberman, and R. Zarate. 2006. Recent advances in social skills training for schizophrenia. *Schizophrenia Bulletin* 32: S12-S23.

Kravitz, R., N. Duan, and J. Braslow. 2004. Evidence-based medicine, heterogeneity of treatment effects, and the trouble with averages. *Millbank Quarterly* 82: 661-87.

Kruger, A. 2000. Schizophrenia: Recovery and hope. *Psychiatric Rehabilitation Journal* 24: 29-37.

Krupa, T. 2008. Part of the solution ... or part of the problem? Addressing the stigma of mental illness in our midst. *Canadian Journal of Occupational Therapy* 75: 198-207.

Krupa, T., and C. Clark. 2004. Occupational therapy in the field of mental health: Promoting occupational perspectives on health and well-being. *Canadian Journal of Occupational Therapy* 71: 69-71.

Krupa, T., et al. 2005. How do people who receive ACT experience this service? *Psychiatric Rehabilitation Journal* 29: 18-24.

–. 2009. Doing daily life: How occupational therapy can inform psychiatric rehabilitation practice. *Psychiatric Rehabilitation Journal* 32: 155-61.

Kulig, J., and A. Williams. 2012. *Health in Rural Canada*. Vancouver: UBC Press.

Kushner, H., and C. Sterk. 2005. The limits of social capital: Durkheim, suicide and social cohesion. *American Journal of Public Health* 95: 1-5.

Kuyken, W., T. Dalgleish, and E. Holden. 2007. Advances in cognitive-behavioural therapy for unipolar depression. *Canadian Journal of Psychiatry* 52: 5-12.

Lacasse, J., and J. Leo. 2005. Serotonin and depression: A disconnect between the advertisements and the scientific literature. National Center for Biothechnology Information. http://www.ncbi.nlm.nih.gov/pmc/articles/PMC1277931/.

Lacey, M. 2011. Suspect in shooting of Giffords ruled unfit for trial. *New York Times*. http://www.nytimes.com/2011/05/26/us/26loughner.html?_r=1.

Lafave, H., H. deSouza, and G. Gerber. 1996. Assertive community treatment of severe mental illness: A Canadian experience. *Psychiatric Services* 47: 757-59.

Laird, G. 2004. The politics of homelessness. *Georgia Straight*, 5-12 February, 19-21.

Lam D., et al. 2003. A randomized controlled study of cognitive therapy for relapse prevention for bipolar affective disorder: Outcome of the first year. *Archives of General Psychiatry* 60: 145–52.

Lam, R., et al. 2008. RTMS for treatment resistant depression: A systematic review and meta-analysis. *Canadian Journal of Psychiatry* 53: 621-31.

Lambert, M., and D. Barley. 2001. Research summary on the therapeutic relationship and psychotherapy outcome. *Psychotherapy: Theory, Research, Practice, Training* 38: 357-61.

Lambert, M., et al. 1996. The reliability and validity of the Outcome Questionnaire. *Clinical Psychology and Psychotherapy* 3: 249-58.

Lancet. 2004. Editorial: Is GSK guilty of fraud? *Lancet* 363: 1919.

–. 2012. Psychiatry's identity crisis. *Lancet* 379: 1274.

Langley, J., et al. 2009. Suicidality in seriously mentally ill clients of two intensive community mental health programs. *Canadian Journal of Community Mental Health* 28: 151-64.

Larimer, M., et al. 2009. Health care and public service use and costs before and after provision of housing for chronically homeless persons with severe alcohol problems. *Journal of the American Medical Association* 301: 1349-57.

Latimer, E. 1999. Economic impacts of assertive community treatment: A review of the literature. *Canadian Journal of Psychiatry* 44: 443-54.

–. 2005. Community-based care for people with severe mental illness in Canada. *International Journal of Law and Psychiatry* 28: 561-73.

Lau, M., and M. Monro. 2008. Promoting mentally health communities in the workplace. http://secure.cihi.ca/cihiweb/products/mentally_healthy_communities_en.pdf.

Lauber, C., et al. 2004. Factors influencing social distance toward people with mental illness. *Community Mental Health Journal* 40: 265-74.

LaVeque, P. 2012. Johnson & Johnson fined 1.2 billion in Arkansas Risperdal case. 24 Medica. http://www.24medica.com/content/view/2717/2/.

Lavoie, K., and R. Fleet. 2002. Should psychologists be granted prescription privileges? A review of the prescription privilege debate for psychiatrists. *Canadian Journal of Psychiatry* 47: 443-49.

Lawrence, D., S. Kisely, and J. Pais. 2010. The epidemiology of excess mortality in people with mental illness. *Canadian Journal of Psychiatry* 55: 752-60.

Lawrie, S., et al. 2008. Brain structure and function changes during the development of schizophrenia. *Schizophrenia Bulletin* 34: 330-40.

Lawton-Smith, S. 2008. Community treatment orders are not a good thing. *British Journal of Psychiatry.* http://bjp.rcpsych.org/cgi/content/full/193/2/96#REF29.

Layard, R., et al. 2007. Cost-benefit analysis of psychological therapy. *National Institute Economic Review* 201: 90-98.

Lechky, O. 1999. Bringing health care to the homeless. *Canadian Medical Association Journal* 161: 13.

Lecomte, T., and C. Lecomte. 2002. Toward uncovering robust principles of change inherent to cognitive-behavioral therapy for psychosis. *American Journal of Orthopsychiatry* 72: 50-57.

Lederbogen, F., et al. 2011. City living and urban upbringing affect neural social stress processing in humans. *Nature* 474: 498-501.

Lee, J. 2011. Number of homeless living on Metro Vancouver streets dropping. *Vancouver Sun.* http://www.vancouversun.com/news/Number+homeless+living+Metro+Vancouver+streets+dropping/4832515/story.html.

Leenars, A. 2000. Suicide prevention in Canada: A history of a community approach. *Canadian Journal of Community Mental Health* 19: 57-71.

Lefley, H. 1997. Mandatory treatment from the family's perspective. *New Directions in Mental Health Services* 75: 7-15.

Lemstra, M. 2009. Suicidal ideation: The role of economic and Aboriginal cultural status after multivariate adjustment. *Canadian Journal of Psychiatry* 54: 589-95.

Lesage, A. 2010. Contribution of psychiatric epidemiology to the study of the adult severely mentally ill. In *Mental Disorder in Canada: An Epidemiological Perspective,* ed. J. Cairney and D. Streiner, 145-69. Toronto: University of Toronto Press.

Lesage, A., and R. Morissette. 2002. Editorial: Chronic my ass. *Canadian Journal of Psychiatry* 47: 617-20.

Lesage, A., et al. 2003. Toward benchmarks for tertiary care for adults with severe and persistent mental disorders. *Canadian Journal of Psychiatry* 48: 485-92.

Lester, H., et al. 2011. Views of young people in early intervention services for first-episode psychosis in England. *Psychiatric Services* 62: 882-87.

Leucht, S. 2006. Translating research into clinical practice: Critical interpretation of clinical trials in schizophrenia. *International Clinical Psychopharmacology* 21 (suppl. 2): S1-S10.

Leucht, S., et al. 2003. Relapse prevention in schizophrenia with new-generation antipsychotics: A systematic review and exploratory meta-analysis of randomized, controlled trials. *American Journal of Psychiatry* 160: 1209-22.

Lev, A. 1998. Feminism and mental illness. http://www.choicesconsulting.com/aboutarlene/articles/feminism.html.

Levinson, W., et al. 2005. Not all patients want to participate in decision making: A national study of public preferences. *Journal of General Internal Medicine* 20: 531-35.

Li, H., and A. Browne. 2000. Defining mental illness and accessing mental health services: Perspectives of Asian Canadians. *Canadian Journal of Community Mental Health* 19: 143-57.

Liberman, R. 1998. International perspectives on skills training for the mentally disabled. *International Review of Psychiatry* 10: 5-8.

Liberman, R., and A. Kopelowicz. 2005. Recovery from schizophrenia: A concept in search of research. *Psychiatric Services* 56: 735-42.

Lieberman, J. 2011. Psychiatric diagnosis in the lab: How far off are we? Medscape. http://www.medscape.com/viewarticle/750288.

Lieberman, J., et al. 2008. Science and recovery in schizophrenia. *Psychiatric Services* 59: 487-96.

Lim, K., P. Jacobs, and C. Dewa, 2008. How much should we spend on mental health? Institute of Health Economics, Alberta. http://www.ihe.ca/documents/Spending%20on%20Mental%20Health%20Final.pdf.

Linehan, M. 1993a. *Cognitive-Behavioral Treatment of Borderline Personality Disorder*. New York: Guildford Press.

–. 1993b. *Skills Training Manual for Treating Borderline Personality Disorder*. New York: Guildford Press.

Linehan, M., et al. 1991. Cognitive-behavioral treatment of chronically parasuicidal borderline patients. *Archives of General Psychiatry* 48: 1060-64.

–. 2006. Two-year randomized controlled trial and follow-up of dialectical behavior therapy vs. therapy by experts for suicidal behaviors and borderline personality disorder. *Archives of General Psychiatry*. 63: 757-66.

Lines, E. 2000. An introduction to early psychosis intervention: Some relevant findings and emerging practices. Canadian Mental Health Association. http://www.cmha.ca.

Link, B., et al. 1999. Public conceptions of mental illness: Labels, causes, dangerousness and social distance. *American Journal of Public Health* 89: 1328-33.

–. 2011. Arrest outcomes associated with outpatient commitment in New York State. *Psychiatric Services* 62: 504-8.

Ling, P. 2010. People with mental health issues tasered more by police: Report. *Vancouver Sun*. http://www.vancouversun.com/health/People+with+mental+health+issues+tasered+more+police+Report/3197380/story.html.

Livesley, W. 1998. Suggestions for a framework for an empirically based classification of personality disorder. *Canadian Journal of Psychiatry* 43: 137-47.

Livingston, J., and J. Boyd. 2010. Correlates and consequences of internalized stigma for people living with mental illness: A systematic review and meta-analysis. *Social Science and Medicine* 71: 2150-61.

Livingston, J., T. Nicholls, and J. Brink. 2011. The impact of realigning a tertiary psychiatric hospital in British Columbia on other institutional sectors. *Psychiatric Services* 62: 200-5.

Livingston, J., et al. 2009. Cognitive-behavioural therapy for adults with mental health problems: Working to improve access in BC. *Visions Journal* 6: 25-26.

Lo, H., and K. Fung. 2003. Culturally competent psychotherapy. *Canadian Journal of Psychiatry* 48: 161-70.

Lorentz, W., J. Scanlan, and S. Borson. 2002. Brief screening tests for dementia. *Canadian Journal of Psychiatry* 47: 723-33.

Lott, D. 2001. New developments in treating anxiety disorders. *Psychiatric Times*. http://www.psychiatrictimes.com/p010946.html.

Lovell, A. 1992. Classification and its risks: How psychiatric status contributes to homelessness policy. *New England Journal of Public Policy* 8: 247-63.

Lowry, F. 2011. Schizophrenia gene mutation discovered. http://www.medscape.com/viewarticle/736798.

Loy, I. 2006. James slams housing gap. *24 Hours*, 2 October.

–. 2008. In your backyard? Streams of Justice, Vancouver. http://www.streamsofjustice.org/2008/07/in-your-backyard.html.

Loukidelis, D., and A. Cavoukian. 2008. Emergency disclosure of personal information by universities, colleges and other educational institutions. Office of the Information and Privacy Commissioner. http://www.oipc.bc.ca/pdfs/Policy/ipc-bc-disclosure-edu.pdf.

Lu, W., et al. 2008. Correlates of adverse child experiences among adults with severe mood disorders. *Psychiatric Services* 59: 1018-26.

Luo, Z., et al. 2010. Birth outcomes in the Inuit-inhabited areas of Canada. *Canadian Medical Association Journal* 182: 235-42.

Lurie, S., B. Kirsh, and S. Hodge. 2007. Can ACT lead to more work? The Ontario experience. *Canadian Journal of Community Mental Health* 26: 161-71.

Lynch, T., et al. 2007. Dialectical behavior therapy for borderline personality disorder. *Annual Review of Clinical Psychology* 3: 181-205.

Lynch, D., K. Laws, and P. McKenna. 2010. Cognitive behavioural therapy for major psychiatric disorders: Does it really work? *Psychological Medicine* 40: 9-24.

Lysaker, P., D. Roe, and P. Yanos. 2007. Toward understanding the insight paradox: Internalized stigma moderates the association between insight and social functioning, hope and self-esteem among people with schizophrenia spectrum disorders. *Schizophrenia Bulletin* 33: 192-99.

MacCourt, P., K. Wilson, and M. Tourgny-Rivard. 2011. *Guidelines for Comprehensive Services for Older Adults.* Ottawa: Mental Health Commission of Canada.

MacDonald, Z. 2002. Virtually facing real fears. *Visions: BC's Mental Health Journal* 14: 20.

MacNaughton, E. 2000. Cultural competence and the "knowledge resource base." *Visions: BC's Mental Health Journal* 9: 14-15.

MacPhee, K. 2002. No safe refuge: Barriers to accessing transition houses and women's shelters from a hospital emergency department. Master's graduating essay, School of Social Work and Family Studies, University of British Columbia.

MacPherson, D., and B. Gushulak. 2010. Migrants and epidemiology of psychiatric disorders in Canada. In *Mental Disorder in Canada: An Epidemiological Perspective*, ed. J. Cairney and D. Streiner, 286-303. Toronto: University of Toronto Press.

Maggie, S., et al. 2010. Rural-urban migration patterns and mental health diagnoses of adolescents and young adults in British Columbia, Canada: A case-control study. *Child and Adolescent Psychiatry and Mental Health* 4: 1-11.

Magliano, L., et al. 2008. Views of persons with schizophrenia on their own disorder: An Italian participatory study. *Psychiatric Services* 59: 795-99.

Maguire, L. 2002. *Clinical Social Work: Beyond Generalist Practice with Individuals, Groups and Families.* Pacific Grove, CA: Brooks/Cole.

Malla, A., and A. Pelosi. 2010. Is treating patients with first-episode psychosis cost-effective? *Canadian Journal of Psychiatry* 55: 3-8.

Mamo, D. 2007. Managing suicidality in schizophrenia. *Canadian Journal of Psychiatry* 52 (suppl. 1): 59s-70s.

Mandel, C., and K. Meaney. 2007. Man's jail death prompts review of tasers in NS. *Vancouver Sun*, 23 November.

Margolese, H., et al. 2005. Tardive dyskinesia in the era of typical and atypical antipsychotics. *Canadian Journal of Psychiatry* 50: 703-14.

Marie-Albert, J. 2002. The psychiatrist and the clinical practice of psychiatry in an uncertain environment: Looking ahead. *Canadian Journal of Psychiatry* 47: 913-20.

Marsh, D., and D. Johnson. 1997. The family experience of mental illness: Implications for intervention. *Professional Psychology* 28: 229-37.

Marshall, M. 2003. Acute psychiatric day hospitals. *British Medical Journal* 327: 116-17.

Marshall, M., and J. Rathbone. 2011. Early intervention for psychosis. *Schizophrenia Bulletin* 37: 1111-14.

Marshall, T., et al. 2008. Key factors for implementing supported employment. *Psychiatric Services* 59: 886-92.

Mathew, B., et al. 2007. Psychosocial outcomes following ECT in a community setting: Retrospective chart review with 2-year follow-up. *Canadian Journal of Psychiatry* 52: 598-604.

Matsui, D., et al. 2003. The trials and tribulations of doing drug research in children. *Canadian Medical Association Journal* 169: 1033-34.

Mauri, M., et al. 2008. Depression in schizophrenia: Comparison of first and second-generation antipsychotic drugs. *Schizophrenia Research* 99: 7-12.

Maxwell, V. 2012. Families falling apart: When adult children with mental illness don't want help. *Psychology Today*. http://www.psychologytoday.com/blog/crazy-life/201202/families-falling-apart-when-adult-children-mental-illness-dont-want-help.

McAlister, F. 2008. The "number needed to treat" turns 20 – and continues to be used and misused. *Canadian Medical Association Journal*. http://www.cmaj.ca/content/179/6/549.full.

McAndrew, B. 1999. Innu suicide rate highest in the world: British report blames Ottawa, Catholic Priests. *Toronto Star*, 8 November.

McCabe, L., D. Butterill, and P. Goering. 2004. Residential crisis units: Are we missing out on a good idea? *Canadian Journal of Community Mental Health* 23: 65-74.

McCabe, R., and S. Priebe. 2004. Explanatory models of illness in schizophrenia: Comparison of four ethnic groups. *British Journal of Psychiatry* 185: 25-30.

McCaldon, R., G. Conacher, and B. Clark. 1991. The right to remain psychotic. *Canadian Medical Association Journal* 145: 777-80.

McCann, E. 2010. Investigating mental health service user views regarding sexual and relationship issues. *Journal of Psychiatric and Mental Health Nursing* 17: 251-59.

McCann, T., D. Lubman, and E. Clark. 2011. First-time primary caregivers' experience of caring for young adults with first-episode psychosis. *Schizophrenia Bulletin* 37: 381-88.

McClellan, J., and J. Werry. 2003. Evidence-based treatments in child and adolescent psychiatry: An inventory. *Journal of the American Academy of Child and Adolescent Psychiatry*. 42: 1388-400.

McCormick, T. 1998. Principles of bioethics. http://depts.washington.edu/bioethx/tools/princpl.html.

McEwan, K., and E. Goldner. 2001. *Accountability and Performance Indicators for Mental Health Services and Supports: A Resource Kit*. Ottawa: Health Canada.

McCoy, M., et al. 2004. Jail linkage assertive community treatment services for individuals with mental illnesses. *Psychiatric Rehabilitation Journal* 27: 243-50.

McCrone, P., et al. 2009. The REACT study: Cost-effectiveness analysis of ACT in North London. *Psychiatric Services* 60: 908-13.

McDonell, M., et al. 2009. Global Appraisal of Individual Needs Short Screener (GSS): Psychometric properties and performance as a screening measure in adolescents. *American Journal of Drug and Alcohol Abuse* 35: 157-60.

McGrath, J. 2006. Variations in the incidence of schizophrenia: Data vs. dogma. *Schizophrenia Bulletin* 32: 195-97.

McGrew, J., R. Wilson, and G. Bond. 2002. An exploratory study of what clients like least about assertive community treatment. *Psychiatric Services* 53: 761-63.

McGrew, J., B. Pescosolido, and E. Wright. 2003. Case managers' perspectives on critical ingredients of assertive community treatment and on its implementation. *Psychiatric Services* 54: 370-76.

McGuffin, P., et al. 2003. The heritability of bipolar affective disorder and the genetic relationship to unipolar depression. *Archives of General Psychiatry* 60: 497-502.

McKnight, P. 2007. What if most medical research is mostly wrong? *Vancouver Sun*, 27 October.

McLaren, N. 2002. The myth of the biopsychosocial model. *Australian and New Zealand Journal of Psychiatry* 36: 701.

McMain, S., et al. 2009. A randomized trial of dialectical behavior therapy versus general psychiatric management for borderline personality disorder. *American Journal of Psychiatry*. 166: 1365-74.

McNiel, D., et al. 2008. Effects of training on suicide risk assessment. *Psychiatric Services* 59: 1462-65.

Mead, S., D. Hilton, and L. Curtis. 2001. Peer support: A theoretical perspective. *Psychiatric Rehabilitation Journal* 25: 134-41.

Medalia, A., N. Revheim, and T. Herlands. 2009. *Cognitive Remediation for Psychological Disorders.* New York: Oxford University Press.

Mee, J., T. Sumison, and C. Craik. 2004. Mental health clients confirm the value of occupation in building competence and self-identity. *British Journal of Occupational Therapy* 67: 225-33.

Meehan, T., et al. 2008. Recovery-based practice: Do we know what we mean or mean what we know? *Australian and New Zealand Journal of Psychiatry* 42: 177-82.

Mehta, D. 2013. Taser 'key factor' in mentally ill man's death, top pathologist tells inquest. *Vancouver Sun.* http://www.vancouversun.com/news/national/Inquest+into+mentally+mans+death+returns+spotlight+police/8488292/story.html.

Menear, M., et al. 2011. Organizational analysis of Canadian supported employment programs for people with psychiatric disabilities. *Social Science and Medicine* 72: 1028-35.

Mental Health America of Los Angeles. 2005. Milestones of recovery scale (MORS): Executive summary. http://www.mhala.org/MORS-Executive-Summary-11-09.pdf.

Mental Health Center of Greater Manchester. 1998. Integrating dialectical behaviour therapy into a community mental health program. *Psychiatric Services* 49: 1338-40.

Mental Health Commission of Canada 2009. *Toward Recovery and Well-Being: A Framework for a Mental Health Strategy for Canada.* http://www.mentalhealthcommission.ca/Site CollectionDocuments/boarddocs/15507_MHCC_EN_final.pdf.

–. 2011. *Mental Health Strategy for Canada* (Draft). http://thetyee.ca/Documents/2011/08/28/Drafmhcc-draft-June7-2011-FINAL.pdf.

–. 2012. *Changing Directions, Changing Lives: The Mental Health Strategy for Canada.* http://strategy.mentalhealthcommission.ca/pdf/strategy-images-en.pdf.

Mental Health Evaluation and Community Consultation Unit. 2000. *Emergency Mental Health: Education Manual.* Vancouver: Department of Psychiatry, University of British Columbia.

–. 2002. *Early Psychosis: A Care Guide Summary.* Vancouver: Department of Psychiatry, University of British Columbia.

Menzies, R. 1989. *Survival of the Sanest: Order and Disorder in a Pre-Trial Psychiatric Clinic.* Toronto: University of Toronto Press.

Meredith, L., et al. 2007. Factors associated with primary care clinicians' choice of a watchful waiting approach to managing depression. *Psychiatric Services* 58: 72-78.

Merskey, H., and A. Piper. 2007. Posttraumatic stress disorder is overloaded. *Canadian Journal of Psychiatry* 52: 499-500.

Metherell, M. 2011. Changing the mental health blame game. Sarasota Memorial Health Care System. http://www.smh.com.au/national/changing-the-mental-health-blame-game 20111011-1lj1z.html.

Michel, K., et al. 2002. Discovering the truth in attempted suicide. *American Journal of Psychotherapy* 56: 424-37.

Mickelburgh, R. 2011. Patient-based funding breathes new life into hospitals. *Globe and Mail.* http://www.theglobeandmail.com/life/health/patient-based-funding-breathes-new-life -into-hospitals/article2266746/singlepage/.

Miller, A., J. Rathus, and M. Linehan. 2007. *Dialectical Behavior Therapy with Suicidal Adolescents.* New York: Guilford Press.

Miller, B., C. Paschall, and D. Svendsen. 2006. Mortality and medical comorbidity among patients with serious mental illness. *Psychiatric Services* 57: 1482-87.

Miller, W., and S. Rollnick. 2002. *Motivational Interviewing: Preparing People for Change,* 2nd ed. New York: Guilford Press.

–. 2009. Ten things that motivational interviewing is not. *Behavioural and Cognitive Psychotherapy* 37: 129-40.

Miller, W., and G. Rose. 2009. Toward a theory of motivational interviewing. *American Psychologist* 64: 527-37.

Minkoff, K. 2001. Developing standards of care for individuals with co-occurring psychiatric and substance use disorders. *Psychiatric Services* 52: 597-600.

Minsky, A. 2011. Canada to receive new standards to protect workers' mental health. Canada. com (*Postmedia News*). http://www.canada.com/health/Canada+receive+standards+ protect+workers+mental+health/4959926/story.html.

Mintzes, B., et al. 2001. *An Assessment of the Health System Impacts of Direct-To-Consumer Advertising of Prescription Medicines*. Vancouver: Centre for Health Services and Policy Research.

–. 2002. Influence of DTC pharmaceutical advertising and patients' requests on prescribing decisions: Two-site cross-sectional survey. *British Medical Journal* 324: 278-79.

Mitchell, A., and S. Malladi. 2010. Screening and case finding tools for the detection of dementia. Part 1: Evidence-based meta-analysis of multidomain tests. *American Journal of Geriatric Psychiatry* 18: 759-82.

Mitchell, A., et al. 2013. Prevalence of metabolic syndrome and metabolic abnormalities in schizophrenia and related disorders: A systematic review and meta-analysis. *Schizophrenia Bulletin* 39: 306-18.

Mitchell, B., et al. 2008. Trends in psychostimulant and antidepressant use by children in two Canadian provinces. *Canadian Journal of Psychiatry* 53: 152-59.

Mittal, V., W. Brown, and E. Shorter. 2009. Are patients with depression at heightened risk of suicide as they begin to recover? *Psychiatric Services* 60: 384-86.

Mojtabai, R. 2007. Americans' attitudes toward mental health treatment-seeking: 1990-2003. *Psychiatric Services* 58: 642-51.

–. 2009. Americans' attitudes toward psychiatric medications: 1998-2006. *Psychiatric Services* 60: 1015-23.

Mojtabai, R., and R. Olfson. 2006. Treatment seeking for depression in Canada and the United States. *Psychiatric Services* 57: 631-39.

Mok, K. 2006. Cross-cultural treatment issues in patients with mood and anxiety disorders. Paper presented at the Clinical Neurosciences Conference, Vancouver, BC, 24 February.

Molloy, D., T. Standish, and D. Lewis. 2005. Screening for mild cognitive impairment: Comparing the SMMSE and the ABCS. *Canadian Journal of Psychiatry* 50: 52-58.

Molnar, F. 2004. Recovery is in the eye of the beholder. *The Bulletin: Official Publication of the Vancouver/Richmond Mental Health Network Society* 9: 7.

Monahan, J. 2003. Violence risk assessment. *Handbook of Psychology*. 2nd ed. http://online library.wiley.com/doi/10.1002/9781118133880.hop211022/full.

Monahan, J., et al. 1996. Coercion to inpatient treatment: Initial results and implications for assertive community treatment in the community. In *Coercion and Aggressive Community Treatment*, ed. D. Dennis and J. Monahan, 13-28. New York: Plenum Press.

Moncrieff, J. 2009. The pharmaceutical industry and the construction of psychiatric diagnoses. *Journal of Ethics in Mental Health* 4 (suppl.): 1-4.

Monette, M. 2012. Rural life hardly healthier. *Canadian Medical Association Journal* 184: E889-90.

Mood Disorders Society of Canada. 2011a. House of Commons Standing Committee on Finance Pre-Budget Submission. http://www.mooddisorderscanada.ca/documents/ Advocacy/MDSC%20Finance%20Committee%20Pre-budget%20Consultation%20 Brief%202011.pdf.

–. 2011b. Pan-Canadian Opinion Survey. http://www.mooddisorderscanada.ca/documents/ Survey/Key%20Findings%20of%20MDSC%20Mental%20Health%20Survey_EN.pdf.

–. 2011c. MDSC & CMA completing work on web-based anti-stigma program. http://www. mooddisorderscanada.ca/documents/About%20Us/August_2011.pdf.

–. 2012. News release: Improving care for post-traumatic stress disorder. http://www. mooddisorderscanada.ca/documents/Advocacy/PTSD_Report_News_Release_EN.pdf.

Morrison, A., and S. Barratt. 2010. What are the components of CBT for psychosis? A Delphi study. *Schizophrenia Bulletin* 36: 136-42.

Morrison, A., et al. 2004. *Cognitive Therapy for Psychosis: A Formulation-Based Approach.* New York: Brunner-Routledge.

Morrison, J. 2006. *DSM-IV Made Easy: The Clinician's Guide to Diagnosis.* New York: The Guilford Press.

Morrison, L. 2005. *Talking Back to Psychiatry: The Psychiatric Consumer/Survivor/Ex-Patient Movement.* New York: Routledge.

Morrow, M., P. Dagg, and A. Pederson. 2008. Is deinstitutionalization a "failed experiment"? The ethics of re-institutionalization. *Journal of Ethics in Mental Health* 3: 1-7.

Motluck, A. 2001. Placebo produces surprise biological effect. *New Scientist.* http://www. newscientist.com/article/dn1137-placebo-produces-surprise-biological-effect.html#. UcThzaTn-ic.

Mottaghipour, Y., and A. Bickerton. 2005. The pyramid of family care: A framework for family involvement with adult mental health services. Australian Network for Promotion, Prevention, and Early Intervention for Mental Health. http://www.psychodyssey.net/wp-content/ uploads/2012/05/The-Pyramid-of-Family-Care.pdf.

Mourra, S. 2013. Lost in medication. *The Atlantic.* http://www.theatlantic.com/health/ archive/2013/05/lost-in-medication/275612/.

Moynihan, R., and A. Cassels. 2005. *Selling Sickness: How the World's Biggest Pharmaceutical Companies Are Turning Us All into Patients.* Vancouver: Greystone Books.

MPA Society. 2011. History. http://www.mpa-society.org/history.php.

Mueser, K. 2004. Clinical interventions for severe mental illness and co-occurring substance use disorder. *Acta Neuropsychiatrica* 16: 26-35.

–. 2006. Concurrent disorders: Issues of management. Paper presented at the Annual UBC Faculty of Medicine Clinical Neurosciences Conference, Vancouver, 24 February.

Mueser, K., et al. 1998. Models of community care for severe mental illness: A review of research on case management. *Schizophrenia Bulletin* 24: 37-74

–. 2002. Illness management and recovery: A review of the research. *Psychiatric Services* 53: 1272-84.

Mulvale, G., J. Abelson, and P. Goering. 2007. Mental health service delivery in Ontario, Canada: How do policy legacies shape prospects for reform? *Health Economics, Policy and Law* 2: 363-89.

Mulvey, E., A. Blumstein, and J. Cohen. 1986. Reframing the research question of mental patient criminality. *International Journal of Law and Psychiatry* 9: 57-65.

Mushquash, C., and D. Bova. 2007. Cross-cultural assessment and measurement issues. *Journal on Developmental Disabilities* 13: 53-65.

Mussell, B., K. Cardiff, and J. White. 2004. *The Mental Health and Well-Being of Aboriginal Children and Youth: Guidance for New Approaches and Services.* Report prepared for the British Columbia Ministry of Children and Family Development.

Myhr, G., and K. Payne. 2006. Cost-effectiveness of CBT for mental disorders: Implications for public health care funding policy in Canada. *Canadian Journal of Psychiatry* 51: 662-70.

Naar-King, S., and M. Suarez. 2011. *Motivational Interviewing with Adolescents and Young Adults.* New York: Guilford Press.

Naccarato, T., E. DeLorenzo, and A, Park. 2008. A rapid instrument review (RIR) of independent living program (ILP) evaluation tools. *Journal of Public Child Welfare* 2: 253-67.

Nakhai-Pour, H., P. Broy, and A. Berard. 2010. Use of antidepressants during pregnancy and the risk of spontaneous abortion. *Canadian Medical Association Journal* 182: 1031-37.

Narrow, W., et al. 2002. Revised prevalence rates of mental disorders in the United States. *Archives of General Psychiatry* 59: 115-23.

Nathan, P., J. Gordon, and N. Salkind. 1999. *Treating Mental Disorders: A Guide to What Works.* New York: Oxford University Press.

National Council of Welfare. 2011. Interactive welfare incomes map. http://www.ncw.gc.ca/h.4m.2%40-eng.jsp.

National Housing and Homelessness Network. 2001. *State of the Crisis, 2001: A Report on Housing and Homelessness in Canada*. Ottawa: National Housing and Homelessness Network.

Negrette, J. 2003. Clinical aspects of substance abuse in persons with schizophrenia. *Canadian Journal of Psychiatry* 48: 14-21.

Neilson, G. 2002. The 1996 Canadian Medical Association Code of Ethics annotated for psychiatrists. Ottawa: Canadian Psychiatric Association.

Nelson, G., G. Hall, and C. Forchuk. 2003. Current and preferred housing of psychiatric consumers/survivors. *Canadian Journal of Community Mental Health* 22: 5-19.

Nelson, G., et al. 2007. A review of the literature on the effectiveness of housing and support, assertive community treatment, and Intensive Case Management interventions for persons with mental illness who have been homeless. *American Journal of Orthopsychiatry* 77: 350-61.

New York State Office of Mental Health. 2005. Kendra's law: Final report on the status of assisted outpatient treatment. Office of Mental Health, New York. http://mentalillnesspolicy.org/kendras-law/research/kendras-law-study-2005.pdf.

Newbold, B. 2009. The short-term health of Canada's new immigrant arrivals: Evidence from LSIC. *Ethnicity and Health* 19: 315-36.

Newman, S., and D. Schopflocher. 2008. Trends in antidepressant prescriptions among the elderly in Alberta during 1997 to 2004. *Canadian Journal of Psychiatry* 53: 704-7.

Newton, J., and P. Yardley. 2007. Evaluation of CBT training of clinicians in routine clinical practice. *Psychiatric Services* 58: 1497.

Newton-Howes, G., and R. Mullen. 2011. Coercion in psychiatric care: Systematic review of correlates and themes. *Psychiatric Services* 62: 465-70.

Nielssen, O., et al. 2011. Homicide of strangers by people with a psychotic illness. *Schizophrenia Bulletin* 37: 572-79.

Nietzel, M., D. Bernstein, and R. Milich. 1998. *Introduction to Clinical Psychology*. 5th ed. Upper Saddle River: Prentice Hall.

Niezen, R. 2009. Suicide as a way of belonging: Causes and consequences of cluster suicides in Aboriginal communities. In *Healing Traditions: The Mental Health of Aboriginal Peoples in Canada*, ed. L. Kirmayer and G. Valaskakis, 178-95. Vancouver: UBC Press.

Norko, M., and M. Baranoski. 2005. The state of contemporary risk assessment research. *Canadian Journal of Psychiatry* 50: 18-26.

Norman, R., and L. Townsend. 1999. Cognitive-behavioral therapy for psychosis: A status report. *Canadian Journal of Psychiatry* 44: 245-52.

Norman, R., et al. 2008. Are personal values of importance in the stigmatization of people with mental illness? *Canadian Journal of Psychiatry* 53: 848-56.

North Shore Schizophrenia Society. 2009. Unprofessional faddism can end in tragedy. http://www.northshoreschizophrenia.org/images/2009%20May%20Advocacy%20Bulletin.pdf.

–. 2010. Family involvement means information sharing. http://www.northshoreschizophrenia.org/images/2010%20November%20Advocacy%20Bulletin.pdf.

–. 2011. Legislative and government. http://www.northshoreschizophrenia.org/legislative.htm.

– 2012. Cosmetic anti-stigma campaigns miss the point. http://www.northshoreschizophrenia.org/images/2012%20Feb%20Advocacy%20Bulletin.pdf.

Nurnberg, H., et al 2003. Treatment of antidepressant associated sexual dysfunction with sildenafil. *Journal of the American Medical Association* 289: 56-64.

Oakes, D. 2003. Drug companies help fund drive for forced outpatient treatment. Straight Goods News Online. http://www.straightgoods.com/item341.shtml.

O'Brian, A. 2004. Why wasn't I told my daughter was suicidal? *Vancouver Sun*, 9 July.

O'Connell, M., W. Kasprow, and R. Rosenheck. 2008. Rates and risk factors for homelessness after successful housing in a sample of formerly homeless veterans. *Psychiatric Services* 59: 268-75.

O'Connor, D. 2010. Understanding and assessing incapacity. *Perspectives*, September 4-9.

O'Connor, D., M. Hall, and M. Donnelly. 2009. Assessing capacity within a context of abuse or neglect. *Journal of Elder Abuse and Neglect* 21: 156-69.

O'Connor, K. 2009. Cognitive and meta-cognitive dimensions of psychosis. *Canadian Journal of Psychiatry* 54: 152-58.

O'Connor, N. 2003. Pharma care. *Vancouver Courier*, 3 September, 5-7.

Ogrodniczuk, J. 2011. Psychotherapies for borderline personality disorder. *Visions* 7: 21-23.

O'Hagan, M., et al. 2010. Making the case for peer support. Mental Health Commission of Canada. http://www.mentalhealthcommission.ca/SiteCollectionDocuments/Peer%20Support/Service%20Systems%20AC%20-%20Peer%20support%20report%20EN.pdf.

Ohayan, M., et al. 1998. Fitness, responsibility and judicially ordered assessments. *Canadian Journal of Psychiatry* 43: 491-95.

Olfson, M., and S. Marcus. 2009. National patterns in antidepressant medication treatment. *Archives of General Psychiatry* 66: 848-56.

Olfson, M., S. Marcus, and F. Ascher-Svanum. 2007. Treatment of schizophrenia with long-acting fluphenazine, haloperidol or risperidone. *Schizophrenia Bulletin* 33: 1379-87.

Olfson, M., et al. 2006a. National trends in the outpatient treatment of children and adolescents with antipsychotic drugs. *Archives of General Psychiatry* 63: 679-85.

–. 2006b. Awareness of illness and nonadherence to antipsychotic medications among persons with schizophrenia. *Psychiatric Services* 57: 205-11.

–. 2009. Dropout from outpatient mental health care in the US. *Psychiatric Services* 60: 898-907.

Olivier, C. 2010. Teach officers how to deal with the mentally ill: Jury. *Vancouver Province*, 19 December.

Olson, G. 2007. Addictions often fester after cultures collapse. *Vancouver Courier*, 16 November, 11.

Ontario Human Rights Commission. 2010. Annual Report. http://www.ohrc.on.ca/en/resources/annualreports/0910/pdf.

Ontario Ministry of Health and Long-Term Care. 2005. *Intensive Case Management Service Standards*. http://www.ontla.on.ca/library/repository/mon/10000/252444.pdf.

O'Reilly, R. 2008. The capacity to execute an advance directive for psychiatric treatment. *International Journal of Law and Psychiatry* 31: 66-71.

O'Reilly, R., et al. 2003. A survey of Canadian psychiatrists' experiences and opinions on using videoconferencing for assessments required by mental health legislation. *Canadian Psychiatric Association Bulletin* 35: 18-20.

–. 2006. A qualitative analysis of the use of community treatment orders in Saskatchewan. *International Journal of Law and Psychiatry* 29: 516-24.

Orford, J., et al. 2002. How is excessive drinking maintained? Untreated heavy drinkers experiences of the personal benefits and drawbacks of their drinking. *Addiction Research and Theory* 10: 347-72.

Owens, D. 1999. *A Guide to the Extrapyramidal Side-Effects of Antipsychotic Drugs*. Cambridge, UK: Cambridge University Press.

Oyebode, F. 2004. Invited commentary on the rediscovery of recovery. *Advances in Psychiatric Treatment* 10: 48-49.

Pablo, C. 2007. Nurse troubled by tasers. *Georgia Straight*, 22-28 November, 13.

–. 2008. Metro Vancouver homeless count hides many. *Georgia Straight*. http://www.straight.com/article-140217/homeless-count-hides-many.

–. 2010. Critics blast housing policy. *Georgia Straight*, 13-20 April, 17.

Page, S., and M. King. 2008. No suicide agreements: Current practices and opinions in a Canadian urban health region. *Canadian Journal of Psychiatry* 53: 169-76.

Palmer, B., S. Pankratz, and J. Bostwick. 2005. The lifetime risk of suicide in schizophrenia. *Archives of General Psychiatry* 62: 247-53.

Parboosing, R., et al. 2013. Gestational influenza and bipolar disorder in adult offspring. *JAMA Psychiatry*. http://archpsyc.jamanetwork.com/article.aspx?articleid=1686037.

Parens, E., and J. Johnston. 2008. Understanding the agreements and controversies surrounding childhood psychopharmacology. *Child and Adolescent Psychiatry and Mental Health* 2: 5.

Parent, R. 1996. "Aspects of police use of deadly force in BC: The phenomenon of victim-precipitated homicide." MA thesis, Simon Fraser University.

–. 2004. "Aspects of police use of deadly force in North America: The phenomenon of victim-precipitated homicide." PhD diss., Simon Fraser University.

Parikh, S., et al. 2012. A randomized controlled trial of psychoeducation or cognitive-behavioral therapy in bipolar disorder: A Canadian Network for Mood and Anxiety Treatments (CANMAT) study. *Journal of Clinical Psychiatry* 73: 803-10.

Paris, J. 1998. Editorial. Personality disorders: Psychiatry's stepchildren. *Canadian Journal of Psychiatry* 43: 135.

–. 2000. Canadian psychiatry across five decades: From clinical inference to evidence-based practice. *Canadian Journal of Psychiatry*: 45: 34-39.

–. 2005a. *The Fall of an Icon: Psychoanalysis and Academic Psychiatry*. Toronto: University of Toronto Press.

–. 2005b. Borderline personality disorder. *Canadian Medical Association Journal* 172: 1579-83.

Parkinson, S., G. Nelson, and S. Horgan. 1999. From housing to homes: A review of the literature on housing approaches for psychiatric consumer/survivors. *Canadian Journal of Community Mental Health* 18: 145-63.

Parnes, B., et al. 2009. Lack of impact of direct-to-consumer advertising on the physician-patient encounter in primary care. *Annals of Family Medicine* 7: 41-46.

Paterson, R. 1997. *The Changeways Core Program: Trainers Manual*. Vancouver: Changeways Clinic.

Paterson, R., and D. Bilsker. 2002. *Self-Care Depression Program: Patient Guide*. Vancouver: Mental Health Evaluation and Community Consultation Unit, Department of Psychiatry, University of British Columbia.

Pathak, P., et al. 2010. Evidence-based use of second generation antipsychotics in a state Medicaid pediatric population. *Psychiatric Services* 61: 123-29.

Patten, S. 2006. Does almost everybody suffer from a bipolar disorder? *Canadian Journal of Psychiatry*. 51: 6-9.

–. 2008. Major depression prevalence is very high, but the syndrome is a poor proxy for community populations' clinical treatment needs. *Canadian Journal of Psychiatry*. 53: 411-18.

Patten, S., and C. Beck. 2004. Major depression and health care utilization in Canada, 1994 to 2000. *Canadian Journal of Psychiatry* 49: 303-9.

Patterson, M. 2007. The faces of homelessness across BC. *Visions Journal* 4: 7-8.

Paulsen, M., and T. Sandborn. 2008. BC's homeless death toll: 56 or more in two years. *Tyee*. http://thetyee.ca/News/2008/04/17/BCHomeless/.

Pearson, C., et al. 2007. *The Applicability of Housing First Models to Homeless Persons with Serious Mental Illness: Final Report*. Report prepared for the US Department of Housing and Urban Development. http://www.huduser.org/portal/publications/hsgfirst.pdf.

Peele, R., and S. Kadekar. 2007. Dimensional models of personality disorders: Refining the research agenda for DSM-V. *Psychiatric Services* 58: 1016-17.

Peen, J., and J. Dekker. 2004. Is urbanicity a risk factor for psychiatric disorders? *Lancet* 363: 2012-13.

Penrose, L. 1939. Mental disease and crime: Outline of a comparative study of European statistics. *British Journal of Medical Psychology* 18: 1-15.

Perkins, M., et al. 2007. Applying theory-driven approaches to understanding and modifying clinicians' behavior: What do we know? *Psychiatric Services* 58: 342-48.

Perrault, M., et al. 2011. Predictors of caregiver satisfaction with mental health services. Springer Link. http://www.springerlink.com.ezproxy.library.ubc.ca/content/21p8m 168161125w8/fulltext.pdf.

Perseius, K., et al. 2007. Stress and burnout in psychiatric professionals when starting to use DBT in the work with young self-harming women showing borderline personality symptoms. *Journal of Psychiatric and Mental Health Nursing* 14: 635-43.

Pescosolido, B., et al. 2010. "A disease like any other?" A decade of change in public reactions to schizophrenia, depression and alcohol dependence. *American Journal of Psychiatry* 167: 1321-30.

Petrila, J. 2009. Law and psychiatry: Congress restores the Americans with Disabilities Act to its original intent. *Psychiatric Services* 60: 878-79.

Peyser, H. 2004. What is normal? What is sick? *Psychiatric Services* 55: 7.

Phares, E., and T. Trull. 1997. *Clinical Psychology: Concepts, Methods and Profession*. 5th ed. Pacific Grove, CA: Brooks/Cole Publishing.

Phelan, J., et al. 2000. Public conceptions of mental illness in 1950 and 1996: What is mental illness and is it to be feared? *Journal of Health and Social Behavior* 41: 188-207.

Phelan, J., L. Yang, and R. Cruz-Rojas. 2006. Effects of attributing serious mental illnesses to genetic causes on orientations to treatment. *Psychiatric Services* 57: 382-87.

Phillips, P., and S. Johnson. 2001. How does alcohol and drug misuse develop among people with psychotic illness? *Social Psychiatry and Psychiatric Epidemiology* 36: 269-76.

Phillips, S., et al. 2001. Moving assertive community treatment into standard practice. *Psychiatric Services* 52: 771-78.

Piat, M., J. Sabetti, and D. Bloom. 2009. The importance of medication in consumer definitions of recovery from serious mental illness: A qualitative study. *Issues in Mental Health Nursing* 30: 482-90.

Piat, M., et al. 2008. Housing for persons with serious mental illness: Consumer and service provider preferences. *Psychiatric Services* 59: 1011-17.

–. 2009. What does recovery mean for me? Perspectives of Canadian mental health consumers. *Psychiatric Rehabilitation Journal* 32: 199-207.

Picard, A. 2008a. The orphans of medicare. *Globe and Mail*, 24 June. http://v1.theglobeand mail.com/servlet/story/RTGAM.20080623.wmhhospitals24/BNStory/mentalhealth/.

–. 2008b. Centralization: A step back for Alberta health care? *Globe and Mail*. http://www. theglobeandmail.com/life/centralization-a-step-back-for-alberta-health-care/article 686741/.

–. 2009a. Should pregnant women take antidepressants? *Globe and Mail*, 24 October.

–. 2009b. The future of medicare is in his hands. *Globe and Mail*. http://www.theglobeandmail. com/life/health/the-future-of-medicare-is-in-his-hands/article1177345/.

–. 2011. Mental health strategy draft doesn't go far enough. *Globe and Mail*. http://www. theglobeandmail.com/life/health/new-health/andre-picard/mental-health-strategy-draft -doesnt-go-far-enough/article2149012/.

Picchioni, M., and R. Murray. 2007. Schizophrenia. *British Medical Journal* 335: 91-95.

Pierre, J. 2010. The borders of mental disorder in psychiatry and the DSM: Past, present and future. *Journal of Psychiatric Practice* 16: 375-86.

Pierson, R. 2009. Depression pill OK'd for kids but probe goes on. Canada.com. http://www. canada.com/health/Depression+pill+kids+probe+goes/1418735/story.html.

Pietrini, P. 2003. Toward a biochemistry of mind? *American Journal of Psychiatry* 160: 1907-8.

Pignatiello, A., et al. 2008. Supporting primary care through pediatric telepsychiatry. *Canadian Journal of Community Mental Health* 27: 139-51.

Pilgrim, D. 2002. The biopsychosocial model in Anglo-American psychiatry: Past, present and future? *Journal of Mental Health* 11: 585-94.

Pinfold, V., and G. Thornicroft. 2006. Influencing the public perception of mental illness. In *Choosing Methods in Mental Health Research*, ed. M. Slade and S. Priebe, 147-56. London: Routledge.

Pitschel-Walz, G., et al. 2001. The effect of family interventions on relapse and rehospitalization in schizophrenia: A meta-analysis. *Schizophrenia Bulletin* 27: 73-92.

Pollack, D., et al. 2009. Show me the evidence: The ethical aspects of pharmaceutical marketing, evidence-based medicine and rational prescribing. *Journal of Ethics in Mental Health* 4: 1-8.

Pope, M., and J. Scott. 2003. Do clinicians understand why individuals stop taking lithium? *Journal of Affective Disorders* 74: 287-91.

Potter, N. 2006. What is manipulative behavior anyway? *Journal of Personality Disorders* 20: 139-56.

–. 2011. Blaming and stereotyping and their effects on healing for patients with borderline personality disorder. *Journal of Ethics and Mental Health.* http://www.jemh.ca/conferences/2011/documents/1-PotterBritishColumbia2011BlamingandStereotypingandTheirEffects onHealingHandout.pdf.

Pound, P., et al. 2005. Resisting medicines: A synthesis of qualitative studies of medicine taking. *Social Science and Medicine* 61: 133-55.

Powers, M., et al. 2010. A meta-analytic review of prolonged exposure for posttraumatic stress disorder. *Clinical Psychology Review* 30: 635-41.

Praxis Information Intelligence, Gartner, Inc. 2011. Telehealth benefits and adoption: Connecting people and providers across Canada. Stamford, CT: Gartner Inc.

Priebe, S., et al. 2010. Patients' views of involuntary hospital admission after 1 and 3 months: Prospective study in 11 European countries. *British Journal of Psychiatry* 196: 179-85.

Prince, M., et al. 2007. No health without mental health. *Lancet* 370: 859-77.

Pritchard, D. 2011. Beheader's docs seek freedoms. *Winnipeg Sun.* http://www.winnipegsun.com/2011/05/30/exit-privileges-for-greyhound-killer-vince-li.

Prochaska, J., and C. DiClemente. 1984. *The Transtheoretical Approach: Crossing Traditional Boundaries of Therapy.* Homewood, IL: Dow/Jones Irwin.

Proudfoot, S. 2007. Depression still seen as career damaging, poll suggests. *Windsor Star.* http://www.canada.com/windsorstar/story.html?id=aed2acbb-c98b-48e4-b01d-17e53011d785&k=8063.

Provincial Diversion Program Working Committee. 2003. Implementing the Provincial Diversion Program in Alberta Communities: Guidelines and Standards. Alberta: Provincial Forensic Psychiatry Program

Public Health Agency of Canada. 2006. *The Human Face of Mental Health and Mental Illness in Canada.* Ottawa: Public Health Agency of Canada.

Public Safety Canada. 2008. *Corrections and Conditional Release Statistical Overview: Annual Report.* Ottawa: Public Safety Canada.

Pyke, J., et al. 2001. Improving accessibility: The experience of a Canadian mental health agency. *Psychiatric Rehabilitation Journal* 25: 180-85.

Pyne, J., et al. 2006. Agreement between patients with schizophrenia and providers on factors of antipsychotic medication adherence. *Psychiatric Services* 57: 1170-78.

Quan, D. 2011. More programs needed for prisoners with mental health issues: Watchdog. *Vancouver Sun,* 11 September.

Quan, H., and J. Arboleda-Florez. 1999. Elderly suicide in Alberta: Difference by gender. *Canadian Journal of Psychiatry* 44: 762-68.

Queensland Alliance for Mental Health. 2010. *From Discrimination to Social Inclusion: A Review of the Literature on Anti-Stigma Initiatives in Mental Health.* http://www.mhcc.org.au/documents/From-discrimination-to-social-inclusion-Lit-review.pdf.

Radke, A., J. Parks, and T. Ruter. 2010. A call for improved prevention and reduction of obesity among persons with serious mental illness. *Psychiatric Services* 61: 617-19.

Rae-Grant, Q. 2002. Editorial. The role of pharmaceutical companies in research and development: plaudits and cautions. *Canadian Journal of Psychiatry* 47: 513.

Ragins, M. n.d. A recovery based program inventory. The Village Integrated Service Agency. http://www.village-isa.org/Ragin's%20Papers/inventory.htm.

Rai, R. 2006. Addiction: A shared shame. *Visions Journal* 3: 12.

Ralph, I. 2009. *Addictions and Mental Health.* 5th ed. Grand Forks, BC: IGR Publications.

Ralph, R., K. Kidder, and D. Phillips. 2000. *Can We Measure Recovery? A Compendium of Recovery and Recovery-Related Instruments.* Human Services Research Institute, Cambridge, MA. http://www.tecathsri.org/pub_pickup/pn/pn-43.pdf.

Rapoport, M., M. Mamdani, and H. Herrman. 2006. Electroconvulsive therapy in older adults: 13 year trends. *Canadian Journal of Psychiatry* 51: 616-19.

Rapp, C. 1998. The active ingredients of effective case management: A research synthesis. *Community Mental Health Journal* 34: 363-380.

Rapp, C., and R. Goscha. 2012. *The Strengths Model.* 3rd ed. New York: Oxford University Press.

Rappolt, S. 2003. The role of professional expertise in evidence-based occupational therapy. *American Journal of Occupational Therapy* 57: 589-93.

Ratnasingham et al. 2012. *Opening Eyes, Opening Minds: The Ontario Burden of Mental Illness Report.* Toronto: Institute for Clinical Evaluative Sciences and Public Health Ontario.

Raue, P., et al. 2009. Patients' depression treatment preferences and initiation, adherence and outcome: A randomized primary care study. *Psychiatric Services* 60: 337-43.

Raune, D., E. Kuipers, and P. Bebbington. 2004. Expressed emotion at first-episode psychosis: Investigating a carer appraisal model. *British Journal of Psychiatry* 184: 321-26.

Raymond, C., S. Morgan, and P. Caetano. 2007. Antidepressant utilization in BC from 1996 to 2004: Increasing prevalence but not incidence. *Canadian Journal of Psychiatry* 58: 79-84.

Reaume, G. 1997. Accounts of abuse of patients at the Toronto Hospital for the Insane, 1883-1937. *Canadian Bulletin of Medical History* 14: 65-106.

Rector, N., A. Beck, and N. Stolar. 2005. The negative symptoms of schizophrenia: A cognitive perspective. *Canadian Journal of Psychiatry* 50: 247-57.

Redwood-Campbell, L., et al. 2003. How are new refugees doing in Canada? Comparison of the health and settlement of the Kosovars and Czech Roma. *Canadian Journal of Public Health* 94: 381-85.

–. 2008. Understanding the health of refugee women in host countries: Lessons from the Kosovar resettlement in Canada. *Prehospital and Disaster Medicine* 23: 322-27.

Reesal, R., and R. Lam. 2001. Clinical guidelines for the treatment of depressive disorders: Principles of management. *Canadian Journal of Psychiatry* 46 (suppl. 1): 21S-28S.

Regehr, C., and G. Glancy. 2010. *Mental Health Social Work Practice in Canada.* Don Mills, ON: Oxford University Press.

Regehr, C., and K. Kanani. 2006. *Essential Law for Social Work Practice in Canada.* Don Mills, ON: Oxford University Press.

Reger, M., and G. Gahm. 2009. A meta-analysis of the effects of internet- and computer-based cognitive-behavioral treatments for anxiety. *Journal of Clinical Psychology* 65: 53-75.

Reid, S., H. Berman, and C. Forchuk. 2005. Living on the streets in Canada: A feminist narrative study of girls and young women. *Issues in Comprehensive Pediatric Nursing* 28: 237-56.

Reiling, D. 2002. Boundary maintenance as a barrier to mental health help-seeking for depression among the Old Order Amish. *Journal of Rural Health* 18: 428-36.

Remund, L. 2007. Housing first: The Triage experience. *Visions Journal* 4: 30-31.

Repper, J., and T. Carter. 2011. A review of the literature on peer support in mental health. *Journal of Mental Health* 20: 392-411.

Reyers, C. 2011. Altering the course of schizophrenia. National Alliance on Mental Illness. http://www.nami.org/ADVTemplate.cfm?Section=Advocate_Magazine&template=/Content Management/ContentDisplay.cfm&ContentID=126586.

Rhodes, A., and J. Bethell. 2008. Suicidal ideators without major depression: Whom are we not reaching? *Canadian Journal of Psychiatry* 53: 125-30.

Rhodes, A., et al. 2010. Depression and mental health supports and services in Canada. In *Mental Disorder in Canada: An Epidemiological Perspective*, ed. J. Cairney and D. Streiner, 393-413. Toronto: University of Toronto Press.

Richard, A., L. Jongbloed, and A. MacFarlane. 2009. Integration of peer support workers into community mental health teams. *International Journal of Psychosocial Rehabilitation* 14: 99-110.

Robertson, G. 1994. *Mental Disability and the Law in Canada*. 2nd ed. Toronto: Carswell.

Robinson, J. 2001. *Prescription Games*. Toronto: McClelland and Stewart.

Robotham, J. 2011. Genetics may link mental illnesses. *Canberra Times.* http://www.canberratimes.com.au/news/national/national/general/genetics-may-link-mental-illnesses/2295924.aspx.

Rochefort, D. 1992. More lessons, of a different kind: Canadian mental health policy in comparative perspective. *Hospital and Community Psychiatry* 43: 1083-90.

Roll, J., et al. 2006. A comparison of five reinforcement schedules for use in contingency management-based treatment of methamphetamine abuse. *Psychological Record* 56: 67-81.

Rollinson, R., et al. 2007. The application of cognitive-behavioral therapy for psychosis in clinical and research settings. *Psychiatric Services* 58: 1297-302.

Romans, S., and L. Ross. 2010. Gender and depression. In *Mental Disorder in Canada: An Epidemiological Perspective*, ed. J. Cairney and D. Streiner, 259-85. Toronto: University of Toronto Press.

Rooney, J., and L. Heuvel. 2004. Root cause analysis for beginners. Webspace, University of Texas. https://webspace.utexas.edu/mae548/www/research/digital%20forensics/qp0704rooney.pdf.

Rosengren, D. 2009. *Building Motivational Interviewing Skills: A Practitioner Workbook*. New York: Guilford.

Rosenhan, D. 1973. On being sane in insane places. *Science* 179: 250-57.

Rosenheck, R. 2005. The growth of psychopharmacology in the 1990s: Evidence-based practice or irrational exuberance. *International Journal of Law and Psychiatry* 28: 467-83.

Rosenheck, R., et al. 2003. Effectiveness and cost of olanzapine and haloperidol in the treatment of schizophrenia: A randomized control trial. *Journal of the American Medical Association* 290: 2693-702.

Roslin, A. 2008. The pill pushers. *Georgia Straight.* http://www.straight.com/article-160083/pill-pushers.

Ross, M. 2011a. Serious mental illness, care-giver stress and the Mental Health Commission of Canada. Huffington Post. http://www.huffingtonpost.ca/marvin-ross/mental-health-canada_b_877791.html.

–. 2011b. Many inoculated against science in understanding schizophrenia. Huffington Post. http://www.huffingtonpost.ca/marvin-ross/schizophrenia_b_1023721.html.

–. 2012. Why the media shuns mental illness. http://www.huffingtonpost.ca/marvin-ross/bell-talk-mental-illness_b_1256863.html.

Rossi, C. 2006. Mental illness fastest growing workplace disability. *Vancouver Courier*, 3 March.

–. 2007. Controversial Fraser Street residence slated for Aug. 1 opening. *Vancouver Courier*, 6 June.

Rossi, P. 2003. *Case Management in Health Care*. 2nd ed. Philadelphia: Norton.

Row, C. 2003. Hearing voices that are not real. *Visions: BC's Mental Health Journal* 18: 27-28.

Rueve, M., and R. Welton. 2008. Violence and mental illness. *Psychiatry* 5: 34-48.

Ruggeri, M., et al. 2000. Definition and prevalence of severe and persistent mental illness. *British Journal of Psychiatry* 177: 149-55.

Ruo, B., et al. 2003. Depressive symptoms and health-related quality of life: The heart and soul study. *Journal of the American Medical Association* 290: 215-21.

Rusch, N., et al. 2008. Predictors of dropout from inpatient dialectical behavior therapy among women with borderline personality disorder. *Journal of Behavior Therapy and Experimental Psychiatry* 39: 497-503.

–. 2010. Biogenetic models of psychopathology, implicit guilt, and mental illness stigma. *Psychiatry Research* 179: 328-32.

Rush, B., and J. Koegl. 2008. Prevalence and profile of people with co-occurring mental and substance use disorders within a comprehensive mental health system. *Canadian Journal of Psychiatry* 53: 810-20.

Rush, B., et al. 2008. Prevalence of co-occurring substance use and other mental disorders in the Canadian population. *Canadian Journal of Psychiatry* 53: 800-8.

Russell, D. 1986. *The Secret Trauma: Incest in the Lives of Girls and Women*. New York: Basic Books.

Russinova, Z., P. Bloch, and A. Lyass. 2007. Patterns of employment among individuals with mental illness in vocational recovery. *Journal of Psychosocial Nursing* 45: 48-54.

Saari, K., et al. 2004. Serum lipids in schizophrenia and other functional psychoses. *Acta Psychiatrica Scandinavica* 110: 279-85.

Sackett, D. 2000. *Evidence Based Medicine*. London, UK: Churchill Livingstone.

Sadavoy, J., R. Meier, and A. Ong. 2004. Barriers to access for mental health services for ethnic seniors: The Toronto study. *Canadian Journal of Psychiatry* 49: 192-99.

Sadock, B., and V. Sadock, V. 2007. *Kaplan and Sadock's Synopsis of Psychiatry*. 10th ed. Philadelphia, PA: Lippincott, Williams and Wilkins.

St. Clair, D., et al. 2005. Rates of adult schizophrenia following prenatal exposure to the Chinese famine of 1959-61. *Journal of the American Medical Association* 294: 557-62.

Saks, E. 2013. Successful and schizophrenic. *New York Times*. http://www.nytimes.com/2013/01/27/opinion/sunday/schizophrenic-not-stupid.html?_r=0.

Salkever, D., et al. 2007. Measures and predictors of community-based employment and earnings of persons with schizophrenia in a multisite study. *Psychiatric Services* 58: 315-24.

Salyers, M. et al. 2004. A ten-year follow-up of a supported employment program. *Psychiatric Services* 55: 302-8.

Salzer, M., L. Wick. and J. Rogers. 2008. Familiarity with and use of accommodations and supports among postsecondary students with mental illness. *Psychiatric Services* 59: 370-75.

Samson, C. 2009. A colonial double-bind: Social and historical contexts of Innu mental health. In *Healing Traditions: The Mental Health of Aboriginal Peoples in Canada*, ed. L. Kirmayer and G. Valaskakis, 109-39. Vancouver: UBC Press.

Sanchez, N. 2000. Stigmatized views of mental illness in the Latin American community. *Visions: B.C.'s Mental Health Journal* 9: 10.

Sands, R., and B. Angell. 2002. Social workers as collaborators on interagency and interdisciplinary teams. In *Social Work Practice in Mental Health*, ed. K Bentley, 254-80. Pacific Grove, CA: Brooks/Cole.

Sareen, J., et al. 2005a. Perceived need for mental health treatment in a nationally representative Canadian sample. *Canadian Journal of Psychiatry* 50: 643-51.

–. 2005b. The relationship between perceived need for mental health treatment, DSM diagnosis, and quality of life. *Canadian Journal of Psychiatry* 50: 87-94.

Satel, S. 1999. Editorial: What should we expect from drug abusers? *Psychiatric Services* 50: 861.

Satel, S., and K. Humphreys, K. 2003. Mind games. http://www.sallysatelmd.com/html/a-ws2.html.

Satel, S., and M. Zdanowicz. M. 2003. Commission's omission. *National Review Online*. http://www.nationalreview.com/articles/207650/commissions-omission/sally-satel.

Scardillo, N. 2012. Mental health clubhouses: The road to nowhere. *Networker* (newsletter of the West Coast Mental Health Network) 17, 12.

Schaedle, R., et al. 2002. A comparison of experts' perspectives on assertive community treatment and intensive case management. *Psychiatric Services* 53: 207-10.

Scheid, T., and C. Anderson. 1995. Living with chronic mental illness: Understanding the role of work. *Community Mental Health Journal* 31: 163-76.

Schiff, J., H. Coleman, and D. Miner. 2008. Voluntary participation in rehabilitation: Lessons learned from a clubhouse environment. *Canadian Journal of Community Mental Health* 27: 65-76.

Schizophrenia Commission. 2012. *The Abandoned Illness: A Report by the Schizophrenia Commission* (U.K.). http://www.rethink.org/media/514093/TSC_main_report_14_nov.pdf.

Schinnar, A., et al. 1990. An empirical literature review of definitions of severe and persistent mental illness. *American Journal of Psychiatry* 147: 1602-8.

Schneider, B. 2010. *Hearing (Our) Voices: Participatory Research in Mental Health*. Toronto: University of Toronto Press.

Schneider, S., H. Bloom, and M. Heerema. 2007. *Mental Health Courts: Decriminalizing the Mentally Ill*. Toronto: Irwin Law.

Scholten, D. et al. 2003. Removing barriers to treatment of first-episode psychotic disorders. *Canadian Journal of Psychiatry* 48: 561-65.

Schrank, B., and M. Slade. 2007. Recovery in psychiatry. *Psychiatric Bulletin* 31: 321-25.

Schwartz, M., et al. 2006. Substance use in persons with schizophrenia. *Journal of Nervous and Mental Disease* 194: 164-72.

Schwarz, E., et al. 2010. Validation of a blood-based laboratory test to aid in the confirmation of a diagnosis of schizophrenia. *Biomarker Insights* 5: 39-47.

Schwenk, T., L. Davis, and L. Wimsatt. 2010. Depression, stigma and suicidal ideation in medical students. *Journal of the American Medical Association* 304: 1181-90.

Scott, M. 2007. Overcoming cultural stigma is a tough task. *Vancouver Sun*, 24 February.

Scull, A. 1977. *Decarceration: Community Treatment and the Deviant – A Radical View*. Englewood Cliffs, NJ: Prentice Hall.

Scully, J. 2004. Should psychologists have prescribing authority? A great leap backwards. *Psychiatric Services* 55: 1,424.

Seale, C., et al. 2006. Sharing decisions in consultations involving anti-psychotic medication: A qualitative study of psychiatrists' experiences. *Social Science and Medicine* 62: 2861-73.

Sealey, P., and P. Whitehead. 2004. Forty years of deinstitutionalization of psychiatric services in Canada: An empirical assessment. *Canadian Journal of Psychiatry* 49: 249-57.

Seeman, M. 2007. An outcome measure in schizophrenia: Mortality. *Canadian Journal of Psychiatry* 52: 55-59.

Sells, D., et al. 2008. Beyond generic support: Incidence and impact of invalidation in peer support services for clients with severe mental illness. *Psychiatric Services* 59: 1322-27.

Sernyak, M., and R. Rosenheck. 2004. System-wide costs associated with second-generation antipsychotics in the treatment of schizophrenia. *Psychiatric Services* 55: 1361-62.

Shah, P., and D. Mountain. 2007. The medical model is dead – long live the medical model. *British Journal of Psychiatry* 191: 375-77.

Shain, M. 2008. The mentally safe workplace: What it means and why we need it. https://secure.cihi.ca/free_products/mentally_healthy_communities_en.pdf.

Shankar, J., J. Martin, and C. McDonald. 2009. Emerging areas of practice for mental health social workers: Education and employment. *Australian Social Work* 62: 28-44.

Shapcott, M. 2010. Controversial TO street needs assessment reports sharp drop in street homelessness. Wellesley Institute. http://www.wellesleyinstitute.com/blog/controversial-to-street-needs-assessment-reports-sharp-drop-in-street-homelessness/.

Sharma, V., et al. 2000. Preferred terms for users of mental health services among service providers and recipients. *Psychiatric Services* 51: 205-9.

Shattuck, P. 2006. Diagnostic substitution and changing autism prevalence. *Pediatrics* 117: 1438-39.

Shaw, G. 2007. What happens to our aging seniors with too few doctors to provide medical care? *Vancouver Sun*, 2 November.

Shaw, R. 2012. B.C. police officers afraid to use Tasers says RCMP official. *Vancouver Sun*. http://www.vancouversun.com/news/Police+afraid+Tasers+says+RCMP+official/7397471/story.html.

Sheehan, K., and T. Burns. 2011. Perceived coercion and therapeutic relationship: A neglected association? *Psychiatric Services* 62: 471-76.

Shevlin, M., et al. 2008. Cumulative traumas and psychosis: An analysis of the National Comorbidity Survey and the British Psychiatric Morbidity Survey. *Schizophrenia Bulletin* 34: 193-99.

Shimrat, I. 2011. The Mental Patients Association and the Vancouver Emotional Emergency Centre. http://www.wcmhn.org/bulletin_files/Networker-FALL%202011%20wcmhn.pdf.

Shinn, M., et al. 1998. Predictors of homelessness among families in New York City: From shelter request to housing stability. *American Journal of Public Health* 88: 1651-57.

Shorter, E., 1997. *A History of Psychiatry*. New York: John Wiley and Sons.

Sibitz, I., et al. 2011. Stigma resistance in patients with schizophrenia. *Schizophrenia Bulletin* 37: 316-23.

Silberfeld, M., and A. Fish. 1994. *When the Mind Fails*. Toronto: University of Toronto Press.

Silver, T. 2004. Staff in mental health agencies: Coping with the dual challenges as providers with psychiatric disabilities. *Psychiatric Rehabilitation Journal* 28: 165-71.

Simmie, S., and J. Nunes. 2001. *The Last Taboo: A Survival Guide to Mental Health Care in Canada*. Toronto: McClelland and Stewart.

Sinnema, J. 2008. Pharmacists get power of prescriptions. Canada.com. http://www2.canada.com/topics/lifestyle/parenting/story.html?id=a4e3fa27-0236-42f9-bfeb-e88fe1fe54ac.

Skeem, J., and J. Loudon. 2006. Toward evidence-based practice for probationers and parolees mandated to mental health treatment. *Psychiatric Services* 57: 333-42.

Skodol, A., and B. Bender. 2009. Editorial: The future of personality disorders in *DSM*-V. *American Journal of Psychiatry* 166: 388-91.

Skodol, A., et al. 2002. The borderline diagnosis I: Psychopathology, comorbidity, and personality structure. *Biological Psychiatry* 51: 936-50.

Slade, M. 2009. 100 ways to support recovery. Mental Health Shop. http://www.mentalhealthshop.org/products/rethink_publications/100_ways_to_support.html#.

Slade, M., et al. 2005. Patient-rated mental health needs and quality of life improvement. *British Journal of Psychiatry* 187: 256-61.

Sledge, W., et al. 2011. Effectiveness of peer support in reducing readmissions of persons with multiple psychiatric hospitalizations. *Psychiatric Services* 62: 541-44.

Slomp, M., et al. 2009. Three year physician treated prevalence rate of mental disorders in Alberta. *Canadian Journal of Psychiatry* 54: 199-202.

Smiderle, W. 2003. Stand up and be heard: Unified voice putting mental health on the government radar screen. *Schizophrenia Digest* (Summer): 32-34.

Smith, C. 2003. Martin's care cure questioned. *Georgia Straight*, 23 October, 33.

–. 2007a. Liberals leave expert off stacked drug panel. *Georgia Straight*. http://www.straight.com/node/124451/print.

–. 2007b. Guardian protects us from the drug pushers. *Georgia Straight*. http://www.straight.com/article-110424/guardian-protects-us-from-the-drug-pushers.

–. 2011. Meds aren't required to get through midlife. *Georgia Straight*, 24 November, 38.

Smith, K. 2007. Highlights of the census of immigration, citizenship and language. *CanWest News Service*. http://www2.canada.com/montreal/francais/story.html?id=29e32201-c5bf-43e5-861e-ff902d725344.

Smyth, M., and J. Hoult. 2000. The home treatment enigma. *British Medical Journal* 320: 305-8.

Söderberg, P., S. Tungström, and B. Armelius. 2005. Reliability of global assessment of functioning ratings made by clinical psychiatric staff. *Psychiatric Services* 56: 434-38.

Solomon, P. 2001. The cultural context of interventions for family members with a seriously mentally ill relative. *New Directions for Mental Health Services* 91: 67-78.

Somers, J. 2007. Cognitive behavioural therapy: Core information document. Vancouver: Centre for Applied Research in Mental Health and Addictions.

Somers, J., et al. 2011. Drug treatment court of Vancouver: an empirical evaluation of recidivism. *Addiction Research and Therapy* 2: 1-7.

Sorensen, H., et al. 2011. Association between prepartum maternal iron deficiency and offspring risk of schizophrenia. *Schizophrenia Bulletin* 37: 982-87.

Sowers, W., and R. Benacci. 2010. *Locus Training Manual: Level of Care Utilization System for Psychiatric and Addiction Services Adult Version 2010.* Erie, PA: Deerfield Behavioral Health Inc.

Spaeth-Rublee, B., et al. 2010. Measuring quality of mental health care: A review of initiatives and programs in selected countries. *Canadian Journal of Psychiatry* 55: 539-48.

Sparks, J., and B. Duncan. 2008. Do no harm: A critical risk/benefit analysis of child psychotropic medication. *Journal of Family Psychotherapy* 19: 1-19.

Spataro, J. 2004. Impact of child sexual abuse on mental health: Prospective study in males and females. *British Journal of Psychiatry* 184: 416-21.

Spiegel, A. 2005. Dictionary of disorder. *New Yorker*, 3 January, 56-62.

Spindel, P., and J. Nugent. 1999. The trouble with PACT: Questioning the increasing use of assertive community treatment teams in community mental health. People Who. http://www.peoplewho.org/readingroom/spindel.nugent.htm.

Sporn, A., et al. 2003. Progressive brain volume loss during adolescence in childhood-onset schizophrenia. *American Journal of Psychiatry* 160: 2181-89.

Srinivasan, J., N. Cohen, and S. Parikh. 2003. Patient attitudes regarding causes of depression: Implications for psychoeducation. *Canadian Journal of Psychiatry* 48: 493-95.

Stainsby, J. 2000. Extended leave. *Canadian Journal of Community Mental Health* 19: 152-55.

Standing Senate Committee on Social Affairs, Science and Technology. 2002. *The Health of Canadians: The Federal Role.* http://www.parl.gc.ca/Content/SEN/Committee/372/SOCI/rep/repoct02vol6-e.pdf.

–. 2004. *Mental Health, Mental Illness and Addiction: Overview of Policies and Programs in Canada.* http://www.parl.gc.ca/Content/SEN/Committee/381/soci/rep/report1/repintnov04vol1table-e.htm.

–. 2006. *Out of the Shadows at Last: Transforming Mental Health, Mental Illness and Addiction Services in Canada.* Ottawa: Government of Canada.

Statistics Canada 2003. Canadian community health survey: Mental health and well-being. http://www.statcan.gc.ca/pub/82-617-x/index-eng.htm.

–. 2006. *A Portrait of Seniors in Canada.* http://www.statcan.gc.ca/pub/89-519-x/89-519-x2006001-eng.pdf.

–. 2010. *Projections of the Diversity of the Canadian Population, 2006-2031.* http://www.statcan.gc.ca/pub/91-551-x/91-551-x2010001-eng.htm.

Steadman, H., et al. 1998. Violence by people discharged from acute psychiatric inpatient facilities and by others in the same neighborhoods. *Archives of General Psychiatry* 55: 393-401.

Stefan, S. 2002. *Hollow Promises: Employment Discrimination against People with Mental Disabilities.* Washington, DC: American Psychological Association.

Stein, L., and M. Test. 1980. Alternatives to mental hospital treatment: Conceptual model, treatment programs and clinical evaluation. *Archives of General Psychiatry* 37: 392-97.

Steinberg, P. 2012. Our failed approach to schizophrenia. *New York Times.* http://www.nytimes.com/2012/12/26/opinion/our-failed-approach-to-schizophrenia.html?_r=0.

Steiner, W., and E. Amir. 2003. Depression screening day: A mental illness awareness week project. *Canadian Psychiatric Association Bulletin* 35: 14-15.

Steingard, S. 2012. Anosognosia: How conjecture becomes medical "fact." Mad in America. http://www.madinamerica.com/2012/08/anosognosia-how-conjecture-becomes-medical-fact/.

Steinke, C., and A. Dastmalchian. 2009. The economic impacts: Workplace mental illness and substance abuse. *Visions: BC's Mental Health and Addictions Journal*. http://www.heretohelp.bc.ca/sites/default/files/visions_workplaces.pdf.

Sterle, F. 2006. Compassion by law enforcers: More common than may be expected. *Visions Journal* 2: 24-26.

Stip, E. 2009. Psychosis: A category or a dimension? *Canadian Journal of Psychiatry* 54: 137.

Stip, E., and G. Letourneau. 2009. Psychotic symptoms as a continuum between normality and pathology. *Canadian Journal of Psychiatry* 54: 140-51.

Stobbe, M. 2007. Autism "epidemic" may be all in the label. http://www.msnbc.msn.com/id/21600784/.

Stone, J., et al. 2010. Review: The biological basis of antipsychotic response in schizophrenia. *Journal of Psychopharmacology* 24: 953-64.

Straus, S., J. Tetroe, and I. Graham. 2009. Defining knowledge translation. *Canadian Medical Association Journal* 181: 165-68.

Strauss, J. 2008. Is prognosis in the individual, the environment, the disease, or what? *Schizophrenia Bulletin* 34: 245-46.

Stuart, H. 2003. Stigma and the daily news: Evaluation of a newspaper intervention. *Canadian Journal of Psychiatry* 48: 651-55.

–. 2006. Reaching out to high school youth: The effectiveness of a video-based antistigma campaign. *Canadian Journal of Psychiatry* 51: 647-53.

–. 2008. Fighting the stigma caused by mental disorders: Past perspectives, present activities and future directions. *World Psychiatry* 7: 185-88.

–. 2010. Mental disorders and social stigma: Three moments in Canadian history. In *Mental Disorder in Canada: An Epidemiological Perspective*, ed. J. Cairney and D. Streiner, 304-30. Toronto: University of Toronto Press.

Stuart, H., and J. Arboleda-Florez. 2000. Homeless shelter users in the post-deinstitutionalization era. *Canadian Journal of Psychiatry* 45: 55-62.

Stuart, H., and J. Arboleda-Florez. 2001. Community attitudes toward people with schizophrenia. *Canadian Journal of Psychiatry* 46: 245–52

Subramaniam, K., et al. 2012. Computerized cognitive training restores neural activity within the reality monitoring network in schizophrenia. *Neuron* 73: 842-53.

Sue, D., P. Arredondo, and R. McDavis. 1992. Multicultural counseling competencies and standards: A call to the profession. *Journal of Counseling and Development* 70: 484-86.

Sullivan, W., and C. Rapp, C. 2002. Social workers as case managers. In *Social Work Practice in Mental Health*, ed. K. Bentley, 180-210. Pacific Grove, CA: Brooks/Cole.

Sussman, S. 1998. The first asylums in Canada: A response to neglectful community care and current trends. *Canadian Journal of Psychiatry* 43: 260-64.

Sutton, B. 2008. Lessons to be learned from CATIE and CUTLASS. *Psychiatric Services* 59: 473.

Swaminath, R., et al. 2002. Experiments in change: Pretrial diversion of offenders with mental illness. *Canadian Journal of Psychiatry* 47: 450-58.

Swartz, M. 2010. Introduction to the special section on assisted outpatient treatment in New York State. *Psychiatric Services* 61: 967-69.

Swartz, M., et al. 2006. Substance use in persons with schizophrenia. *The Journal of Nervous and Mental Disease* 194: 164-173.

–. 2007. Effects of antipsychotic medications on psychosocial functioning in patients with chronic schizophrenia. *American Journal of Psychiatry* 164: 428-36.

Szasz, T. 1974. *The Myth of Mental Illness*, rev. ed. New York: Harper and Row.

–. 1976. *Schizophrenia: The Sacred Symbol of Psychiatry.* New York: Basic Books.

–. 1977. *Psychiatric Slavery.* New York: Free Press.

Szmuckler, G. 1999. Ethics in community psychiatry. *Australian and New Zealand Journal of Psychiatry* 33: 328-38.

Szmukler, G., and F. Holloway. 1998. Mental health legislation is now a harmful anachronism. *Psychiatric Bulletin* 22: 662-65.

Takeuchi, C. 2012. Choosing to see the future – or maybe not. *Georgia Straight,* 3-10 May, 24.

Tam, C., and S. Law. 2007. A systematic approach to the management of patients who refuse medications in an ACT team setting. *Psychiatric Services* 58: 457-59.

Taylor, L. 2012. Canada's health ministers call for VBP for generics. *PharmaTimes Online.* http://pharmatimes.com/Article/12-07-30/Canada_s_health_ministers_call_for_VBP_for_generics.aspx.

Taylor, P. 2008. Psychosis and violence: Stories, fears and reality. *Canadian Journal of Psychiatry* 53: 647-59.

Tee, K., and L. Hanson. 2004. Fraser South early psychosis intervention program. In *Best Practice in Early Psychosis Intervention,* ed. T. Ehmann, W. MacEwan, and W. Honer, 131-40. London, UK: Taylor and Francis.

Teotonio, I. 2011. Canadian woman denied entry to US because of suicide attempt. Toronto Star. http://www.thestar.com/news/article/930110–canadian-woman-denied-entry-to-u-s-because-of-suicide-attempt.

Teplin, L. 1984. Criminalizing mental disorder: The comparative arrest rate of the mentally ill. *American Psychologist* 39: 794-803.

Teplin, L., and N. Pruett. 1992. Police as streetcorner psychiatrist: Managing the mentally ill. *International Journal of Law and Psychiatry* 15: 139-56.

Tervalon, M., and J. Murray-Garcia. 1998. Cultural humility versus cultural competence: A critical distinction in defining physician training outcomes in multicultural education. *Journal of Health Care for the Poor and Underserved* 9: 117-25.

Thara, R. 2004. Twenty-year course of schizophrenia: The Madras longitudinal study. *Canadian Journal of Psychiatry* 49: 564-69.

Thomas, C., et al. 2006. Trends in the use of psychotropic medication among adolescents, 1994-2001. *Psychiatric Services* 57: 63-69.

Thomas, L. 2000. What "best practices" means for mental health housing. *Visions: BC's Mental Health Journal* 10: 5.

–. 2007. Mental health supported housing means less time in hospital. *Visions Journal* 4: 27-28.

Thompson, S. 2010. Policing Vancouver's mentally ill: The disturbing truth. Vancouver Police Board. http://vancouver.ca/police/assets/pdf/reports-policies/vpd-lost-in-transition-part-2-draft.pdf.

Thomson, H. 2003. Drug costs may soar for Canada's seniors. *UBC Reports,* 5 June, 3.

–. 2010. Harmful if swallowed. Alumni Affairs. *Trek* Magazine Archives. http://www.alumni.ubc.ca/trekmagazine/27-summer2010/harmful.php.

Thor-Larsen, L. 2002. Changing the paradigm. *Bulletin: Official Publication of the Vancouver/Richmond Mental Health Network Society* 7: 4.

Tibbetts, J. 2003. Physicist wins no-drug fight. *Vancouver Sun,* 7 June.

Tienari, P., et al. 2003. Genetic boundaries of the schizophrenia spectrum: Evidence from the Finnish adoptive family study of schizophrenia. *American Journal of Psychiatry* 160: 1587-94.

Tiwari, S., and J. Wang. 2006. The epidemiology of mental and substance use use-related disorders among white, Chinese and other Asian populations in Canada. *Canadian Journal of Psychiatry* 51: 904-12.

Todd, D. 2004. Schizophrenia: Two steps forward, one step back. *Vancouver Sun,* 4 December.

–. 2008. Chinese people suffer in silence, shunning therapy. *Vancouver Sun,* 23 February.

–. 2009. Aboriginals, churches share a mutual respect. *Vancouver Sun,* 28 August.

–. 2012. The "giggle factor" is gone. *Vancouver Sun*, 9 October.

Tollefson, G., et al. 1997. Blind, controlled, long-term study of the comparative incidence of treatment emergent tardive dyskinesia with olanzapine or haloperidol. *American Journal of Psychiatry* 154: 1248-54.

Tolomiczenko, G., P. Goering, and J. Durbin. 2001. Educating the public about mental illness and homelessness: A cautionary note. *Canadian Journal of Psychiatry* 46: 253-57.

Tolson, M. 2006. Community engagement report: Multicultural mental health liaison program. Report prepared for Vancouver Community Mental Health Services, Vancouver, BC.

Tondora, J., R. Miller, and L. Davidson. 2012. The top ten concerns about person-centered care planning in mental health systems. *International Journal of Person-Centered Medicine* 2: 410-20.

Toneguzzi, M. 2005. Superbug takes its toll on homeless. *Vancouver Sun*, 1 April.

Torrey, E. 1988. *Surviving Schizophrenia*. New York: Harper and Row.

–. 1997. *Out of the Shadows: Confronting America's Mental Illness Crisis*. New York: John Wiley and Sons.

–. 2011a. Patients, clients, consumers, survivors et al: What's in a name? *Schizophrenia Bulletin* 37: 466-68.

–. 2011b. Schizophrenia as a brain disease: Studies of individuals who have never been treated. Treatment Advocacy Center, Arlington, VA. http://www.treatmentadvocacycenter. org/resources/briefing-papers-and-fact-sheets/159/466.

–. 2011c. Stigma and violence: Isn't it time to connect the dots? *Schizophrenia Bulletin* 37: 892-96.

–. 2012. Anosognosia, denial and the new antipsychiatry. Treatment Advocacy Center, Arlington, VA. http://www.treatmentadvocacycenter.org/problem/anosognosia/2178.

Torrey, E., et al. 2010. More mentally ill persons are in prisons and jails than hospitals: A survey of the states. Treatment Advocacy Center, Arlington, VA. http://www.treatment advocacycenter.org/storage/tac/documents/final_jails_v_hospitals_study.pdf.

Torrible, S., et al. 2006. Improving recruitment into geriatric medicine in Canada: Findings and recommendations from the geriatric recruitment study." *Journal of the American Geriatrics Society* 54: 1453-62.

Tracy, B. 2003. Evidence-based practices or value-based services? *Psychiatric Services* 54: 1437.

Trainor, J., E. Pomeroy, and B. Pape. 1993. *A New Framework for Support for People with Serious Mental Health Problems*. Toronto: Canadian Mental Health Association.

Trauer, T., G. Tobias, and M. Slade. 2008. Development and evaluation of a patient-rated version of the CANSAS-P. *Community Mental Health Journal* 44: 113-24.

Treatment Advocacy Center. 2005. Anosognosia (impaired awareness of illness): A major problem for individuals with schizophrenia and bipolar disorder. National Alliance on Mental Illness. http://www.nami.org/Content/Microsites86/NAMI_Albuquerque/Home82/ Current_Activities/NAMIWalks6/Briefing-anosognosia_(05).pdf.

–. 2009a. Assisted outpatient treatment laws. http://www.treatmentadvocacycenter.org/index. php?option=com_content&task=view&id=39&Itemid=68.

–. 2009b. Why individuals with severe psychiatric disorders often do not take their medications. http://www.treatmentadvocacycenter.org/index.php?option=com_content&task= view&id=1375&Itemid=234.

–. 2011. Dr. Torrey takes questions about SAMHSA. http://www.treatmentadvocacycenter. org/problem/SAMHSA/1965.

–. 2012. The problem with saying 20% of people have mental illnesses. http://treatment advocacycenter.org/about-us/our-blog/69-no-state/2003-feds-say-20-of-us-residents -suffer-mental-illness.

Tremayne-Lloyd, T. 2003. Right to confidentiality vs. duty to disclose: The Supreme Court of Canada in Smith vs. Jones. National Center for Biotechnology Information. http://www. ncbi.nlm.nih.gov/pmc/articles/PMC2018400/pdf/11281081.pdf.

Tschopp, M., M. Berven, and F. Chan. 2011. Consumer perceptions of assertive community treatment interventions. *Community Mental Health Journal* 47: 408-14.

Tsemberis, S., L. Gulcur, and M. Nakae. 2004. Housing first, consumer choice, and harm reduction for homeless individuals with a dual diagnosis. *American Journal of Public Health* 94: 651-56.

Turbett, H. 2000. The mental health system ... as racist? *Visions: BC's Mental Health Journal* 9: 28-29.

Turcotte, M., and G. Schellenberg. 2007. *A Portrait of Seniors in Canada 2006*. Ottawa: Statistics Canada.

Turner, E., et al. 2008. Selective publication of antidepressant trials and its influence on apparent efficacy. *New England Journal of Medicine* 358: 252-60.

Turney, J., and J. Turner. 2000. Predictive medicine, genetics and schizophrenia. *New Genetics and Society* 19: 5-22.

Tyrer, P., and K. Kendall. 2009. The spurious advance of antipsychotic drug therapy. *Lancet* 373: 4-5.

Ucok, A., et al. 2004. Attitudes of psychiatrists toward patients with schizophrenia. *Psychiatry and Clinical Neurosciences* 58: 89-91.

United States Department of Health and Human services. 2007. The National CLAS Standards. http://minorityhealth.hhs.gov/templates/browse.aspx?lvl=2&lvlID=15.

United States Substance Abuse and Mental Health Services Administration. 2012. SAMHSA's Working Definition of Recovery Updated. http://blog.samhsa.gov/2012/03/23/defintion -of-recovery-updated/.

University of Toronto Psychiatric Outreach Program. 2002. Telepsychiatry: Guidelines and procedures for clinical activities. http://www.psychiatry.med.uwo.ca/ecp/info/toronto/ telepsych/.

Urness, D. 2003. Telepsychiatry and doctor-patient communication: A tale of two interviews. *Canadian Psychiatric Association Bulletin* 35: 21-25.

Uttal, W. 2003. *Psychomythics: Sources of Artifacts and Misconceptions in Scientific Psychology.* Mahwah, NJ: Lawrence Erlbaum Associates.

Vagnerova, P. 2003a. Self-management of psychosis and schizophrenia. *Visions: BC's Mental Health Journal* 18: 18-19.

–. 2003b. What BC campus disability centres can offer students. *Visions: BC's Mental Health Journal* 17: 28-29.

Vahia, I., et al. 2008. Adequacy of medical treatment among older persons with schizophrenia. *Psychiatric Services* 59: 853-59.

Valenstein, M., et al. 2004. Benzodiazepine use among depressed patients treated in mental health settings. *American Journal of Psychiatry* 161: 654-61.

–. 2011. Using a pharmacy-based intervention to improve antipsychotic adherence among patients with serious mental illness. *Schizophrenia Bulletin* 37: 727-36.

Valmaggia, L., et al. 2009. Economic impact of early intervention in people at high risk of psychosis. *Psychological Medicine* 39: 1617-26.

Vancouver at Home Research Team. 2012. The Vancouver At Home Project: Synopsis of findings after one year. Vancouver: Mental Health Commission of Canada.

Van der Kolk, B. 2002. The assessment and treatment of complex PTSD. In *Psychological Trauma*, ed. R. Yehuda, 127-56. Washington, DC: American Psychiatric Press.

Vandermark, L. 2007. Promoting the sense of self, place and belonging in displaced persons: The example of homelessness. *Archives of Psychiatric Nursing* 21: 241-48.

Van Le, C. 2000. Stigma and mental illness in the Vietnamese culture. *Visions: BC's Mental Health Journal* 9: 9.

van Minnen, A., et al. 2003. Treatment of trichotillomania with behavioral therapy or fluoxetine: a randomized, waiting-list controlled study. *Archives of General Psychiatry* 60: 517-22.

Van Os, J. 2004. Does the urban environment cause psychosis? *British Journal of Psychiatry* 184: 287-88.

Vasiliadis, H., et al. 2005. Service use for mental health reasons: Cross-provincial differences in rates, determinants and equity of access. *Canadian Journal of Psychiatry* 50: 614-19.

VanAndel, M., and H. Oetter. 2008. Message from the Registrar: Pharmacists' expanded scope of practice. College of Physicians and Surgeons of British Columbia. https://www.cpsbc.ca/files/u6/CQ_Sept_2008_Web.pdf.

Vatnaland, T., et al. 2007. Are GAF scores reliable in routine clinical use? *Acta Psychiatrica Scandinavica* 115: 326-30.

Vedantam, S. 2006. Comparison of schizophrenia drugs often favors firm funding study. *Washington Post*, 12 April.

Verdun-Jones, S. 2010. *Criminal Law in Canada: Cases, Questions, and the Code*. Toronto: Nelson Education.

Vieta, E., and M. Phillips. 2007. Deconstructing bipolar disorder: A critical review of its diagnostic validity and a proposal for DSM-V and ICD-11. *Schizophrenia Bulletin* 33: 886-92.

Viljoen, J., R. Roesch, and P. Zapf. 2002. Interrater reliability of the Fitness Interview Test across four professional groups. *Canadian Journal of Psychiatry* 47: 945-52.

Volkow, N., et al. 2008. Methylphenidate decreased the amount of glucose needed by the brain to perform a cognitive task. *PLoS ONE* 3: e2017.

Votta, E., and I. Manion. 2003. Factors in the psychological adjustment of homeless adolescent males: The role of coping style. *Journal of the American Academy of Child and Adolescent Psychiatry* 42: 778-85.

Waddell. C., et al. 2004. Preventing and treating anxiety disorders in children. Research report prepared for the BC Ministry of Children and Family Development.

Wakefield, J., A. Horwitz, and M. Schmitz. 2005. Are we overpathologizing the socially anxious? Social phobia from a harmful dysfunction perspective. *Canadian Journal of Psychiatry* 50: 317-19.

Waldron, D., et al. 1999. Quality-of-life measurement in advanced cancer. *Journal of Clinical Oncology* 17: 3603-11.

Walker, F. 2007. Huntington's disease. *Lancet* 369: 212-28.

Wallace, B., S. Klein, and M. Reitsma-Steet. 2006. Denied assistance: Closing the door on welfare in BC. Vancouver: Canadian Centre for Policy Alternatives.

Wallace, C., P. Mullen, and P. Burgess. 2004. Criminal offending in schizophrenia over a 25-year period marked by deinstitutionalization and increasing prevalence of comorbid substance use disorders. *American Journal of Psychiatry* 161: 716-27.

Wang, P., et al. 2008. The impact of cost sharing on antidepressant use among older adults in British Columbia. *Psychiatric Services* 59: 377-83.

Wasylenki, D., et al. 1997. A home-based program for the treatment of acute psychosis. *Community Mental Health Journal* 33: 151-62.

Watson, A., P. Corrigan, and V. Ottati. 2004. Police officers' attitudes toward and decisions about persons with mental illness. *Psychiatric Services* 55: 49-53.

Watson, A., et al. 2001. Mental health courts and the complex issue of mentally ill offenders. *Psychiatric Services* 52: 477-81.

Watson, D., et al. 2005. Population-based use of mental health services and patterns of delivery among family physicians. *Canadian Journal of Psychiatry* 50: 398-406.

Watters, E. 2010. The Americanization of mental illness. *New York Times.* http://www.nytimes.com/2010/01/10/magazine/10psyche-t.html?pagewanted=all.

Wazana, A. 2000. Physicians and the pharmaceutical industry: Is a gift ever just a gift? *Journal of the American Medical Association* 283: 373-80.

Webb, S. 2001. Some considerations on the validity of evidence-based practice in social work. *British Journal of Social Work*, 31: 57-79.

Webster, C., et al. 1997. *The HCR-20: Assessing the Risk for Violence.* Version 2. Burnaby, BC: Mental Health Law and Policy Institute, Simon Fraser University.

Wehring, H., and W. Carpenter. 2011. Violence and schizophrenia. *Schizophrenia Bulletin* 37: 877-78.

Weiden, P. 2010. Is recovery attainable in schizophrenia? *Medscape.* http://www.medscape.com/viewarticle/729750.

Weiner, E. 2008. Accommodating students with ongoing mental health issues. *Visions Journal* 4: 24-25.

Welch, K., et al. 2011. The impact of substance use on brain structure in people at high risk of developing schizophrenia. *Schizophrenia Bulletin* 37: 1066-76.

Wente, M. 2009. Is your sanity at stake? *Globe and Mail,* 4 July.

Werner, S., D. Malaspina, and J. Rabinowitz. 2007. Socioeconomic status at birth is associated with risk of schizophrenia: Population-based multilevel study. *Schizophrenia Bulletin* 33: 1373-78.

Westra, H., A. Aviram, and F. Doell. 2011. Extending motivational interviewing to the treatment of major mental health problems: Current directions and evidence. *Canadian Journal of Psychiatry* 56: 643-50.

Whitaker, R. 2010. *Anatomy of an Epidemic: Magic Bullets, Psychiatric Drugs, and the Astonishing Rise of Mental Illness in America.* New York: Crown Publishers.

White, C. 2011. Self-management: A close companion to recovery in mental illness. *Occupational Therapy Now* 13 (5): 26-27.

White, H., et al. 2003. Survey of consumer and non-consumer mental health service providers on assertive community treatment teams in Ontario. *Community Mental Health Journal* 39: 265-76.

Whiting, P. 2008. Student mental health at Simon Fraser University. *Visions Journal* 4: 10-11.

Whitley, R., and R. Drake. 2010. Recovery: A dimensional approach. 61: *Psychiatric Services* 1248-50.

Whitley, R., and W. Lawson. 2010. The psychiatric rehabilitation of African Americans with severe mental illness. *Psychiatric Services* 61: 508-11.

Whitley, R., L. Kirmayer, and D. Groleau. 2006. Understanding immigrants' reluctance to use mental health services: A qualitative study from Montreal. *Canadian Journal of Psychiatry* 51: 205-9.

Wiggins, J., and N. Cummings. 1998. National study of the experience of psychologists with psychotropic medication and psychotherapy. *Professional Psychology: Research and Practice* 29: 549-52.

Wilk, J., et al. 2006. Patterns of adult psychotherapy in psychiatric practice. *Psychiatric Services* 57: 472-76.

Williams, C. 2001. Increasing access and building equity into mental health services: An examination of the potential for change. *Canadian Journal of Community Mental Health* 20: 37-49.

–. 2008. Insight, stigma, and post-diagnosis identities in schizophrenia. *Psychiatry: Interpersonal and Biological Processes* 71: 246-56.

Williams, L. 1998. Personal accounts: A "classic" case of borderline personality disorder. *Psychiatric Services* 49: 173-74.

Wilson, D. 2011. Drug firms face billions in losses in '11 as patents end. *New York Times.* http://www.nytimes.com/2011/03/07/business/07drug.html?_r=2&pagewanted=all.

Wilson, D., G. Tien, and D. Eaves. 1995. Increasing the community tenure of mentally disordered offenders: An assertive case management program. *International Journal of Law and Psychiatry* 18: 61-69.

Wilson, M. 2005. Getting there from here: next steps. *Canadian Public Policy* 31, supplement: S69-S74.

Wilson-Bates, F. 2008. Lost in transition: How a lack of capacity in the mental health system is failing Vancouver's mentally ill and draining police resources. BC Schizophrenia Society. http://www.bcss.org/wp-content/uploads/2008/02/vpd-lost-in-transition.pdf.

Wilton, R. 2003. Poverty and mental health: A qualitative study of residential care facility clients. *Canadian Journal of Community Mental Health* 39: 139-56.

Winram, R. 2002. Managing bipolar disorder: A patient's perspective. Presentation at the Annual Riverview Hospital Mood and Anxiety Disorders Conference, Port Coquitlam, BC, 3 April.

Witheridge, T. 1991. The "active ingredients" of assertive outreach. *New Directions in Mental Health Services* 52: 47-64.

Wittek, S. 2001. Enough is enough: Joe Ribeiro wants the Vancouver police to stop shooting people with mental illnesses. *Terminal City*, 3-9 August, 10.

Womack, J., and D. Jones. 2003. *Lean Thinking: Banish Waste and Create Wealth in Your Corporation*. New York: Free Press.

Wong, K., et al. 2008. A randomized controlled trial of a supported employment program for persons with long-term mental illness in Hong Kong. *Psychiatric Services* 59: 84-90.

Wood, E., et al. 2008. Burden of HIV infection among Aboriginal injection drug users in Vancouver, BC. *American Journal of Public Health* 98: 515-19.

Woodward, N., et al. 2005. A meta-analysis of neuropsychological change to clozapine, olanzapine, quetiapine and risperidone in schizophrenia. *International Journal of Neuropsychopharmacology* 8: 457-72.

Woollaston, K., and P. Hixenbaugh 2008. "Destructive whirlwind": Nurses perceptions of patients diagnosed with borderline personality disorder. *Journal of Psychiatric and Mental Health Nursing* 15: 703-9.

Working Group for a Nunavut Suicide Prevention Strategy. 2011. Nunavut Suicide Prevention Strategy Action Plan. http://www.tunngavik.com/wp-content/uploads/2011/09/nsps-action -plan-eng4.pdf.

World Health Organization. 2002. *Prevention and Promotion in Mental Health*. http://www. who.int/mental_health/media/en/545.pdf.

–. 2010. Mental health: Strengthening our response. http://www.who.int/mediacentre/ factsheets/fs220/en/.

Wykes, T., et al. 2007. Cognitive remediation therapy in schizophrenia. *British Journal of Psychiatry* 190: 421-27.

–. 2008. Cognitive behavior therapy for schizophrenia: Effect sizes, clinical models and methodological rigor. *Schizophrenia Bulletin* 34: 523-37.

–. 2011. A meta-analysis of cognitive remediation for schizophrenia: Methodology and effect sizes. *American Journal of Psychiatry*. http://ajp.psychiatryonline.org/cgi/content/abstract/ appi.ajp.2010.10060855v1.

Xia, J., L. Merinder, and M. Belgamwar. 2011. Psychoeducation for schizophrenia. *Schizophrenia Bulletin* 37: 21-22.

Yanos, P., and Ziedonis, D. 2006. The patient-oriented clinician-researcher: Advantages and challenges of being a double agent. *Psychiatric Services* 57: 249-53.

Yanos, P., et al. 2008. Pathways between internalized stigma and outcomes related to recovery in schizophrenia spectrum disorders. *Psychiatric Services* 59: 1437-42.

Yates, D. 2004. Should psychologists have prescribing authority? A psychologist's perspective. *Psychiatric Services* 55: 1420-21.

Yehuda, R., ed. 2002. *Psychological Trauma*. Washington, DC: American Psychiatric Press.

Young, A., et al. 2001. The quality of care for depressive and anxiety disorders in the US. *Archives of General Psychiatry* 58: 55-61.

Young, J. 2008. Why pharmacists should not refill. *Vancouver Sun*, 12 September.

Zanarini, M. 2000. Childhood experiences associated with the development of borderline personality disorder. *Psychiatric Clinics of North America* 23: 89-101.

Zaretsky, A., et al. 2008. Is cognitive-behavioural therapy more effective than psycho-education in bipolar disorder? *Canadian Journal of Psychiatry* 53: 441-48.

Ziguras, S., et al. 2003. Ethnic matching of clients and clinicians and use of mental health services by ethnic minority clients. *Psychiatric Services* 54: 535-41.

Zippay, A. 2007. Psychiatric residences: Notification, NIMBY, and neighborhood relations. *Psychiatric Services* 58: 109-13.

Zosky, J., et al. 2010. Supporting recovery by capturing consumers' complex needs. Psychological Rehabilitation Canada/Réadaptation Psychosociale Canada. http://www. psrrpscanada.ca/clientuploads/documents/OCAN%20Presentation_PSRConference _20100920_v1.0_CMHCAP.PPT#257,1,OCAN.

Zubin, J., and B. Spring. 1977. Vulnerability: A new view on schizophrenia. *Journal of Abnormal Psychology* 86: 103-26.

Index

deinstitutionalization and, 196, 201, 202, 204-6; as early/premature, 169, 205, 225, 276, 340*n*2, 421; family involvement in, 162, 168-69, 246, 277; housing and, 288-89, 292, 298, 301; outcomes after, 97-98, 202; planning for, 140, 162, 173*n*5, 202, 276-77; problems of, 43*n*9, 204-5, 225, 246, 281*n*11, 421; re-hospitalization after, 204, 225, 269, 425

disclosure, of mental health issues: cultural barriers to, 115; by peer support workers, 408-9; by practitioners, 62, 85*n*1, 409; by students, 412-13; in workplace, 61-62, 409. *See also* confidentiality

disease mongering, 29, **179-82**, 191*n*2

diversion of mentally ill, from criminal justice system, **314**; court programs for, 314, 316, 317-18

"do no harm" principle, 117, 237, 353, **438**

doctors (general practitioners). *See* family physicians; physicians; practitioners, *and entries following*

domestic violence/abuse, 8-12, 14, 121, 288, 311, 324, 330, 391

Dominion Mental Health Grants Program, 201

Drug Abuse Screening Test (DAST), 259

drug addiction, 31-33, 37, 67, 258-59, 308. *See also* substance misuse/abuse, *and entry following*

drug companies, **175-91**; advertising/promotions by, 17, 177, 178, 182-85; costs incurred by, 176-79, 190-91; disease mongering by, 29, 179-82; and evidence base/drug trials, 185-89, 190, 219, 234, 348; and off-label prescriptions, 176, 191*n*2, 220, 355-57, 363*n*12; patents of, 177-78, 181-82, 186, 346; and pharmacare, 176, 190-91; and practitioners, 149, 175, 176-77, 182-83, 188-90; profitability of, 175-78; social media use by, 185; studies independent of, 190, 348

drug courts, 316-17

drug trials. *See* randomized controlled trials

drugs. *See* medications, *and entry following*

Druss, Benjamin, 39, 245

DSM. See *Diagnostic and Statistical Manual*

Duncan, Barry, Scott Miller, and Jacqueline Sparks: *The Heroic Client*, 6, 221, 226, 336

duration: and seriousness, 34

Durkheim, Emile, 9, 123

duty of care, 107, 141, **143-44**, 147, 193, 436

duty to warn/protect, 146-47

dysthymia, 30, 31

Dziekanski, Robert, 311

early intervention programs, 211, 239(f), 240, **251-56**, 410; factors in implementing, 45, 251-52; for psychosis treatment, 52-54, 253-56; relapse prevention and, 370-72

early psychosis intervention (EPI), 52-54, **253-56**; at day hospitals, 267; and difficulties of identification, 53, 58, 73, 254; economic arguments for, 53-54, 58; ethical issues of, 53, 254-55; evidence base for, 254, 255, 256; examples of programs in, 256; family involvement/education and, 255-56; side effects of, 53, 366; young people and, 252, 253-56

eating disorders, 27, 37, 46, 239(f), 240, 278, 375

education, as affected by mental illness, 411-13

education, public. *See* mental health literacy; public education

education and skills training, **367-78**; and assertiveness skills, 373-74; BRIDGES program in, 375-76, 392; and cognitive remediation, 377-78; group delivery of, 378; and relapse prevention, 370-72; relaxation techniques of, 372-73; structured problem solving in, 374-75; WRAP program in, 376-77, 392

educational and counselling psychologists, 139

elderly, **50-51**, 205, 301, 328, 377, 429-30; as caregivers, 159-61; and dementia, 50-51, 55, 301, 325, 326-27; depression in, 50-51, 55, 267, 351; hospital care for, 278; prescription drug use by, 351, 354, 355; prevention/health promotion and, 55

electroconvulsive therapy (ECT), 198, 275, **361-62**, 428

Eli Lilly, 17, 182, 186, 188, 220

eligibility for programs/services, factors determining, **26-38**, 442; agency mandates and, 34-35; anxiety disorders and, 37-38; diagnosis, 27-29, 33, 37, 40-41, 442; disability, 29-31, 34, 37; duration, 34; personality disorders, 27, 31-33, 35,

fluvoxamine (Luvox), 350
Food and Drug Administration, US (FDA), 187, 191*n*4, 352, 356; approval of medications by, 182, 236*n*1, 363*n*12
Forchuk, Cheryl, 289
forensic psychiatry, 144, 239(f), 240, 305, 315-16, **319-21**; and assessment process, 314, 319-20, 330; facilities for, 70, 239(f), 314, 319, 435; non-forensic psychiatry and, 315-16, 320-21; and sex offenders, 320
Fountain House (New York), 90, 155, 400
Freedom of Information and Protection of Privacy Acts: BC, 168-69; Ontario, 145
Freud, Sigmund, 10, 164, 170, 365. *See also* psychodynamic treatments
functional assessment, 331-32

GAIN-SS (addiction screening instrument), 259
general hospital psychiatric units (GHPUs), 274. *See also* hospitals
genetic factors, 6, 7, 9-10, 12-14, 15, 32, 68, 71, 337, 441; and drug response, 345; in schizophrenia, 18-20, 52, 81, 83-84, 171, 212. *See also* "biomarkers"
geriatric units, in hospitals, 278
Gerstein Centre (Toronto), 251, 300
Glannon, Walter, 8, 15
GlaxoSmithKline (GSK), 187-88, 220
Glenmullen, Joseph, 350-51
Global Assessment of Functioning (GAF), 30, 34, 338
Goffman, Erving: *Asylums*, 90-91, 199
Goldacre, Ben, 178-79, 181, 185, 186, 187, 190, 191*n*2, 353
Gray, John (New York State Asylum), 6
Gray, John E., Margaret A. Shone, and Peter F. Liddle: *Canadian Mental Health Law and Policy*, 418, 419-20, 422, 424, 428, 429, 433
group delivery, of education/skills training, 378
group homes, 292, 294-96. *See also* residential housing
Gumpp, Ruth, 361, 446

half-life, of medications, **344**, 354
Hamid, Sarah, 295-96
Hare, Robert, 330
Harper, Stephen, 210
Hart, Stephen, 305, 309, 330

HCR-20 violence risk assessment tool, 330
Health and Human Services, US Department of, 130, 269
health care, public, 242. *See also* medicare
Health Care Consent Act (Ontario), 424, 439*n*7
Health Care Consent and Care Facility Admission Act (BC), 432
Health of the Nation Outcome Scales (HoNOS), 30, 205, 326, 338
health-adjusted life years (HALYs), 31, 47
health-related quality of life (HRQOL), 46
Healy, David, 148, 188-89
help-seeking, **38-42**; cultural issues of, 112, 114-20, 127-34; depression and, 83, 185, 350; increased comfort with, 68; and perceived need, 38-42; in rural areas, 264; stigma and, 38, 58-59, 61, 63-65, 74-77, 251; by young people, 54, 84
HIV, 48, 121, 127, 178
hoarding, 1-2, 37, 340
Home Treatment Program for Acute Psychosis (Toronto), 273
homelessness, 30, **283-91**; causes of, 287-91; definitions of, 282, 283; deinstitutionalization and, 201, 305; demographics of, 284-85; episodic vs chronic, 285; health service use and, 287; hospitalization and, 288-89; impact of, 286-87; of mentally ill, 48, 49, 72, 285-87, 308; negativity toward, 80, 84-85; prevalence of, 283-86; socio-economic factors and, 48, 289-91; substance misuse/abuse and, 257, 261, 285, 288, 290, 292, 293, 298
hopefulness/optimism, 93-95
Hospital for Sick Children (Toronto), 266
hospitals, 239(f), 240, **274-79**; admission to/discharge from, 275-77; day, 239(f), 240, 267; homeless and, 288-89; in-patient programs at, 277-78; involuntary admission to, 419-29; and suicide, 76, 442; tertiary care at, 238, 239(f), 240, 278-79; utilization of programs at, 274-75. *See also* discharge, from hospital; involuntary hospital admission, *and entry following*
hospitals/facilities, forensic, 70, 239(f), 314, 319, 435
hospitals/facilities, psychiatric. *See* asylums/psychiatric hospitals; deinstitutionalization

needs assessment, and tools for, 332-33
Neglected Adults Welfare Act (Newfoundland and Labrador), 429
Nelson, Geoff, 229-30, 272
neurotransmitters, **344**, 346-47, 349-50, 354; as discussed on "Depression Hurts" website, 17, 182
"nervios," 116, 134*n*3
A New Framework for Support for People with Serious Mental Health Problems (CMHA report), 136-37, 280
Niezen, Ronald, 122
NIMBY (not in my back yard) syndrome, **65-66**, 86*n*4, 201, 295-96, 300
"no wrong door" approach, to mental health care access, 246
non-adherence, to medications/prescriptions, 269, **357-61**
non-maleficence ("do no harm"), as ethical principle, 117, 237, 353, **438**
non-medical treatments. *See* counselling and educational approaches, *and entry following*
non-profit sector, 250, **279-80**, 295, 408; client-controlled organizations in, 155, 157-59, 400
noradrenaline dopamine modulators (NDMs), 350
North American Free Trade Agreement, 177
North Shore Schizophrenia Society (Vancouver), 84, 144, 164, 173, 174*n*19
Northern Ontario, health services in, 263-64, 267
Northern Ontario School of Medicine, 267
not criminally responsible on account of mental disorder (NCRMD), persons found to be, 70, 73, 319, 330, **433-35**; discharge of, 319, 322*n*10, 434-35; recent government legislation on, 322*n*10, 435
"not otherwise specified" (NOS), diagnosis of, 181, 339
nurse practitioners (NPs), 140, 142, 421
nurses, 37, **139-40**, 246, 273, 299-300, 421; CBT experience of, 248-49; and police, in crisis units, 250-51, 313; psychiatric, 133, 140, 277

obsessive-compulsive disorder (OCD), 1-2, 350, 362-63
occupation, **397-413**; and education deficit, 411-13; and employment, 399, 401-5;

and peer support initiatives, 405-9; and personal life/life skills, 397-99; and workplace mental illness, 409-11. *See also* employment; unemployment; workplace, mental illness in
occupational therapists (OTs), 77, **140**, 255, 331-32, 399
off-label prescriptions, 176, 191*n*2, 220, **355-57**, 363*n*12
olanzapine, 48, 345, 347, 348, 349, 355; Zyprexa, 186, 188, 220
Olivieri, Nancy, 188
One Flew Over the Cuckoo's Nest (novel/film), 198, 419
Ontario Association of Chiefs of Police, 309
Ontario Common Assessment of Need (OCAN), 24, 332-33
Opening Minds (MHCC anti-stigma initiative), 78, 85
Out of Sight, Not Out of Mind (Mood Disorders Society of Canada report), 38
Out of the Shadows at Last. See Kirby Report
Outcome Rating Scale (ORS), 30, 205
outpatient programs, 98, 155, 198, 247, 279, 387, 395; after deinstitutionalization, 201; forensic psychiatry and, 144, 240, 319-20; physical treatments as, 362; specialized, 239(f). *See also* community treatment orders; mandatory outpatient treatment
outpatient services, specialized, 239(f)
outreach services, 57, 239(f), 240, 245, 261, 263, 265, 275, 278, 444; geriatric, 278; in housing, 292, 293, 297; risk of dependency on, 438; by shelters, 299-300. *See also* acute home-based treatment; assertive community treatment; Intensive Case Management
oxazepam (Serax), 353

paliperidone, 347, 348; compared to risperidone, 179, 179(f), 347, 363*n*7
Parent, Richard, 310-11
participatory research, 227-30
Pathways to Housing (New York), 292
paroxetine (Paxil), 191*n*2, 350
patents, of drug companies, 177-78, 346; and strategies for expiration of, 181-82, 186
paternalism, of practitioners/system, 137, 381, 399, 437; case management and,

Printed and bound and Canada by Friesens

Set in Giovanni Book and Garamond Condensed
by Artegraphica Design Co. Ltd.

Text design: Irma Rodriguez

Copy editor: Joanne Richardson

Proofreader: Julie Sedger

Indexer: Cheryl Lemmens